Principles of Genitourinary Radiology

Principles of Genitourinary Radiology

Zoran L. Barbaric, M.D.
Professor of Radiology
Department of Radiological Sciences
UCLA School of Medicine
Los Angeles, California

1991
Thieme Medical Publishers, Inc., New York
Georg Thieme Verlag, Stuttgart • New York

Thieme Medical Publishers, Inc.
381 Park Avenue South
New York, New York 10016

Principles of Genitourinary Radiology
Zoran L. Barbaric, M.D.

Library of Congress Cataloging-in-Publication Data
Barbaric, Zoran L.
    Principles of genitourinary radiology / Zoran L. Barbaric.
        p.   cm.
    Includes index.
    ISBN 0-86577-347-5 (TMP). — ISBN 3-13-752001-0 (GTV)
    1. Genitourinary organs—Radiography—Atlases.   I. Title.
    [DNLM: 1. Diagnostic Imaging—atlases. 2. Genital Diseases,
Female—diagnosis—atlases. 3. Genital Diseases, Male—diagnosis—
atlases. 4. Urography—methods—atlases. 5. Urologic Diseases—
diagnosis—atlases.   WJ 17 B229p]
RC874.B37   1991
616.6'0757—dc20
DNLM/DLC
for Library of Congress   90-11200
                                                            CIP

Important note: Medicine is an ever-changing science. Research and clinical experience are continually broadening our knowledge, in particular our knowledge of proper treatment and drug therapy. Insofar as this book mentions any dosage or application, readers may rest assured that the authors, editors, and publishers have made every effort to ensure that such references are strictly in accordance with the state of knowledge at the time of production of the book. Nevertheless, every user is requested to carefully examine the manufacturers' leaflets accompanying each drug to check on his own responsibility whether the dosage schedules recommended therein or the contraindications stated by the manufacturers differ from the statements made in the present book. Such examination is particularly important with drugs that are either rarely used or have been newly released on the market.

Some of the product names, patents, and registered designs referred to in this book are in fact registered trademarks or proprietary names even though specific reference to this fact is not always made in the text. Therefore, the appearance of a name without designation as proprietary is not to be construed as a representation by the publisher that it is in the public domain.

Printed in the United States of America.

5   4   3   2   1

TMP ISBN 0-86577-347-5
GTV ISBN 3-13-752001-0

This book is dedicated to my loving family—
Erika, Adrian, and Evan.

Contents

Preface

This book is primarily written for general radiologists in need of concise, consolidated, and pertinent updates in genitourinary radiology; radiology residents during their uroradiology rotation and when preparing for boards; urology residents and fellows; urologists; medical students during their urology rotation or elective; and nephrologists.

An attempt was made to consolidate relevant material concerning genitourinary radiology in one volume. The subject headings are organized according to organ systems and diseases rather than technologies. It is this author's feeling that books relating to technology, such as "CT of this. . ." and "MR of that. . ." leave the reader with uncertainty as to what is the proper imaging procedure needed for evaluation of a particular clinical entity. The only exception to this approach is sonography, which cannot be learned without "hands on" experience. In most radiology departments sonography is a separate subspecialty, therefore the space devoted to this subject is mostly descriptive.

Most beginning radiology residents, some practicing radiologists, and practitioners in all clinical specialties are in need of a simplified view of the physics involved in imaging. To be sure, what is presented in this book will not be sufficient to pass the Radiology Boards, but it will give the reader a clear understanding of how images are acquired.

Interventional radiology is presented in terms of what it can accomplish rather than in detailed "how to" descriptions. A radiology resident should, for example, be able to perform a simple percutaneous nephrostomy. The more difficult procedures, such as establishing and dilating a tract for staghorn removal, require additional training.

Zoran L. Barbaric, M.D.

Acknowledgments

The completion of this book caused me to pause and reflect upon the numerous individuals who imparted their knowledge to me and influenced my career as a radiologist. Among many luminaries, Stanley Rogoff, M.D., Harry Fisher, M.D., Eliot Lipchik, M.D., Lionel Young, M.D., Jim Usselman, M.D., Victor Hegedus, M.D., Paul Ross, M.D., John Thornberry, M.D., Anthony Lalli, M.D., Thomas Sherwood, M.D., Irwin Frank M.D., Charles Linke, M.D., Donald Sun, M.D., and Philip Rubin, M.D., stand out most as the ones who taught me the fundamentals. To them I am forever grateful.

Many more bestowed a fraction of their wisdom through personal interactions. Among those are Lee Theros, M.D., Leo Rigler, M.D., William Hanafee, M.D., Joseph J. Kauffman, M.D., Willard Goodwin, M.D., Shlomo Raz, M.D., Robert Smith, M.D., Richard Erlich, M.D., Jean deKernion, M.D., Arthur Segal, M.D., William Hare, M.D., Geoffrey Benness, M.D., Richard Friedenberg, M.D., George Foote, M.D., Martti Kormano, M.D., Richard Katzberg, M.D., Robert Spataro, M.D., Robert Nelson, Ph.D., Christian Chaussy, M.D., Gerhard Fuchs, M.D., Donald Skinner, M.D., Gerald Lim, M.D., Anthony House, M.D., Francis Burgener, M.D., Nancy Curry, M.D., Bernie Huang, Ph.D., Andrew LeRoy, M.D., Howard Mindell, M.D., Ines Boechat, M.D., Franklin Tessler, M.D., Hooshang Kangarloo, M.D., Lawrence Bassett, M.D., Poonam Batra, M.D., Sachiko Cochran, M.D., and Richard Gold, M.D.

Many thanks to Rita Perella, M.D., David Cho, M.D., and Barbara Kadell, M.D., for allowing me to use some of their unpublished material, and to Julie Lee Short, R.N., Nancy A. Little, M.D., and Kenneth Linden, M.D., for reviewing parts of the manuscript. Also, sincere thanks to Hooshang Kangarloo, M.D., chairman of the UCLA Department of Radiological Sciences, for his support. Many illustrations appearing throughout the book were conceived and drawn during teaching and reviewing sessions with University of Rochester and UCLA residents. Their inquisitiveness and enthusiasm were the driving force for much of my work.

Many of the fine radiographs presented in the book were created by dedicated radiology technologists Virgia Gardner, R.T., Gennie Acosta, R.T., Larry Argnosa, R.T., Richard Padilla, R.T., and Barbara Calander, R.T.

My secretary Cynthia Shirley has braved many trips to photographic and printing shops and has helped immeasurably in the preparation of the manuscript.

Most of the laborious editing was done by my wife Erika. Without her support and assistance throughout two arduous years, the book would not be completed.

Special thanks to Steve Jobs and Jeff Raskins for creating Macintosh, Mike Schuster and his group for developing Adobe Illustrator, and to Gil Iwamoto, a friend and master boat builder, for teaching me not only how to build a boat, but also that there is life beyond radiology.

Zoran L. Barbaric, M.D.

Historical Perspective

1826	Niepce	Permanent photograph
1842	Doppler	Doppler shift
1880	Curie brothers	Piezoelectric effect
1895	Roentgen	Discovery of X-ray
1896	Becquerel	Discovery of radioactivity
1896	Pupin	Film-screen combination
1896	MacIntyre; Adams	Radiologic diagnosis of renal calculus
1898	Pierre & Marie Curie	Discovery of radium and polonium
1904	Klose	Pyelogram (bismuth emulsion)
1906	Völcker & Lichtenberg	Retrograde pyelography (colloidal silver)
1907	Bukhardt & Polano	"Negative" pyelography (oxygen)
1918	Cameron, Graves, Davidoff	Retrograde pyelography & cystography (NaI)
1919	Braash & Olson	Radiographic diagnosis of renal tuberculosis
1923	Osborne & Rowntree	Principle of excretory urography (sodium iodide)
1929	Swick	Intravenous pyelography (Uroselectan)
1929	Dos Santos	Lumbar aortography
1931	Lawrence	Cyclotron
1934	F. Joliot & I. Curie	Discovery of artificial radioactivity
1937	Langmuir	Principle of fluoroscopic image intensifier
1940	Firestone	Pulsed-echo principle
1945	Bloch & Purcell	Magnetic resonance
1947	Kolman	Scintillation counter
1948	Coltman	Modern fluoroscopic image intensifier
1949	Cassen	Rectilinear scanner
1950	Pierce	Transfemoral angiography
1950	Howry & Bliss	B-mode scanner
1953	Wallingford	Hippuran and acetrizoate
1953	Seldinger	Seldinger technique of arterial puncture
1953	Goodwin & Casey	Percutaneous nephrostomy
1954	Evans	Bolus nephrotomography
1954	Winter & Taplin	Radionuclide renogram
1954	Howry & Holms	Compound sonograms
1956	Hoppe et al	Diatrizoate
1956	Odman, Edholm, Seldinger	Selective renal angiography
1957	Richards	M99/Tc-99m generator
1958	Anger	Scintillation camera
1958	Donald & Brown	Direct-contact, manually operated scanner
1959	Odman	Radiopaque angiographic catheter
1963	Kuhl & Edwards	Principles of single photon emission tomography (SPECT)
1964	Dotter & Judkins	Transluminal angioplasty
1964	Maxwell et al.	Rapid sequence urogram

1970	Bates et al.	Videourodynamics
1971	Watanabe et al.	Transrectal ultrasound of the prostate
1971	Damadian	MR tumor detection
1972	Nyegaard Labs & Almen	Metrizamide (first nonionic contrast)
1972	Hounsfield	CT scan
1973	Lauterbur	MR imaging
1974	Phelps, Hoffman, Mullani, Ter-Pogossian	PET camera
1976	Fernström & Johannson	Percutaneous pyelolithotomy
1977	Jaszczak	SPECT camera
1978	Grüntzig	Renal artery angioplasty
1981	Chaussy, Brendel, Schmiedt	ESWL
1983	Whitfield et al.	Percutaneous pyelolysis

REFERENCES

Röntgen WC. Eine neue art von Strahlen. Sitzungsberichte. Phys Med Ges Wurzburg 1895; 137:132–141.

Becquerel H. Emission de radiations nouvelles par l'uranium metallique. C.R. Acad Sci 1896; 122:1086–1088.

Curie P, (Mme) Curie S. Sur une substance nouvelle radioactive, contenue dans la pechblende. C.R. Acad Sci 1898; 127:175–178.

Curie I, Joliot F. Artificial production of a new kind of radio-element. Nature (London) 1934; 133:201–202.

Swick M. Darstellung der Niere und Harnwege im Rontgenbild durch intravenose einbringgung eines neuen Kontraststoffes, des Uroselectans. Klin Wochenschr 1929; 8:2087–2089.

Swick M. The discovery of intravenous urography: historical and developmental aspects of the urographic media and their role in other diagnostic and therapeutic areas. Bull NY Acad Med 1966; 42:128.

Wallingford VH. The development of organic iodine compounds as x-ray contrast media. J Am Pharm Assoc 1953; 42:721–729.

Maxwell MH, Gonick HC, Wiita R, Kaufman JJ. Use of the rapid sequence intravenous pyelogram in the diagnosis of renovascular hypertension. N Engl J Med 1964; 279:213–215.

Bates CP, Whiteside CG, Turner-Warvick R. Synchronous cine/pressure/flow/cystourethrography with special reference to stress and urge incontinence. Br J Urol 1970; 42:714.

Watanabe H, Kaiho H, Tanaka M, Terasawa Y. Diagnostic application of ultrasonotomography to the prostate. Invest Urol 1971; 8:548–549.

Metrizamide: a nonionic water soluble contrast medium. Acta Radiol (Suppl) 1973.

Lauterbur PC. Image formation of induced local interactions: examples employing NMR. Nature 1973; 242:190–191.

Fernstrom I, Johannson B. Percutaneous pyelolithotomy: A new extraction technique. Scand J Urol Nephrol 1976; 10:257–260.

Grüntzig A, Vetter W, Meier B, et al. Treatment of renovascular hypertension with percutaneous transluminal dilatation of a renal artery stenosis. Lancet 1978; 1:801–802.

Damadian R. Tumor detection by nuclear magnetic resonance. Science 1971; 171: 1151–1153.

Chaussy C, Schmiedt E, Jocham D, et al. First clinical experience with extracorporeally induced destruction of kidney stones by shock-waves. J Urol 1981; 127:417–420.

Whitfield HN, Mills V, Miller RA, Wickham JEA. Percutaneous pyelolysis: an alternative to pyeloplasty. Br J Urol 1983; 55(Suppl):93–96.

Principles of
Genitourinary
Radiology

Instrumentation

PROJECTIONAL RADIOGRAPHY

X-ray Production

X-rays are produced in an x-ray tube when high velocity electrons are drawn across a vacuum from a cathode to a tungsten anode (Fig. 1–1). Colliding with the anode, their energy is converted to heat and x-rays (Fig. 1–2).

The number of x-rays produced is proportional to the number of electrons colliding with the tungsten anode. The number of electrons is proportional to the current (mA) allowed to flow through the cathode heating coil (where the electrons are "boiled" off) and to the length of time (s) the electrons are allowed to continually flow to the anode.

The penetrating ability of the x-rays is proportional to electron velocity at the time of impact with the tungsten anode. Electron velocity is proportional to the potential difference (voltage) between the cathode and the anode (kVp).

In summary, the higher the kVp, the more penetrating the x-rays; the higher the multiple of mA and s (mAs), the greater the number of x-rays.

X-ray Attenuation

As x-rays transverse the body, most are absorbed. This absorption is nonuniform. Bones, calcifications, and metallic foreign objects attenuate an x-ray beam the most, parenchymal organs and water less, fat far less than water, and air almost not at all. There are several physical ways the x-ray photons interact with the body's atoms, but only two are important in diagnostic radiology:

1. *Photoelectric effect:* incoming x-rays collide with tightly bound K-shell electrons, thereby losing all of their energy. In the process the K-electron is ejected from its orbit, leaving a vacancy. The vacancy is filled by L-shell electron during which process a *characteristic x-ray* is emitted (Fig. 1–3).

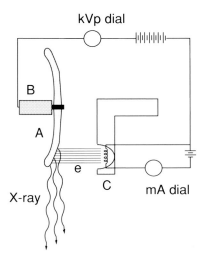

Figure 1–1.   Schematic drawing of an x-ray tube. **(A)** Rotating anode. **(B)** Rotor. **(C)** Cathode filament. "Boiled-off" electrons (e) are accelerated in vacuum and collide with anode.

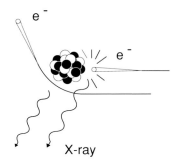

Figure 1–2.   Some electrons collide "head-on" with the tungsten atom and all their energy is converted into x-rays. Other electrons that are deflected and deaccelerated also produce x-rays, although of lower energy compared with "head-on" colliders.

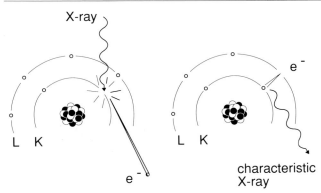

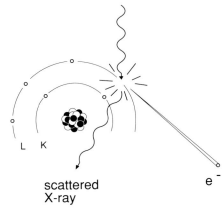

Figure 1–3.   Photoelectric effect.

Figure 1–4.   Compton effect.

2. *Compton effect:* incoming x-ray collides with a free electron or a loosely bound outer shell electron (Fig. 1–4). If the collision is head-on, the x-ray photon loses all of its energy to the electron in the form of kinetic energy. More frequently, the collision with the electron is at an angle and only a partial transfer of energy occurs. The x-ray photon loses some of its energy and in the process also changes its direction. A single photon in this type of interaction may experience multiple collisions and directional change.

X-ray Detection

Only a small fraction of x-rays escape absorption in the patient and are available for detection and analysis on exiting the body. Detection is accomplished by the use of a film sandwiched between two phosphor screens. When exposed to x-rays, the screen glows light (luminescence) and exposes the film (Fig. 1–5). The glow is proportional to the number and energy of the x-rays, and since these have been modulated through interaction with different structures in the body, the latent image is imprinted on the film. Once developed in the film processor, it is no longer called a film, but a radiograph.

Radiographic Contrast

Projectional radiography can distinguish only five conspicuous densities within the human body. These are *air density* (lungs, intestinal gas), *fat density* (subcutaneous and retroperitoneal fat, some fatty tumors), *water density* (urine, solid organs, walls of viscus organs, muscles, ligaments), *metallic density* (surgical clips, prosthesis), and *contrast material density* (iodinated contrast, barium sulfate).

The x-ray attenuations of soft tissues and fat differ sufficiently to permit organ visualization. For exam-

ple, the kidney is seen (barely) on a radiograph because it is "contrasted" by surrounding fat. On the other hand, the attenuations of soft tissue and water differ negligibly and that is why, for example, on the plain radiograph of the abdomen the collecting system cannot be seen within the kidney, or a bladder tumor cannot be seen in the bladder full of urine. The attenuation differences between soft tissues and water are just not sufficient enough to be recorded with this imaging technique.

Radiographic contrast materials are specifically designed to overcome this shortcoming. Because radiographic contrast materials strongly attenuate the x-ray beam, anatomical structures filled with contrast (ureters, bladder, collecting system) will be easily visualized. Iodinated contrast materials used in radiographic examinations of the urinary tract system attenuate best the x-rays produced under 70 kVp. Higher energy x-rays pass through radiographic contrast with ease, resulting in a gray, "non-contrasty" image.

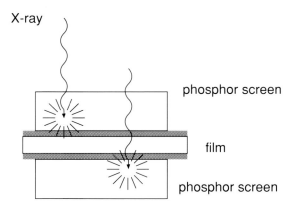

Figure 1–5.   Radiographic film is coated with emulsion on each side. Sandwiched between two phosphor screens, the detection efficiency of such a film-screen system is nearly double that of single emulsion systems, since more x-rays are captured with two screens.

Strongly attenuating materials such as radiographic contrasts, metals, and bone are labeled *radiopaque* and appear white on radiographs. Poorly attenuating materials are referred to as *radiolucent* and are black or dark.

Scattered Radiation

Scattered radiation adds baseline fog to the film and decreases image quality by decreasing contrast. Sources of scattered radiation are the patient, x-ray tube, table top, cassette, and screen; the culprits are the Compton effect and characteristic radiation. Scatter increases proportionally with higher energy x-rays and with patient thickness. To eliminate unwanted scatter, a grid is placed in front of the film-screen cassette. The grid permits passage of the modulated primary beam only, thereby significantly reducing the scatter and improving radiographic contrast (Fig. 1–6).

FLUOROSCOPY

Real time visualization of happenings in the body allows functional examination of organ systems and execution of various diagnostic and interventional procedures, where "seeing" what one is doing is imperative. The conversion of the x-ray into visible light is accomplished by an electronic device called an *image intensifier*.

Instead of a film-screen combination, the attenuated x-rays exiting the body are captured by a cesium iodide (input) screen and converted into electrons. Electrons are accelerated across the vacuum tube and focused onto a smaller (output) phosphor screen. Because the accelerated electrons carry more energy and because the output screen is so much smaller, it luminesces many times brighter compared with the input screen. The brightness gain is several thousandfold. A closed-circuit television camera is focused at the output screen and displays the resultant real time image on a CRT monitor (Fig. 1–7).

DIGITAL RADIOGRAPHY

Digital Subtraction Angiography (DSA)

Principle of subtraction is explained in Fig. 1–8. Because two radiographic images are taken at slightly different times, the process is called temporal subtraction. Subtraction may be accomplished through analog film processing in the dark room or electronically using digital image manipulation (see also Fig. 12–46).

Images are digitized by assigning gray level value from 0 to 256 to the incoming TV signal from the fluoroscope. These numerical values are spread over a matrix containing 512×512 picture elements (pixels), which are stored in digital memory. Temporal subtraction of grabbed TV frames containing no

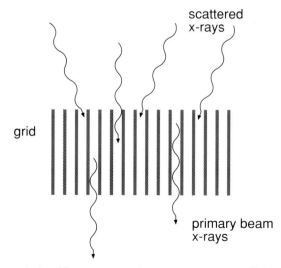

Figure 1–6. Most scattered x-rays are not parallel to the primary beam and can be prevented from reaching film-screen combination by a grid placed between the object and the cassette. Some of the primary beams are also attenuated by the grid, requiring an increase in dose to compensate for the loss.

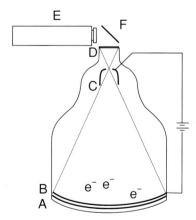

Figure 1–7. Schematic drawing of an image intensifier. On exiting the patient, the modulated x-rays hit the input phosphorus (**A**) causing luminescence. The light liberates electrons from adjacent photocathode (**B**) proportionally to its intensity. Potential difference between the cathode (**B**) and anode (**C**) accelerates electrons which eventually crash onto output phosphor (**D**) and produce a very bright image that is captured through a reflecting mirror (**F**) by a TV camera (**E**).

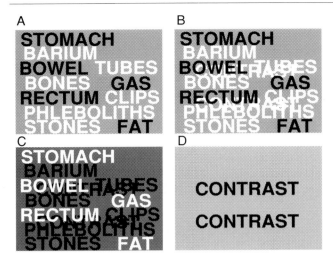

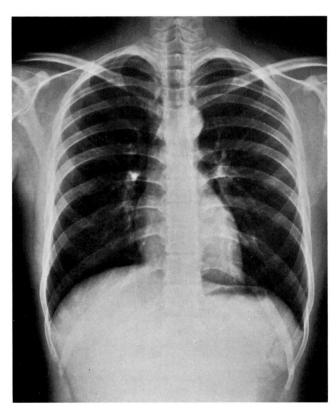

Figure 1–8. **(A)** Schematic representation of a scout radiograph. **(B)** A few seconds later radiographic contrast is injected but is obscured by unwanted shadows. **(C)** Image B is made into a negative. **(D)** Image A (scout) and image C (negative with contrast) are superimposed together and transilluminated on a final film. All unwanted shadows have cancelled each other out, but there was nothing to cancel introduced contrast, which is thus clearly visible against a uniform background.

intravascular contrast from those containing intravascular contrast will yield the same result as subtraction of the images recorded on film, except there is no need for the darkroom, since the whole process is electronic.

Digital Projection Radiography

The breakthroughs in the computer industry make it feasible to adopt computerized digital projection radiography (Figs. 1–9, 1–10). This type of image acquisition, archiving, and viewing is probably the way radiology will be practiced in the future. Several "digital-only" radiology departments are already operating in Japan. There are many advantages to digital general radiography, such as decreased radiation exposure to the general population, uniformity of exposure, generation of monochromatic x-ray beam, dual energy subtraction, convenience of image retrieval, no lost radiographs, and smaller format (Fig. 1–11). After all, more than half of the images generated in the average radiology department are already in digital form (CT, MR imaging, ultrasound,

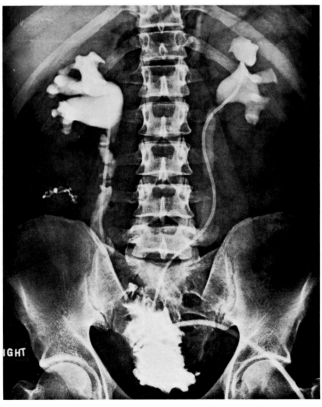

Figure 1–9. Example of a digital chest radiograph on 2000 × 2000 pixel matrix.

Figure 1–10. Example of a digital radiograph of the abdomen in a patient with a neobladder, bilateral ureteral stents, and suprapubic cystostomy tube.

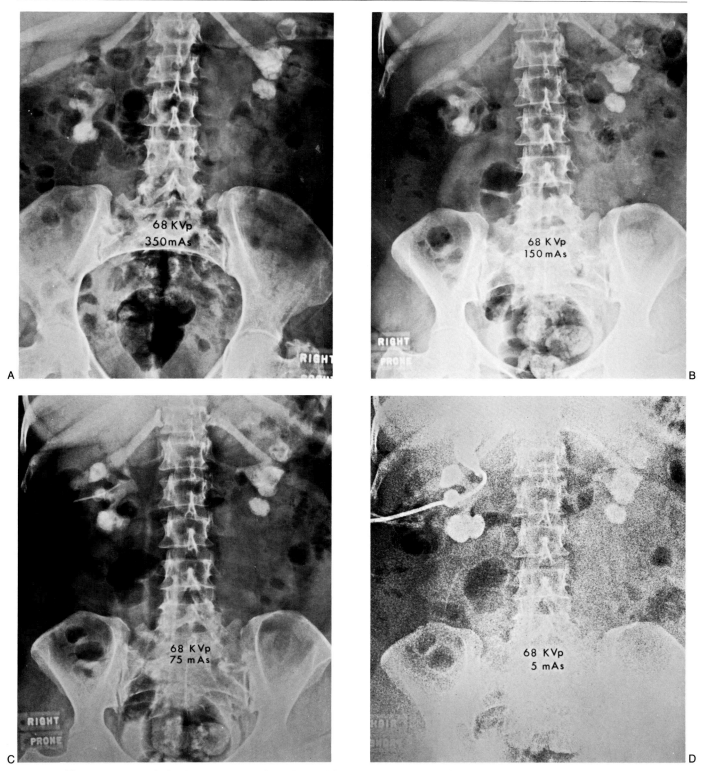

Figure 1–11 (A,B,C,D). A series of radiographic exposures were obtained during nephrostomy tube placement in a morbidly obese patient with bilateral staghorn calculi. The kVp was kept constant for each exposure while the mAs was progressively decreased. Despite decreasing exposure, all images, except the last one, are of diagnostic quality.

nuclear medicine). Development is somewhat hampered by uncertainty as to whether the large film manufacturers will respond by introducing a self-developing film ten times cheaper than current silver halide films.

Several types of x-ray image receptors for general projection radiography are already in use. *Linear receptor* technology employs an array of linear receptors that move in unison with the x-ray tube across the width (90° to long axis) of the patient through a narrow slit or slot. To match resolution of the radiographic films, the output signals from the receptors are digitized and displayed on a 2000 × 2000 matrix and at least 256 or more gray levels. *Area receptors* utilize a screen made of a special type of phosphor material that when exposed to x-rays retains a latent image. When the screen is scanned by a pinpoint laser beam, it emits light of a different wavelength proportional to the amount of radiation received. This emitted light is captured, amplified, converted into an electronic signal, and digitized. A fluoroscopic tube could also be used as an area receptor but the resolution matrix cannot exceed 1000 × 1000.

COMPUTERIZED AXIAL TOMOGRAPHY (CT)

Scanners

CT images are acquired while the x-ray tube is rotating 360° around the patient. The x-ray beam is collimated in axial orientation, and divergent to encompass the patient's width in the other. The intensity of attenuated x-rays emerging from the patient is measured with an array of minute detectors. The detector array simultaneously rotates around the patient in unison with the x-ray tube (third generation CT), or is arranged in a stationary ring (fourth generation CT) (Fig. 1–12). Multiple

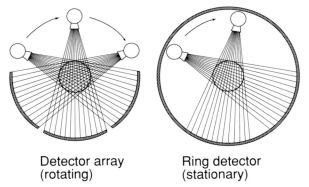

Detector array   Ring detector
(rotating)   (stationary)

Figure 1–12.   Two most common CT scan configurations.

angular views of a 10 mm thick slice (or less) are obtained, and from the numerous attenuation values measured, a computer image is reconstructed using Fourier transform functions.

The images in CT are displayed in a two dimensional plane on a 512 × 512 matrix of image elements or pixels. The tissue volume that a *pixel* represents is called a *voxel*, which usually measures 1 × 1 × 10 mm. The longest dimension of the voxel is oriented parallel to the long axis of the patient and represents *slice thickness*. The slice may be as thin as 5, 2, or even 1 mm for "high resolution" imaging.

While projectional radiography can only discriminate air, water, and calcifications as separate densities, CT is capable of differentiating minute differences of x-ray attenuation within the tissues. Attenuation differences between blood and clotted blood, between urine and bladder tumor, and between kidney and liver, for example, are discernable. However, intravenous contrast is still needed, since the attenuation differences between parenchymal organs and solid tumors may not be large enough to allow adequate discrimination.

Hounsfield Units (CT Numbers)

X-ray attenuation values are measured in Hounsfield units (HU) and are represented on the *Hounsfield scale*. Arbitrarily, water was assigned a value of 0 HU, air, of −1000 HU, and dense cortical bone, +1000 HU. The scale is not limited but extends above and below these values, depending on the quality of a particular machine.

Numerical readout of the attenuation values from specific areas is obtained by placing a cursor anywhere on the image matrix while monitoring the image on the CRT. Renal mass with attenuation value between 0 and 20 HU is likely a cyst, while a value of −50 HU is characteristic of a lipomatous tumor. Since x-ray attenuation is directly proportional to the atomic number (Z) of the material through which it passes, the CT number in a circuitous way measures the specific weight of different tissues, at least on precontrast scans.

Window Width and Window Level

The human eye is capable of distinguishing up to 64 levels of gray and, when presented with an image of 2000 levels of gray or more (such as the Hounsfield scale), it cannot discriminate such small density differences (Fig. 1–13).

Two controls provide for selection of *window width* and *window level*. These allow high-contrast

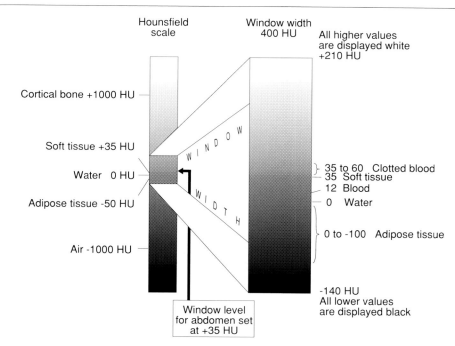

Figure 1–13. Hounsfield scale.

viewing around the area of interest. For instance, the window level is set at +35 HU when examining soft tissues of the abdomen, above +100 HU when examining bones, and −700 HU when examining air-filled lungs (Fig. 1–14). The window width selects only a segment of the Hounsfield scale and displays that "window" at the full 256 gray levels. All values above the window width are displayed as white, and all values below are displayed as black (Fig. 1–15).

Archiving and Viewing

The acquired images are then photographed from a CRT monitor or are laser printed on a film for interpretation and archiving. Alternative type of archiving is on an optical disc. The images may be recalled and viewed on an image-viewing station composed of one or several CRT monitors.

MAGNETIC RESONANCE IMAGING

Nucleus as a Dipole

A spinning atomic nucleus possessing a magnetic field is called a dipole. Similar to our planet, a spinning nucleus has opposing magnetic poles of

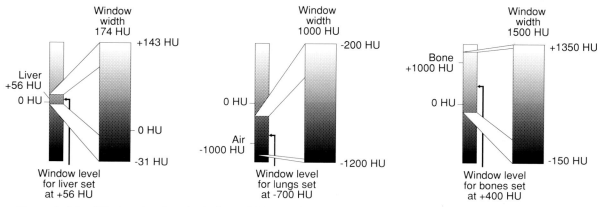

Figure 1–14. Window level and window width are chosen for viewing and printing of an already acquired digital image, depending on which area of the body is viewed and on the amount of contrast needed to best display pathological processes.

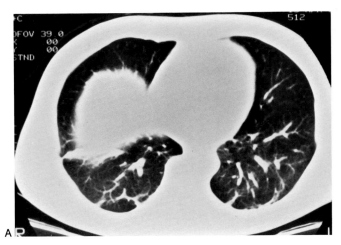
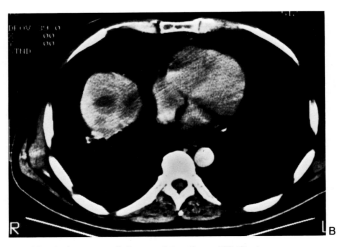

Figure 1–15.   CT scan obtained through the lower thorax and includes part of dome of the liver. **(A)** On lung window even the small vessels are well visualized at the lung bases. The heart, liver, bones, and muscles all appear white. **(B)** When the liver window is chosen, lung detail is gone and displayed as black. Within the liver, however, a hypodense metastasis becomes visible.

equal magnitude. All nuclei of hydrogen (proton), sodium, and phosphorus exhibit this phenomenon.

Magnetic Moment (Mo)

The strength and direction of the magnetic field created by the spinning nucleus is called *magnetic moment* (Mo). Like any other vector, magnetic moment is graphically represented by an arrow. The arrow size is proportional to the magnetic field strength and the arrow orientation to its direction.

Net Magnetization Vector (M)

Dipoles in our bodies are randomly oriented and their vectors (Mo) point every which way. When placed in an *external magnetic field* (H) all dipoles align with the external field's magnetic lines of force. Sum total of all Mo of the aligned dipoles is a *net magnetization vector* (M) and is also represented by an arrow (Fig. 1–16).

Precession

The dipoles are never perfectly aligned with H and rotate along the axis of H, much as a spinning top wobbles around a vertical line representing gravitational line of pull. This random and out-of-phase motion is induced by dipole spin and misalignment torque and is called *precession*.

Larmor Frequency

The frequency by which the nucleus wobbles is referred to as *precession frequency* or *Larmor frequency*. This frequency is dependent on the external magnetic field strength and on a *gyromagnetic constant*. The gyromagnetic constant is a known value and is specific for each element (gyromagnetic constant for hydrogen is 42.58 MHz). It follows that in the same magnetic field different types of nuclides have precession frequencies that are unique for them. It also follows that Larmor frequency for hydrogen is different in imagers with dissimilar magnetic field strengths.

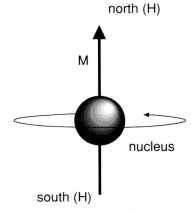

Figure 1–16.   Net magnetization vector.

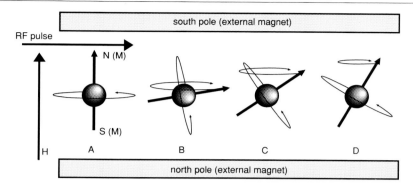

Figure 1–17. The 90° RF pulse knocks aligned dipoles (**A**) to a 90° orientation to H (**B**), where they continue to wobble and induce a signal as they pass by antenna coil. Eventually, they realign with the external magnetic field (**C,D**) and the signal becomes progressively weaker.

RF Pulse

The stable orientation of M in H may be changed by subjecting all dipoles to a radio frequency (RF) pulse through an antenna coil surrounding the patient. The RF pulse must have a frequency that matches the Larmor frequency (multiple of external magnetic field strength and gyromagnetic constant [example: 0.5 T × 42.58 MHz = 21.29 MHz]).

RF pulse is applied perpendicular to H long enough to change the orientation of M from a vertical axis (along H) to tranverse plane (perpendicular to H). An RF pulse of appropriate duration to accomplish this is referred to as "90° pulse." In some instances M need not reach the transverse plane and may be at any angle *(flip angle)* in relation to H.

MR Signal

Once the RF pulse is turned off, rotating M returns in a spiral fashion into alignment with H (Fig. 1–17). RF coils now assume the function of a receiving antenna. Rotating M induces current in the antenna, which is sinusoidal and of decreasing amplitude as it spirals into H orientation. If M is allowed to return to H axis free of any interference, the signal produced is called *free induction decay (FID) signal* (Fig. 1–18). This in essence is magnetic resonance signal. The time for this decay is characterized by a time constant T1 or *T1 relaxation time.*

Phase

Ninety degree RF pulse does more than just orient M in transverse plane. It also forces all Mo to spin in phase, all together and aligned. After the pulse, and when in phase, FID signal is the strongest. Dephasing eventually takes place as individual Mo slow down at a different rate and the signal becomes weaker. They are brought back together, in phase, by a 180° RF pulse by reversing the spin direction of Mo. Several

dephasing episodes are corrected and brought into phase by 180° RF pulses so that most of MR signal possible is generated before M had a chance to realign with H and before the next 90° pulse is initiated.

The time needed for the dephasing process to transpire (loss of nuclear spin coherence) is characterized by a time constant T2 or better known as *T2 relaxation time.*

MR Signal Intensity

Lack of signal from the sample (body, tissue, organ, mass) is represented as black (hypointense) while maximum signal is represented as white (hyperintense) on MR image. Signal intensity is proportional to:

1. Hydrogen concentration in the specimen. Since hydrogen is the most abundant nucleus in living tissue, MR imaging visually displays differences in hydrogen concentration in the body. The rate of signal decay, however, is markedly influenced by the bonds the water molecules have within different tissues. Most of the hydrogen nuclei in living tissues are present in water and lipids and yet these have a very different appearance on the final

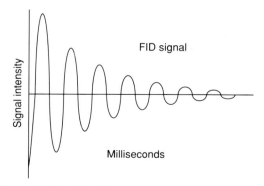

Figure 1–18. Graphic representation of FID signal.

image. The reconstructed MR image in reality represents *water bonding characteristics* in different tissues.

2. T2 relaxation time. The longer T2 relaxation time of the specimen (the longer dipoles stay in phase), the stronger the MR signal.

Signal intensity is inversely proportional to T1 relaxation time. Dipoles with short T1 relaxation time rapidly recover from the 90° RF pulse (M rapidly realigns with H). One hundred eighty degree pulse does nothing to them so that there are no phasing episodes to produce more signal.

Spatial Orientation

Three additional magnetic fields, called *gradient fields,* are introduced in various planes within H. Gradient fields change the strength of H and along their narrow planes of influence force dipoles to: 1) precess at a different Larmor frequency; 2) respond to slightly different RF pulse frequency; and 3) emit MR signal of different frequency. Of course, the RF pulse, instead of being a single frequency, is purposely made of a narrow band of frequencies to match these differences in Larmor frequencies. Since the rate of change along the gradient is known, and the frequency from a specific voxel is known, it is possible to assign that voxel a specific depth on two-dimensional representation. In addition, gradient fields also determine slice thickness and size of the active imaging area.

Pulse Sequences

The timing and character of the RF pulse are known as pulse sequences.

REPETITION TIME (TR)

TR is the time interval between two pulse sequences, usually between 200 and 2000 ms.

ECHO TIME (TE)

TE is the time interval between the first 90° pulse and the moment at which the MR signal is read, usually 18 to 120 ms.

SPIN ECHO T1-WEIGHTED SEQUENCE

The sequence starts with a 90° pulse, followed by 180° pulse, and signal readout (Fig. 1–19).

Repetition time (TR) is the time between two 90° pulses and is kept short. Sequences employing short TR and TE times, for example 300/28, bring out T1 characteristics of the tissues and are called *T1 weighted.*

On T1-weighted MR images, subcutaneous and retroperitoneal fat, a strong signal producer, is presented as white. Muscle, urine, and calcium are depicted dark on the image as they emit a signal of low intensity. Liver, spleen, pancreas, adrenal glands, and lymph nodes emit signals of medium intensity and are shown as gray. Renal cortex is of medium signal intensity while renal medulla is relatively more hypointense than cortex and appears darker. Corticomedullary differentiation is therefore possible even without contrast (Fig. 1–20).

SPIN ECHO T2-WEIGHTED SEQUENCE

The sequence starts with a 90° pulse followed by a series of rephasing 180° pulses. Number of readouts are obtained in between 180° pulses. These sequences employ long TR and TE times, for example, 2000/80, place emphasis on T2 characteristics, and are referred to as *T2 weighted.*

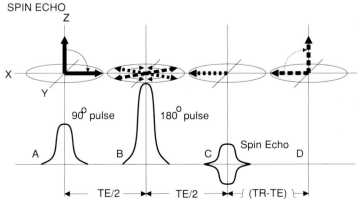

Figure 1–19. Schematic presentation of T1-weighted spin echo sequence. After a 90° pulse brings M into horizontal plane (**A**), a 180° pulse brings all rotating M into phase (**B**). This is when the signal is the strongest (**C**) but it soon decays as M realigns with the external magnetic field (**D**).

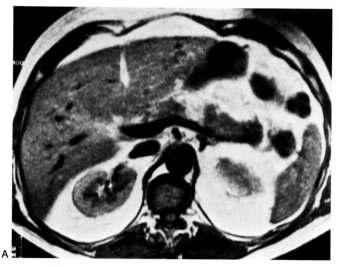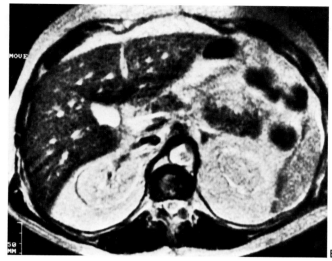

Figure 1–20. **(A)** T1-weighted image is easily recognized because spinal fluid is always of low signal intensity (dark) on this sequence. The gallbladder on this particular image is almost invisible. **(B)** T2-weighted sequence is recognized because of strong signal (bright) produced by the spinal fluid. Note changes in signal intensity between the two sequences. Gallbladder is now clearly seen as a bright area in an otherwise dark liver. The kidneys are now almost isointense to the retroperitoneal fat.

On T2-weighted images, the same tissues appear totally different compared with T1-weighted images. Liver and muscle become much darker (hypointense), while the spleen and kidneys become bright (hyperintense). Fluid tends to be hyperintense, air and calcium hypointense. Gas appears the same on both.

Tumors usually have different appearances on T1- and T2-weighted sequences and usually appear hyperintense (bright) on T2-weighted images.

INVERSION RECOVERY

The sequence starts with a 180° pulse, followed after an interval by a 90° pulse, followed by another 180° pulse. The sequence emphasizes T1 characteristics. If the interval between the initiating 180° and 90° pulse (inverting pulse time, or TI) is made short, the sequence is known as *short pulse time inversion recovery or STIR,* for short. In STIR images the signal from fat is markedly diminished and motion artefacts are reduced.

GRADIENT OR FIELD-ECHO SEQUENCES

The sequence starts with a pulse between 5° and 90° (flip angle) followed by rephasing, which is accomplished by reversing the gradient field rather than by 180° pulses. These sequences may use very short repetition times (TR) and readout times (TE), requiring little time for completion of examination.

These sequences are T1 weighted if the flip angle is between 45° and 90°, TR is short, and TE very, very short (200/8).

These sequences are known as *proton density weighted* if the flip angle is between 5° and 20°, TR is short, and TE very, very short (200/8).

Gradient echo images are particularly useful in depicting blood vessels, since flowing blood presents with an extremely strong signal.

Field Strength and Type of Magnets

The strength of the magnetic field is measured in *tesla (T).* Commercially available magnets range between 0.3 and 2 T. Mid-strength field magnets are adequate and perhaps better in depicting abdominal organs than high field. Permanent and hybrid magnets have a contained magnetic field. Cryogenic magnets have a magnetic field extending beyond the gantry, thus requiring extra precaution regarding admittance of metallic objects into the examining room.

Surface Coils

Resolution may be significantly improved by employing a surface coil placed as close to the anatomical area of interest as possible (Fig. 1–21). Surface coils only image a small field of view comparable to

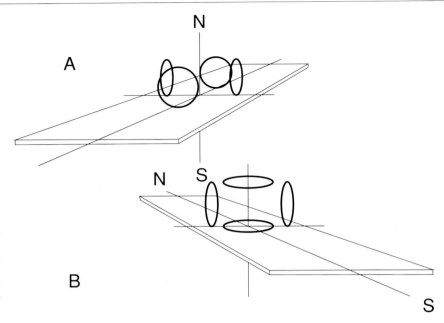

Figure 1–21. Orientation of the surface coil in relation to the magnetic field and table top is different for the permanent magnet (**A**) and superconductive tubular magnet (**B**). The latter is more conducive to performing examinations such as scrotal and endorectal prostatic MR imaging.

their size. In uroradiology there are excellent uses for surface coils, particularly for examination of the scrotum and its contents. An endorectal surface coil has been developed for the prostate.[1]

MR Imaging of Abdomen and Pelvis

MR images are continually acquired over a period of time, usually spanning 10 to 20 minutes per pulse sequence. Any motion during image acquisition adversely affects image quality. Respiration, bowel peristalsis, vascular and cardiac pulsation, and voluntary and involuntary muscular movements all contribute to degradation of the final image. Patient cooperation is essential for obtaining good images. Glucagon (0.1 mg IV) may decrease bowel peristalsis and improve image quality. Motion is less noticeable in the pelvis compared with the upper abdomen.

MR imaging of abdomen and pelvis usually requires both T1- and T2-weighted pulse sequences in the same or different planes. Choice of imaging planes depends largely on the indication and specific organ being evaluated.

Precautions

Metal objects can be attracted to the magnet; thus, oxygen tanks, IV poles, etc., cannot be brought into the examining room.

Patients with surgical clips in the head and heart, metallic ear prostheses, orthopedic prostheses, etc., are at risk. Surgical clips in the abdomen older than 6

weeks pose no danger but may introduce artefacts and interfere with image quality.

Some patients develop claustrophobia within the confined gantry space. Infants have to be sedated.

NUCLEAR MEDICINE

Principles

Unlike radiography, which relies on x-ray transmission *through* the patient, nuclear medicine relies on gamma-ray emission *from* the patient. This is achieved by injecting the patient with a pharmaceutical compound labeled with a radioisotope. The behavior of the radiopharmaceutical compound, such as concentration in different parts of the body, accumulation, and excretion rates, can be documented by tracing the tagged-on radioactive element. This allows functional assessment of various organs, particularly the kidneys.

Detection and spatial presentation are carried out using a multitude of detectors arranged in a lead-shielded container called a *gamma camera*. Only parallel gamma rays are admitted to the receptor. All others are rejected by a multihole collimator installed in front of the gamma camera. A 256 × 256 matrix is used and images are presented in the coronal plane, either as the anterior or posterior view. The printed image is called a scintigram. Resolution of the system is below those of other imaging modalities. The primary application in the urinary tract is the functional assessment of the kidneys followed by radionuclide cystography and detection of bone metastases in patients with carcinoma of the prostate.

Radiopharmaceuticals

The radioisotope used almost exclusively for labeling radiopharmaceuticals in urinary tract examinations is Tc-99m (technetium). The half-life of this radiolabel is 6 hours (after six half-lives no detectable radioactivity remains) and it emits 143 keV gamma rays.

Many radiopharmaceuticals have been developed for evaluation of the urinary tract but only those listed below are in common use today.

Renal Radiopharmaceuticals

Renal radiopharmaceuticals are conveniently divided according to their mechanism of excretion by the kidneys.

GLOMERULAR FILTRATION

Tc-99m DTPA (diethylenetriaminepentaacetic acid) is eliminated from the body by glomerular filtration. There is no tubular cell reabsorption, retention, or secretion.

Following rapid intravenous injection of a compact bolus, there is rapid transit through the kidney. Early sequential imaging, obtained a few seconds apart, demonstrates blood flow to the kidney.

Within minutes the tracer is seen in the cortex during tubular transit and eventually it appears in the collecting system (Fig. 1–22). Delayed images provide information regarding the collecting system, such as hydronephrosis.

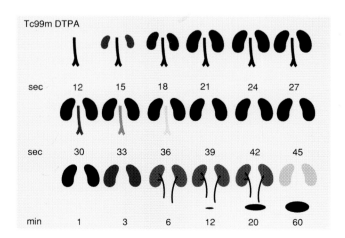

Figure 1–22. Schematic presentation of Tc-99m scintigraphy. Increased activity is represented as dark.

In all respects the behavior of this radiopharmaceutical parallels that of radiographic contrast materials. However, only a miniscule amount of the tracer is needed to crudely visualize the vascular system, and compare relative function of both kidneys.

Because of the rapid imaging necessary to visualize blood flow, the dose administered should be relatively high, 12–15 mCi. Because the tracer is present in the upper urinary tract system for only a limited time, the dose to the kidney is low. An exception, of course, is ureteral obstruction where the dose to the obstructed kidney is higher because of prolonged retention of the radionuclide.

The main application of Tc-99m DTPA is in evaluation of relative renal perfusion, such as in renal transplants, suspected renovascular hypertension, and exclusion of vascular occlusion in patients with acute anuria.

TUBULAR SECRETION

I-131 OIH (o-iodohippurate) is cleared from plasma primarily by tubular secretion and to a lesser degree by glomerular filtration. Extraction efficiency is about 80%. High gamma energy of 364 keV, presence of beta emission, and long half-life, make it an unattractive imaging agent. Its clearance reflects effective renal plasma flow (ERPF).

Tc-99m MAG₃ (mercaptoacetyltriglycine) is cleared from plasma primarily by tubular secretion, with a total extraction efficiency of 70–90%. It is likely to replace I-131 OIH (o-iodohippurate) and Tc-99m DMSA.[2] Estimate of ERPF is possible. Excellent images of the kidney are possible, unlike those obtained with higher energy I-131 OIH.[2–5]

TUBULAR BINDING

Tc-99m DMSA (dimercaptosuccinate) is bound by the tubules and accumulates up to several hours in the renal cortex. Pharmacologically, this compound behaves much like the mercurial diuretic chlormerodin. Prolonged cortical retention provides for excellent morphological imaging of the renal parenchyma.

Because of prolonged retention by the tubular cells, the total dose should not exceed 2–6 mCi because radiation dose to the kidney will be unacceptably high. This limitation does not permit renal blood flow studies (radionuclide angiography) with this tracer.

The main application of Tc-99m DMSA is in differentiating renal pseudotumors from tumors, and in quantitative analysis of renal function. For example, activity in each kidney can be expressed as a percentage of total renal function after correction for background activity.

COMPLEX RENAL HANDLING

Tc-99m GHA (glucoheptonate) undergoes glomerular filtration, tubular secretion, tubular binding, and tubular reabsorption. Because of moderate excretion rate, the collecting system can be evaluated in the first 30 minutes. Tubular binding of the tracer allows assessment of cortical morphology on images obtained at 1 hour.

Other Radiopharmaceuticals

- Tc-99m pertechnetate is injected as a bolus for diagnosis of testicular torsion.
- I-131-6-iodomethyl-19-norcholesterol concentrates in functioning adrenal cortical adenomas such as aldosteronomas.
- Tc-99m diphosphonate is the bone scanning agent for detection and follow-up of bone metastases.
- In-111 labeled leukocytes are used to detect obscure focus of infection, such as infected cyst in polycystic disease.[6]

Archiving

Images obtained by most imaging methods are conventionally viewed as if the patient were facing the examiner. Scintigrams, however, are viewed the way they were obtained, pretending that the eye is the gamma camera. Since almost all renal nuclear medicine imaging is a posterior view, that is, the image is obtained with the gamma camera close to the patient's back, the scintigrams are also viewed from the back.

SONOGRAPHY

Audible sound (to humans) ranges from 16 to 20,000 Hz. Ultrasound is any sound with frequency greater than audible sound. Depth and fish finders in the marine environment use ultrasound in 50 to 250 KHz range. Medical imaging uses ultrasound ranging in frequencies from 2 to 10 MHz.

Production and Detection of Ultrasound

Piezoelectric crystals expand or contract when crossed by electric current, depending on polarity. The reverse is also true. Piezoelectric crystals produce electricity when their volume is changed, for example, when deformed by a reflected ultrasound wave.

Ultrasound may be generated by oscillating piezoelectric crystals by alternating electrical current with specific frequency. More commonly, however, ultrasound in medical imaging is produced by "jolting" the crystal with a single short electrical pulse and allowing it to resonate for a very short period of time, much like a guitar string. In this situation ultrasound frequency is determined by the crystal thickness.

Most transducers send 1000 pulses per second. Ultrasound transducer serves both as an ultrasound generator and detector. In fact, most of the time the transducer "listens" for returning echoes from the body after an extremely short pulse. Returning echoes deform the piezoelectric crystal ever so slightly and thus generate minute electrical signals.

Since the velocity of ultrasound in the body is known (1.5 mm/μsec), the time it takes for ultrasound pulse to reflect (echo) can be converted into distance (or depth) of the reflective surfaces from the transducer.

Reflection

Reflection occurs at interfaces where the tissues on two sides are of different densities, i.e., have different *acoustic impedance*. The greater the density difference, the greater the reflection. Very small differences in densities are needed for reflection to occur, in which case a very small portion of the beam is reflected. The main beam continues through the body and parts of it are reflected at each subsequent interface. On its way back to the transducer a portion of the returning beam may again be reflected away from the transducer.

Reflection may be specular and nonspecular. For *specular reflection* to occur, the interface surface must be larger than the sound beam. The incidence angle and the reflection angle in specular reflection are equal. The echo at the transducer is the strongest when the interface (specular reflector) is 90° to the primary beam. It follows that the strength (or the amplitude) of the return beam is dependent not only on the difference in acoustical impedance at the interface, but also on the angle of incidence or "dependence angle." Examples of specular reflectors are surfaces of liver, kidney, spleen, prostate, and great vessels.

Reflection is *nonspecular* if the interface is smaller than the sound beam. The strength of a nonspecular echo is independent of the primary beam direction. The small interface is surrounded by the beam and incidence angle is nonexistent. Examples of nonspecular reflectors are cells, intercellular spaces, renal tubules, capillaries, and small vessels. Although smaller in amplitude than head-on specular reflections, the nonspecular echoes make gray scale sonography, or visual representation of different tissue textures, possible.

Attenuation

Multiple to and fro reflections, reflections at an angle away from the transducer, tissue absorption, scatter (by interface surfaces smaller than the primary beam), refraction, and diffraction all contribute to marked attenuation of the primary and also of the returning beam. The beam is attenuated by approximately 1 dB/cm/MHz. Higher frequency beam is attenuated much more readily than a beam of lower frequency. By the time a beam reaches several centimeters into the body, most of the higher frequencies are attenuated or filtered out. The beam has been "softened."

It follows that for imaging deeper in the body a high-frequency beam is impossible to use. Usually 3 or 3.5 MHz is more practical. More superficial structures may be imaged with a 5 MHz beam, while small parts (such as testicle and prostate transrectal probe) may be imaged with 7 MHz or even higher frequency beam.

Resolution

Axial resolution is resolution along the pathway of the beam. Axial resolution cannot exceed half the pulse length. Since the speed of ultrasound in the tissues is 1.5 mm/μsec and since each pulse generation is limited typically to 1 or 2 μsec, it follows that a typical pulse is about 2 mm long. Half of this value is the best possible axial resolution expressed in millimeters (Fig. 1–23).

Pulse length cannot be shorter than one wavelength. The only way to shorten pulse length (generate it for a shorter period of time) is to use higher frequency sounds, since their wave lengths are shorter. This is why a 7 MHz "small parts" transducer provides better resolution than a 3 MHz transducer.

Lateral resolution refers to resolution in a plane 90° to the beam and is limited by the beam width. The thinner the beam, the smaller the distances between separate interfaces in this plane that can be resolved. A beam may be made thinner by focusing.

Focused Transducers

The simplest way to focus the beam is to interpose an acoustical lens in front of the piezoelectric crystal.

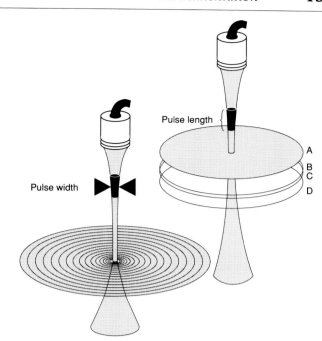

Figure 1–23. It is visually obvious that a pulse length (depicted black) cannot resolve planes B and C from each other. It is also obvious that beam focusing is not uniform along the entire depth, and lateral resolution will be the best where the beam is the narrowest.

The area where the beam is focused the narrowest (2–3 mm) and where lateral resolution is the best is referred to as *focal zone*. The distance between focal zone and the transducer is referred to as *focal length*. The focal length of the transducer may be short for imaging of near field or made longer for imaging at any particular depth.

Phased-array transducers, as the name implies, are made of a number of crystal elements, each independently controlled by its own circuitry. These can be arranged in a single line (linear phased-array transducers) or in concentric rings (annular phased-array transducers). If each individual crystal is activated in a phased sequence, slightly apart, the outer crystals first, the net effect resembles that of an acoustical lens. Some such transducers can be electronically focused during the examination for optimal resolution at the depth required.

Real-Time Imaging

A sweeping beam is created mechanically by rocking or rotating the crystal within the transducer or bouncing the beam from an oscillating acoustical mirror. The beam may also be made to sweep electronically from phased linear array transducers.

Returning echoes are amplified and digitized and displayed on a video format. The operator may make certain adjustments regarding the video display, such as brightness and contrast levels, but these should be optimally adjusted and thereafter left alone (Fig. 1–24).

More importantly, the operator has control of the *time compensated gain (TCG)* function, which is differential amplification of returning echoes. Those echoes returning from deeper areas of the body are disproportionately attenuated compared with more superficial echoes. To make the final image more balanced, these late echoes need to be proportionately amplified. The operator should adjust TCG knob while looking at the liver until the near field and far field are the same shade of gray and the density of echoes is uniform throughout the image.

The other operating button is *gain control,* which increases all the echoes uniformly and should be set high enough for all solid tissues to produce echoes. Only clear fluid, such as urine, is echo-free.

Shadowing and Enhancement

When an interface is between two areas with marked difference in densities (acoustic impedance) such as between soft tissues and renal calculus, or between soft tissue and gas, the sound beam is almost completely reflected. Without a sound beam left to produce echoes in the tissues behind the acoustically grossly mismatched regions, a "shadow" is seen on the monitor. Stones, gas, rib, or foreign material such as clips and tubes are the most common "shadow" producers. This phenomenon allows detection of renal stones or gallstones, but it may also hide important pathological findings within the shadow.

Where there are no interfaces, such as in a simple renal cyst, for example, the sound beam is not attenuated and has greater amplitude (or intensity) as it emerges from the cyst compared to a parallel beam that has propagated through the tissues. The tissues under the cyst, having unattenuated sound beam available, produce more intense echoes and appear "enhanced."

Reverberations and Refractions

These are some important sources of artefacts on sonographic images. *Reverberation* occurs when the returning beam reflects from the transducer back into the tissues. Upon echoing back into the transducer, it produces spurious signals portraying one or more tissue interfaces that in reality do not exist.

Refraction refers to bending of the beam at the edges of acoustically mismatched interfaces. The tissues from which the beam is refracted away are echo-free and resemble acoustical "shadowing."

Duplex Doppler Sonography

Doppler shift refers to the magnitude of frequency change when sound and observer are in relative motion to each other. In medical sonography this effect has been successfully applied to detect blood flow. Compared to the original beam transmitted from an ultrasound transducer, a returning ultrasound beam will have changed frequency when reflected by flowing blood. The magnitude of the frequency change is proportional to the flow velocity.

Continuous wave Doppler instruments employ separate transducers, one for continuous transmission and the other for uninterrupted reception of reflected echoes. Changes in frequency over time may be listened to in audible tone. Doppler flow meters use this technique.

Pulsed Doppler uses a single transducer to send short pulses. The returning echoes are detected by the same transducer and analyzed for the Doppler shift frequency.

Duplex Doppler instruments combine pulsed Doppler and real-time sonographic imaging. An electronic gate allows the operator to choose a small area of interest for analysis and to aim the interrogating

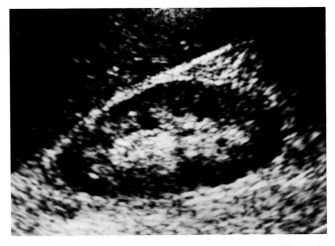

Figure 1–24. Typical appearance of a sonogram of the right kidney.

beam appropriately. The source of the vascular signal and its place relative to other anatomical structures in the body is discerned on real-time imaging. The returning echo is processed by a spectrum analyzer and graphically displayed as shift frequency (or velocity) over time. The shape of this graphic display is influenced by resistance to flow in the distal vascular bed. High or low vascular resistance can be defined by utilizing different pulsatility indices. One such pulsatility index is defined as the height of the peak systolic component minus the height of end-diastolic component divided by the height of the peak systolic component.

Color Doppler displays motion in color. Different colors are chosen to symbolize different velocities. Flow toward the transducer may also be assigned color to differentiate it from the flow away from the transducer.

REFERENCES

1. Schnall MD, Lenkinski RE, Pollack HM, et al. Prostate: MR imaging with an endorectal surface coil. Radiology 1989; 172:570–574.
2. Taylor A Jr, Ziffer JA, Steves A, et al. Clinical comparison of I-131 ortoiodohippurate and the kit formulation of Tc-99m mercaptoacetyltriglycine. Radiology 1989; 170:721–725.
3. McAfee JG. Update on radiopharmaceuticals for medical imaging. Radiology 1989; 171:593–601.
4. Schaap GH, Alferink THR, deJong RBJ, et al. Tc-99m MAG3: dynamic studies in patients with renal disease. Eur J Nucl Med 1988; 14:28–31.
5. Russell CD, Thorstad BL, Stutzman ME, et al. The kidney: imaging with Tc-99m mercaptoacetyltriglycine, a technetium-labeled analog of iodohippurate. Radiology 1989; 172:427–430.
6. McAfee JG, Samin A. In-111 labeled leucocytes: review of problems in image interpretation. Radiology 1985; 155:221–223.

2

Procedures and Anatomy

EXCRETORY UROGRAPHY (INTRAVENOUS PYELOGRAPHY)

Excretory urography (EXU) is one of the basic methods of urinary tract imaging and is presented here as an example of projectional imaging. After the development of modern intravenous radiographic contrasts, this examination replaced retrograde pyelography for the majority of patients with urinary tract problems and was appropriately named intravenous pyelography (IVP). When it became evident that other parts of the urinary tract system, including renal parenchyma, ureters, bladder, and even urethra, could be visualized after intravenous administration of contrast, and, that in a crude way, one could determine the difference in renal function between two kidneys, an effort was made to change the name to excretory urography (EXU) so that these additional imaging capabilities would be more accurately reflected.

With the development of sonography and CT, the role of EXU has somewhat diminished. This is primarily because renal parenchyma is better visualized with these two imaging modalities. Even small renal masses are detected and characterized with greater frequency and accuracy than ever before possible on EXU.[1] Presence of a retroperitoneal tumor or lymph node enlargement could previously only be inferred indirectly, by the amount of renal or ureteral displacement on EXU. Direct visualization of these abnormalities is the norm on cross-sectional imaging modalities.

Nevertheless, EXU remains an important radiological imaging method by which the collecting system and ureters (the plumbing part of the system, if you will) are rendered visible. Spatial resolution far ex-

ceeds that of cross-sectional methods so that small filling defects (which may represent epithelial neoplasm) or other discrete pathological entities, such as papillary necrosis, small calculi, and ureteral pathology, are better seen. EXU is a quick and efficient method for evaluating patients with suspected urolithiasis, obstruction, hematuria, and recurrent infection. Attention to technical details, such as using low kVp and appropriately matched film-screen combinations, adequate dose of contrast material, patient preparation, ureteral compression, proper exposure, and monitoring progress of examination, are absolutely necessary for performing a successful examination.[2]

Patient Preparation

Most radiologists prefer to administer a laxative one night prior to examination. No solid food should be consumed after supper. The patient is allowed liquids until several hours before the procedure. Dehydration should be avoided. Empty stomach at the time of the examination diminishes the possibility of aspiration should the patient vomit after contrast injection.

Preliminary Radiograph ("Scout Film")

Preliminary (scout) radiograph is always obtained prior to administration of intravenous, intra-arterial, or intracavitary radiographic contrast for the following reasons:

1. *To check on the technical quality of the examination.* It is improper to administer radiographic contrast to the patient if the positioning is not correct, or

if the radiograph is over- or underexposed. A proper preliminary radiograph for contrast examination of the urinary tract must include the areas of both adrenal glands on the top and 2 cm below the inferior margin of the symphysis pubis on the bottom. Frequently, it is impossible to fit this large area on a single radiograph and two different film formats will have to be used.

2. *To detect urinary tract calculi.* Contrast in the collecting system may make urinary calculi invisible. Without the preliminary radiograph, many renal calculi cannot be diagnosed. Frequently, it is impossible from a single preliminary radiograph to determine whether a calcific density is in the expected anatomical distribution of the urinary tract. An additional oblique projection is often needed to take a second look at the calcification to see if it "moves" with the kidney.

3. *To determine whether a contraindication to abdominal compression exists.* Compression is frequently used in the course of an excretory urogram in order to distend the upper urinary tract system, thus better visualizing the collecting system. Contraindications to compression are: abdominal aorta or iliac artery aneurysm (Fig. 2–1), ileus, bowel obstruction, ascites, acute abdomen, recent abdominal surgery,

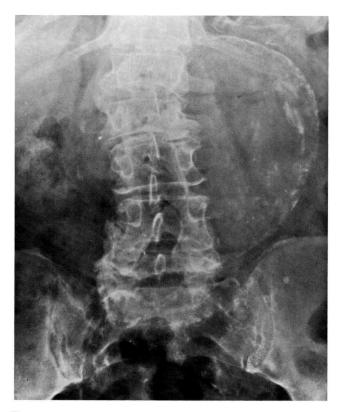

Figure 2–1. Large abdominal aorta aneurysm is an absolute contraindication to external ureteral compression.

various types of urinary tract diversions, stomas, abdominal trauma, Greenfield filter or umbrella in the inferior vena cava, and acute renal colic. Many of the radiographic signs contributing to diagnosis of the conditions just enumerated are present on the preliminary radiograph. This, of course, does not imply other pathological entities are being ignored, just that, if need be, they can be detected on all of the other radiographs obtained in the course of urographic contrast examination.

4. *To determine if bowel preparation is adequate.* Residual contrast, usually barium from an earlier radiological examination, is frequently discovered. Whether or not to proceed with the contrast examination is a decision that has to be made for each patient individually, depending on indications.

5. *To detect other pathological processes* (see Chapter 3, "Abdomen.")

Contraindications to Radiographic Contrast Injection

There are no absolute contraindications to intravenous administration of contrast material. The risks must always be weighed against the benefits.

A past history of major contrast reactions will certainly influence the radiologist to use other imaging modalities, but even in these patients pretreatment with steroids may allow a contrast examination to be performed (with some assistance from an anesthesiologist) if there are absolutely no other alternatives.

Patients with serum creatinine above 1.2 mg/dl are at higher risk of contrast nephropathy if large doses of contrast are used, such as in cardioangiography. However, in a patient with bilateral partial obstruction the site and the cause of obstruction may be identified even if creatinine is 2 mg/dl and even if a lower than standard dose of contrast is used.

The risks, prophylaxis, and treatment regimens relating to radiographic contrast are addressed in more detail in Chapter 4.

Administration of Contrast Material

Bolus technique: Contrast is delivered as a bolus through a needle appropriately sized to the patient's vein. Injection rate must also be adjusted to the vessel's size. Antecubital vein is the best. Dorsal veins of the hand should be avoided.

Arm pain may occasionally develop during the injection. In the absence of extravasation into the soft tissues the pain is most likely due to hyperosmolar effect of the contrast upon the vessel wall. The rate of injection should be decreased or injection stopped. The arm should be elevated and the venous system flushed with normal saline.

Usual dose is 1 cc/kg body weight of 60–76% contrast. This translates into 75 ml of contrast or a total of 20–22 g of iodine for a 75 kg patient.

Drip infusion: This technique has been largely abandoned but may be employed if the vessel is so small that administration of contrast may require more than 10 minutes. Contrast for drip infusion is available as a 30% concentration in 300 ml bottles. Half of this amount represents the "usual dose." The entire bottle is the "double dose."

Filming Sequence

Each urogram should be tailored to the patient's needs. A single large (14 × 17″) radiograph at 15 minutes after the injection, for example, may be adequate for the follow-up of a previously known condition and may be the only postcontrast exposure needed.

The more usual sequence is a radiograph over the kidneys within 10–20 seconds after completion of the injection during the early (and the most radiopaque) nephrographic phase (Fig. 2–2). This allows easy detection of the renal outline and avascular space-occupying lesions (Fig. 2–3). Next exposure is made at 5 minutes, at which time both collecting systems should be opacified (Fig. 2–4). Differences in renal function between the two kidneys or delay in excretion by both kidneys is determined on this radiograph. The next radiograph may be obtained with abdominal compression. The purpose is to compress the ureters against the pelvic brim, creating mild obstruction. The upper system becomes mildly distended and, as it is filled with more contrast, it is that much better seen on the radiograph (Fig. 2–5). Thereafter the compression is released and a full abdominal radiograph is obtained. Ureters are usually well seen on this "10 minute" radiograph.

Oblique radiographs may be obtained, either coned views or full views, depending on whether the collecting system or ureters deserve more attention (Fig. 2–6). Finally, a postvoid radiograph is obtained specifically to uncover any pathological process that might have gone unnoticed while the bladder was full.

An endless variety in the appearance of the pelvocalyceal system is encountered, appearances considered as diverse as are fingerprints. Anatomical nomenclature of various parts of the kidney as seen on projectional radiography is presented in Figure 2–7.

Peristalsis of the collecting system and ureter oc-

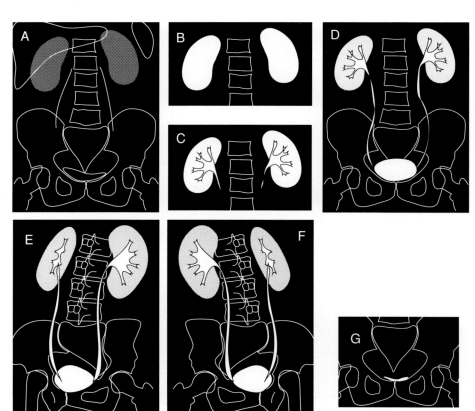

Figure 2–2. Schematic drawing of the usual filming sequence during excretory urography. **(A)** "Scout." **(B)** Early nephrogram phase when the parenchyma is the most radiopaque. **(C)** A 5-minute radiograph to detect differential in function. **(D)** Large abdominal radiograph to visualize the kidneys, ureters, and bladder is usually obtained at 10 to 15 minutes. **(E,F)** Two oblique projections may be obtained over the kidneys only or encompass ureter and bladder. **(G)** Postvoid radiograph may disclose unsuspected pathology besides providing information about residual urine. This sequence is by no means a rule and should be tailored to suit the individual patient.

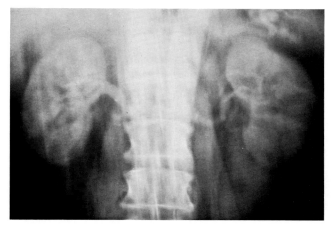

Figure 2–3. Injection of compact bolus of radiographic contrast may provide excellent visualization of the renal outline. On occasion, even the aorta and renal vessels are seen.

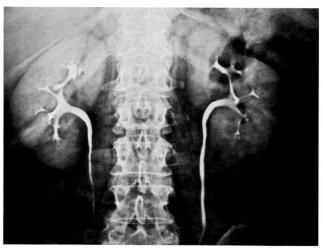

Figure 2–4. Normal excretory urogram at 5 minutes after contrast injection.

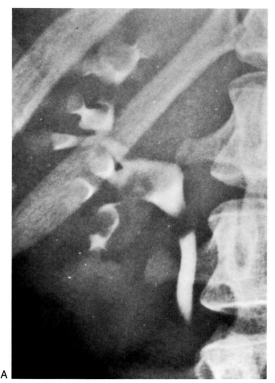

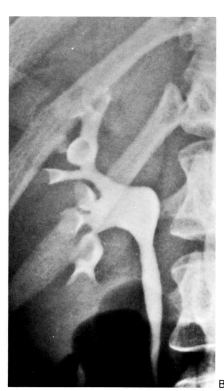

A   B

Figure 2–5. Value of external ureteral compression during urography. **(A)** Vascular impressions upon the collecting system may be misinterpreted as "filling defects" representing various pathological processes. **(B)** By applying external compression upon the ureters, relative obstruction is created so that the collecting system and ureters distend. The "filling defects" have disappeared.

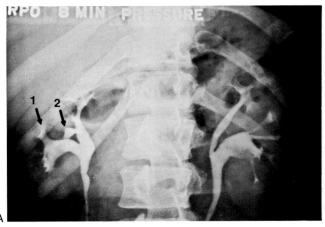
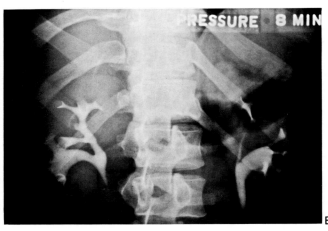

Figure 2–6. **(A)** Right posterior oblique and **(B)** left posterior oblique coned views of the kidney with compression on. Note relational change of different calyces with each other on two projections. For instance, one should be able to determine that calyx "1" is anterior to calyx "2." Understanding relative motion of two anatomical structures on different projections is of fundamental importance in mastering projectional radiography.

curs several times a minute, more if the system is burdened by diuretic effect or overfilling. Bizarre appearances may be encountered occasionally (Fig. 2–8).

Tomography

Tomography is a method that eliminates unwanted superimposing radiographic densities, such as bowel gas, which deter visualization of an area of interest. This is achieved by simultaneously moving the x-ray tube and the film cassette in opposite directions and around an imaginary fulcrum in the body. Every structure above and below the plane of the focal point will become an unrecognizable blur that will no longer interfere with visualization of the area of interest. The plane in the fulcrum will remain sharp.

During the course of examination several tomographic cuts may be obtained over the kidney, preferably in the early nephrographic phase (Fig. 2–3). By eliminating bowel gas from the image, kidneys are seen that much better. Later in the examination, tomography may help clarify any other ill-defined observation. In more obese patients excellent visualization of the kidneys is possible. In very thin patients tomography is not as pleasing.

Scoliosis and low-positioned kidney require spe-

Figure 2–7. Nomenclature and schematic presentation of renal anatomy.

- Upper pole
- Medulla
- Papilla
- Minor infundibulum
- Major infundibulum
- Septum of Bertin
- Cortex
- Fornix
- Renal capsule
- Lower pole
- Sinus fat
- Pelvis
- UPJ

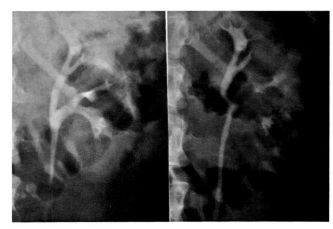

Figure 2–8. Pelvocalyceal peristalsis. Left: during relaxation. Right: during peristaltic wave.

cial attention. In both instances the two kidneys are likely in different planes and more tomographic cuts are required to visualize both. Total radiation dose is somewhat higher for the tomogram compared with the conventional radiograph. This is because the slanted x-ray beam travels diagonally through a greater volume of tissue, so that more x-rays are absorbed, and more are also needed to properly expose the film-screen combination.

PYELOGRAPHY

Retrograde Pyelography

Retrograde pyelography is the oldest in vivo radiological imaging method employed to visualize the collecting system of the kidney and ureters. Ureteral orifice is catheterized under visual control provided by a cystoscope placed in the bladder. The catheter may either be wedged in the ureterovesical orifice or it may be inserted in a retrograde manner all the way up into the collecting system.

Contrast is injected against the natural flow of urine, in a retrograde manner, hence the name. The major indication for retrograde pyelography as an imaging procedure is to render visible the parts of the collecting system and ureters that cannot be satisfactorily examined by excretory urography, particularly in those instances where a urothelial tumor is suspected.

Contrast is injected, preferably under fluoroscopic control, although "blind" retrograde injections are perfectly acceptable. Contrast concentration of 30% is adequate. Inadvertently injected bubbles of air are a common finding and interfere with diagnosis. Multiple projections, particularly oblique, make the study easier to interpret. However, because the patient is in the supine position, in the stirrups, and usually under anesthesia, obtaining oblique projections may be difficult. If such is the case, the retrograde catheter may be left in place for several hours. A perfect study, with multiple spot films, may be obtained in the radiology department when the patient is awake.

In patients with known sensitivity, iodinated contrast may be substituted with air or carbon dioxide.[3]

Retrograde catheter placement serves other useful purposes, such as selective collection of urine samples for cytology. A number of endoscopic interventional procedures are performed using the same route, such as retrograde stent placement (Fig. 2–9), retrograde brush biopsy, retrograde ureteroscopy (Fig. 2–10) and renoscopy (Fig. 2–11), retrograde

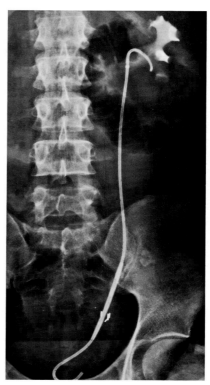

Figure 2–9. Retrograde "double J" stent placed to allow urine flow through the stricture that formed at the site of prior ureteral surgery (see surgical clips).

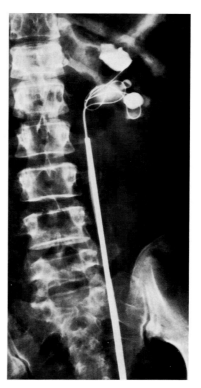

Figure 2–10. Rigid ureteroscope is introduced over a guidewire almost to the level of ureteropelvic junction.

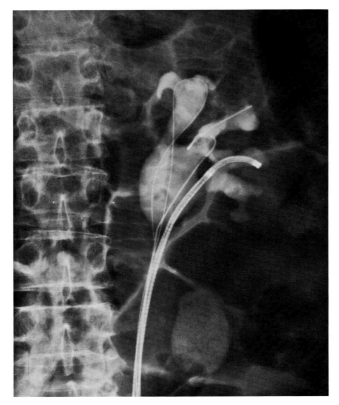

Figure 2–11. Flexible fiberoptic ureteroscope/renoscope may be selectively introduced in every calyx for visual observation, biopsy, or stone manipulation.

balloon dilatation of ureteral strictures, and endoscopic removal of ureteral calculi.

Antegrade Pyelography

Contrast may be inserted into the collecting system through an already present nephrostomy tube *(nephrostogram)*, or the collecting system may be percutaneously punctured with the sole purpose of injecting contrast *(percutaneous antegrade pyelogram)*. (See Chapter 7, "Urinary Tract Obstruction.") Antegrade pyelography is usually performed to determine the presence or absence, cause, site, and severity of ureteral obstruction.

Complications

Artificially increased pressure in the collecting system during injection of contrast material may result in complications unique to the urinary tract. These relate to contrast entering into various parts of the kidney in a backward way and are referred to as "backflows." The "backflows" indubitably occur in

cases of ureteral obstruction but are seldom identified on urography.

Pyelosinus backflow occurs when the collecting system ruptures under pressure and the contrast spills into the renal sinus (Fig. 2–12). The rupture occurs at the weakest point, which is the fornix of a calyx *(forniceal rupture)*, and the contrast assumes a streaky appearance within the sinus fat, frequently encompassing the ureter and extending into the retroperitoneum. This type of extravasation is the only one that may be identified during contrast examination of the kidney during acute obstruction.

Pyelotubular backflow refers to retrograde flow of contrast from the collecting system into the collecting tubules.[4] This is not to be confused with normal papillary blush or even distinct visualization of the collecting tubules on excretory urography.[5]

Pyelolymphatic backflow is rupture of the collecting system into the lymphatics. Since lymphatic channels drain the interstitial spaces, simultaneous *pyelointerstitial backflow* is also frequently seen (Fig. 2–13).

Pyelovenous backflow is usually most difficult to discern because rapid venous flow dilutes the small amount of contrast injected. The common site for pyelovenous intravasation is also at forniceal areas (Fig. 2–14).

Obviously, such backflows are the main venues for bacterial entrance into the bloodstream and a cause for sepsis. During performance of either retrograde or antegrade pyelography, intrapelvic pressure should not exceed 30 cm H$_2$O.

Other complications are related to inappropriate catheter placement, intravasation into bladder mucosa (Fig. 2–15), vascular intravasation (Fig. 2–16), ureteral and calyceal perforation (Fig. 2–17), etc.

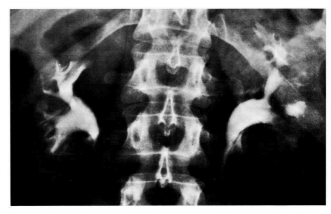

Figure 2–12. Bilateral pyelosinus backflow is seen as streaks of contrast outside collecting system.

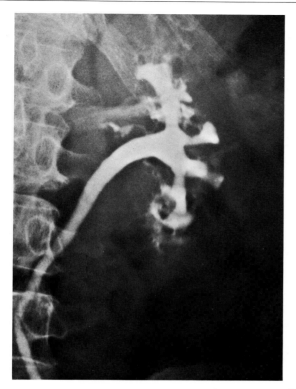

Figure 2–13. Pyelointerstitial and pyelolymphatic backflow.

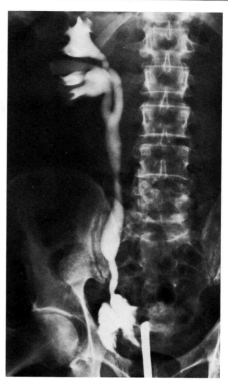

Figure 2–15. Submucosal injection of radiographic contrast into the bladder during retrograde pyelography. Although the appearance may be alarming, the consequences are negligible.

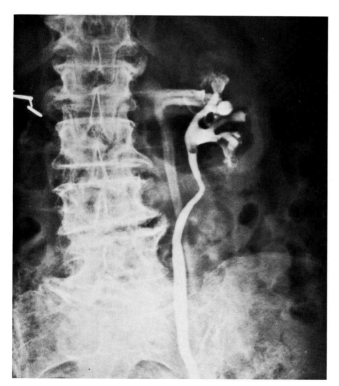

Figure 2–14. Pyelovenous backflow. Contrast is seen entering the left renal vein and is flowing in a retrograde direction in the large gonadal vein. (Photograph courtesy of Dr. E. Augustine.)

RENAL ANGIOGRAPHY

Diagnostic Renal Angiography

This is a procedure whereby a vascular radiopaque catheter is placed in the aorta at or just above the takeoff of the renal arteries. A bolus of radiographic contrast material is then injected. Simultaneously, rapid serial film exposures are made following the compact bolus on its transit through the kidneys. Because the contrast is injected into the abdominal aorta, the study is called *abdominal aortogram*. With a single contrast injection, both kidneys and their vascular supply are seen on what is a series of radiographs.

Unfortunately, many other vessels in the abdomen are simultaneously opacified so that it is frequently necessary to exchange the aortic catheter with one that may be placed directly into the renal artery under fluoroscopic control. Serial filming is again simultaneously performed with contrast injection, and the result is the *selective renal arteriogram* (Fig. 2–18). The contrast volume for selective injections is appropriately reduced.

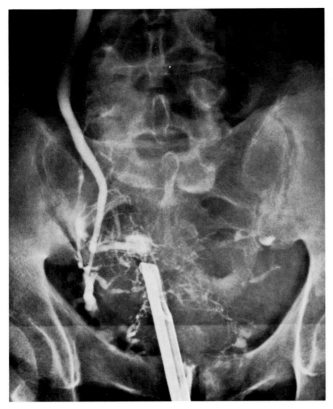

Figure 2–16. Intravasation into the pelvic veins during an attempted retrograde pyelography.

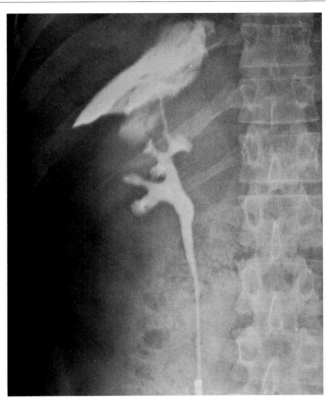

Figure 2–17. Perforation of the upper pole calyx and renal parenchyma. The injection of radiographic contrast is made in the perinephric space.

ANATOMY

Two renal arteries suppling a single kidney are seen in 20–30% of the population. The smaller artery is usually, but not always, distal.

Main renal artery divides into the *ventral and dorsal rami* and these further subdivide into *segmental arteries,* which transverse through the renal sinus (Fig. 2–19). In the next division, the *interlobar arteries* penetrate into the renal parenchyma between septum of Bertin and medullary pyramid. They give rise to *arcuate arteries* which are situated between renal cortex and medulla and toward the end become parallel to renal outline. In the next division, the *interlobular arteries* which run perpendicular to the renal outline give rise to *afferent arteries* to the glomerulus. Because the interlobular and afferent arteries are so small and there are so many of them, they are beyond resolution capability of radiographic equipment. They coalesce and contribute to the overall nephrogram.

The renal lobe is usually supplied by several interlobar arteries (Fig. 2–20) with sharp demarcation between perfused areas.

Renal arteries are not the end-arteries, since they provide blood supply to tissues other than kidneys.

Inferior adrenal arteries, capsular arteries, recursive capsular arteries, ureteric arteries, perforating capsular arteries, and pelvocalyceal rami are the vessels that originate either from the main renal artery or

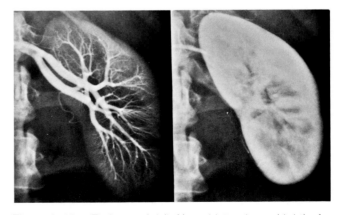

Figure 2–18. Early arterial (left) and late phase (right) of a normal selective left renal arteriogram. Most contrast is already in the proximal convoluted tubules or in glomerular tuft. Corticomedullary differentiation may be observed. Since contrast did not reach the medullar tubular structures, medulla is relatively radiolucent. Careful inspection reveals left renal vein which contains only a fraction of contrast injected into the artery and is barely visible.

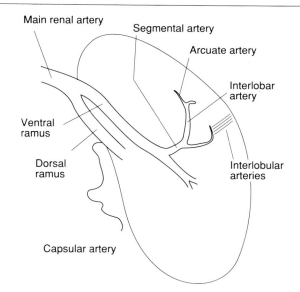

Figure 2–19. Schematic drawing of renal arterial blood supply (from Figure 2–18).

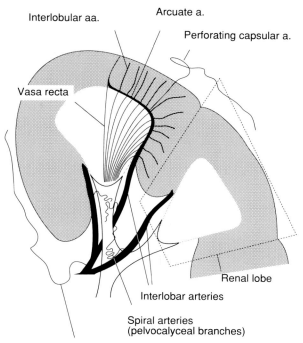

Recursive capsular a.

Figure 2–20. Renal lobe is made of all the parenchyma draining into a single calyx (dotted lines). An interlobar artery supplies only a part of a renal lobe. It pierces parenchyma in between the pyramid and septum of Bertin, thereafter becoming the arcuate artery. The arcuate eventually interposes itself between cortex and medulla and runs parallel to the kidney surface. Interlobular arteries supply cortex, including one half of the septum of Bertin. The other half is supplied by another interlobar artery. At the division between two different interlobar vascular beds, an indentation is frequently seen on the kidney surface, referred to as fetal lobation. Perforating capsular arteries may originate from the interlobar or arcuate arteries. Small spiral arteries may enlarge to provide collateral circulation to an occluded segment and produce pelvocalyceal notching.

later divisions up to and including arcuate arteries. These arteries become important collateral pathways to the kidney in the presence of renal artery stenosis.

However, renal arterial branches do not cross-communicate. Acute occlusion of any branch at any level causes complete distal infarction. This is in contrast to the venous renal circulation where there is communication at the level of segmental or arcuate veins between different segments of the kidney (Fig. 2–21).[6] Renal veins in general parallel arterial distribution.

Lymphatic drainage of the cortical and medullary interstitial spaces accompanies renal veins. Lymphatics enlarge in the presence of ureteral obstruction and some drain via the perinephric spaces, causing thickening of the bridging septa and renal fascia. Continual production of lymph by a transplanted kidney and leakage through lymphatics severed during harvest may result in a lymphocele. There are no lymph nodes in the renal sinus. First barrier is at the renal vein/gonadal vein junction on the left, and paracaval nodes on the right.

POSITIONS AND PROJECTIONS

The patient may assume several different positions for projectional radiologic examination. For a chest radiograph, for example, the patient is usually situated in the *upright* position, while for most abdominal examinations the patient's position is recumbent, usually *supine* and occasionally *prone*.

Projection is determined by the relative positions of the x-ray tube, patient, and the image receptor (film-screen cassette or image intensifier) (Fig. 2–22). *Anteroposterior (AP)* projection implies that the x-ray tube is in front of the patient and the receptor behind. In the *posteroanterior (PA)* projection the opposite is true.

If the patient is positioned sideways to the x-ray beam the projection is *lateral*. When the right side of the patient is closer to the image receptor, the projection is the *right lateral*, and if the left side is closer to the image receptor, it is the *left lateral*. There are also *upright lateral* if the patient is standing and *overhead lateral* if the patient is horizontal.

When the right side is closer to the receptor, the projection is *right overhead lateral* (Fig. 2–23) and

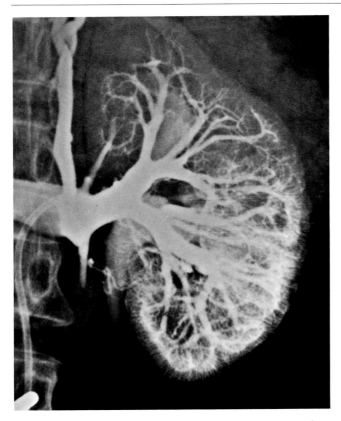

Figure 2–21. Selective retrograde left renal venogram. Arcuate veins are particularly well seen in the lower pole and likely communicate. Occlusion of one segmental venous branch does not result in venous infarct.

right anterior oblique (RAO) and *left anterior oblique (LAO)* the right or left anterior aspect of the patient, respectively, is closer to the image receptor.

If the patient continues to be on his side in the recumbent position and if the x-ray beam is horizontal, the projection is called *cross-table lateral decubitus.* When the patient is on his right side, then it is a *right cross-table decubitus,* and when the patient is lying on his left, it is *left cross-table lateral decubitus.*

Any of the above projections can be modified by angling the tube *cephalad* or *caudad.* Caudad AP projection of the pelvis, for example, "opens" the bony pelvis, while the cephalad angulation will demonstrate bladder elevation by an enlarged prostate.

Radiographic Markers

To help orient the viewer, a lead letter "R" or "L" is placed on the cassette and permanently registered on the radiograph. If only a small part of the abdomen is imaged, such as right kidney, the right marker must be on the right side of the anatomical structure imaged.

As a rule, the markers should not be trusted. Many mistakes in labeling are bound to occur, leading to incorrect diagnosis. One should practice orienting oneself without markers and question any discrepancies (Fig. 1–11A).

when the left side is closer to the film, it is *left overhead lateral.*

There are four possible oblique projections. If the right posterior aspect of the patient is closer to the image receptor, projection is the *right posterior oblique (RPO),* and if the left side of the patient is closer to the receptor, it is the *left posterior oblique (LPO).* In

CT OF ABDOMEN AND PELVIS

For the purposes of requesting radiological consultation (and billing), CT of abdomen and CT of pelvis are considered two different examinations.

If no radiographic contrast is injected, the study is referred to as *nonenhanced* or *precontrast.* On CT images, there should be a label indicating that no intravenous contrast was administered.

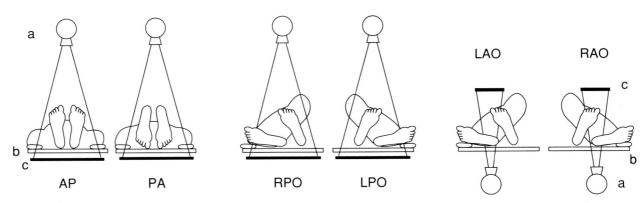

Figure 2–22. Projections in conventional radiography; a: x-ray source, b: table top, c: image receptor (e.g., film-screen combination or fluoroscope).

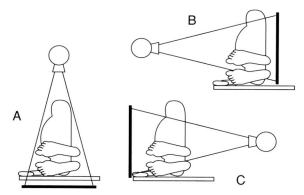

Figure 2–23. (A) Right overhead lateral projection; (B) AP right lateral decubitus; (C) PA right lateral decubitus.

If radiographic contrast is given, the study is referred to as *enhanced* or *postcontrast* and an appropriate label should be affixed on the image.

Patients undergoing CT examination routinely drink diluted barium to help differentiate enlarged lymph nodes or other mass lesions from loops of bowel. It may take several hours of intermittent drinking before the entire digestive tract is completely opacified.

Thin cuts refer to slice thickness of 2, 3, or 5 mm, the latter usually reserved for examination of adrenal glands and small renal tumors. *Thick cuts* refer to slice thickness of 10 mm or more. Slices may be *contiguous,* meaning each slice is adjacent to another, or *spaced* where areas between the slices are not imaged.

Dynamic CT scanning refers to rapid repeated acquisition of the same slice over a period of time, usually after a bolus injection of contrast material.

CT images may be *reconstructed* in any plane. Resolution in the reconstructed plane is determined by the original slice thickness. If thin contiguous slices are used for reconstruction, the resultant images have higher resolution compared with images reconstructed from thick slices.

Cross-Sectional Anatomy

Without in-depth knowledge of cross-sectional (and projectional) anatomy, it is impossible to practice good radiology. One semester at the beginning of a physician's medical education seems woefully inadequate.

Radiographic cross-sectional anatomy of the abdomen and pelvis is provided to introduce the subject and serve as a quick reference in the future (Figs. 2–24–2–45).

Perinephric and paranephric spaces and adjoining fascial layers deserve special attention (Fig. 2–46). The kidney and adrenal gland are enclosed within perinephric space boundaries, which are comprised of anterior leaf (Gerota fascia) and posterior leaf (Zukerkandl fascia) of the renal fascia (RF).[7–9] Medially, RF blends with connective tissues around great vessels. Laterally and distally, anterior and posterior leaves usually fuse. Such an enclosed space limits propagation of perinephric fluid and helps contain and arrest acute hemorrhage from the kidney. Perinephric space is filled with fat (adipose capsule of the

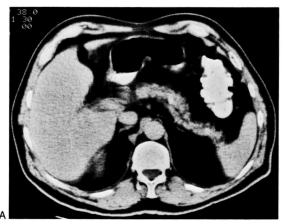

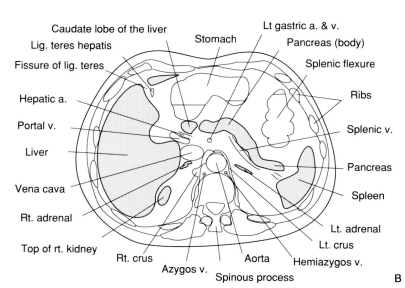

Caudate lobe of the liver
Lig. teres hepatis
Fissure of lig. teres
Hepatic a.
Portal v.
Liver
Vena cava
Rt. adrenal
Top of rt. kidney
Rt. crus
Azygos v.
Spinous process
Aorta
Hemiazygos v.
Lt. crus
Lt. adrenal
Spleen
Pancreas
Splenic v.
Ribs
Splenic flexure
Pancreas (body)
Lt gastric a. & v.
Stomach

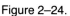

Figure 2–24.

Figures 2-24–2-35. Cross-sectional anatomy of the abdomen in a middle-aged man. The cuts are 0.5 cm thick and spaced 0.5 cm apart.

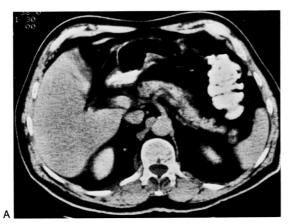

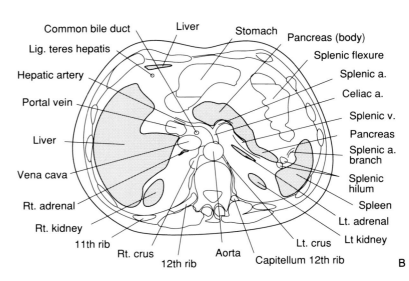

Figure 2–25.

Common bile duct — Liver — Stomach — Pancreas (body)
Lig. teres hepatis — Splenic flexure
Hepatic artery — Splenic a.
— Celiac a.
Portal vein — Splenic v.
— Pancreas
Liver — Splenic a. branch
— Splenic hilum
Vena cava — Spleen
Rt. adrenal — Lt. adrenal
Rt. kidney — Lt kidney
11th rib — Lt. crus
Rt. crus — Aorta — Capitellum 12th rib
12th rib

B

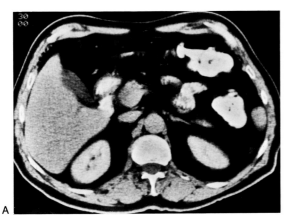

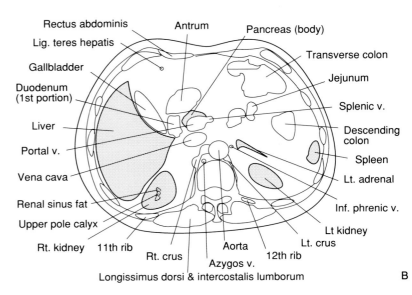

Figure 2–26.

Rectus abdominis — Antrum — Pancreas (body)
Lig. teres hepatis — Transverse colon
Gallbladder — Jejunum
Duodenum (1st portion) — Splenic v.
Liver — Descending colon
Portal v. — Spleen
Vena cava — Lt. adrenal
Renal sinus fat — Inf. phrenic v.
Upper pole calyx — Lt kidney
— Lt. crus
Rt. kidney — 11th rib — Aorta — 12th rib
Rt. crus — Azygos v.
Longissimus dorsi & intercostalis lumborum

B

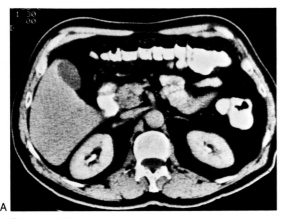

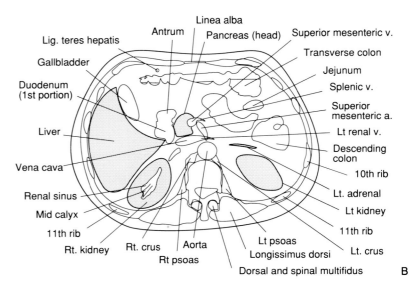

Figure 2–27.

Linea alba
Lig. teres hepatis — Antrum — Pancreas (head) — Superior mesenteric v.
Gallbladder — Transverse colon
— Jejunum
Duodenum (1st portion) — Splenic v.
— Superior mesenteric a.
Liver — Lt renal v.
— Descending colon
Vena cava — 10th rib
Renal sinus — Lt. adrenal
Mid calyx — Lt kidney
11th rib — 11th rib
Rt. kidney — Rt. crus — Aorta — Lt psoas — Lt. crus
Rt psoas — Longissimus dorsi
Dorsal and spinal multifidus

B

30

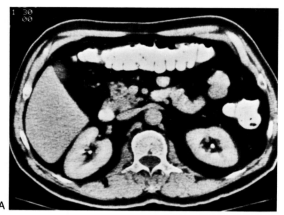

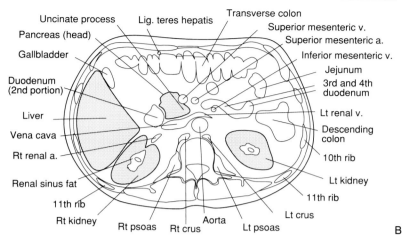

Uncinate process
Pancreas (head)
Gallbladder
Duodenum (2nd portion)
Liver
Vena cava
Rt renal a.
Renal sinus fat
11th rib
Rt kidney
Rt psoas
Rt crus
Lig. teres hepatis
Transverse colon
Superior mesenteric v.
Superior mesenteric a.
Inferior mesenteric v.
Jejunum
3rd and 4th duodenum
Lt renal v.
Descending colon
10th rib
Lt kidney
11th rib
Lt crus
Aorta
Lt psoas

A
Figure 2–28.
B

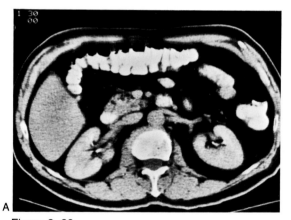

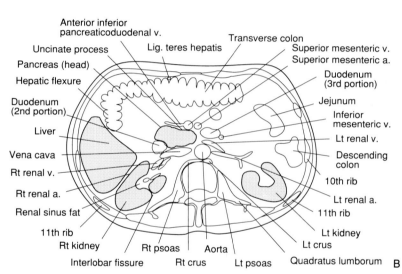

Anterior inferior pancreaticoduodenal v.
Uncinate process
Pancreas (head)
Hepatic flexure
Duodenum (2nd portion)
Liver
Vena cava
Rt renal v.
Rt renal a.
Renal sinus fat
11th rib
Rt kidney
Interlobar fissure
Rt psoas
Rt crus
Lig. teres hepatis
Transverse colon
Superior mesenteric v.
Superior mesenteric a.
Duodenum (3rd portion)
Jejunum
Inferior mesenteric v.
Lt renal v.
Descending colon
10th rib
Lt renal a.
11th rib
Lt kidney
Lt crus
Aorta
Lt psoas
Quadratus lumborum

A
Figure 2–29.
B

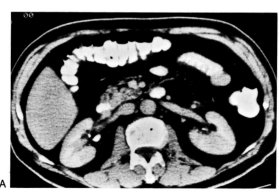

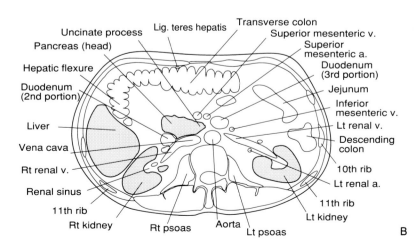

Uncinate process
Pancreas (head)
Hepatic flexure
Duodenum (2nd portion)
Liver
Vena cava
Rt renal v.
Renal sinus
11th rib
Rt kidney
Rt psoas
Lig. teres hepatis
Transverse colon
Superior mesenteric v.
Superior mesenteric a.
Duodenum (3rd portion)
Jejunum
Inferior mesenteric v.
Lt renal v.
Descending colon
10th rib
Lt renal a.
11th rib
Lt kidney
Aorta
Lt psoas

A
Figure 2–30.
B

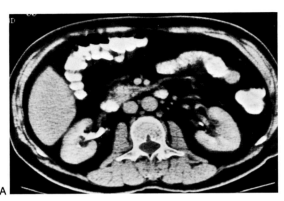

A

Figure 2–31.

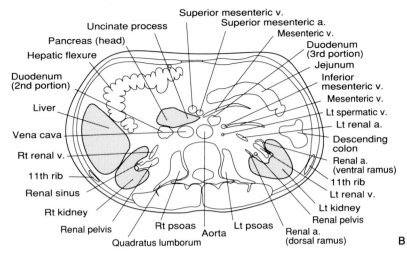

B

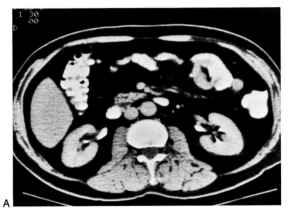

A

Figure 2–32.

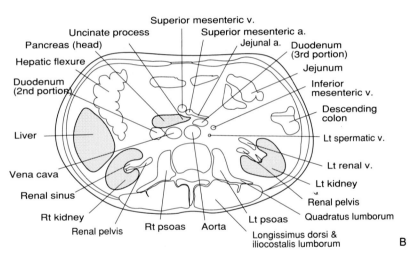

B

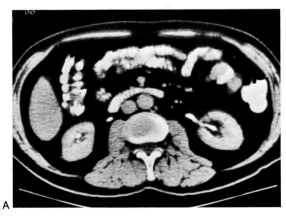

A

Figure 2–33.

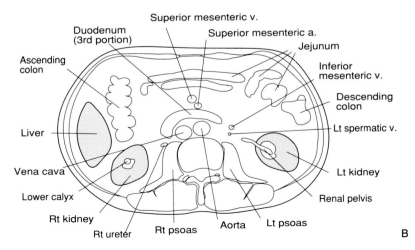

B

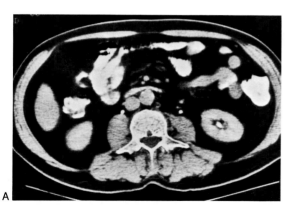

Figure 2–34.

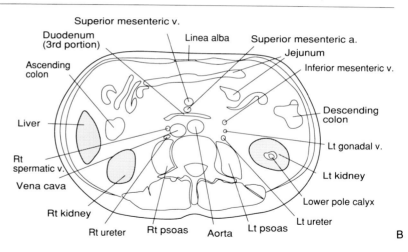

Superior mesenteric v.
Duodenum (3rd portion)
Linea alba
Superior mesenteric a.
Jejunum
Ascending colon
Inferior mesenteric v.
Liver
Descending colon
Rt spermatic v.
Lt gonadal v.
Vena cava
Lt kidney
Rt kidney
Lower pole calyx
Rt ureter
Rt psoas
Aorta
Lt psoas
Lt ureter

B

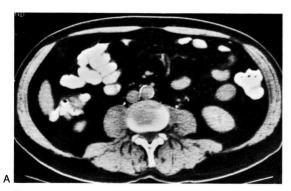

Figure 2–35.

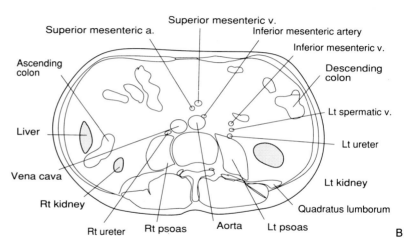

Superior mesenteric v.
Superior mesenteric a.
Inferior mesenteric artery
Inferior mesenteric v.
Ascending colon
Descending colon
Liver
Lt spermatic v.
Vena cava
Lt ureter
Rt kidney
Lt kidney
Quadratus lumborum
Rt ureter
Rt psoas
Aorta
Lt psoas

B

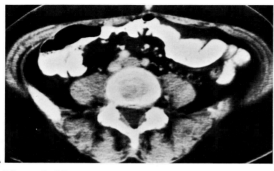

Figure 2–36.

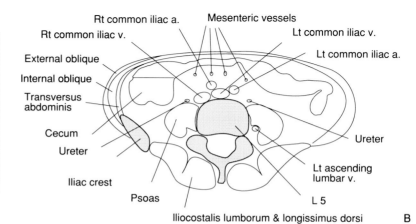

Rt common iliac a.
Mesenteric vessels
Rt common iliac v.
Lt common iliac v.
External oblique
Lt common iliac a.
Internal oblique
Transversus abdominis
Cecum
Ureter
Ureter
Iliac crest
Lt ascending lumbar v.
Psoas
L 5
Iliocostalis lumborum & longissimus dorsi

B

Figures 2–36–2–44.   Cross-sectional anatomy of the female pelvis. The cuts are 1 cm thick and spaced 1 cm apart.

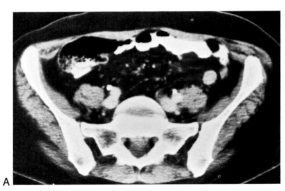

Figure 2–37.

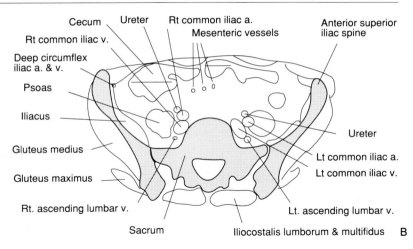

Cecum
Ureter
Rt common iliac a.
Mesenteric vessels
Anterior superior iliac spine
Rt common iliac v.
Deep circumflex iliac a. & v.
Psoas
Iliacus
Ureter
Gluteus medius
Lt common iliac a.
Gluteus maximus
Lt common iliac v.
Rt. ascending lumbar v.
Lt. ascending lumbar v.
Sacrum
Iliocostalis lumborum & multifidus
B

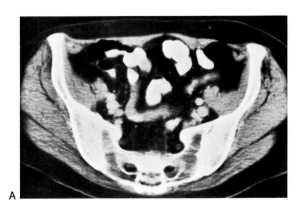

Figure 2–38.

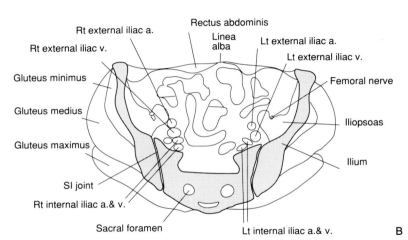

Rt external iliac a.
Rectus abdominis
Rt external iliac v.
Linea alba
Lt external iliac a.
Lt external iliac v.
Gluteus minimus
Femoral nerve
Gluteus medius
Iliopsoas
Gluteus maximus
Ilium
SI joint
Rt internal iliac a.& v.
Sacral foramen
Lt internal iliac a.& v.
B

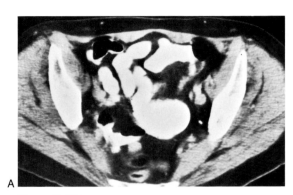

Figure 2–39.

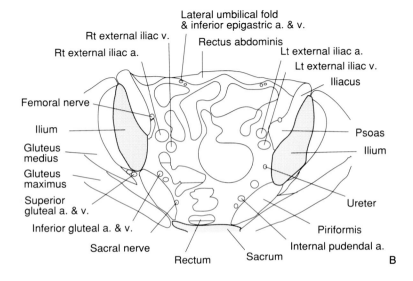

Lateral umbilical fold & inferior epigastric a. & v.
Rt external iliac v.
Rectus abdominis
Rt external iliac a.
Lt external iliac a.
Lt external iliac v.
Iliacus
Femoral nerve
Ilium
Psoas
Gluteus medius
Ilium
Gluteus maximus
Superior gluteal a. & v.
Ureter
Inferior gluteal a. & v.
Piriformis
Sacral nerve
Internal pudendal a.
Rectum
Sacrum
B

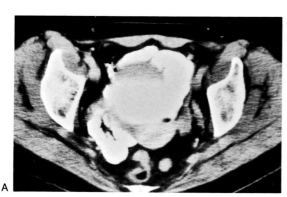

Figure 2–40.

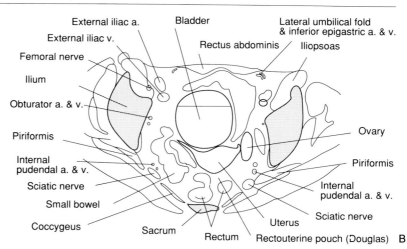

External iliac a.
External iliac v.
Femoral nerve
Ilium
Obturator a. & v.
Piriformis
Internal pudendal a. & v.
Sciatic nerve
Small bowel
Coccygeus
Bladder
Rectus abdominis
Sacrum
Rectum
Uterus
Lateral umbilical fold & inferior epigastric a. & v.
Iliopsoas
Ovary
Piriformis
Internal pudendal a. & v.
Sciatic nerve
Rectouterine pouch (Douglas)   B

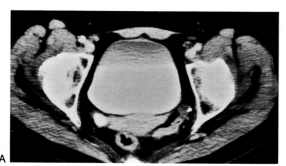

Figure 2–41.

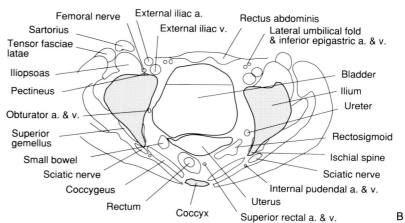

Femoral nerve
Sartorius
Tensor fasciae latae
Iliopsoas
Pectineus
Obturator a. & v.
Superior gemellus
Small bowel
Sciatic nerve
Coccygeus
Rectum
External iliac a.
External iliac v.
Rectus abdominis
Lateral umbilical fold & inferior epigastric a. & v.
Bladder
Ilium
Ureter
Rectosigmoid
Ischial spine
Sciatic nerve
Internal pudendal a. & v.
Uterus
Coccyx
Superior rectal a. & v.   B

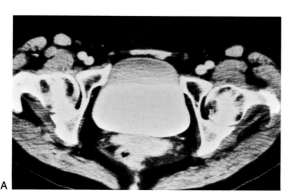

Figure 2–42

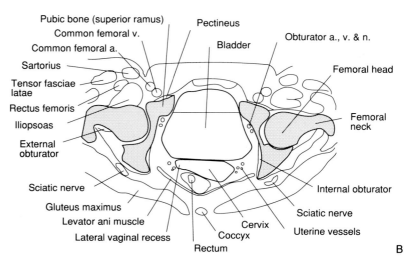

Pubic bone (superior ramus)
Common femoral v.
Common femoral a.
Sartorius
Tensor fasciae latae
Rectus femoris
Iliopsoas
External obturator
Sciatic nerve
Gluteus maximus
Levator ani muscle
Lateral vaginal recess
Pectineus
Bladder
Obturator a., v. & n.
Femoral head
Femoral neck
Internal obturator
Sciatic nerve
Uterine vessels
Cervix
Coccyx
Rectum   B

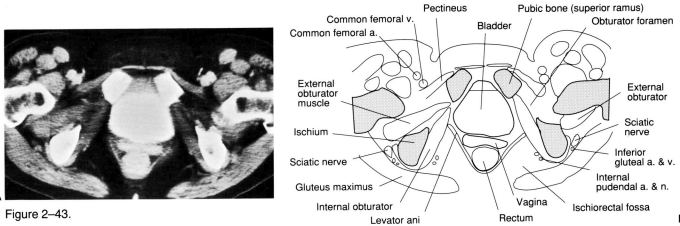

Figure 2–43.

Figure 2–43 B labels:
Common femoral v.
Common femoral a.
Pectineus
Bladder
Pubic bone (superior ramus)
Obturator foramen
External obturator muscle
Ischium
Sciatic nerve
Gluteus maximus
Internal obturator
Levator ani
External obturator
Sciatic nerve
Inferior gluteal a. & v.
Internal pudendal a. & n.
Ischiorectal fossa
Vagina
Rectum

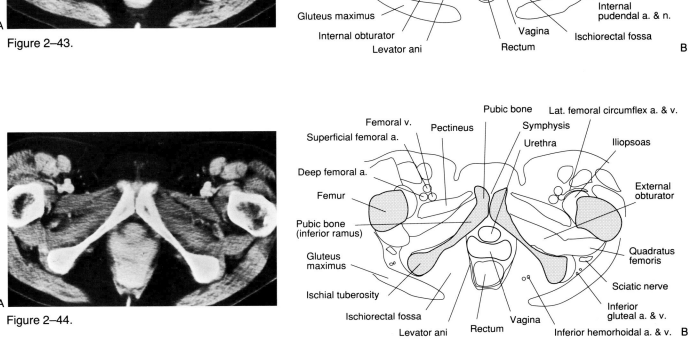

Figure 2–44.

Figure 2–44 B labels:
Femoral v.
Superficial femoral a.
Pectineus
Pubic bone
Symphysis
Lat. femoral circumflex a. & v.
Urethra
Iliopsoas
Deep femoral a.
Femur
Pubic bone (inferior ramus)
Gluteus maximus
Ischial tuberosity
Ischiorectal fossa
Levator ani
Rectum
Vagina
External obturator
Quadratus femoris
Sciatic nerve
Inferior gluteal a. & v.
Inferior hemorhoidal a. & v.

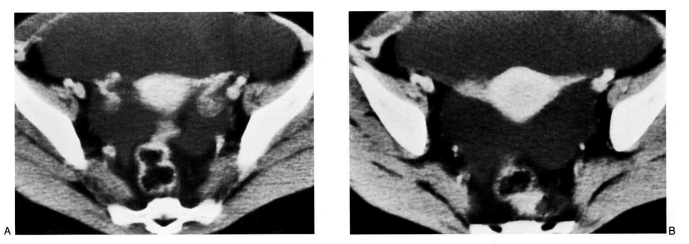

Figure 2–45. Contiguous 1 cm cuts from a contrast-enhanced CT scan in a female patient on peritoneal dialysis with large amount of intraperitoneal fluid. (A) Uterus, broad ligaments, and ovaries are suspended in the fluid. (B) More distally, fluid fills pouch of Douglas. The extraperitoneal space is seen as radiolucent areas along the pelvic wall and contains ureters, internal pudendal artery, and inferior gluteal artery and vein along piriformis. More superiorly, one can identify external iliac and internal iliac (hypogastric) arteries and veins.

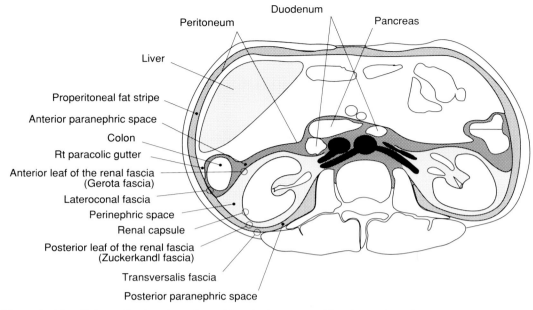

Figure 2–46. Schematic drawing of renal fascia, lateroconal fascia, perirenal and pararenal spaces.

kidney in old literature) and also contains bridging septa and lamela, which help support the kidney and hamper propagation of fluid within that space.[10,11] Vascular supply to the perinephric fat is from recursive and perforating renal capsular vessels and from branches of the lumbar arteries.

Posterior paranephric space continues laterally as *properitoneal fat stripe.* Posterior boundary of this space is *transversalis fascia;* anterior boundary is formed by posterior leaf of the renal fascia.[12]

Anterior boundary of *anterior paranephric space* is formed by posterior parietal peritoneum and the posterior boundary is made of anterior leaf of the renal fascia. On the left, pancreatic capsule fuses with anterior leaf of the renal fascia.

Anterior paranephric space also contains ascending and descending colon as well as the second part of the duodenum. Anterior and posterior paranephric spaces are separated by *lateroconal fascia.*

There are variations to the idealized anatomical appearance of the renal and lateroconal fascias. In some individuals lateroconal fascia may be partially absent, possibly explaining the presence of fluid in acute pancreatitis in the posterior paranephric space or retrorenal position of the colon.[13] Peritoneal recesses may extend deeply in the retrorenal area and intraperitoneal organs, such as spleen and liver, may partially extend posterior to the kidney (Fig. 2–47).[12]

Potential communication between two perinephric spaces exists along a narrow plane anterior to great vessels caudad to renal vessels.[14]

Midline sagittal anatomy in a male is presented in Fig. 2–48.

Additional radiological procedures and more detailed anatomy are provided in appropriate chapters throughout the book.

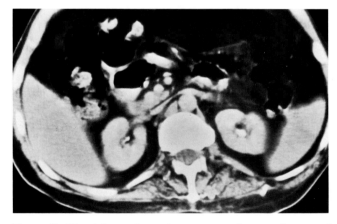

Figure 2–47. Intraperitoneal organs such as spleen and liver may extend posterior to the kidneys, showing how far posteriorly peritoneal cavity may extend. This, of course, has implications during percutaneous placement of nephrostomy catheters, etc.

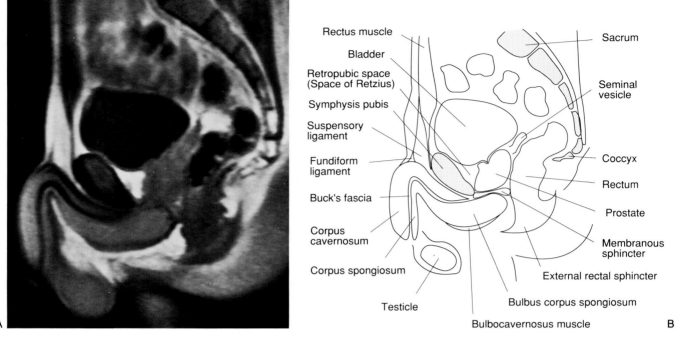

Figure 2–48A,B. Midline sagittal plane on MR image (400/28). (A: From Holliday J, Saxon R, Lufkin RB, et al. Anatomic correlations of magnetic resonance images with cadaver cryosections. Radiographics 1985; 5:887–921. Reprinted with permission.)

REFERENCES

1. Warshauer DM, McCarthy SM, Street L. Detection of renal masses: sensitivities and specificities of excretory urography/linear tomography, US, and CT. Radiology 1988; 169:363–365.
2. Hattery RR, Williamson B Jr, Hartman GW, et al. Intravenous urographic technique. Radiology 1988; 167:593–599.
3. Christiansen J. Retrograde pyelography with gas (carbon dioxide) as contrast medium. Acta Chir Scand 1970; 136:441–445.
4. Thomsen HS, Dorph S. Pyelorenal backflow during retrograde pyelography in adult patients. Scand J Urol Nephrol 1981; 15:63–68.
5. Ohlson L. Normal collecting ducts: visualization at urography. Radiology 1989; 170:33–37.
6. Clark RL, Klein S. Renal arcuate veins: new angiographic observations. AJR 1983; 141:755–759.
7. Chesbrough RM, Burkhard TK, Martinez AJ, Burks DD. Gerota versus Zuckerkandl: the renal fascia revisited. Radiology 1989; 173:845–846.
8. Meyers MA, Whalen JP, Peelle K, et al. Radiologic features of extraperitoneal effusions: an anatomic approach. Radiology 1972; 104:249–257.
9. Love L, Meyers MA, Churchill RJ, et al. Computed tomography of the extraperitoneal spaces. AJR 1981; 136:781–786.
10. Kunin M. Bridging septa of the perinephric space: anatomic, pathologic and diagnostic considerations. Radiology 1986; 158:361–365.
11. McClennan BL, Lee JKT, Peterson RR. Anatomy of the perirenal area. Radiology 1986; 158:555–557.
12. Love L, Demos TC, Posniak H. CT of retrorenal fluid collections. AJR 1985; 145:87–91.
13. Hopper KD, Sherman JL, Luethke JM, Ghaerd N. The retrorenal colon in the supine and prone patient. Radiology 1987; 162:443–445.
14. Kneeland JB, Auh YH, Rubenstein WA, et al. Perirenal spaces: CT evidence for communication across the midline. Radiology 1987; 164:657–661.

3

Abdomen

CALCIFICATIONS

All extraosseous calcifications within the abdomen are pathologic. Some are clinically important, some are irrelevant, but all should be familiar to the radiologist.

CT is more sensitive in detecting miniscule calcific deposits than is plain radiography, but small calcifications may be missed, depending on slice thickness and spacing.

Sonography may detect renal and other calculi larger than 3 mm and also may suggest nephrocalcinosis, sometimes even before it is seen on radiographs. Increased echogenicity within the pyramids is the principal finding, although nonspecific, since entities not associated with medullary calcifications must be considered. Increased pyramid echogenicity is also seen in gout, primary aldosteronism, Sjögren syndrome, Wilson syndrome, renal tubular ectasia/medullary sponge kidney (with or without calcifications), infantile polycystic kidney, and tubular ectasia with congenital hepatic fibrosis.[1]

MR imaging is perhaps the least sensitive imaging modality for detection of calcifications. Heavy calcification, such as large renal or bladder calculi, exhibit low signal intensity (dark) on both T1- and T2-weighted images.

Calcifications in the Urinary Tract

Renal Calcifications
A. *Focal Renal Calcifications*

Localized parenchymal calcifications may form within a scar resulting from a focal infectious process such as tuberculosis or a renal abscess, or infarct, and intrarenal hematoma. End-stage renal transplant may also calcify.[2]

Calcifications within the solid renal mass are almost always associated with renal cell carcinoma until proven otherwise (Fig. 3–1). Other malignant masses with calcifications are osteosarcoma, metastases to the kidney from mucinous adenocarcinomas, and Wilms tumor.

Benign renal masses may also calcify. Linear calcifications may be seen in the wall of a renal cyst (but also in renal carcinoma). Diffuse calcifications may be present in renal fibroma.

Vascular calcifications are associated with renal artery atherosclerosis and renal artery aneurysm (Fig. 3–2).

B. *Intraluminal Renal Calcifications*

Most common calcifications visible on radiography or sonography are renal calculi. *Milk of calcium urine* and *milk of calcium renal cyst* are rare conditions where a suspension of small calcified crystals shifts and layers within the lumen

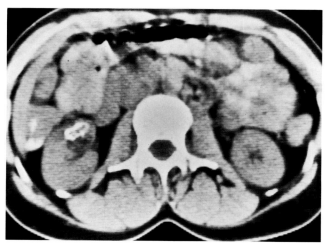

Figure 3–1. Focal renal calcification of unknown etiology in a young woman. Altered nephrogram immediately posterior to the calcification is suggestive of a mass; renal carcinoma enters into differential diagnosis.

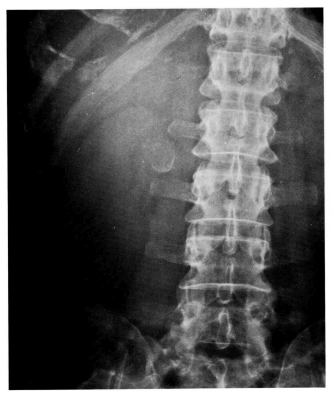

Figure 3–2. Calcified renal artery aneurysm masquerading as a gallstone.

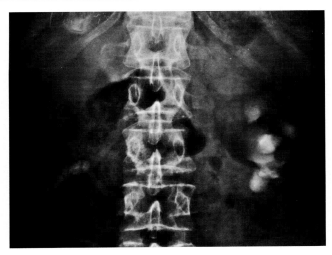

Figure 3–3. On plain radiograph radiopaque milk of calcium urine is seen in the left renal pelvis. In the supine position differentiation from a staghorn calculus is impossible. Layering occurred on upright radiograph.

of an obstructed renal pelvis or obstructed calyceal diverticulum (Fig. 3–3).[3]

C. *Intratubular Renal Calcifications*

The prime example of intratubular calcifications is medullary sponge kidney.

D. *Interstitial Renal Calcifications (Nephrocalcinosis)*

1. *Medullary nephrocalcinosis* is the most common type of nephrocalcinosis. Calcific deposits are in the interstitial spaces, although intratubular increments may be concomitantly present (Fig. 3–4). Medullary nephrocalcinosis is most frequently the result of a metabolic disease such as renal tubular acidosis,[4,5] milk alkali syndrome, hypervitaminosis D, hyperparathyroidism, primary hypercalciuria, primary and secondary oxalosis, Cushing disease, antacid abuse, and rheumatoid arthritis associated with Sjögren syndrome.[6] Hypercalcemia such as in sarcoidosis,[7,8] postimmobilization, and idiopathic hypercalcemia form the other large group.

2. *Cortical nephrocalcinosis* is usually dystrophic calcification, a consequence of a destructive type of cortical disease such as glomerulonephritis,[9] renal cortical necrosis,[10,11] Alport syndrome, and transplant rejection.[2,12] Cortical nephrocalcinosis in a functionally normal kidney is rare.[13]

3. *Combined medullary and cortical nephrocalcinosis* may be seen in primary and secondary oxalosis,[14,15] infection with *Mycobacterium avium-intracellulare* (seen in AIDS),[16] and preterm infants.[17]

Uroepithelial Calcifications

Schistosomiasis, tuberculosis, adenocarcinoma, and amyloidosis are the main causes of rather rare uroepithelial calcifications.

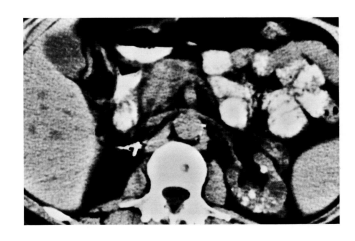

Calcifications in Male Genitalia

Prostatic intratubular calcifications are very common. Calcification of vas deferens is usually seen in diabetics but also in nondiabetics.[18] Scrotal calcifications are usually the result of trauma. Calcification of corpora cavernosa may occur in sickle cell disease. Plaques in Peyronie's disease may be seen to be calcified on CT scan.

Calcifications Outside Urinary Tract

Numerous calcific densities in different organ systems and of different etiologies are found in the abdomen (Table 3–1; Figs. 3–5–3–9).

SOFT TISSUE DENSITIES

Organomegaly, such as hepatomegaly, splenomegaly, nephromegaly, and uterine enlargement (Fig. 3–10), may be detected, although with some difficulty, on projectional radiography. CT is more useful in this regard. Sonography is generally unreliable in estimating renal size but otherwise an excellent "first look" modality.

A spleen measuring more than 14 cm in the longest axis on plain radiograph may be considered abnormal. Fundus of the stomach and the left kidney may be displaced medially and anteromedially (Fig. 3–11). Occasionally, the left kidney may be displaced, at least partially, across the midline by an enormous spleen.

Abnormal thickness of the bowel wall can be observed on the plain radiograph or CT. Presence of Crohn's disease or ulcerative colitis may be suspected.

X-ray attenuation differences between parenchymal organs and "water" densities, such as urine, cyst fluid, and bile are miniscule and cannot be discriminated on a plain radiograph. A mass, just like an organ, is visible only if contrasted by surrounding fat

Table 3-1. Calcifications Outside the Urinary Tract

Location	Curvilinear	Amorphous/Solid
Liver	Hepatic artery aneurysm; hydatid cysts; simple cysts; capsular	Metastatic mucinous adenocarcinoma; alveolar hydatid disease; tuberculosis; hepatoblastoma; giant hemangioma; portal vein thrombosis; granulomatous diseases
Gallbladder	Porcelain gallbladder; gallstones	Gallstone; milk of calcium bile
Spleen	Splenic cyst; echinococcal cyst; splenic artery aneurysm	Histoplasmosis; tuberculosis; infarct; hematoma; sickle-cell disease; phleboliths
Pancreas	Pseudocyst	Ch. pancreatitis (intraductal-calcium carbonate); ch. pancreatitis (fat necrosis-calcium hydroxyapetite); hereditary pancreatitis; cystic fibrosis
Adrenal glands	Adrenal cyst; adenocarcinoma	Hemorrhage; tuberculosis; metastases; neuroblastoma; adenocarcinoma; pheochromocytoma; Wolman's disease
Lymph nodes		Inflammatory; tuberculosis; metastases
Arterial	Atherosclerosis; aortic aneurysm; other large vessels aneurysm	
Venous	Inferior vena cava thrombus; phleboliths	Phleboliths
Intestinal		Appenicolith; meckolith; fecolith; schistosomiasis (rare)
Uterus/ovaries		Uterine leiomyoma; lithopedion; dermoid; endometriosis; pelvic inflammatory disease; cystadenoma and cystadenocarcinoma of the ovary
Muscles, ligaments, and cartilage		Injection granulomas; myositis ossificans; rib cartilage retroperitoneal hematoma; psoas abscess
Intraperitoneal	Appendices epiploicae; globules of mineral oil	Cystadenocarcinoma of the ovary; gallstones (perforated gallbladder); peritonitis (meconium, tuberculous)

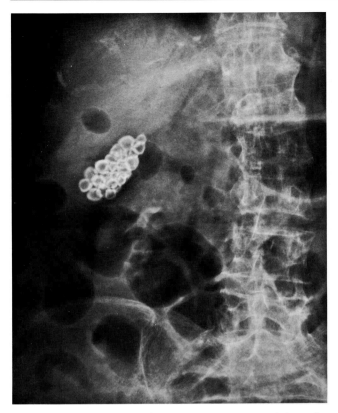

Figure 3–5. Gallstones. Only 15% are seen on plain radiograph.

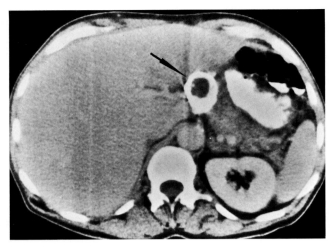

Figure 3–7. Calcified splenic artery aneurysm (arrow).

or air and is usually visible as an abnormality in organ contour. Deformity of the renal contour, for example, may suggest a renal tumor.

Poor discrimination of x-ray attenuation differences between various soft tissues on plain radiographs led to the development of radiographic contrast material-assisted examinations, as well as CT, ultrasound, and MR imaging.

CT, MR imaging, and ultrasound provide for much easier detection of a hypothetical mass, and in many instances will characterize the mass further (Fig. 3–12). For instance, it is possible to determine presence of blood, necrotic tissues, fluid levels, hemorrhage and minute calcification, and to determine if the mass is solid or cystic (Fig. 3–13).

Soft tissue masses protruding from the skin, such as moles, stomas, neurofibromas, and anterior wall hernias, are surrounded and contrasted by atmospheric air and thus made visible on abdominal radiograph.

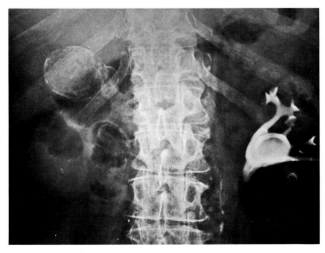

Figure 3–6. Porcelain gallbladder, calcification in the aortic wall, and left nephrostomy tube.

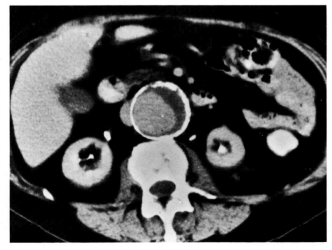

Figure 3–8. Calcified aneurysm of the abdominal aorta. Lucency between intraluminal contrast and calcified wall is a thrombus.

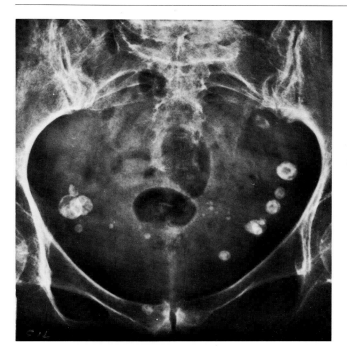

Figure 3–9. Phleboliths.

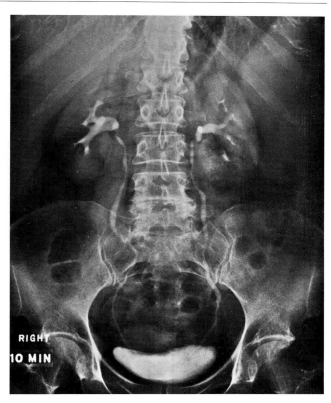

Figure 3–11. Enlarged spleen may displace left kidney medially. This can occur despite the fact that the kidney is a retroperitoneal organ, while the spleen is intraperitoneal.

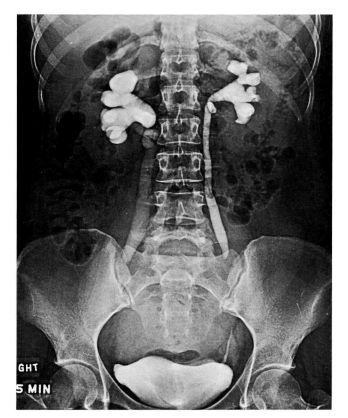

Figure 3–10. Superior outline of a pelvic mass is difficult to perceive even on a properly exposed radiograph. Note mild bilateral obstruction caused by the mass compressing ureters upon the pelvic brim.

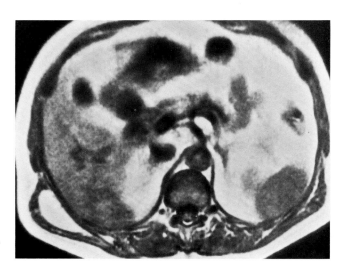

Figure 3–12. Right flank lipoma is easily recognized and characterized on this T1-weighted MR sequence. The same would be true for CT. On projectional radiography, however, such a tumor will go unrecognized.

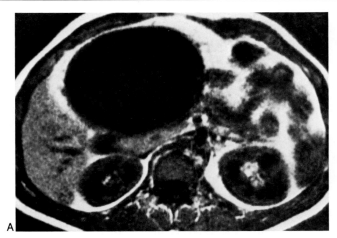
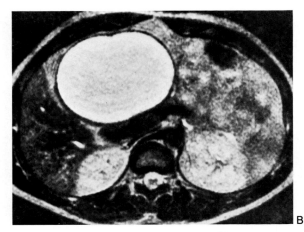

Figure 3–13. T1- (A) and T2-weighted (B) sequences of a large transverse colon mesenteric cyst. Change in signal intensities from one sequence to the other is similar to changes that are exhibited by the spinal fluid and is suggestive of fluid.

Displacement of various organs may suggest the anatomical origin of a mass. A retroperitoneal tumor may displace the ureter or the inferior vena cava, or if sufficiently large, loops of bowel.

FOREIGN MATERIAL

Metallic fragments, such as surgical clips, bullets, shotgun pellets, ingested metallic objects, surgical needles, hip prostheses, inferior vena cava umbrella, Gianturco occlusive steel coils, and lost needle holders are all clearly visible because of their marked x-ray attenuation (Fig. 3–14).

A whole variety of draining tubes may be encountered. These include nasogastric tubes, Kantor tube, Foley catheter, nephrostomy tubes, "double J" ureteral stents, suprapubic tubes, van Sonnenberg tubes, and many more.

Barium may be retained in the large bowel diverticula or appendix for a long period of time. Droplets of oily myelographic contrast are retained for years in the subarachnoidal space, and so is lymphangiographic contrast in the lymph nodes. Ablation of the renal cysts used to be accomplished by percutaneous installation of oily myelographic contrast.

During total hip replacement, orthopedic cement may leak into the pelvis through a defect created in the medial acetabular wall (Fig. 3–15). A tantalum mesh may be seen after hernia repair (Fig. 3–16).

Intrauterine contraceptive devices (Figs. 3–17, 3–18), vaginal tampons, pessaries, diaphragms, tubal ligation clips, and, occasionally, vasectomy clips may be seen.

Illegal drugs are occasionally smuggled in ingested condoms. Precipitating finding may be acute small or large bowel obstruction or symptoms of drug overdose.

Battery-operated sexual implements have been lost in the rectum. Various foreign bodies have been lost in male and female urethra.

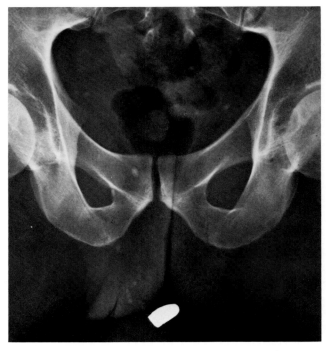

Figure 3–14. Bullet lodged in the soft tissues of the perineum.

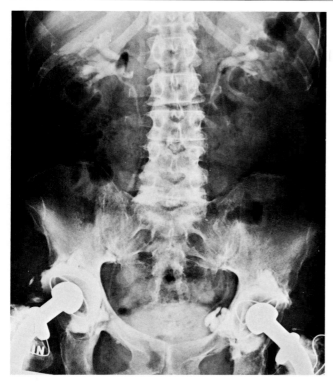

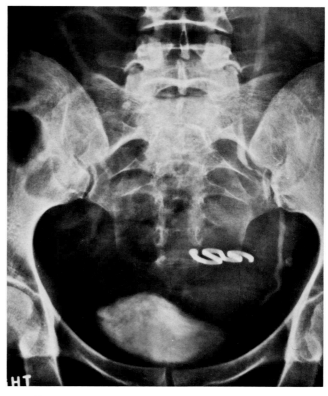

Figure 3–15. Bilateral total hip replacement. Radiopaque cement has leaked and solidified in the true pelvis.

Figure 3–17. Lippes loop contraceptive device.

A variety of anti-incontinence and anti-impotence prosthetic devices and testicular prostheses are encountered in male patients.

Ingested food, such as caraway seeds, bones, tablets, and capsules may cast confusing shadows on the radiograph. Rectal suppositories in various stages of dissolution may be seen.

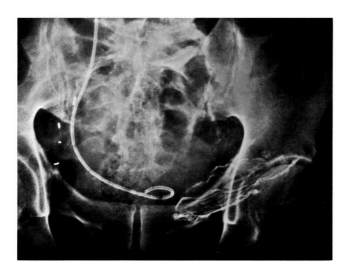

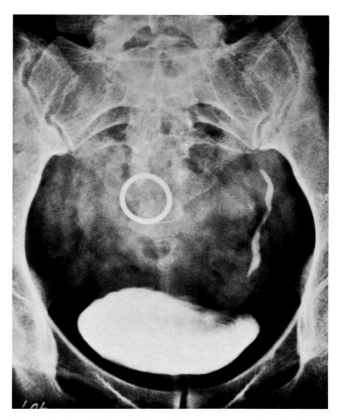

Figure 3–16. Tantalum mesh after left hernia repair. Ureteral stent is in the left ureter.

Figure 3–18. Unusual intrauterine contraceptive device in an immigrant.

A skin fold, stoma bag, smudge of contrast on the skin, clothing, or items in pockets may all cast peculiar shadows on the radiograph.

ILEUS

Etiology. Numerous causes have been described, including postoperative ileus, systemic diseases, uremia, hypokalemia, drugs, scleroderma, diabetes, ischemic bowel disease, and many more. Postoperative ileus is common after abdominal surgery.

Radiological Findings. Lack of peristaltic activity is also likely to cause bowel dilatation. The important differentiating finding from acute small bowel obstruction is that in a dynamic ileus both small and large bowel are proportionally distended.

Inflammatory process in the abdomen such as pancreatitis or acute cholecystitis may inhibit peristalsis in an adjacent bowel loop and cause localized distention, a radiographic sign known as *sentinel loop* (Fig. 3–19).

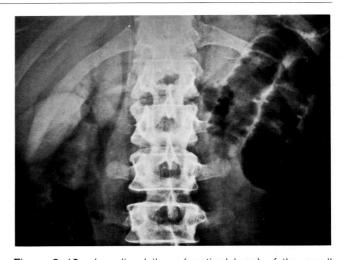

Figure 3–19. Localized ileus (sentinel loop) of the small bowel in the left upper quadrant due to extravasation of urine in the adjacent retroperitoneum. Extravasation (forniceal rupture) was caused by acute ureteral obstruction. Note excretion and concentration of radiographic contrast material in the gallbladder 24 hours after urography.

ACUTE ABDOMEN

Intestinal Obstruction

SMALL BOWEL OBSTRUCTION

Etiology. Postsurgical edema, adhesions, intussusception, hernia, gallstone ileus, metastases, primary tumor, tumor extension, duodenal ulcer, primary carcinoma of the duodenum, duodenal hematoma, cast syndrome,[19] congenital.

Radiological Findings. Soon after the obstruction has occurred, small bowel proximal to the point of obstruction may not have had a chance to dilate and the distal intestine may not have had a chance to empty. Gas and fecal material may still be present and serial radiographs may be necessary to confirm the diagnosis.

The intestine above the point of obstruction eventually becomes dilated and contains gas, intestinal fluid, and perhaps food material. Air-fluid levels are seen on the upright radiograph and are more numerous if the site of the obstruction is more distant (Fig. 3–20).

Possibility of a hernia should not be overlooked (Fig. 3–21). Soft tissue densities, perhaps containing air, may be found at the groin or incision sites.

The *double bubble* sign is seen in duodenal obstruc-

tion and is formed by separate stomach and duodenal air pockets. The *triple bubble* sign may be seen in proximal jejunal obstruction.

COLONIC OBSTRUCTION

Etiology. Carcinoma, metastases, volvulus, diverticulitis, fecal impaction, hernia in adults, meconium plug syndrome, colon atresia, and anal atresia in neonates.

Radiological Findings. Small and large bowel dilatation is present. Disproportional distention of the cecum may occur with distal colonic obstruction. Perforation is likely when the diameter of the distended colon is over 10 cm.

Gastrointestinal Perforation

Etiology. Ulcer, infarction, strangulation, inflammation, disruption of bowel anastomosis. Aside from gastrointestinal perforation, air in the peritoneal cavity can be due to surgery, percutaneous instrumentation, and transvaginal/transtubular insufflation.

Radiological Findings. On plain radiographs free intraperitoneal air is best seen on left cross-table lateral decubitus. In this position air that might have collected in the lesser sac (posterior gastric wall perforation) will escape through the gastroepiploic

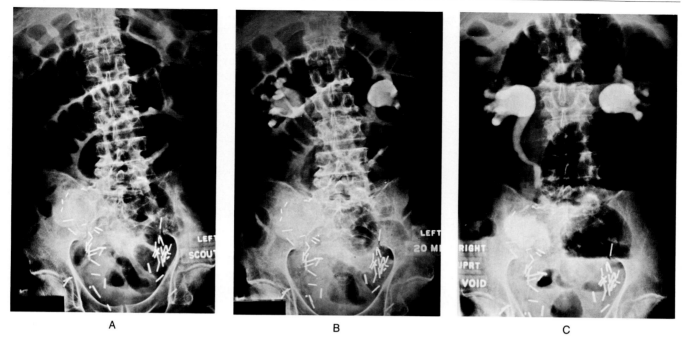

A   B   C

Figure 3–20. Small bowel and ureteral obstruction following ileal loop diversion. **(A)** Plain radiograph demonstrates disproportional dilatation of the small bowel as compared with transverse and sigmoid colon compatible with either partial or early small bowel obstruction. Differentiation from small bowel and colon is possible since valvulae conniventes span across the entire width of the small bowel while thick colonic haustra do not. **(B)** Urogram on the same patient demonstrates dilatation and delayed filling of the collecting system compatible with urinary obstruction. **(C)** On the upright radiograph multiple air-fluid levels are seen in dilated small bowel. Bilateral ureteral obstruction is present at the anastomotic site with the conduit.

foramen into the greater peritoneal cavity.[20] There it is detected between the liver and abdominal wall. An upright chest radiograph frequently discloses minute amounts of free air under the diaphragm.

Intraperitoneal structures, such as the bowel *(double wall sign)* (Fig. 3–22),[21] the falciform ligament *(falciform ligament sign)*,[22] or even intraperitoneal fluid *(football sign)*,[23,24] may be outlined by free air. Air trapped between loops of small bowel may assume a triangular appearance *(triangle sign)*,[25] or in children air may be seen in the scrotum.

Intestine interposed between diaphragm and liver *(Chilaiditi's syndrome)* and subdiaphragmatic fat may simulate free air.[26]

Intraperitoneal air is relatively easily seen on CT imaging. The air tends to rise under the anterior abdominal wall and again the bowel wall is outlined from both sides.[27,28]

On MR imaging air generates almost no signal and appears dark (hypointense) on both T1- and T2-weighted spin echo sequences.

Acute Appendicitis

Radiographic signs specific or suggestive for acute appendicitis are:[29,30]

a) *Appendicolith* which is more common in children (overall incidence of 14%) and found more commonly in the retrocecal appendix.
b) *Soft tissue mass* in right lower quadrant representing abscess or edema. Cecum may be displaced medially.

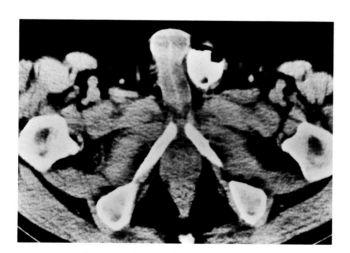

Figure 3–21. Left inguinal hernia.

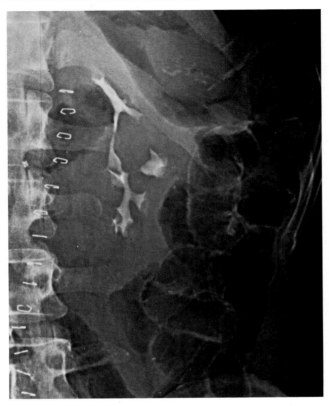

Figure 3–22. Intraperitoneal gas "contrasts" bowel wall from outside, intraluminal gas from inside.

c) *Dilated transverse colon* sign is suggestive of perforation.[31] Ascending colon is in spasm and therefore gasless, while transverse colon is dilated due to reflex ileus.

Ureteral obstruction may be caused by retrocecal appendicitis.

Acute Cholecystitis

Etiology.   Cystic duct obstruction by a stone. Cholelithiasis.

Radiological Findings.   Most patients with acute cholecystitis harbor gallstones, although only 10 to 20% are visible on the plain radiograph. Detection rate is much higher on CT and ultrasound. Thickening of the gallbladder wall is the principal finding on sonography. Fluid sometimes may be present in the gallbladder fossa.

MR imaging may also disclose thickened gallbladder wall. Bile is usually of strong signal intensity (bright) on T2-weighted sequences and obscures equally bright edematous wall. On the same se-quence, gallstones are seen as dark (hypointense) areas within the bright bile.

Emphysematous cholecystitis is a form of acute cholecystitis characterized by the presence of intramural and/or intraluminal gas. Gas is most easily seen on a CT scan. Acoustical shadowing and hyperechoic gallbladder wall are seen on ultrasound.[32]

Perforation into the peritoneal cavity or small bowel is possible, the result of which may be small bowel obstruction *(gallstone ileus)*.[33] Gas may be present in the biliary system.

Peritoneal Fluid

Etiology.   Peritonitis, congestive heart failure, nutritional edema, obstruction to portal circulation, peritoneal metastases, peritoneal dialysis, intraperitoneal bladder rupture, etc.

Radiological Findings.   Centrally positioned "floating" bowel loops and an overall haze and increased density are indicative of a large ascites.

Smaller amounts of fluid are more difficult to detect on plain radiographs. The most dependent parts of the intraperitoneal cavity fill first: a) pouch of Douglas and peritoneal recesses in the pelvis; b) right pericolic gutter; and c) Morison's pouch (hepatorenal angle).[34,35]

Radiographic density in the pelvis increases as the fluid accumulates, often assuming a characteristic appearance resembling "dog ears" as the fluid fills the lateral pelvic recesses.

Because the right pericolic gutter is tangential to the x-ray beam on projectional radiography, detection of fluid in that area is easier. The fluid is contrasted from the outside by properitoneal fat and from the inside by the air in the ascending colon. Distance of 4 mm between these two structures is diagnostic of fluid (Fig. 3–23).

As the fluid continues to accumulate, the tip of the liver becomes surrounded and obliterated, since mesenteric fat no longer provides contrast.

Presence of retroperitoneal fluid is suggested if there is obliteration of the psoas outline, although the psoas need not be seen in a number of normal patients.[36] Very large amounts of fluid are needed to fill the space along the psoas for it to become obliterated.

Renal outline is obliterated by perinephric fluid. Perinephric fat may be outlined on the plain radiograph by fluid in paranephric space.[37,38]

Very small amounts of peritoneal fluid may be detected with ultrasound in the pelvis, particularly in females.

Because of cross-sectional display, CT is very sen-

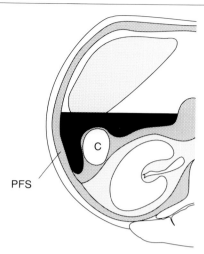

Figure 3–23. Schematic drawing of intraperitoneal fluid (black) filling pericolic gutter. Ascending colon (C), despite being retroperitoneal, is displaced medially and away from properitoneal fat stripe (PFS). Tip of the liver is also silhouetted by the fluid.

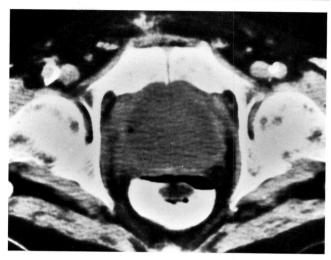

Figure 3–24. CT scan of a pelvic abscess after cystectomy.

sitive in detecting very small amounts of peritoneal fluid.[39] Fluid in the pouch of Douglas is readily seen, as are the pericolic gutters and hepatorenal angle.

On MR imaging small amounts of intraperitoneal fluid may be detected, particularly on the sagittal plane in the pouch of Douglas. Fluid is of low signal intensity (dark) on T1-weighted images and of strong signal intensity (bright) on T2-weighted sequences.

Abdominal and Pelvic Abscess

Etiology. Postoperative, colonic diverticulitis, perforated appendix, cholecystitis, pancreatitis, etc.

Radiological Findings. An abscess may frequently be seen on plain abdominal radiograph or sonography, but CT is the imaging method of choice for detecting presence, location, and extension of intra-abdominal and pelvic abscesses. Fluid collection, sometimes with gas, is seen.

The most dependent parts of the peritoneal cavity are the common location sites for abscesses to develop. Pelvis, subphrenic spaces, pericolic gutter, Morison's pouch, and lesser sac are frequent locations (Fig. 3–24). In the retroperitoneum, pararenal spaces, perivesical space, and ischiorectal fossa are the common sites. Renal and perirenal abscesses will be discussed elsewhere.

Needle aspiration of the fluid collection may be needed to determine whether or not infection is present.

Percutaneous catheter drainage is the preferred method of treatment for the majority of abdominal abscesses. The abscess should be liquified for the percutaneous method to be successful.

ABSCESS DRAINAGE

Percutaneous drainage of abdominal and pelvic abscesses is performed under CT or ultrasound guidance.[40–43] Sonography is preferred when large, easily accessible fluid collections are present, while CT is the better method for drainage of smaller, deeply situated abscesses where it is necessary to avoid injury to adjacent organs. The entry site is chosen from a preliminary cut, and angle and length of the puncture needle are determined. Placement is achieved under local anesthesia and mild sedation. The exact placement of the needle is verified on additional CT cuts. Over an exchange guidewire, the tract is dilated using progressively larger dilators, and finally a single or double bore 14 F, 16 F, or larger catheter is placed. If the abscess cavity is septated, several catheters may have to be placed in different locations within the abscess. The abscess cavity may be irrigated, drained by gravity, or the draining port may be connected to a sump.

UNUSUAL GAS COLLECTIONS IN THE ABDOMEN

The following are causes of gas collections in the abdomen:

- *Pneumatosis intestinalis.* Pneumatosis intestinalis is intramural bowel wall gas involving the colon *(pneumatosis coli)* (Fig. 3–25), small bowel, and occasionally stomach *(emphysematous gastri-*

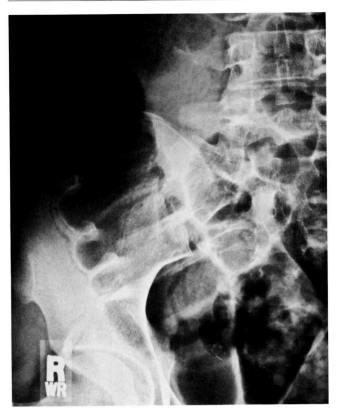

Figure 3–25. Pneumatosis coli in an asymptomatic patient. Radiolucent gas is seen in the wall of the ascending colon.

tis).[44,45] Necrotizing enterocolitis, intestinal obstruction, mesenteric vessels occlusion, intestinal surgery, obstructive pulmonary disease, and pneumomediastinum have all been described as causative factors. Air in the portal system may occasionally be seen and is a grave prognostic sign.

- *Pneumatobilia.* Pneumatobilia is the presence of air in the biliary system. Causes are neocholedochoduodenostomy, gallbladder perforation, and acute cholangitis.
- *Subcutaneous emphysema.* Collection of air in the abdominal wall is seen after surgery, chest tube placement, rib fractures, tracheostomy, pneumomediastinum, and liposuction.
- *Emphysematous cystitis.* This is an acute bladder infection, usually seen in diabetics where gas is present in the bladder wall and lumen. Frequency, dysuria, and pneumaturia may be present.
- *Urinary diversions.* Urinary tract diversions, such as ureterosigmoidostomy and ileal loop diversion, can be associated with gas reflux into the upper system.
- *Catheters.* Catheters commonly allow some air into the urinary tract system.

- *Renal artery embolization or infarction.* After embolization of renal carcinoma, gas may be seen in the infarcted tissues even without presence of infection.
- *Dead fetus.* Gas formation sometimes occurs in a dead fetus without presence of infection.
- *Vaginal tampon.* Vaginal tampon and vaginal packing may produce confusing shadows on a plain radiograph.
- *Epidural anesthesia.* Needle placement into the epidural space is facilitated by small incremental injections of air, which may remain in the soft tissues of the back (Fig. 3–26).[46]

SKELETAL ABNORMALITIES

Degenerative Changes of the Spine

Radiographic findings are narrowing of the intervertebral disc space, osteophytic spurs, osteosclerosis, facetal joint narrowing, and disc "vacuum phenomenon."

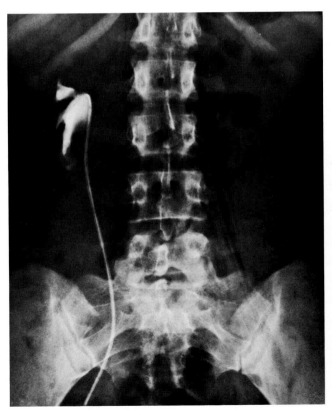

Figure 3–26. Air is frequently present in the soft tissues during needle positioning for epidural anesthesia. Here the air is seen as radiolucent strands to the left of the spine.

Spondylolisthesis and Spondyloliasis

Anterior slippage of one vertebral body over the other is called spondylolisthesis and is usually caused by degenerative disease of the spine and degenerative disease of the facetal joints. This condition on frontal radiographs resembles *inverted Napoleon's hat.* Spondyloliasis is unilateral or bilateral. Disruption of the pars interarticularis, usually of L5, is best seen on oblique projections.

Paget's Disease

This is a skeletal disease characterized by concurrent destructive and reparative process. Radiographic findings on plain radiograph or CT are: a) trabeculae are fewer and coarse; b) cortical thickening; c) bone expansion; and d) bone deformity (Fig. 3–27).

Ileopectineal line is the site of earliest involvement. *Acetabular protrusion* may occur in advanced stages due to bone remodeling. Enlargement of the vertebral body and the thickened cortex resembles a *picture frame.* Pedicles and spinous processes may be involved.

Large calcium content makes the lesion appear hypointense on MR images.

Complete obliteration of the bone trabeculae occurs in the sclerotic phase and it becomes difficult to differentiate this disease from osteoblastic bone metastases.

Osteoblastic metastases into Paget-involved bone have been described. Osteogenic sarcoma and fibrosarcoma may complicate Paget's disease and present as areas of lytic bone destruction.

Osteoblastic Metastases

Carcinoma of the prostate and breast are the most common osteoblastic metastases. Other carcinomas and lymphomas may also produce various degrees of osteoblastic reaction. There is obliteration of the trabecula and the inner cortical margin once the marrow fat is replaced by the tumor (Fig. 3–28).

Ivory vertebra is a solitary vertebra with an osteoblastic metastasis. A solitary metastasis may sometimes be found in the pedicle and nowhere else (Fig. 3–29, A,B). Renal carcinoma only exceptionally may produce an osteoblastic metastasis.

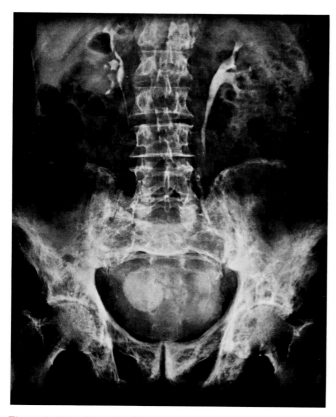

Figure 3–27. Paget's disease in a patient with carcinoma of the prostate. Compare with Figure 3–28.

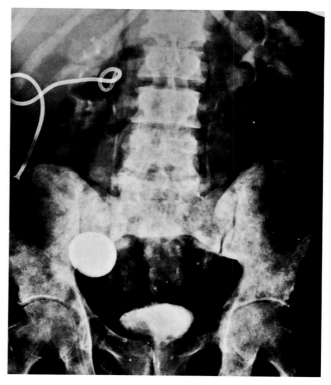

Figure 3–28. Osteoblastic metastases from carcinoma of the prostate. Note also right percutaneous nephrostomy tube and anti-incontinence prosthesis with contrast-filled reservoir.

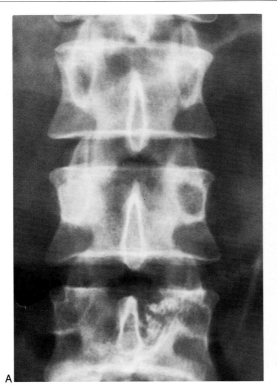
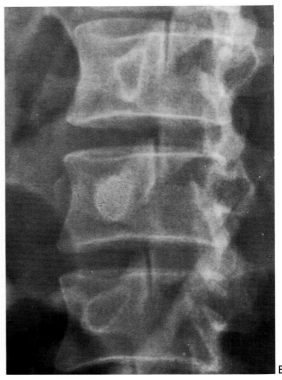

Figure 3–29. **(A)** Right pedicle of the vertebra in the center is radiodense and the cortical margins are obliterated. **(B)** RPO projection confirms the presence of an osteoblastic lesion in the pedicle.

Bony Island

Compact cortical bone within a cancellous bone is known as a bony island (Fig. 3–30). Rarely, it may show growth on serial examinations. Also, rarely, it shows uptake on a bone scan. MR imaging will disclose a hypointense lesion on T1- and T2-weighted images.

Myelofibrosis

Because of osteosclerotic changes involving the bones, this disease should be considered in differential diagnosis in a patient suspected of having osteoblastic metastases. Myelofibrosis is usually seen in patients over 50 years of age and is characterized by progressive fibrosis of the bone marrow. Pelvis and spine are commonly involved with osteosclerotic lesions. Associated findings are normochromatic normocytic anemia, leukemoid blood disorder, and marked splenomegaly.

Tuberous Sclerosis

In addition to renal angiomyolipoma, other benign tumors, adenoma sebaceum, mental retardation, calcification in the brain ganglia, etc., solitary or multi-

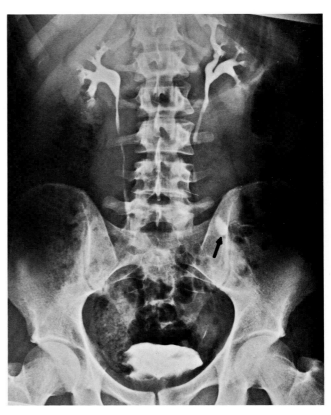

Figure 3–30. A 1 cm osteoblastic lesion in the left iliac crest medially has been unchanged for several years and represents a bony island.

ple osteosclerotic lesions are all seen in the spine and pelvis.

Vertebral Hemangioma

This is a common finding on a plain radiograph, CT, and MR imaging and may be confused with Paget's and osteoblastic metastases. Coarse trabecular pattern is present with vertical orientation (corduroy). Unlike Paget's disease, there is no bone expansion nor cortical thickening. On MR images hemangiomas are hyperintense on both T1- and T2-weighted images.[47]

Osteitis Condensans Ilii

Osteosclerosis involving triangular area of bone on the ileal side of the sacroiliac joints is thought to represent an aftermath of childbirth and has no clinical significance (Fig. 3–31).

Other Osteosclerotic Bone Diseases

Numerous other causes of osteosclerotic bone lesions exist. These include osteopetrosis, osteo-

poikilosis, hypervitaminosis D, idiopathic hypercalcemia, Ewing's sarcoma, osteoid osteoma, fluorosis, and mastocytosis.

Osteolytic Metastases

Lytic bone metastases from the urinary tract are seen in renal carcinoma, transitional cell carcinoma, carcinoma of the urethra, renal and retroperitoneal sarcomas, and occasionally carcinoma of the prostate and carcinoma of the seminal vesicle. Bone expansion may be seen in metastases from renal carcinoma. Metastases are likely to be hypervascular if the primary renal neoplasm is hypervascular. Radiographic findings are cortical discontinuity, scalloping of the inner cortex, loss of bony trabecula, and disappearing pedicle or spinous process. Pathological fractures may occur.

Osteitis Pubis

Osteitis pubis is a complication of any pelvic surgery and presents with intense and incapacitating pain over the symphysis pubis. It is probably infectious in origin and treatment consists of bed rest and antibiotics. Rarefaction of the pubic bone is seen in the acute stage and eventually is replaced by osteosclerosis (Fig. 3–32).

Avascular Necrosis of the Femoral Head

Osseous necrosis of the femoral head is thought to result from a vascular infarct, possibly venous.

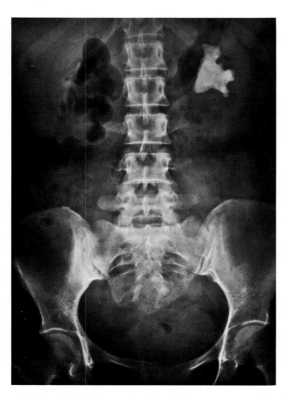

Figure 3–31. Osteitis condensans ilii is present on the ileal side of the right sacroileal joint. Comparing paired structures is the best way to detect any lesion on radiographs. Note staghorn calculus in the left kidney.

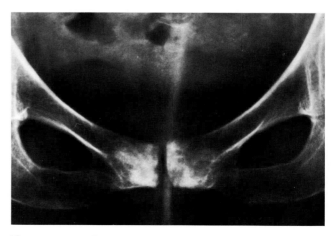

Figure 3–32. Old osteitis pubis with sclerotic changes in both pubic bones. Degenerative changes have also developed since a radiolucent "vacuum phenomenon" is present in symphysis.

Radiographic findings are osteosclerosis and a radiolucent subcortical band (rim sign) under the weight-bearing area of the femoral head and hypointense area on MR image. Cortical disruption, bone fragmentation and sclerosis are seen in later stages.

Spina Bifida

Spina bifida is incomplete fusion of the posterior neural arches. A small and asymptomatic defect is called *spina bifida occulta*. Meningomyelocele may be associated with large defects.

Diseases of the Sacrum

Sacral agenesis has a characteristic appearance where the iliac bones fill the void. Associated deformities of other bones may be present. Anterior meningomyelocele may be associated with anterior bone defect. A common primary neoplasm of the sacrum is chordoma, which presents as an osteolytic destructive process. Other tumors of the sacrum are rare.

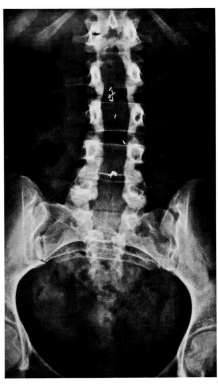

Figure 3–33.   Laminectomy has been performed from L1 to S1. Note absence of spinous processes and posterior elements.

Postoperative Changes

Many postoperative skeletal changes may be evident on abdominal radiograph, CT, or MR imaging. These include laminectomy (Fig. 3–33), rib resection, bone biopsy defects, resection of symphysis pubis, bone defects associated with Pereyra urethral suspension, posterior spinal fusion, Harrington rods, and many more.

REFERENCES

1. Toyoda K, Miyamoto Y, Ida M, et al. Hyperechoic medulla of the kidneys. Radiology 1989; 173:431–434.
2. Harrison RB, Vaughan ED. Diffuse cortical calcification in rejected renal transplants. Radiology 1978; 126:635–636.
3. Berg RA. Milk of calcium renal disease. Am J Roentgenol 1967; 101:708–713.
4. Buckalew VM Jr. Nephrolithiasis in renal tubular acidosis. J Urol 1989; 141:731–737.
5. Courey WR, Pfister RC. The radiographic findings in renal tubular acidosis. Radiology 1972; 105:497–503.
6. Grindulis KA, Roy S. Renal and pancreatic calcification in rheumatoid arthritis with Sjögren's syndrome. Br J Rheumat 1987; 26:212–215.
7. Hughes JJ, Wilder WM. Computed tomography of renal sarcoidosis. J Comput Assist Tomogr 1988; 12:1057–1058.
8. Bear RA, Handelsman S, Lang A, et al. Clinical and pathological features of six cases of sarcoidosis presenting with renal failure. Can Med Assoc J 1979; 121:1367–1371.
9. Arons WL, Christensen WR, Sosman MC. Nephrocalcinosis visible by X-ray associated with chronic glomerulonephritis. Ann Intern Med 1955; 42:260–282.
10. Brennan RP, Pearlstein AE, Miller SA. Computed tomography of the kidneys in a patient with methoxyflurane abuse. J Comput Assist Tomogr 1988; 12:155–156.
11. Riesz PB, Wagner CW Jr. Unusual renal calcification following acute bilateral cortical necrosis. Am J Roentgenol 1967; 101:705–707.
12. Lamkin N, Raval B, Carey LS. CT appearance of long-term renal transplant rejection. CT 1981; 5:340–342.
13. Hoffbrand BI, Oppenheimer SM, Sachs ML, Wrong OM. Nodular cortical nephrocalcinosis: a benign and hitherto undescribed form of renal calcification. Nephron 1987; 46:370–372.
14. Billimoria PE, Fabian TM, Schultz EE, Chase DR. Case report. Acquired renal oxalosis. J Comput Assist Tomogr 1983; 7:158–160.
15. Luers PR, Lester PD, Siegler RL. CT demonstration of cortical nephrocalcinosis in congenital oxalosis. Pediatr Radiol 1980; 10:116–118.
16. Falkoff GE, Rigsby CM, Rosenfield AT. Partial, combined cortical and medullary nephrocalcinosis: US and CT patterns in AIDS-associated MAI infection. Radiology 1987; 162:343–344.
17. Ezzedeen F, Adelman RD, Ahlfors CE. Renal calcification in preterm infants: pathophysiology and long-term sequelae. J Pediatr 1988; 113:532–539.

18. King JC, Rosenbaum HD. Calcification of the vasa deferentia in non-diabetics. Radiology 1971; 100:603–606.

19. Bisla RS, Louis HJ. Acute vascular compression of the duodenum following cast application. Surg Gynecol Obstet 1975; 140:563–567.

20. Johnson CD, Rice RP. Acute abdomen: plain radiographic evaluation. Radiographics 1985; 5:259–270.

21. Rigler LG. Spontaneous pneumoperitoneum. A roentgenologic sign found in the supine position. Radiology 1941; 37:604–607.

22. Schultz EH. An aid to the diagnosis of pneumoperitoneum from supine abdominal films. Radiology 1958; 70:728–731.

23. Miller RE. Perforated viscus in infants: a new roentgen sign. Radiology 1960; 74:65–67.

24. Han SY, Shin MS, Tishler JM. Plain film findings of hydropneumoperitoneum. AJR 1981; 136:1195–1197.

25. Miller RE, Nelson SW. The roentgenologic demonstration of tiny amounts of free intraperitoneal gas: experimental and clinical studies. AJR 1971; 112:574–585.

26. Miller RE. The radiologic evaluation of intraperitoneal gas (pneumoperitoneum). CRC Crit Rev Radiol Sci 1973; 4:61–85.

27. Sturman MF, Perez M. Computer-assisted diagnosis of acute abdominal pain. Compr Ther 1989; 15:26–35.

28. Shaff MI, Tarr RW, Partain CL, James AE Jr. Computed tomography and magnetic resonance imaging of the acute abdomen. Surg Clin North Am 1988; 68:233–254.

29. Shimkin PM. Radiology of acute appendicitis-commentary. AJR 1978; 130:1001–1004.

30. Vaudagna JS, McCort JJ. Plain film diagnosis of retrocecal appendicitis. Radiology 1975; 117:533–536.

31. Swischuk LE, Hyden Jr. CK. Appendicitis with perforation: the dilated transverse colon sign. AJR 1980; 135:687–689.

32. Campbell EW, Rogers CL. Submucosal gallbladder emphysema. JAMA 1974; 227:790–792.

33. Rigler LG, Borman CW, Nobel JF. Gallstone obstruction pathogenesis and roentgen manifestations. JAMA 1941; 117:1753–1754.

34. Meyers MA. Dynamic Radiology of the Abdomen: Normal and Pathologic Anatomy. New York: Springer-Verlag, 1976.

35. Meyers MA, Oliphant M, Berna AS, Feldberg MAM. The peritoneal ligaments and mesenteries: pathways of intraabdominal spread of disease. Radiology 1987; 163:593–604.

36. Williams SM, Harned RK, Hultman SA, Quaife MA. Psoas sign: reevaluation. Radiographics 1985; 5:525.

37. Fritzsche P, Toomey FB, Ta HN. Alteration of perirenal fat secondary to diffuse retroperitoneal infiltration. Radiology 1979; 131:27–29.

38. Susman N, Hammerman AM, Cohen E. The renal halo sign in pancreatitis. Radiology 1982; 142:323–327.

39. Federle MP. Acute abdomen: Computed tomography. Radiographics 1985; 5:307–320.

40. Hoffer FA, Shamberger RC, Teele RL. Ilio-psoas abscess: diagnosis and management. Pediatr Radiol 1987; 17:23–26.

41. Muller PR, Ferrucci JT Jr, Simeone JF, et al. Lesser sac abscesses and fluid collections: drainage by transhepatic approach. Radiology 1985; 155:615–618.

42. Jeffrey RB Jr, Tolentino CS, Federle MP, et al. Percutaneous drainage of periappendiceal abscesses: review of 20 patients. AJR 1987; 149:59–62.

43. Nosher JL, Winchman HK, Needell GS. Transvaginal pelvic abscess drainage with ultrasound guidance. Radiology 1987; 165:872–874.

44. Meyers MA, et al: Pneumatosis intestinalis. Gastrointest Radiol 1977; 2:91.

45. Bloch C. Natural history of pneumatosis coli. Radiology 1977; 123:311–314.

46. Roberts MC, Pollack HM, Banner MP, et al. Interstitial emphysema associated with epidural anesthesia for extracorporeal shock-wave lithotripsy. AJR 1987; 148:301–302.

47. Ross JF, Masaryk TJ, Modic MT, et al. Vertebral hemangiomas: MR imaging. Radiology 1987; 165:165–169.

4

Radiographic Contrast Material

Gastrointestinal tract, vessels, and most parenchymal organs may be rendered visible if they contain a sufficient amount of contrast material at the time of radiographic exposure. Gastrointestinal radiology, urology, angiography, computerized tomography (CT), and a score of other radiographic examinations owe their existence to contrast materials. Even MR imaging will to a large extent depend on development of better paramagnetic contrasts in its quest to become a dominant imaging modality in the 21st century.

Several different classes of contrast material are used in imaging. Barium contrasts are primarily used to opacify the gastrointestinal tract, as in barium enema or upper gastrointestinal series, or in the diluted form to render gastrointestinal tract visible on CT scan. Oily contrasts are now mostly used for an occasional lymphangiogram or for hysterosalpingography. Iodinated water-soluble contrast materials are the most widely used of any contrast materials. Several thousand metric tons are used worldwide annually, easily outweighing any other pharmaceutical.

The use of iodinated contrast materials is not based on their pharmacological effects but on their distribution in and elimination from the body. The iodine atoms markedly attenuate the primary x-ray beam so that vessels and tissues containing contrast media appear white (radiodense) on the radiograph. They are administered intravenously for excretory urography, CT scanning, venography, and some types of subtraction angiography. Intra-arterial injections are necessary for angiography and angiocardiography. Intracavitary instillation serves the purpose of visualizing the lumen of various organs.

Examples are cystography, urethrography, and hysterosalpingography.

WATER-SOLUBLE IODINATED CONTRAST MATERIALS

Ionic Contrasts

IONIC MONOMERS

Basic contrast materials intended for intravascular administration are salts. Like all salts when dissolved in water, contrast material molecules dissociate and form an electrolyte (Fig. 4–1). Three major groups of contrast material are named after their anions: *diatrizoate*, its structural isomer *iothalamate*, and *metrizoate*.

Diatrizoate, *iothalamate*, and *metrizoate* are benzoic acid derivatives that harbor three iodine atoms. The chemical difference between two anions is in their radicals at the 3 and 5 positions, but concerning their excretion by the kidney, there is no appreciable difference.

Two different cations are found in association with diatrizoate and iothalamate. These are *sodium* and *meglumine* (N-methylglucamine). The difference in tubular handling of these two cations is significant. Tubular reabsorption of sodium (and water) makes for a more concentrated contrast. Meglumine is not absorbed by the tubule and will cause some diuresis. While both types of contrast materials induce diuresis, meglumine salts are more effective in this regard.

Therefore, sodium cations help produce more con-

56

1. Ionic monomers

    Ratio iodine/ions 3 : 2

Diatrizoate Meglumine
(Renografin®, Squibb)

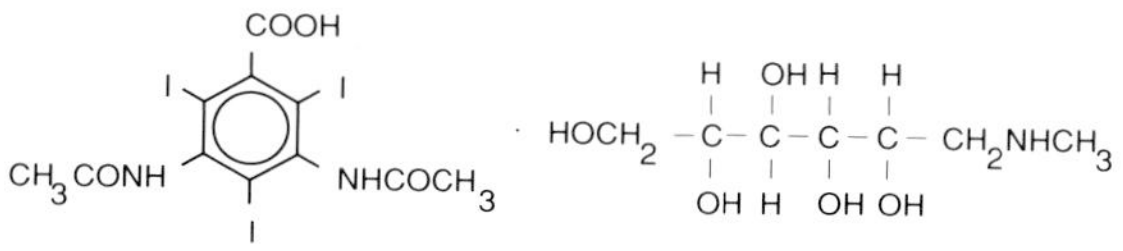

Diatrizoate Sodium
(Hypaque®, Winthrop)

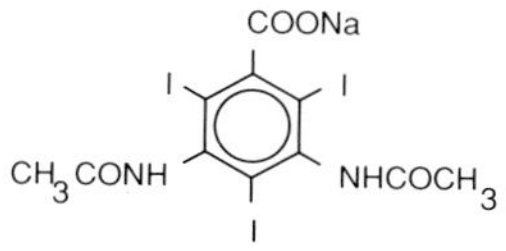

Iothalamate Meglumine
(Conray®, Mallenckrodt)

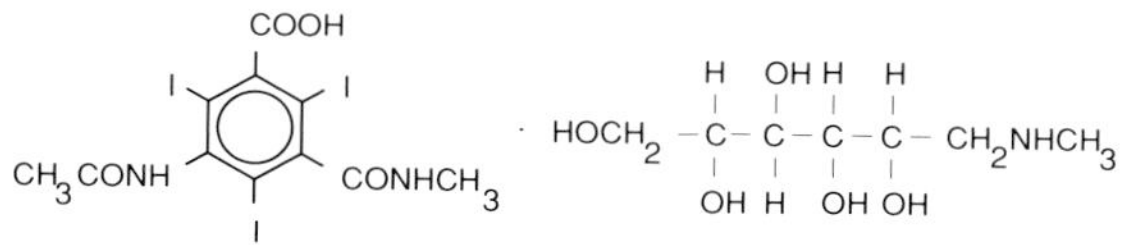

Iothalamate Sodium
(Conray®, Mallenckrodt)

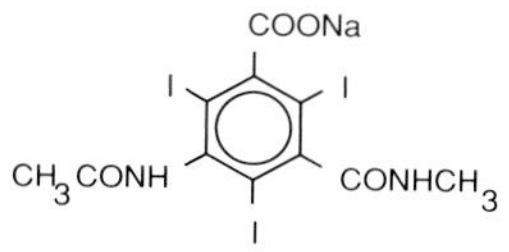

2. Ionic divalent dimer

    Ratio iodine/ions 2 : 1

Iodipamide Meglumine
(in Sinographin® &
Cholographin®, Squibb;
for salpingography
and cholecystography)

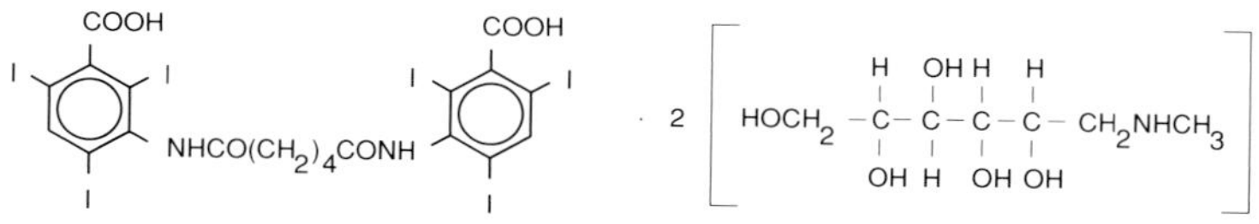

3. Ionic monovalent dimer

    Ratio iodine/ions 3 : 1

Ioxaglate Meglumine
(Hexabrix®, Mallenckrodt)

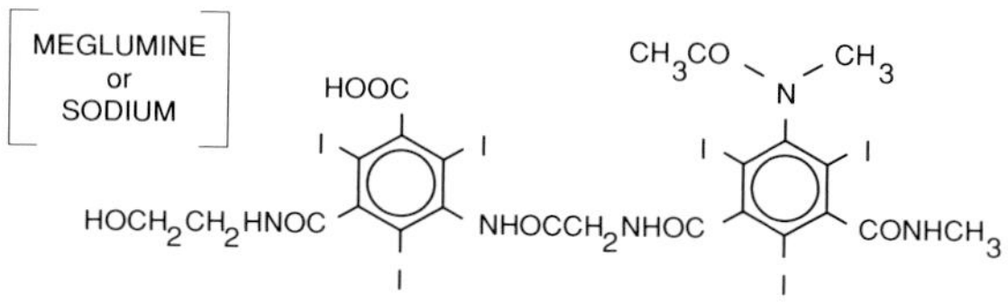

Figure 4–1. Ionic contrast materials.

centrated contrast in the urine while meglumine cations are somewhat better in distending the collecting system, which may be useful in the diagnostic process.

IONIC DIVALENT DIMER

The idea to join two ionic monomers was quite unique. It provided six iodine atoms and three ions per molecule, but unfortunately it was too toxic and was abandoned.

IONIC MONOVALENT DIMER

This molecule dissociates into only two ions. Cation may be either meglumine or sodium, while anion contains six iodine atoms. Osmolality is reduced somewhat from that of ionic monomers.

Nonionic Contrasts

NONIONIC MONOMERS

The new generation of nonionic contrast materials differs from ionic in that these contrasts do not dissociate in water (Fig. 4–2). Diuretic effect is negligible compared with ionic contrast materials, allowing for more concentration in the collecting system. Because of minimal diuretic effect, there may be inadequate distention of the collecting system during urography. In general, there is better tolerance by patients, and fewer side reactions compared with ionic contrasts. Nonionics, unfortunately, are also ten times more expensive than ionic contrasts.

NONIONIC DIMER

The only product in this group is *iotrolan,* which is intended for use in myelography. It has the lowest osmolality of any water-soluble contrast material and highest number of iodine atoms per molecule.[1]

Physical Characteristics

Color.   All radiographic contrasts are clear, colorless fluids. There should be no precipitate in the vial.

4. Nonionic monomers

Ratio iodine/molecule 3 : 1

Iopamidol (Isovue®, Squibb)

Iohexol (Omnipaque®, Winthrop)

Ioversol (Optiray®, Mallenckrodt)

5. Nonionic dimer

Ratio iodine/molecule 6 : 1

Iotrolan (Schering)

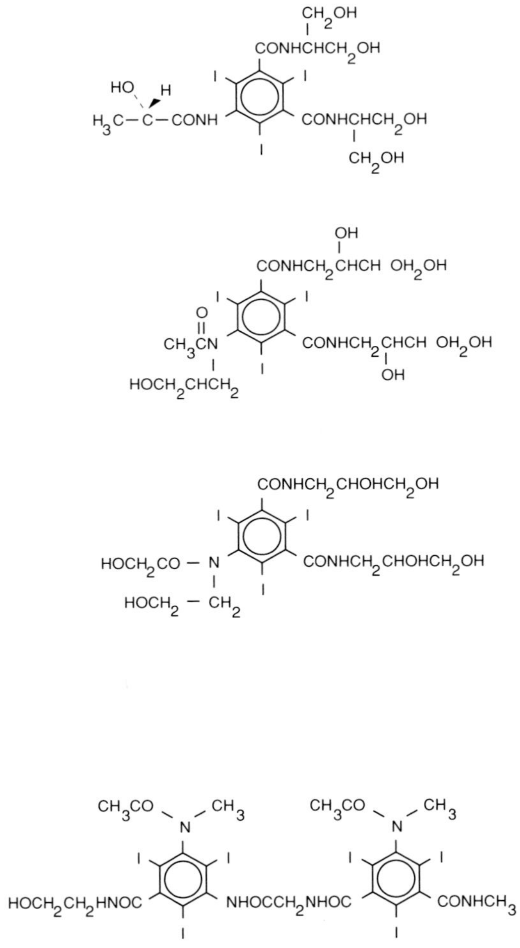

Figure 4–2.   Nonionic contrast materials.

Stabilizing agents such as sodium citrate and edetate sodium may be added.

Viscosity. Low viscosity is an important physical property of injectable contrast material. It assures rapid delivery through small-bore needles and angiographic catheters. Heating contrast to body temperature just prior to injection significantly decreases viscosity. Most automatic power injectors are equipped with a heating coil just for that purpose. Viscosity is influenced by the concentration and basic chemical design of the molecule. Sodium salts are less viscous than meglumine salts.

Osmolality. Ideally, contrast materials should be isotonic. In practice only one compound, a nonionic dimer (iotrolan), has such low osmolality.

The next best are monomeric nonionic contrasts with osmolality about twice physiological value (metrizamide, iohexol, iopamidol, and iopromide).

Some ionic contrast materials such as ionic monovalent dimer (ioxaglate) also have low osmolality. All other conventional ionic monomers (diatrizoate, iothalamate, and metrizoate), which form the bulk of the contrasts used in clinical practice today, have an osmolality five times greater than that of plasma.

High osmolality is responsible for many side effects that patients experience following contrast injection. These include a burning sensation, hot flush, nausea, etc.

Solubility. All ionic contrasts are *hydrophobic* and depend on their being salts for solubility. Nonionic contrasts hide their hydrophobic regions by hydrophilic hydroxyl side chains. Therefore nonionic contrasts are *hydrophilic,* and this is likely what allows for their high biological tolerance.[2]

Protein Binding. Ionic contrasts are very weak serum protein binding agents. Nonionic contrasts are even less so.

Effect on Coagulation. All contrasts inhibit coagulation. Ionic materials have very potent anticoagulant properties and act by inhibiting platelet aggregation and polymerization of fibrinogen.[3,4] Nonionic media are very weak coagulation inhibitors. When blood and nonionic contrast are mixed in the catheter or syringe, coagulation occurs more readily than when ionic contrast is present. In practice this translates into avoiding prolonged contact between nonionic contrast and blood in the syringe or catheter.[5] Contrast tends to stay in arm veins for some time and it is a good practice to elevate the arm after the injection and empty the veins of any residual contrast.

Clinical Pharmacology

Following intravascular injection, contrast materials are immediately diluted in the circulating plasma, thereafter reaching steady-state distribution between intravascular and extravascular spaces. The pharmacokinetics conform to an open two-compartment model with first-order elimination.

In the presence of normal renal function, elimination half-life of the contrast material is between 1 and 2 hours. The half-life is not dose dependent. Within six to eight half-lives, no detectable trace of contrast should be found within the blood or body tissues (some may still be seen in the bladder).

Radiographic contrasts do not cross the blood-brain barrier. There is minimal plasma protein binding, less so with nonionic contrasts.

Tissue Enhancement on CT Scanning

The degree of tissue enhancement is directly related to the iodine concentration (intravascular and extravascular) per unit volume of the tissue. Peak iodine blood levels occur within one circulation time following rapid IV injection of the dose. Equilibrium with extracellular compartments is reached in about 10 minutes.

Since the contrast material does not cross the blood-brain barrier, enhancement (increased x-ray absorption) in the normal brain is due to the presence of radiographic contrast in the blood pool. Pathological processes disrupt the blood-brain barrier and allow interstitial (extravascular) diffusion of contrast into the abnormal area, which then becomes visible compared to the surrounding normal brain.

In non-neural tissues diffusion into the interstitial spaces of normal and abnormal tissues is the same. Contrast enhancement here is due to the relative difference in extravascular diffusion between normal and abnormal tissues.

Excretion

Radiographic contrasts are excreted by *glomerular filtration.* There is no tubular excretion or reabsorption of the iodinated anion or the nonionic molecule. Because of tubular reabsorption of water, the radiographic contrast becomes markedly concentrated and visible on the radiographs (sodium salts slightly more so).

Insignificant amounts of contrast material are excreted by the liver, small intestine, lacrimal glands, salivary glands, and lactating breast. Some of these excretory pathways become important means for ridding the body of administered contrast in the case of renal failure. For instance, in the presence of renal insufficiency, the gallbladder and large intestine may contain sufficient contrast 24 hours after intravascular administration to be readily visible either on plain radiograph or, especially, on CT. This process is known as "vicarious excretion." One can think of the gastrointestinal tract as a huge nephron. The upper tract excretes contrast while the large bowel concentrates it.

Nephrogram

Cortical nephrogram refers to visualization of the renal parenchyma due to contrast in the capillaries, glomerulus, and proximal convoluted tubules. At this very early stage of contrast transit through the kidney, the cortex is very dense and well contrasted with relatively radiolucent medulla. Cortical nephrogram is seen only when a compact bolus of contrast is delivered rapidly, such as dynamic CT scanning, angiography, and, on occasion, urography.

Uniform nephrogram is present within a minute or two after the injection of the contrast material. In a normal individual it only takes 3 minutes for contrast to transit the nephron and the collecting tubules. The radiographic densities of the cortex and medulla become equal and uniform so that corticomedullary differentiation is no longer seen.

Contrast in the capillaries contributes to only 10% of the overall radiodensity. The nephrogram is mostly visible because of the presence of contrast in the convoluted tubules, loops of Henle, and collecting tubules.

The intensity of the nephrogram is directly proportional to the plasma concentration of the contrast material and to the glomerular filtration rate (GFR). It follows that a larger dose and a bolus injection will produce a denser nephrogram.

State of hydration does not affect the concentration of the contrast material in the convoluted tubules and does not affect the quality of the nephrogram.

Pyelogram

Antidiuretic hormone (ADH) affects water reabsorption in the collecting tubules only. Although its action is insufficient to alter overall nephrogram radiodensity, ADH significantly affects the final concentration of contrast material in the urine. Concentration is higher in the mildly dehydrated patient than in well-hydrated patients. Most radiologists prefer patients to abstain from liquids several hours prior to excretory urography, since this results in a better quality pyelogram.

Dehydration is unnecessary for CT scan or angiography and contraindicated in patients with mild (or moderate) renal insufficiency.

Summary

The best quality excretory urogram is obtained on a slightly dehydrated patient with normal GFR, intact tubular function, and normal pituitary using nonionic hydrophilic contrast material, where a large dose is injected as a compact bolus and the best possible radiographic technique is used.

The second best urogram is obtained by substituting the nonionic contrast with sodium salt ionic contrast material.

Ureteral compression distends the upper system so that a larger number of iodine molecules find themselves in the pathway of the x-ray beam. Even though the concentration remains the same, the beam is that much more attenuated. This increases the overall radiodensity of the urine.

SYSTEMIC REACTIONS TO RADIOGRAPHIC CONTRAST MATERIAL

Incidence: Table 4–1 is the composite from several references.[6–14] There is a lower incidence of mild and moderate, and, perhaps more importantly, of severe reactions with nonionic contrast material (Fig. 4–3).[9,10] The largest multi-institutional study includes 169,284 patients given intravenous ionic contrast compared to 168,363 patients given nonionic contrast.[9] Only two deaths were reported, one in the high-osmolar, and one in the low-osmolar group; it is also uncertain if the deaths were contrast related. The incidence of reactions is also dependent on the route of administration;[8] for instance, intra-arterial injections have a lower overall rate.

Etiology. The etiology is probably multifactorial.

Even small amounts of radiographic contrast given intravenously may produce a severe anaphylactoid reaction. There is an immediate release of histamine and a number of other potent substances, such as kinins, leukotrienes, and possibly prostaglandins. The result is dilatation of capillaries and venules, increased vascular permeability, constriction of bronchial smooth muscles, and constriction of coronary arteries leading to ischemia and arrhythmia.

Table 4-1. Incidence of Systemic Reactions to Radiographic Contrast Material

	IONIC (%)	NONIONIC (%)
Overall reactions		
Intravenous	5-12.6	2-3.1
Intra-arterial	2.3	
Severity		
Fatal	0.01-0.00066	
Very severe*	0.04	0.004
Severe†	0.22	0.04
Mild (no treatment)	5-12.6	2.1-3.13
History		
Allergic history (drug, food, asthma, etc.)	20-25	6-8
Prior reaction to contrast	45	11
Prior exposure to contrast without reaction	9	5.5
Very severe reactions		
High-risk patients	0.36	0.03
Underlying cardiac disease	0.53	0.10
Asthma	1.88	0.23
Prior contrast reaction	0.73	0.18
History of allergy	0.53	0.10
Bolus IV injection	0.25	0.04
Male/female ratio	1:1	1:1

*Dyspnea, hypotension, cardiac arrest, loss of consciousness.
†Treatment or hospitalization.

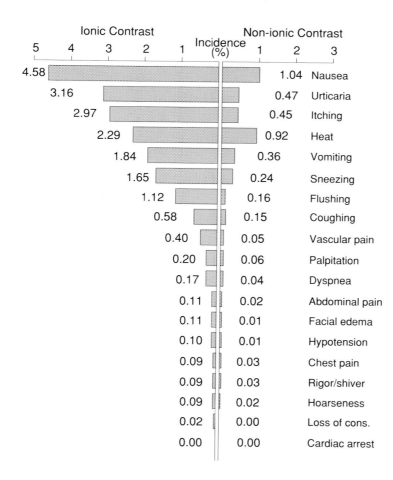

Figure 4-3. Systemic reactions associated with ionic (ioxaglate excluded) and nonionic water-soluble iodinated radiographic contrasts. There is a significant decrease in incidence associated with nonionic contrasts, not only in minor reactions such as urticaria and nausea, but also in serious reactions such as hypotension.

Other reactions are dose-dependent. Contrast hyperosmolality is considered the major contributing factor. Some hypertonic effects are vasodilatation, sensation of heat, increased release of histamine, changes in red blood cell morphology, and vascular endothelial damage with resultant activation of blood coagulation.

Direct toxic effect of the contrast also may contribute to adverse reactions.[3,15] Neurotoxic, cardiotoxic, and nephrotoxic effects are well known. Chemotoxicity of radiographic contrasts appears to be proportional to the serum protein-binding affinity. As expected, low osmolar contrasts have the lowest affinity. Highly hydrophilic contrasts also appear to be better tolerated.

Therefore, systemic adverse reactions to contrast are more than likely: a) an allergic phenomenon; b) a response to hyperosmolality; c) a direct chemotoxic effect of the contrast material; or d) a combination of the above.

Clinical Presentation. Most adverse reactions to contrast material happen within the first 5 minutes after injection. Delayed reactions may occur even after 1 hour.

Urticaria, facial edema, laryngeal edema, bronchospasm, and seizures are easily recognizable either as isolated entities or as a part of anaphylactoid reaction.

Hypotensive episodes, on the other hand, may be due to: a) anaphylaxis; b) vasodilatatory effect of contrast material in a hypovolemic patient; c) myocardial infarction; d) cardiac arrhythmia; e) vasovagal reaction; or f) any combination of several of the above. It is often difficult for the radiologist to be sure of the exact etiology, and the treatment is appropriately dictated by the presenting symptoms and clinical findings.

Radiological Findings. Radiological findings are related to hypotension and to decreases in glomerular perfusion pressure and glomerular filtration rate (Fig. 4–4). Pulmonary edema, if present, may be diagnosed on chest radiograph.

Treatment

URTICARIA

A mild cutaneous reaction consisting of a few hives and pruritus does not require treatment, except perhaps hydration. More severe reactions may be treated with diphenhydramine 50 mg IV, IM, or PO, as well as hydration. Urticaria may be a part of anaphylactoid reaction and all patients should be observed until the symptoms subside.

FACIAL AND LARYNGEAL EDEMA

Swelling of the face may start around the lips or eyelids and may rapidly progress to involve the entire face. Laryngeal edema may be present with or without facial edema. Patients may complain of breathing difficulty. Inspiratory stridor is characteristic. Epinephrine 0.1–0.3 ml 1:1000 SQ given every 15 minutes up to a total of 1 mg is the treatment of choice. Intubation should be considered if the symptoms are moderate or severe. Tracheostomy may be necessary. Adequate oxygen and respiratory assistance should be provided. If there is no improvement from epinephrine alone, cimetidine 300 mg IV in D5W should be given over 15 minutes, and diphenhydramine 50 mg IV.

BRONCHOSPASM

Difficulty in breathing and expiratory stridor are present. Mild bronchospasm may be treated with beta-agonist inhalers such as metoproterenol or albuterol, followed by epinephrine 0.1–0.3 ml 1:1000 SQ given every 15 minutes up to a total of 1 mg if necessary. Oxygen should be provided via nasal cannula or mask. This regimen is effective in the majority of cases.

More difficult cases require terbutaline 0.25–0.5 mg IM or SQ every 6 hours. Alternatively, aminophylline may be given 4–6 mg/kg as a loading dose in D5W for 20 minutes, then 0.4–1.0 mg/kg/hr. Adverse cardiac effects of aminophylline are arrhythmia and hypertension.

HYPOTENSION

Hypotension associated with anaphylactoid reaction may or may not be preceded by mild symptoms such as sneezing, hives, or watery eyes. Hypotension associated with myocardial ischemia and cardiac arrhythmia may be associated with chest pain, palpitations, and shortness of breath. In both groups tachycardia is common. Bradycardia is commonly present in vasovagal reaction with some exceptions. For instance, patients on beta-blockers, such as propranolol, may also be bradycardic in the presence of anaphylactoid reaction.

Anaphylactoid Hypotension. Rapid fluid replacement is the most important therapy. Several liters of 0.9% (normal) saline is administered through one or more large bore needles.[16]

If the hypotensive reaction is mild and not life-threatening, epinephrine 0.1–0.2 mg SQ at a concentration of 1:1000 (1 mg/ml) can be given using 1 ml syringe.

If the hypotensive reaction is severe, epinephrine is

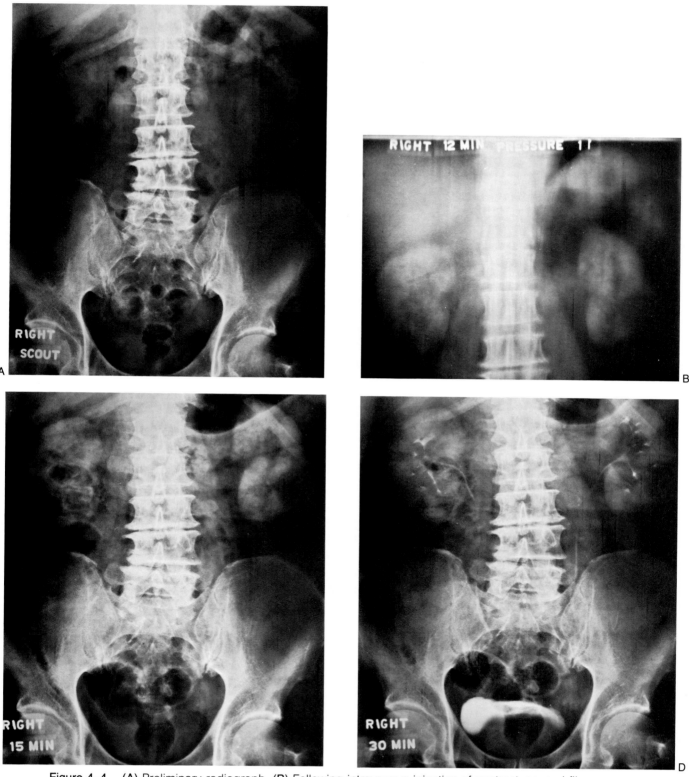

Figure 4–4. **(A)** Preliminary radiograph. **(B)** Following intravenous injection of contrast, several films were obtained. Nephrogram is present but even on 12-minute radiograph there is no excretion into the collecting system. Patient did not appear to be in distress. The technologist applied external compression unaware of developing hypotension. **(C)** Several minutes later there is still no excretion. Radiologist monitoring the films made the diagnosis immediately and started appropriate treatment. Systolic pressure was 80 mm Hg but patient was still responsive and communicating. **(D)** After appropriate therapy, the blood pressure was normal within minutes. Last radiograph shows normal collecting system and ureters, no evidence for obstruction, and enlarged prostate. A simple cyst is in the left kidney.

diluted to 1:10,000 (1 mg/10 ml), in a 10 cc syringe, and given 1–3 ml IV every 5–10 minutes. If venous access is not immediately available epinephrine may be delivered into the trachea after the dose is further diluted to a volume of 10 cc. Undesirable epinephrine side effects are cardiac arrhythmias (beta$_1$ effect) or hypertensive crisis (alpha effect). One should probably start with smaller doses and be particularly careful in patients with known cardiac disease. Electrocardiographic (ECG) monitoring should be instituted.

Oxygen should be provided via nasal cannula or mask as soon as possible.

If there is no response to intravenous administration of fluid and epinephrine, the patient should be placed on vasopressors. Dopamine 2–20 μg/kg/min is infused intravenously.

H$_1$-antihistamine (diphenhydramine) and H$_2$-histamine (cimetidine) may also be added to the regimen.

Cardiogenic Hypotension. Treatment for acute myocardial infarction and cardiac arrhythmias is different from that for anaphylactoid reaction. In fact, if treatment for an allergic-type reaction is instituted in cardiac patients, the situation might well be made much worse. History of angina, chest pain during examination, and shortness of breath point to, but need not necessarily be associated with, cardiac disease.

Patients with angina should be given nitroglycerin 0.4 mg sublingually every 5 minutes, providing that blood pressure and heart rate are closely monitored. ECG should be obtained immediately.

Pulmonary edema is a rare adverse reaction to contrast material. More likely it is due to acute cardiac decompensation in a patient with an underlying cardiac disease. Hydration here is obviously contraindicated. Central venous line and diuretics should be instituted.

Vasovagal Reaction. Restlessness, apprehension, cold sweating, abdominal cramps, and loss of consciousness. Hypotension and bradycardia are found on physical examination.[17] Patients should be placed in the Trendelenburg position, and rapidly infused with normal saline. Atropine in doses of 0.5–2.0 mg may be given intravenously as a bolus. Smaller doses of atropine should be avoided.

Bradycardia may also be associated with anaphylactoid reaction in patients receiving beta-blockers (e.g., propranolol).

SEIZURES

A single episode may be observed while providing for the usual patient protection. Recurrent and generalized seizures (status epilepticus) are controlled with diazepam 5–10 mg IV, a dose that is effective for 15 to 20 minutes. Alternatively, phenytoin 15–18 mg/kg is infused at a rate of less than 50 mg/min. Neurologic consultation should be sought.

PROPHYLAXIS

Pretreatment with steroids 12 hours prior to contrast reduces the frequency of almost all reactions.[18,19] Some suggested regimens are 20 mg of prednisone by mouth or 100 mg hydrocortisone every 6 hours for at least three doses.[20] Since corticosteroids are cheap, they could serve as a substitute for more expensive nonionic contrast. The logistics of administering corticosteroids to patients and feasibility of delivering the pharmaceutical to most patients are the main difficulties. It is still unclear if pretreatment with steroids reduces the frequency of recurrent severe reactions.

Pretreatment with antihistamines reduces the frequency of urticaria, angioedema, and respiratory symptoms.[21,22] The usual dose is diphenhydramine 50 mg, PO, IM, or IV, and cimetidine, 300 mg, PO or IV. The antihistamine and contrast are not to be mixed in the same syringe.

EOSINOPHILIA

Transient benign eosinophilia may be present in up to 21% of the patients 24–48 hours after intravascular contrast examination.[23]

LOCAL REACTIONS TO RADIOGRAPHIC CONTRAST MATERIAL

Ascending Phlebitis

Prolonged contact of contrast material with the vascular endothelium may cause chemical phlebitis and vascular thrombosis. The arm where the injection was made becomes swollen, erythematous, and painful within 24 hours. The symptoms gradually disappear within several days or weeks. Skin ulceration may be seen in more severe cases.

Treatment is symptomatic and includes extremity elevation and warm compresses. Incidence may be reduced by flushing the venous system with isotonic saline after contrast injection or by elevating the arm, thus clearing the venous system of any contrast. After the arm is elevated, the patient usually feels a hot flush, implying that large amounts of contrast have been stored in the arm veins.

Contrast Extravasation

Even small quantities of contrast material inadvertently injected outside of the vessel may cause serious injury. Erythema, swelling, pain, and limitation of motion are the principal findings. In severe cases skin ulceration may develop, requiring debridement and skin grafts.[24–26]

Treatment initially consists of extremity elevation, warm compresses, and dressing. No effective local drug therapy is presently available.

Prevention is of obvious importance in reducing this iatrogenic injury. Injections into the small veins over the dorsum of hand and foot, rapid bolus injections in any small vein, and multiple punctures of the same vein should be avoided. Use of plastic sheaths instead of metallic indwelling needles is also likely to reduce the risk. Meticulous attention to detail is necessary while performing dynamic CT scanning where the injection site cannot be visually inspected during automated mechanical delivery of contrast.

Contact Dermatitis

This is a rare contact skin reaction to contrast-laden urine characterized by cutaneous bullae and surrounding erythema. A predisposing factor may be wet diapers.[27] Avoidance of prolonged contact of skin with contrast-laden urine is appropriate. Treatment is symptomatic.

Salivary Gland Swelling (Iodide Mumps)

Small amounts of free inorganic iodide are frequently found in radiographic contrast solutions and some contrast molecules are probably deiodinated in vivo. Salivary gland swelling is the reaction to this unbound iodine rather than to the contrast molecule itself.[28,29] The incidence may be somewhat higher in azotemic patients.

CONTRAST-INDUCED NEPHROPATHY (CONTRAST NEPHROTOXICITY)

Etiology.   Direct nephrotoxic effect of intravascular radiographic water-soluble contrast material upon renal tubules. Other possible mechanisms are: renal vasoconstriction and ischemic injury to proximal tubular cells, red blood cell sludge, precipitation of Tamm-Horsfall mucoprotein, and intratubular uric acid obstruction.[30,31]

Predisposing Factors (High-Risk Group).   Diabetics with preexisting renal failure are at greatest risk. Other risks are: preexisting renal insufficiency, diabetes mellitus, cardiac disease, elderly patients, proteinuria, hyperuricemia, large dose of contrast material, dehydration, and furosemide.[32] The risk factors may be additive. There is a sharp rise in probability of contrast nephrotoxicity when serum creatinine is at or above 1.2 mg/dl.

Incidence.   Increase in creatinine of 150% of baseline value is detected in 0.15% of patients receiving intravascular radiographic contrast. Increase in serum creatinine over 50% baseline is seen in 1.6% of patients with normal renal function and up to 8.8% of diabetics with preexisting renal failure.

Ionic Versus Nonionic Contrast Material.   There is no difference in nephrotoxicity. Both contrast materials produce nephropathy at identical rates. There is no beneficiary effect of the nonionic contrast in this regard.[33,34] This is despite the fact that nonionic contrasts cause less enzymuria compared with ionic.

Clinical Presentation.   Oliguria occurs 24 to 48 hours after contrast study. There is a gradual recovery to baseline within a week in the majority of patients.

Laboratory Findings.   Rise of at least 0.5 mg/dl occurs in serum creatinine, peaking within 48 hours of exposure.[35] Occasionally, the peak may be reached in 3, 4, or even 10 days after exposure.[36,37] There is low fractional excretion of sodium.

Prophylaxis.   Adequate hydration must be maintained. In high-risk groups pretreatment with mannitol prior to contrast study has been advocated.

Radiological Findings.   Persistent nephrogram may be seen as long as 24 to 48 hours after intravascular administration of contrast material (Fig. 4–5).[35] This prolonged nephrogram is less pronounced compared with the nephrogram seen in acute obstruction. Persistent cortical enhancement is particularly well seen on 24-hour CT scan. Cortical attenuation may be as high as 200 HU and is always associated with nephropathy if above 140 HU.[36] Patients with cortical enhancement without clinical or laboratory evidence for contrast nephropathy are probably at higher risk of developing nephropathy on subsequent contrast examinations.[36]

Vicarious excretion of contrast material by the liver and small bowel may be present. Excreted contrast may be concentrated in the gallbladder and large bowel and rendered visible on plain radiograph or CT scan.

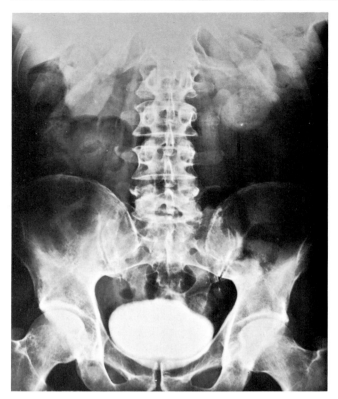

Figure 4–5. Persistent nephrogram 24 hours after intravenous radiographic contrast examination. The bladder did not need to be emptied since the examination (because of oliguria) and still contains contrast.

CONTRAST MATERIALS FOR MAGNETIC RESONANCE IMAGING

Paramagnetic Contrast Materials

Paramagnetic contrasts do not produce MR signals. Rather, they alter the local magnetic field and thereby affect both T1 and T2 relaxation times of adjacent hydrogen nuclei in the tissues where they may transit or concentrate. In their presence the signal intensity on T1-weighted images is generally increased. Higher concentrations eventually result in decreased signal intensity.[38]

The best-known paramagnetic compound, and the only one approved by the FDA so far, is gadolinium-DTPA. This very stable chelate is somewhat hyperosmolar and must be administered intravenously rather slowly. The compound does not cross the blood-brain barrier and is excreted unchanged by the kidney. The recommended dose is 0.1 mmol/kg body weight.

Following injection, normal kidneys will exhibit a rapid decrease in T1 relaxation time, which makes them hyperintense (bright) on T1-weighted sequences. Sequential imaging in 15-second intervals, through the same plane, shows normal procession of the paramagnetic contrast through the cortex, then medulla, and finally accumulation in the collecting

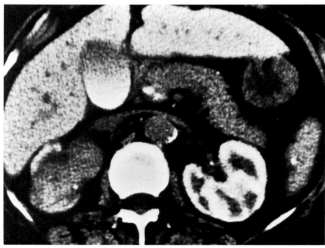
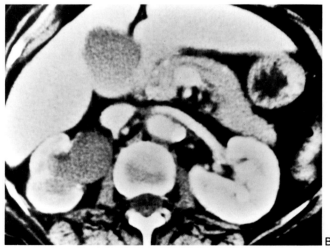

A
B

Figure 4–6. 24 hours after major angiography, a CT scan of the abdomen was obtained looking for a suspected abdominal abscess. **(A)** Precontrast scan (liver window) shows retained contrast in the cortex of the left kidney. The right kidney is a small, hydronephrotic, poorly functioning kidney. There is vicarious excretion of contrast into the gallbladder. This patient is obviously in renal failure even though serum creatinine levels might not show it as yet. The last thing in the world this patient needs is another dose of contrast material. **(B)** Radiologist does not review the precontrast scan and injects the patient with a full dose. The nephrogram becomes more uniform and the renal vein increases in caliber, indicating increase in blood flow. The lesson: intraarterial and intravenous contrast examinations should be scheduled 48 hours apart, CT scans and other contrast radiological examinations should be monitored, and one should be knowledgeable regarding deleterious systemic and renal effects of radiographic contrast.

system. The resemblance to Tc-99m DTPA nuclear medicine flow scan is striking except that the resolution is much better. For instance, in experimental animals in the presence of renal ischemia the affected kidney does not become hyperintense (bright) compared with the normal side.

While the true value of these substances in evaluation of renal disease still remains somewhat elusive, they are the subject of much research and their applications in the urinary tract will be better known.[39-41] There is a wealth of information describing definite benefit in the imaging of brain, spine, and heart.

Free metal ions are potentially the best paramagnetic agents. However, they are either too toxic or are cleared from the body too rapidly for medical imaging. Chelated metal ions have the advantage of marked toxicity reduction and relative tissue specificity.

Since bowel may in some instances simulate abdominal tumors, oral paramagnetic contrast materials are being developed. Ferric (Geritol) or ferrous iron seem to be agents of choice.

REFERENCES

1. Dawson P, Howell M. The non-ionic dimers: a new class of contrast agents. Br J Radiol 1986; 59:987–991.
2. Sovak M, Robertson HJF. Letter to the editor. Radiology 1988; 168:281–282.
3. Dawson P. Chemotoxicity of contrast media and clinical adverse effects: a review. Invest Radiol (Suppl) 1985; 20:84–91.
4. Dawson P, Hewitt P, Mackie IJ, et al. Contrast, coagulation, and fibrinolysis. Invest Radiol 1986; 21:248–252.
5. Robertson HJF. Blood clot formation in angiographic syringes containing nonionic contrast media. Radiology 1987; 163:621–622.
6. Ansell G, Tweedie MCK, West CR, et al. The current status of reactions to intravenous contrast media. Invest Radiol 1980; 15:532–539.
7. Hartman GW, Hattery RR, Witten DM, Williamson B. Mortality during excretory urography. Mayo Clinic experience. AJR 1982; 139:919–922.
8. Shehadi WH. Contrast media adverse reactions: occurrence, recurrence, and distribution patterns. Radiology 1982; 143:11–17.
9. Katayama H. Report of the Japanese committee on the safety of contrast media. Presented at the RSNA 1988.
10. Palmer FJ. The RACR survey of intravenous contrast media reactions: final report. Australas Radiol 1988; 32:426–428.
11. Jacobsson BF, Jorulf H, Kalantar MS, Narasimham DL. Nonionic versus ionic contrast media in intravenous urography: clinical trial in 1,000 consecutive patients. Radiology 1988; 167:601–605.
12. Holtas S. Iohexol in patients with previous severe anaphylactoid reactions to ionic contrast agents. Invest Radiol 1984; 19:563–565.
13. Schrott KM, Behrends B, Clauss W, et al. Iohexol in excretory urography: results of the drug monitoring programme. Fortschr Med 1986; 104:153–156.
14. Kinnison ML, Powe NR, Steinberg EP. Results of randomized controlled trials of low- versus high-osmolality contrast media. Radiology 1989; 170:381–389.
15. Swanson DP, Thrall JH, Shetty PC. Drug review: evaluation of intravascular low-osmolality contrast agents. Clin Pharm 1986; 5:877–891.
16. vanSonnenberg E, Neff CC, Pfister RC. Life-threatening hypotensive reactions to contrast media administration: comparison of pharmacologic and fluid therapy. Radiology 1987; 162:15–19.
17. Poulsen J, Rasmussen F, Georgsen J. Hypotensive shock associated with bradycardia after intravenous injection of contrast medium. Radiology 1987; 164:275–276.
18. Lasser EC, Berry CC, Talner LB, et al. Pretreatment with corticosteroids to alleviate reactions to intravenous cortical material. N Engl J Med 1987; 317:845–849.
19. Lasser EC. Perspective pretreatment with corticosteroids to alleviate reactions to intravenous contrast material: overview and implications. AJR 1988; 150:257–260.
20. Cohan RH, Dunnick NR, Bashore TM. Treatment of reactions to contrast material. AJR 1988; 151:263–270.
21. Ring J, Rothenberger KH, Clauss W. Prevention of anaphylactoid reactions after radiographic contrast media infusion by combined histamine H_1 and H_2 receptor antagonist: results of prospective controlled trial. Int Arch Allergy Appl Immunol 1985; 78:9–14.
22. Small P, Satin R, Palayew MJ, Hyams B. Prophylactic antihistamines in the management of radiographic contrast reactions. Clin Allergy 1982; 12:289–294.
23. Vincent ME, Gerzof SG, Robbins AH. Benign transient eosinophilia following intravenous urography. JAMA 1977; 237:2629.
24. Syre-Smith G. Tissue necrosis following extravasation of contrast material. J Can Assoc Radiol 1982; 33:104.
25. Loth TS, Jones DE. Extravasations of radiographic contrast material in the upper extremity. J Hand Surg [Am] 1988; 13:395–398.
26. Spigos DG, Thane TT, Capek V. Skin necrosis following extravasation during peripheral phlebography. Radiology 1977; 123:605–606.
27. Wood BP, Lane AT, Rabinowitz R. Cutaneous reaction to contrast material. Radiology 1988; 169:739–740.
28. Carter JE. Iodide "mumps." N Engl J Med 1961; 264:987–988.
29. Talner LB, Coel MN, Lang JH. Salivary secretion of iodine after urography. Radiology 1973; 106:263–268.
30. Cohan RH, Dunnick NR. Intravascular contrast media: adverse reactions. AJR 1987; 149:665–670.
31. Gale ME, Robbins AH, Hamburger RJ, Widrich WC. Renal toxicity of contrast agents: iopamidol, iothalamate, and diatrizoate. AJR 1984; 142:333–335.
32. Moore RD, Steinberg EP, Powe NR, et al. Frequency and determinants of adverse reactions induced by high-osmolality contrast media. Radiology 1989; 170:727–732.
33. Schwab SJ, Hlatky MA, Pieper KS, et al. Contrast

nephrotoxicity: a randomized controlled trial of a nonionic and an ionic radiographic contrast agent. N Engl J Med 1989; 320:149–153.

34. Davidson CJ, Hlatky M, Morris KG, et al. Cardiovascular and renal toxicity of a nonionic radiographic contrast agent after cardiac catheterization. Ann Intern Med 1989; 110:119–124.

35. Older RA, Miller JP, Jackson DC, et al. Angiographic induced renal failure and its radiographic detection. AJR 1976; 126:1039–1045.

36. Love L, Lind JA Jr, Olson MC. Persistent CT nephrogram: significance in the diagnosis of contrast nephropathy. Radiology 1989; 172:125–129.

37. Parfrey PS, Griffiths SM, Barrett BJ, et al. Contrast material-induced renal failure in patients with diabetes mellitus, renal insufficiency, or both. A prospective controlled study. N Engl J Med 1989; 320:143–148.

38. Davis PL, Parker DL, Nelson JA, et al. Interactions of paramagnetic contrast agents and the spin echo pulse sequences. Invest Radiol 1988; 23:381–388.

39. Choyke PL, Frank JA, Girton ME, et al. Dynamic Gd-DTPA-enhanced MR imaging of the kidney: experimental results. Radiology 1989; 170:713–720.

40. Kikins R, von Schulthess GK, Jäger P, et al. Normal and hydronephrotic kidney: evaluation of renal function with contrast-enhanced MR imaging. Radiology 1987; 165:837–842.

41. Carvlin MJ, Arger PH, Kundel HL, et al. Use of Gd-DTPA and fast gradient-echo and spin echo MR imaging to demonstrate renal function in the rabbit. Radiology 1989; 170:705–711.

5

Congenital Diseases of the Kidney

RENAL AGENESIS

Bilateral Renal Agenesis

Absence of both kidneys occurs in 0.3% of live newborns and is incompatible with life.

Potter Syndrome

This syndrome consists of bilateral renal agenesis, hypoplastic lungs, oligohydramnios, facial anomalies, and pes equinovarus.[1,2] Newborns with bilateral dysplastic kidney, hydronephrosis, or bilateral multicystic dysplastic kidneys may also present with Potter facies[3] and with all other characteristics of the syndrome. An effort must be made to establish the cause of renal failure, since some entities, such as hydronephrosis, may be treatable.

Unilateral Renal Agenesis

Incidence of congenital absence of one kidney is 1/1000. Ipsilateral ureter is absent in 90% of all cases. Trigone does not form on the side of the absent kidney in 50%. Associated congenital anomalies such as seminal vesicle cyst,[4,5] vaginal agenesis,[6] and colon malposition[7] may be present (Fig. 5–1). A variety of other anomalies involving the reproductive organs may be present.[8–10]

The solitary kidney is hypertrophied, somewhat enlarged (Fig. 5–2), and perhaps somewhat more susceptible to traumatic injury.

Supernumerary Kidney

This is an extremely rare anomaly. The supernumerary kidney has its own independent blood supply and is distinctly separated from the other kidneys.[11]

RENAL HYPOPLASIA

Global Renal Hypoplasia

Renal hypoplasia is an incomplete development of the kidney.[12–14] The kidney is smaller and has fewer calyces and fewer papillae (five or less). Functionally and morphologically the hypoplastic kidney is normal, except that it has proportionally fewer nephrons because of its diminutive size (Fig. 5–3). The hy-

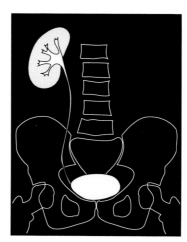

Figure 5–1. Schematic drawing of unilateral renal agenesis.

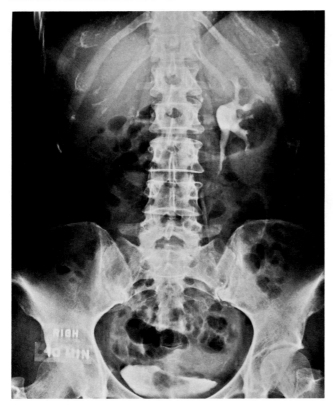

Figure 5–2.   EXU in a patient with congenital absence of the right kidney. The left kidney is enlarged due to compensatory hypertrophy.

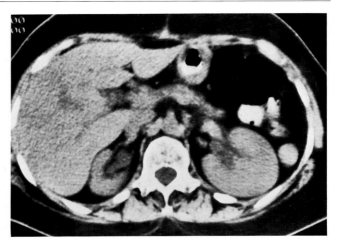

Figure 5–3.   CT scan without contrast in a patient with globally small kidney without prior history of urinary tract infections, hypertension, or obstruction.

poplastic kidney has a smooth outline and rather short infundibula. Calyces may be clubbed. Differential diagnosis with chronic pyelonephritis and renal vascular hypertension may be difficult, since there is increased incidence of both urinary tract infection and hypertension associated with this entity. Short of angiography, differentiation from renal artery stenosis in the presence of hypertension may be impossible.

Unipapillary Kidney

An unbranched renal pelvis is extremely rare.[15–17] Hypertension and other congenital anomalies are common. There are fewer nephrons. Progression to interstitial fibrosis has been reported.

DUPLICATION

In any one of the different types of renal duplication the involved kidney is somewhat larger than usual and contains more functioning renal parenchyma. Usually, there are two distinct renal sinuses separated by normal renal parenchyma.

Bifid Renal Pelvis

This is a common anomaly of the urinary tract and is considered a normal variant (Fig. 5–4A). Trifid renal pelvis is rare, as is multifid.

Incomplete Duplication

Incomplete duplication consists of two ureters and two collecting systems. A single distal ureteral orifice is present (Fig. 5–4B,C). Duplex system is formed because of premature division of the ureteric bud during ascent. The duplicate ureters may join and form a single ureter anywhere between the kidney and the bladder. Such a configuration is also known as "Y"-shaped ureters (Fig. 5–5).

Peristaltic wave in Y-shaped ureters begins in the upper moiety and propagates to the junction and continues toward the bladder. However, a reverse peristaltic wave may propagate up the lower moiety ureter (Fig. 5–6). An extremely rare "yo-yo" phenomenon may be created with alternating reverse peristalsis in both segments, which may result in clinically significant obstruction or infection.[18]

Of clinical significance is the relative difficulty in performing percutaneous nephrostomy, percutaneous stone manipulation, and retrograde endourological procedures, compared with the normal kidney (Fig. 5–7).

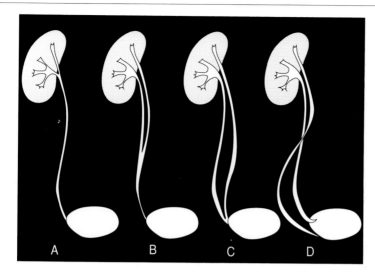

Figure 5–4. Schematic drawing of: **(A)** Bifid renal pelvis; **(B)** incomplete duplication or "Y" ureter; **(C)** incomplete duplication where two ureters join into single ureteral orifice; **(D)** complete duplication where both ureters have a separate insertion into the bladder.

Complete Duplication

Complete duplication presents with two separate ureteral orifices. The ureter of the lower moiety inserts into the bladder more superiorly and laterally in respect to its counterpart. Insertion of the upper system ureter is more distal and medial.

In most instances the two ureteral insertions are in close proximity and in no way interfere with function. However, the intramural portion of the lower moiety ureter is usually short, an anatomical mishap, resulting in increased incidence of vesicoureteral reflux.[19]

Ureteral insertion of the upper moiety may be

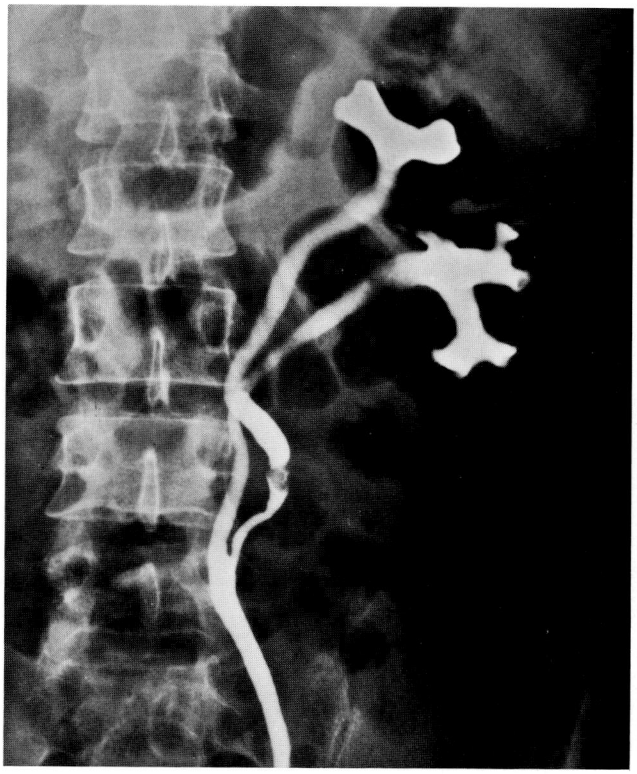

Figure 5–5. Incomplete duplication resulting in a "Y"-shaped ureter. A "filling defect" in the lower moiety ureter is a nonobstructing calculus.

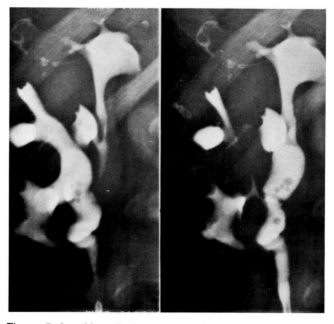

Figure 5–6. "Yo-yo" phenomenon in a bifid renal pelvis. Retrograde pyelogram demonstrates peristaltic activity peculiar to this rare condition. On the left image, the upper moiety is contracted while the lower moiety is relaxed. On the right image taken only a few seconds later, the reverse is true. The upper moiety is distended while the lower moiety is contracted. Fluoroscopic observation of this phenomenon is much more dramatic than can be portrayed with only two spot radiographs.

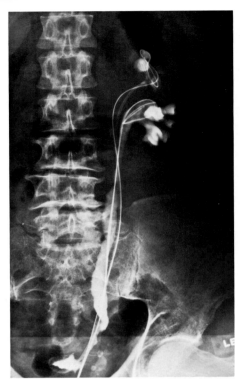

Figure 5–7. Retrograde endoscopic manipulation of renal and ureteral calculi in a patient with incomplete duplication. Each ureter requires its own set of guidewires and catheters.

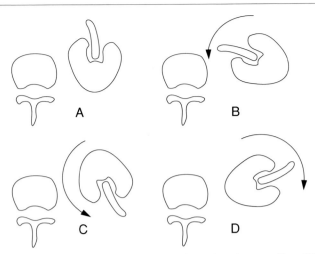

Figure 5–8. Schematic drawing of rotational anomalies: **(A)** Incomplete rotation; **(B)** normal; **(C)** overrotation; **(D)** reversed rotation.

ectopic and may empty low in the bladder, posterior urethra, and vagina. Such an ectopic orifice is more likely to become obstructed or associated with constant urine leak and dribbling.[20,21] Ureterocele is also more frequently seen at the insertion of the upper moiety ureter. More detailed discussion of ectopic ureters is presented in Chapter 15 ("Ureter").

ROTATIONAL ANOMALIES (MALPOSITION)

The most common rotational anomalies happen along the long (vertical) renal axis. During normal development, the kidney during its ascent rotates 90° toward the midline. Failure to do so is called *incomplete rotation* and the renal pelvis will face anteriorly. If the kidney rotates more than the usual 90°, the renal pelvis will face posteriorly, a situation known as *overrotation*. Rotation of the kidney in the direction opposite to normal will result in the renal pelvis facing laterally and is called *reversed rotation* (Fig. 5–8).

Diagnosis of different types of malrotation is very easy on CT and MR imaging studies (Fig. 5–9). On

excretory urography, the pelvis and renal calyces overlap so that some of the calyces are seen closer to the midline than the pelvis. An additional oblique projection will immediately clarify which rotational anomaly is present.

Rotational anomalies along anteroposterior or transverse axis are much less frequent. Rotational anomalies are the rule in renal ectopia and renal fusion.

RENAL ECTOPIA

Ectopic kidneys are more susceptible to infection, obstruction, blunt trauma, and inadvertent intraoperative injury. They present problems for interventional radiologists, since percutaneous catheter placement is difficult.[22] Supernumerary renal ves-

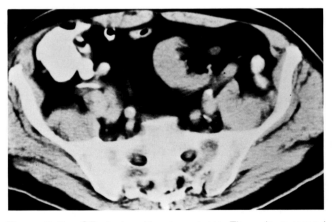

Figure 5–9. CT study without contrast. There is reversed rotation of the left kidney.

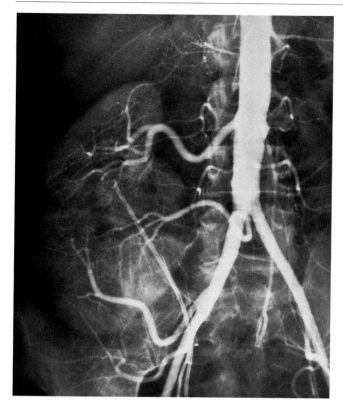

Figure 5–10. Three separate renal arteries supply the low-lying right kidney. The middle and lower arteries take off from the right iliac artery. There is a retrograde catheter in place with the tip in the region of the upper pole.

sels are almost always present, complicating selective renal angiography and surgery (Fig. 5–10).[23]

Pelvic Kidney (Sacral Kidney)

Pelvic kidney is the most common renal ectopia with an incidence of 1/700 of the population (Fig. 5–11). Other congenital anomalies may be present. Pelvic kidney may be difficult to detect on an excretory urogram. It usually does not have normal reniform shape and it may be rotated so that the collecting system readily empties into dependent ureter, leaving little radiographic contrast behind (Fig. 5–12).

Ureteropelvic junction obstruction, reflux, infection, and urolithiasis are common (Fig. 5–13). Detection of renal masses is difficult, since the collecting system and the kidney are usually distorted. Vascular supply to the kidney is from a low-lying renal artery originating from the aorta or iliac artery. Supernumerary renal arteries are frequent.

Bilateral pelvic kidneys are very rare (Fig. 5–14) and incompatible with natural childbirth, unlike unilateral pelvic kidney, where natural childbirth is usually possible (Fig. 5–15).

Under no circumstances should a pelvic kidney be misdiagnosed as a primary pelvic tumor. Central sinus complex and corticomedullary differentiation should be looked for on all pelvic ultrasound examinations. During operations, just as on radiographic examinations, the pelvic kidney may not resemble normal kidney and may not be recognized as such. It could easily be mistaken for a neoplasm and removed, rendering the patient anephric.

Crossed Renal Ectopia

Crossed renal ectopia may be fused or nonfused (Fig. 5–16A), the fused being more common.[24] Vascular supply is frequently anomalous. For instance, the renal artery may originate from contralateral iliac artery, there are supernumerary renal arteries, etc. Varying degrees of rotation are seen.

Thoracic Kidney

This is one of the least common positional anomalies.[25] The kidney is supradiaphragmatic, having

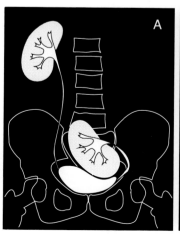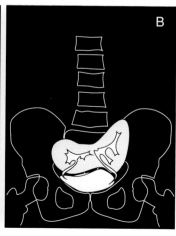

Figure 5–11. Schematic drawing of pelvic kidney **(A)** and bilateral pelvic kidneys **(B)**.

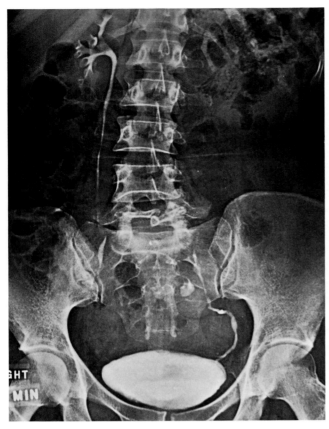

Figure 5–12. Excretory urogram in a patient with left pelvic kidney.

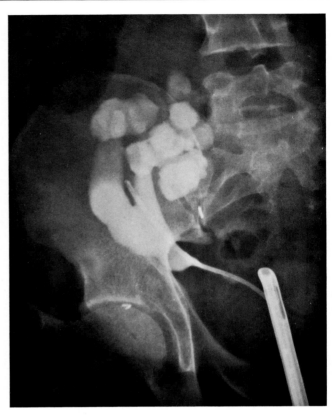

Figure 5–13. Retrograde pyelogram on a pelvic kidney which had several episodes of obstruction due to passing renal calculi and an operation for the same. Calyceal blunting and moderate loss of renal parenchyma resulted.

herniated through the foramen of Bochdalek during development. It should enter in the differential diagnosis of any posterior thoracic or diaphragmatic mass. Vessels originating from high abdominal or thoracic aorta may be present.

RENAL FUSION

Horseshoe Kidney

Incidence of horseshoe kidney is 1/1000. Fusion of the lower poles occurs in over 96% of all cases. The connecting bridge, called "isthmus," is located anterior to the aorta and inferior vena cava, and posterior to the inferior mesenteric artery (Fig. 5–17). In most instances the renal pelvis and ureteropelvic junction are incompletely rotated and are facing forward. The ureters cross the isthmus anteriorly. There are usually supernumerary renal vessels (Fig. 5–18).

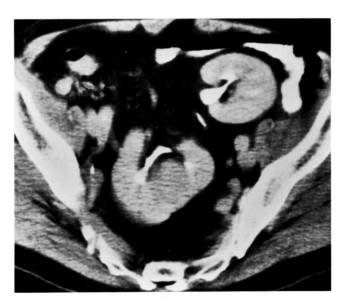

Figure 5–14. Contrast-enhanced CT in a patient with carcinoma of the prostate and unsuspected bilateral pelvic kidneys.

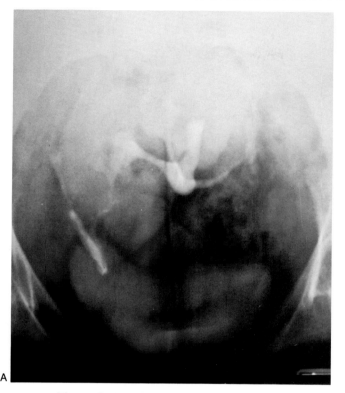
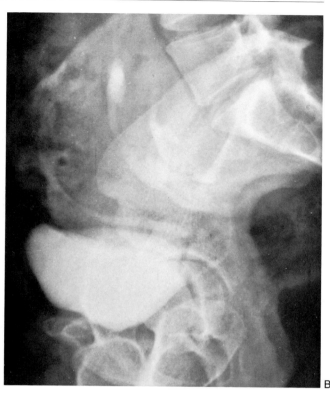

Figure 5–15. Bilateral pelvic kidneys in a woman seen on excretory urogram in AP **(A)** and lateral **(B)** projection. The entire birth canal is occupied by the kidneys and natural childbirth is impossible.

Radiographic diagnosis on plain radiographs, excretory urography, and retrograde pyelography is made by virtue of the long axis of the kidneys, which converge inferiorly. The long axis is determined by connecting the uppermost and the lowest calyces.

On CT, ultrasound, MR imaging, and scintigrams, the isthmus is identified anterior to the major vessels, and crossed by inferior mesenteric artery (Fig. 5–19, 5–20).

Complicating features of the horseshoe kidney are ureteropelvic junction obstruction, urolithiasis (Fig. 5–21), and greater susceptibility to trauma. Other congenital anomalies may be present.

Prior to surgical or percutaneous procedures, it may be desirable to obtain a CT scan, MR, or even a renal angiogram to assess the distribution of multiple renal arteries and anatomical relation of the kidney to liver and spleen (Fig. 5–22).

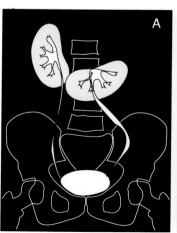
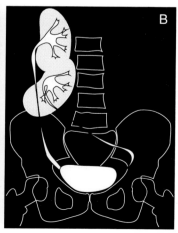

Figure 5–16. Schematic drawing of nonfused **(A)** and fused **(B)** renal ectopia.

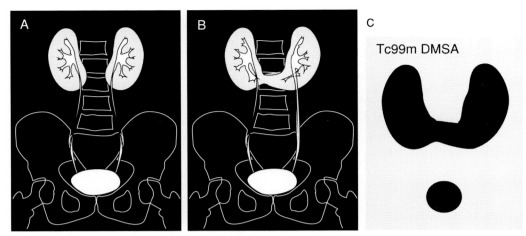

Figure 5–17. Schematic drawing of horseshoe kidney. (A) The connecting isthmus is not visualized; (B) Isthmus is well developed. (C) Tc-99m DMSA scan.

Crossed-Fused Renal Ectopia

Most crossed ectopic kidneys are fused (Fig. 5–16B). The lower kidney is most commonly ectopic (Fig. 5–23), although the reverse may also be true. Varying degrees of rotational anomaly are likely to be present.[26] The pelvis of each kidney may be facing in opposite directions. If the fused kidneys assume an "S" shape, the fused ectopia is called *sigmoid kidney.*

Pancake Kidney

Fusion of both kidneys in front of the lower abdominal aorta and bifurcation results in a flat, nonreniform conglomeration of renal parenchyma, which is called pancake kidney. Multiple renal arteries are the rule.

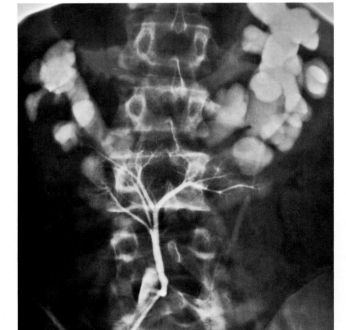

Figure 5–18. Multiple renal arteries are very common in horseshoe kidneys. Here a selective renal arteriogram of the aberrant vessel supplying the isthmus is obtained. The axis of both kidneys is oriented inferomedially and there is bilateral hydronephrosis caused by ureteropelvic junction obstruction.

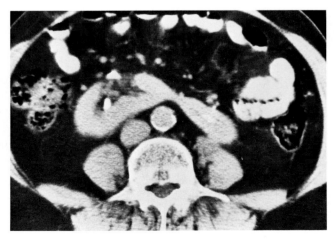

Figure 5–19. Contrast-enhanced CT in the isthmus area. Aorta and vena cava are posterior to the isthmus. Inferior mesenteric artery is seen crossing over the isthmus.

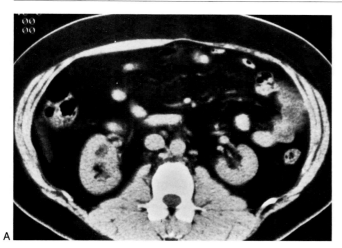
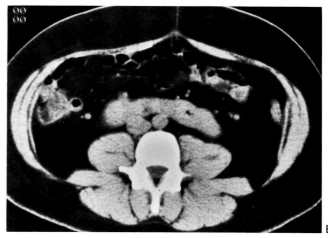

Figure 5–20. CT of a horseshoe kidney. **(A)** A more superior cut through the kidneys; **(B)** cut through the isthmus.

CONGENITAL CYSTIC DISEASES OF THE KIDNEY

Introduction

The unifying concept of congenital cystic dilatation of the urinary tract was proposed by Mellins,[27] based on extensive work of Potter and many others. Most congenital cystic dilatations of the urinary system can be traced to the developmental stages as the ureteral bud ascends, undergoes dichotomous branching, and induces and establishes communication with nephrons.

Any interruption of this process at different stages of development creates a distinct congenital anomaly. These are:

1. *Primary megaureter:* Beginning at the very distal ureter, deficient development of the longitudinal muscle fibers results in narrowing, lack of peristalsis, and dilatation of the ureter above the lesion. (See Chapter 15, Ureter.)
2. *Multicystic dysplastic kidney (MDK):* The next maldevelopment in the ascent of the ureteral bud is atresia of the renal pelvis and infundibula. The ampullary cap of the ureteral bud under normal circumstances stimulates metanephric blastema and induces nephron development. In this disease there is atresia of the pelvoinfundibular system. Thus, the normal influence of the ureteral bud is not felt and development of the nephrons does not materialize. The end result is dysplastic renal parenchyma. Occasionally, only segmental atresia of the upper third of the ureter will be present and will cause a rare hydronephrotic type of multicystic dysplastic kidney. (See p 79.)

3. *Ureteropelvic junction obstruction (UPJ):* This is a very localized lesion that occurs at the site of the first bifurcation of the ureteral bud. Varying degrees of obstruction may be present. Extrarenal pelvis is the rule. This lesion may be con-

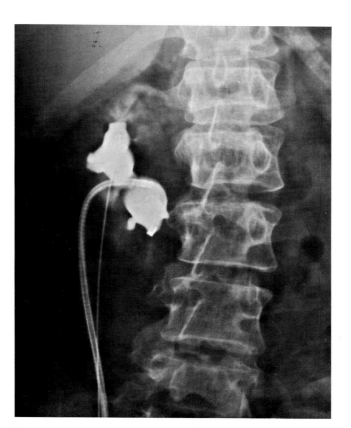

Figure 5–21. Retrograde pelvoureteroscopy in a horseshoe kidney with a flexible ureteroscope. There is partial ureteropelvic junction obstruction. Several calculi are present in the kidney, although obscured with contrast.

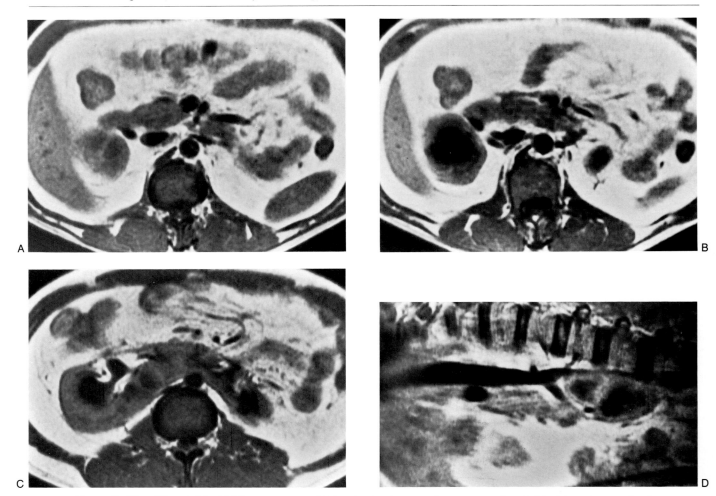

Figure 5–22. T1-weighted MR sequences obtained prior to percutaneous nephrostolithotripsy in a patient with horseshoe kidney. **(A)** The most cephalad image shows the relation of the upper poles of right and left kidneys to the liver and spleen. Percutaneous approach is possible only through the upper pole calyces and attention must be directed toward avoiding injury to the liver and spleen. **(B)** The next cut demonstrates hydronephrotic upper pole on the right and there continues to be unfavorable positional relation with the liver for percutaneous puncture. **(C)** Cut through the isthmus demonstrates bilateral hydronephrosis. The left kidney is smaller than the right. **(D)** Sagittal cut through inferior vena cava. Isthmus is seen anterior to cava. Right renal vein is seen entering the cava. Posterior to the cava the right renal artery is seen as a large dot. Higher up the portal vein is crossing the inferior vena cava anteriorly.

sidered a very mild manifestation in the spectrum of multicystic dysplastic kidney. (See p 124.)

4. *Pelvocalyceal diverticula:* During normal development, the first three to five divisions of the ureteral bud consolidate, fuse, and dilate to form the renal pelvis and infundibula. A few branchings may not assimilate into the collecting system wall and form diverticular outpouchings. (See p 80.)

5. *Congenital megacalyces:* The number of calyces depends on the number of branching generations before the cribriform plate covering the papillae perforates and disappears. A later branching generation than usual may result in increased number of calyces and also in calyces that are flat and polygonal in contour. The medullary rays lack height but cortex above them is of normal thickness. Calyces are usually enlarged at the expense of the short medulla and resemble hydronephrosis. (See p 81.)

6. *Medullary cystic disease:* Ascending farther, a mishap occurring during formation of the collecting tubules results in uniform enlargement of these structures. The dilatation involves only the distal segment of the collecting tubule. There are several diseases in this category:
   a. Medullary sponge kidney

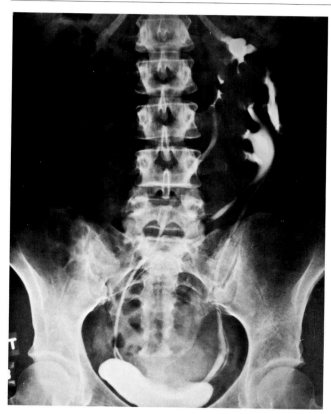

Figure 5–23. Crossed-fused ectopia. There is also complete duplication of both kidneys and four ureters can be counted on this EXU. (Photograph courtesy of Dr. S.T. Cochran.)

    b. Renal tubular ectasia
    c. Renal tubular ectasia with congenital hepatic fibrosis
    d. Juvenile nephronophthisis
    e. Medullary cystic disease (See p 81.)
7. *Infantile polycystic disease:* A more severe malformation at the level of the collecting tubules results in cystic diverticula and fusiform dilatations of the collecting tubules. Even the proximal collecting tubules are dilated. Nephrons (proximal and distal convoluted tubules and loop of Henle), however, are intact. Kidneys are enlarged. (See p 84.)
8. *Adult polycystic kidney disease:* Ascending deeper into the renal parenchyma, cystic dilatation not only of the collecting tubules, but also of the nephrons, is present. Direct communication between the cysts and nephrons or collecting tubules is always present. Kidneys are enlarged. Normal parenchyma is interspersed among the cysts. (See p 85.)
9. *Multilocular renal cyst (cystic nephroma):* Localized, focal failure of a single ureteral bud branch

to stimulate and organize metanephric blastema results in cystic dysplasia. This is a well-demarcated lesion that is surrounded by a fibrous capsule and contains multiple noncommunicating cysts. Differentiated renal parenchyma is not present within the lesion. Remaining renal parenchyma outside the lesion is normal. (See p 162.)
10. *Renal dysplasia:* Renal dysplasia is an expression of urinary tract obstruction. On one end of the spectrum is MDK. On the other end is a small kidney with disorganized and immature tubules, "whorling" mesenchymal tissue, and intrarenal cartilage. Cysts may be present and increase in number, the higher the obstruction. (See p 88.)

Multicystic Dysplastic Kidney

Incidence. The second most common abdominal mass in neonates. There is slight male predominance.

Embryology. Ureteric bud division is arrested. Since ureteric bud normally induces nephron development, this process is arrested as well. The result is transformation of the kidney into a mass of noncommunicating cysts.

Pathology. Pelvoinfundibular atresia is the basic anomaly.[28] The kidney is transformed into a multicystic, dysplastic mass. Lobar disorganization, underdeveloped collecting system, and hypoplastic or absent renal artery are present. Calcification in the cyst wall is possible. Less common is a hydronephrotic form resulting from atresia of the upper third of the ureter.[29]

Clinical Presentation. Palpable abdominal or flank mass in neonates. Asymptomatic in adults. Rarely, symptoms are due to mass effect. Most of the MDK do not change in size over the years. Nine percent of lesions spontaneously disappear within the first 3 years.[30,31] Hypertension is occasionally present. Important contralateral malformations are present in 25%, most commonly UPJ obstruction. Neoplasm within the MKD is rare.[30,32]

Treatment. Nephrectomy if symptomatic or enlarging. Semiannual imaging for first 3 years.[30]

Radiological Findings. Ultrasound is the imaging method of choice in initial examination of any neonatal mass. Typical peripheral cluster of cysts with distinct septa is discovered, replacing most of the renal parenchyma.[33] Renal pelvis and renal sinus are not seen. The most important contribution of ultrasound is the differentiation of MDK from hydronephrosis.[34]

Plain radiography or nonenhanced CT scan may demonstrate curvilinear calcifications.

On excretory urogram, MDK typically does not excrete radiographic contrast material. However, on 24-hour radiograph, "puddling" of contrast may be seen on occasion, depending on the ratio of dysplastic and more normal functioning tissue.[35]

Atretic ureter is demonstrated if cystoscopy and retrograde pyelography are obtained. Angiographic examination is unnecessary, but one would expect an absent or severely hypoplastic renal artery.[36]

MDK is usually a unilateral disease. On occasion, the opposite kidney may be involved with the same process. More frequently, varying degrees of dysplasia, ureteropelvic junction obstruction, or reflux are found on the opposite side. If both kidneys are involved, the neonate may present with all characteristic features of Potter syndrome.

The less common hydronephrotic type of MDK is almost impossible to differentiate from ureteropelvic junction obstruction. Antegrade cyst puncture and contrast injection are said to be diagnostic if filled cystic structures are seen to communicate via small tubular structures.[37]

In rare instances only one half of a duplex kidney may be involved, or only one of the kidneys in crossed renal ectopia.[38,39] Diagnosis of the latter is based on the presence of a multicystic mass of the lower pole of a usually hydronephrotic kidney and on the absence of the contralateral kidney and renal artery.

Bilateral and total MDK has a similar clinical presentation to that of bilateral renal agenesis, i.e., hypoplastic lungs and Potter facies.

Pyelocalyceal Diverticula

Incidence. Infrequent.

Pathology. Urine-filled diverticular outpouching usually arises from calyceal fornix but may originate from renal pelvis or infundibulum. Epithelial lining is transitional epithelium. May contain calculi.

Clinical Presentation. Most are asymptomatic. Stasis of urine may predispose to infection or stone formation. In rare instances transitional cell carcinoma may originate within the diverticulum. Treatment is usually symptomatic.

Radiological Findings. Most pyelocalyceal diverticula communicate with the collecting system and readily fill with contrast material on excretory urog-

raphy (Fig. 5–24),[40,41] retrograde pyelography (Fig. 5–25), or CT. On occasion, the narrow channel connecting the collecting system and the diverticulum may be obstructed and may not fill with contrast. Differentiation with renal cyst under such circumstances is impossible.

If a calculus is present in the "closed-off" calyceal diverticulum, it may appear on CT as a cyst with an intraluminal calcific density. The kidney may be reexamined after placing the patient in the prone position (Fig. 5–26). If free, the calculus will migrate to the dependent part of the cavity. Intramural calcification will not migrate under such circumstances.

Ultrasound will demonstrate a cystic lesion. Typically, the specific diagnosis is difficult to make since the communicating channel is usually too small.

Intradiverticular calculi present special treatment problems when treated with extracorporeal shock wave therapy, since pulverized fragments cannot empty spontaneously (Fig. 5–27). Retrograde endoscopic stone manipulation or percutaneous stone extraction may also be difficult (Fig. 5–28).[42]

On occasion, small calyceal diverticulum may mimic papillary necrosis (Fig. 5–29). Oblique views during an excretory urogram will help determine

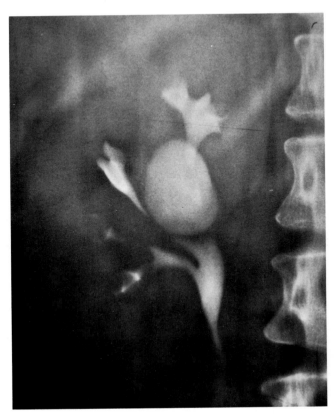

Figure 5–24. Pyelocalyceal diverticulum filling in a retrograde manner during an EXU.

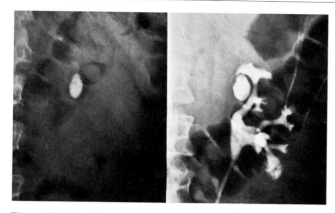

Figure 5–25. Upper calyceal diverticulum containing a calculus fills with contrast on retrograde pyelography.

forniceal origin so characteristic for the diverticulum.

Pelvocalyceal diverticula may be seen in Beckwith-Wiedemann syndrome (exomphalos, macroglossia, gigantism, hypoglycemia).[43]

Congenital Megacalyces

Incidence. Rare. Bilateral in 20%. More common in males.

Pathology. Malformative enlargement of the calyces without obstruction. Medullary rays lack height but cortex above them is of normal thickness. Calyces are usually enlarged at the expense of the short medulla and resemble hydronephrosis.[44,45]

Clinical Presentation. Asymptomatic. The main clinical problem is differentiating this anomaly from

obstruction or from postobstructive dilatation. May be associated with megaureter.

Radiological Findings. In obstructive uropathy the cortex is generally thinned out. In congenital megacalycosis the cortex is of normal thickness.[46] Demonstrating normal cortical thickness is difficult (Fig. 5–30). Perhaps it is more important to conclusively prove the absence of partial obstruction than to try to establish the diagnosis of congenital megacalycosis. An upright projection during excretory urography is perhaps the best. If any doubts remain, other methods described elsewhere should be used (See Chapter 7, "Urinary Tract Obstruction").

Concomitant presence of a megaureter is possible, which further complicates the diagnosis. An element of functional obstruction may be present because of megaureter.[47]

Cystic Diseases of the Renal Medulla

MEDULLARY SPONGE KIDNEY AND TUBULAR ECTASIA

Etiology. Congenital, no definite hereditary pattern.

Incidence. Mild form is seen in 0.5% of patients undergoing excretory urography. Slight male preponderance.

Pathology. One or both kidneys may be involved or the process may be confined to a single papilla.[48,49] Cystic or fusiform dilatation of the collecting tubules. Intratubular calculi are present in more than 50% of cases. Classified as Potter I.

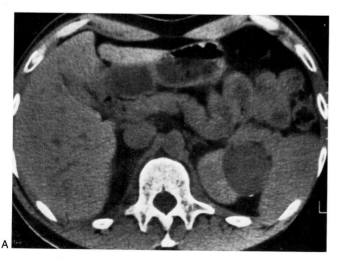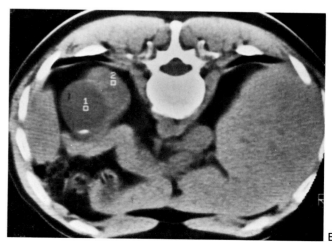

Figure 5–26. Calyceal diverticulum containing a stone seen on nonenhanced CT scan. Supine (**A**) and prone (**B**) positions. The small calculus shifts with the change in position.

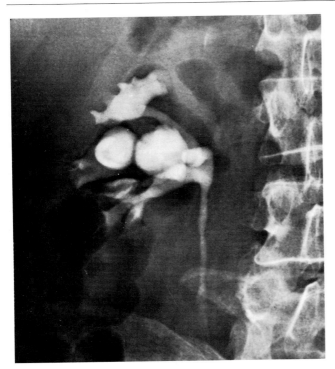

Figure 5–27. Retrograde pyelogram demonstrates two pyeloinfundibular diverticula that contain calculi.

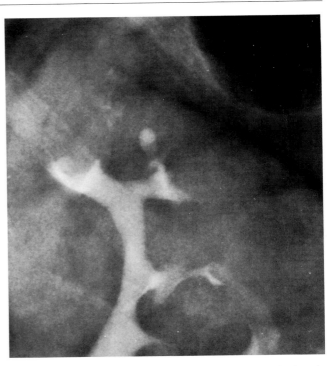

Figure 5–29. A close-up of a small calyceal diverticulum in an upper pole calyx.

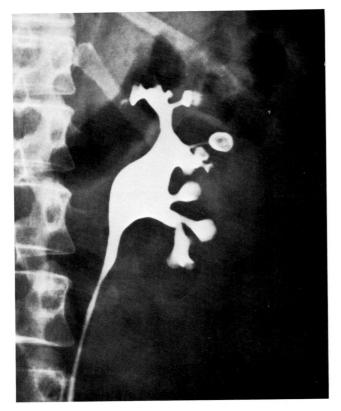

Figure 5–28. Retrograde pyelogram demonstrates a small calyceal diverticulum containing a calculus. Calculus is seen as a relatively radiolucent "filling" defect.

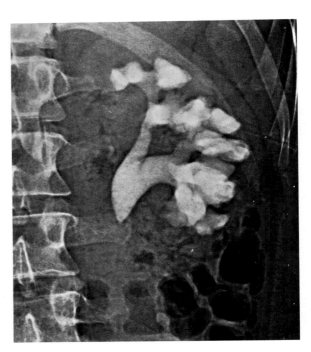

Figure 5–30. Congenital megacalycosis seen on a retrograde pyelogram.

Clinical Presentation. In most instances the symptoms are absent or mild. Hematuria, urinary tract infection, and renal colic may be present. Rarely, limb hemihypertrophy may be seen on the side of unilateral medullary sponge kidney.[50,51] Congenital pyloric stenosis and Ehlers-Danlos syndrome have been described.

Radiological Findings. Renal size and shape are not affected. Since the collecting tubules contain concentrated radiographic contrast, individual dilated tubules are occasionally identified on excretory urography (Fig. 5–31). More likely, however, a streaky brushlike appearance is seen as many dilated collecting tubules superimpose on a radiograph (Fig. 5–32). Contrast may remain within the tubules for some time. Papilla is generally somewhat enlarged (Fig. 5–33). Dilated tubules do not fill during retrograde examination.

Small calculi may be seen in the papillae or pyramids on excretory urography (Figs. 5–34, 5–35) or CT. If numerous, these may be detected on ultrasound as hyperechoic areas associated with acoustical shadowing. Differential diagnosis includes nephrocalcinosis. Unlike calcifications in nephrocalcinosis, which are interstitial, calcifications in medullary sponge kidney are intratubular. Careful comparison with the preliminary radiograph will disclose filling of additional dilated tubules during the course of intravenous urography. This is, of course, not present in nephrocalcinosis.

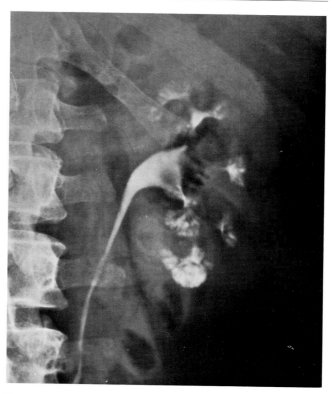

Figure 5–32. Close-up of the left kidney in a patient with medullary sponge disease. Individual dilated tubules may be identified in some papillae. In others, contrast-filled papillae blend into a blush.

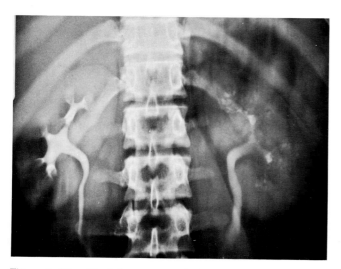

Figure 5–31. Medullary sponge kidney is present on the left. Although both kidneys are usually involved, sometimes only a single kidney, or even only a single papilla, may be involved.

RENAL TUBULAR ECTASIA WITH CONGENITAL HEPATIC FIBROSIS

Inheritance. Autosomal dominant or recessive.

Pathology. Renal tubular ectasia with or without calcifications. Liver involvement is the dominant feature. Fibrosis of the portal triad and bile duct dilatation are present. Cysts are in the liver and may be found in the pancreas. Portal hypertension eventually develops.

Clinical Presentation. The disease is seen in infants and young children. Symptoms related to the liver dominate. These include jaundice, esophageal varices, and gastrointestinal hemorrhage.

Radiological Findings. Findings related to the kidney are the same as in patients with renal tubular ectasia.[52] More dramatic findings relate to the liver. Dilated bile ducts, liver fibrosis, and collateral circulation due to portal hypertension are evident on ultrasound or other examinations.[53]

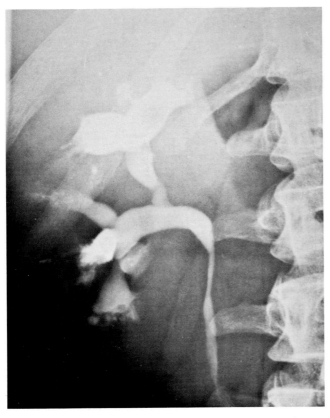

Figure 5–33. Enlargement of renal papillae, and moderate-sized cystic ducts, some of which contain small calculi, are present.

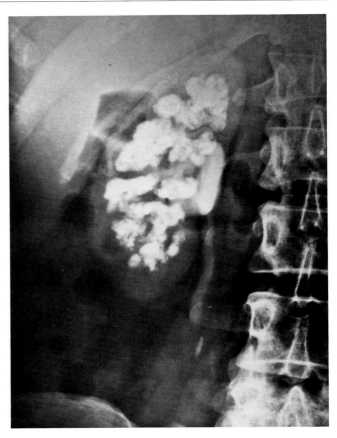

Figure 5–34. Medullary sponge kidney with moderate involvement and calcifications filling most of the dilated tubules. Differentiation from true nephrocalcinosis may be difficult or impossible.

JUVENILE NEPHRONOPHTHISIS AND MEDULLARY CYSTIC DISEASE

Etiology

Juvenile Nephronophthisis. It is uncertain whether this autosomal recessive hereditary disease is an inborn error of metabolism or an anatomic malformation.

Medullary Cystic Disease. Autosomal dominant trait.

Pathology. Cysts measuring several millimeters arise from collecting tubules high in the medullary region of the kidney. There is also proximal tubular dilatation. Cysts abound in the region of corticomedullary junction and medulla (hence the name). Kidneys are sometimes normal in size but are more commonly small.[54–56] Varying amounts of periglomerular and interstitial fibrosis are present.

Clinical Presentation. A disease of adolescents and young adults. Principal presentation is renal failure with polyuria and salt wasting. In childhood, anemia and growth retardation are present, and associated anomalies involving the central nervous system and other organs are frequent.

Laboratory Findings. Hyponatremia, uremia, normochromic, normocytic anemia.

Radiological Findings. Ultrasound is the method of choice.[57] Medullary cysts may be seen if sufficiently large. Otherwise, hyperechoic parenchyma and thin renal cortex are seen. Kidneys are normal or small in size, never large, as in infantile polycystic disease. Same findings are present on CT scan. Streaky parenchyma similar to infantile polycystic disease has been reported on intravenous pyelogram.[57,58]

INFANTILE POLYCYSTIC KIDNEY DISEASE

Incidence. One in 6000 to 14,000 births. Twice as common in females. Transmission is autosomal recessive.

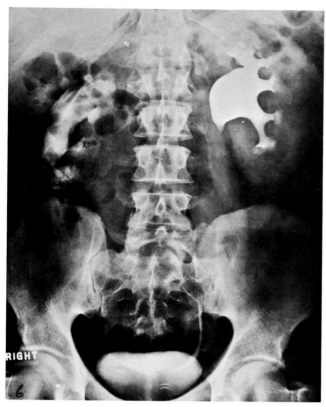

Figure 5–35. Bilateral medullary sponge kidneys and reversed rotation of the right kidney. Right kidney is atrophied because of past obstructions and infections. The left kidney is hypertrophied.

Pathology. Bilaterally enlarged, spongy, smooth kidneys. Small, saccular cystic enlargement of the collecting ducts throughout the medulla. Periportal fibrosis, dilated bile ductules, saccular dilatations of the biliary tree, and epithelial hepatic cysts may be present in the liver. Classified as Potter I.

Clinical Presentation. Presents in two forms:

1. *Newborn form:* Oligohydramnios may be detected in prenatal period. Potter facies is present. The disease is incompatible with life, and patients die of uremia. Pulmonary hypoplasia is common, resulting in respiratory distress. Occasionally, enlarged kidneys may interfere with delivery.
2. *Childhood form:* This is a milder form of the disease in which cystic changes are less pronounced and clinical symptoms become evident at age 3–5 years. Palpable liver and spleen are the common physical findings. Periportal fibrosis may be pronounced, resulting in portal hypertension, varices, and gastrointestinal hemorrhage.

Radiological Findings. Ultrasound is the examination of choice.[59,60] Small diffusely disseminated cysts in symmetrically enlarged kidneys produce a number of interfaces, resulting in brightly increased echogenicity throughout the cortex and medulla.[61] Sonolucent cortical rim may be present. Since the cysts are small, they are seldom detected individually. Cysts may occasionally be seen in the liver. The liver may be enlarged and have increased echogenicity in the presence of fibrosis.

Mottled, "streaky," or "blotchy" nephrogram is seen on excretory urography or CT in the newborn form.

In the childhood form, liver cysts and saccular dilatations are commonly seen on ultrasound.[62] There may be evidence of portal hypertension, splenomegaly, collateral portal circulation, etc.

Renal involvement in the childhood form ranges from severe to mild, and thus varying degrees of expression are seen on ultrasound and contrast examinations. Calyceal splaying and "brush-border" appearance due to medullary tubular ectasia are seen on excretory urography.

ADULT POLYCYSTIC KIDNEY DISEASE

Incidence. One in 1000 of the population is symptomatic. Incidence at autopsy is somewhat higher. Affects 400,000 Americans. Transmission is autosomal dominant with a high penetrance. Males and females are affected equally. May occur in neonates. Rarely unilateral.[63]

Pathology. Bilateral, asymmetrical renal enlargement. Cysts of varying sizes are lined with flat epithelial lining and are randomly scattered within the cortex and medulla. Cysts in other organs are common (liver, 30–50%; pancreas, 9%) (Fig. 5–36). Potter type III.

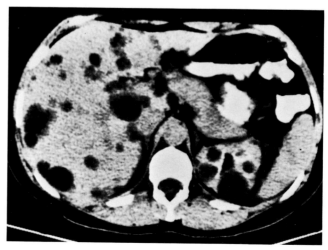

Figure 5–36. Moderate liver involvement in a patient with polycystic renal disease.

Associated Conditions. Cerebral aneurysms are present in 28% at autopsy. Renal calculi are also common (18% at autopsy).[64,65] There is increased incidence of dissecting aortic aneurysms, Marfan syndrome, colonic diverticulosis, and five to ten times increased incidence of renal cell carcinoma compared with normal population has been suggested (Fig. 5–37).[66,67]

Clinical Presentation. In the majority of patients symptoms become manifest at middle age. Adult type of polycystic disease may rarely be seen in children. Progression to renal failure may occur, requiring dialysis and transplantation. Hemorrhage into the cyst or infected cyst may cause pain. Hematuria and hypertension are common. Berry aneurysm occurs at the circle of Willis and may result in intracranial hemorrhage and death in 9% of patients. Spontaneous renal hemorrhage may require embolization or nephrectomy. Grossly enlarged kidneys may cause digestive symptoms by compression of other abdominal organs with their bulk. Cysts may become infected and pyelonephritis may complicate the picture.

Laboratory Findings. Uremia, hematuria.

Radiological Findings. Sonography is the examination of choice for establishing the diagnosis. Multiple cysts of varying size are present in both kidneys. Many cysts contain "sludge" from prior hemorrhage. The kidneys are enlarged and the contours are made irregular by bulging cysts.

The major disadvantage of sonography in evaluating adult polycystic disease is that obstruction and hydronephrosis may be missed, since the dilated calyces are frequently indistinguishable from cysts. One must remember that urolithiasis is common and may cause obstruction (Fig. 5–38).[68] However, symptoms such as hematuria and pain are generally so common in adult polycystic disease that the possibility of ureteral calculus is not seriously entertained.

Many cysts contain blood, which may be seen as "hyperdense" cysts on CT (Figs. 5–39, 5–40).[69,70] Hemorrhagic cysts have varying appearance on MR (Fig. 5–41). They may be hypo-, iso- or hyperintense on T1-weighted images and hyper- or hypointense on T2-weighted images. Fluid-fluid interphase may be

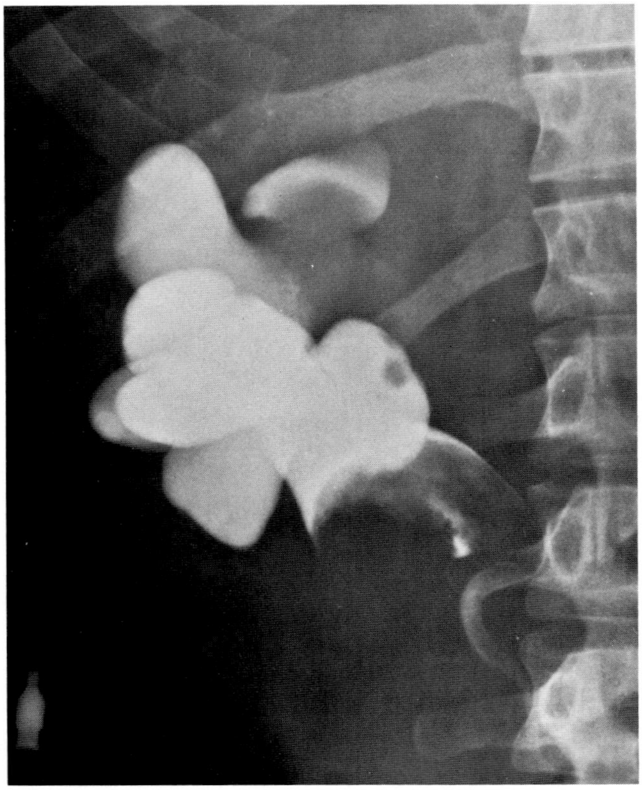

Figure 5–37. Obstruction in a patient with polycystic kidney disease caused by a malignant tumor presenting as a "filling" defect.

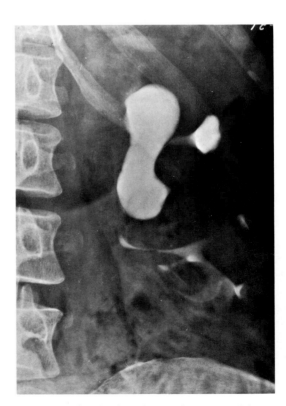

Figure 5–38. Infundibular obstruction caused by a small calculus in a patient with adult polycystic disease. Kidney is enlarged and there is splaying of the pelvis and major infundibula by cystic masses. The upper pole hydrocalyx is caused by obstruction. (From Barbaric et al.[68] reprinted with permission.)

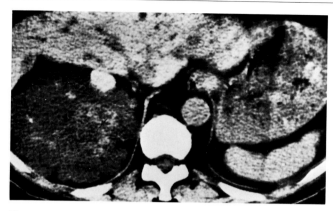

Figure 5–39.   Hyperdense hemorrhagic cyst at the anterior aspect of a massively enlarged polycystic kidney. A small dense calculus is present in a lateral calyx. Liver cysts are also present.

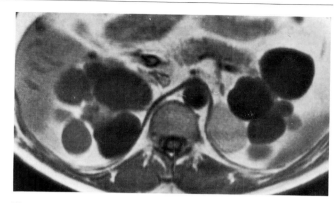

Figure 5–41.   T1-weighted sequences of polycystic kidneys in axial plane. Most cysts are hypointense except for a posteromedial cyst in the left kidney, which is relatively hyperintense. Hemorrhagic cysts show a spectrum of signal intensities, which are more fully explained in Chapter 10, "Renal Cysts."

seen as layering of different components in the hemorrhagic cyst seen in the supine position.[71]

Some cysts may contain curvilinear calcification in the wall, a finding that may be easily seen on CT scan.[72]

Collecting system is splayed by enlarging cysts as seen on excretory urography and retrograde pyelography (Figs. 5–42, 5–43). Nephrogram shows "Swiss cheese" appearance. Since on these examinations it is almost impossible to differentiate solid from cystic masses, differential diagnosis of angiomyolipomas, metastases, lymphomas, and other solid tumors must be considered and excluded by ultrasound.

Angiographic appearance is characteristic of attenuated, splayed vessels. Since so little viable functioning renal parenchyma remains, the need for blood supply diminishes and main renal arteries are of smaller caliber (Fig. 5–44).

Differentiation from multiple benign simple renal cysts may on occasion prove to be difficult. The rule of thumb is: "if you can count them, they are simple cysts; if you can't, it's polycystic."

Diagnosis of infected cysts, which may require percutaneous aspiration, is difficult and perhaps

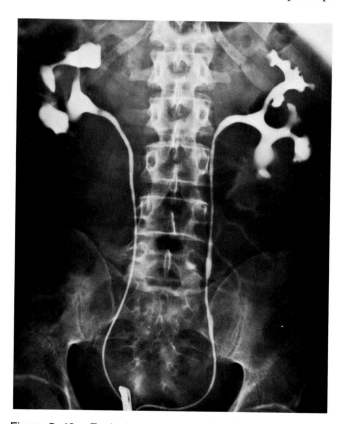

Figure 5–42.   Typical appearance of adult polycystic kidneys on a retrograde pyelogram. Renal enlargement and pelvocalyceal splaying are present. Differential diagnosis includes metastases, angiomyolipomas, and lymphoma. These entities are easily differentiated by sonography and, if necessary, by CT.

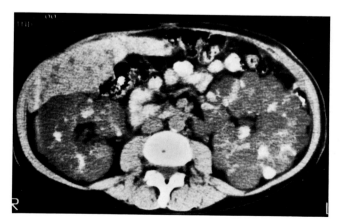

Figure 5–40.   Several hemorrhagic and many simple cysts are present in massively enlarged polycystic kidneys.

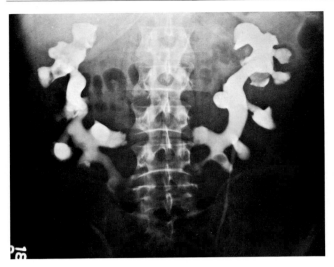

Figure 5–43. Retrograde pyelogram in a patient with polycystic and horseshoe kidneys. The axes of both kidneys are typical for horseshoe while renal enlargement and calyceal splaying suggest the presence of polycystic kidneys. There is a "filling" defect in the upper pole calyx on the right, which proved to be a blood clot.

only possible with the use of In-111 labeled leukocytes,[73] Ga-67 citrate, or Tc-99m glucoheptonate.[74,75] On scintigrams obtained 24 hours following administration of the radiopharmaceutical, increased uptake is seen in the general area of the infected cyst.[76]

Salient points regarding cystic diseases of the kidney are summarized in Table 5–1.

RENAL DYSPLASIA

Etiology. Urinary tract obstruction early in pregnancy. Decreased number of branchings of the ureteric bud.

Pathology. Reduction in number of nephrons and presence of "primitive" immature tubules and whorling mesenchymal tissue.[77] Renal cartilage and cysts may be present.

Clinical Presentation. Urinary tract obstruction may be at any level and of differing severity. If hydronephrosis or obstruction is present, there is a need to determine the presence and severity of dysplasia and remaining renal function. Obstruction need not be present at the time of presentation.

Radiological Findings. Ultrasound is the method of choice in evaluating urinary tract obstruction in neonates, infants, and children. Dilated collecting

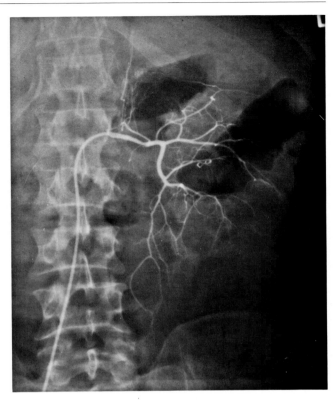

Figure 5–44. Angiographic appearance of a horseshoe kidney. The renal artery is small since most functioning renal parenchyma is gone. Kidney is enlarged and all vessels are splayed around numerous cysts. Renal outline is poorly seen, since it is made of thin and avascular cyst walls.

system is usually found in the majority of cases. This method of examination is also ideal for determining the presence of dysplasia.[78,79]

Dysplastic kidney may be small or large. The large kidney is either hydronephrotic or contains large cysts and is known as multicystic dysplastic kidney (MCDK), an entity that is discussed elsewhere (see "Congenital Cystic Diseases of the Urinary Tract").

A small kidney is the more usual finding. The kidney is usually echogenic. Small cysts may be present. The higher the obstruction, the more numerous the cysts. There need not be any evidence for dilatation of the collecting system and obstruction may not be present at the time of examination.

Segmental dysplasia may involve either the upper or lower pole. A classic example is complete duplication with upper moiety obstruction (ectopic ureterocele).

Bilateral dysplastic kidneys develop in situations where there is outflow bladder obstruction, such as urethral valves or urethral atresia, or if there is simultaneous bilateral ureteral obstruction.

Hydronephrosis and development of the dysplastic

Table 5-1. Cystic Diseases of the Kidney

	Pattern of Inheritance	Diagnostic Features	Complications	Typical Outcome
Multicystic dysplastic kidney	None	Palpable mass, cystic on US	Contralateral UPJ or dysplasia	Benign 9% may disappear
Pelvocalyceal diverticula	None	Solitary or multiple	Calculi, UTI	Benign
Congenital megacalyces	None	Enlarged calyces, flat papillae	Misdiagnosed as hydronephrosis	Benign
Medullary sponge kidney and renal tubular ectasia	None	Medullary cysts, large papillae	Hematuria, UTI, urolithiasis	Benign
Juvenile nephronophthisis	Autosomal recessive	Corticomedullary cysts, normal to small kidneys	Salt wasting, polyuria, anemia growth retardation	Progressive renal failure beginning in childhood
Medullary cystic disease	Autosomal dominant	Corticomedullary cysts, normal to small kidneys	Salt wasting, polyuria	Chronic renal failure beginning in adulthood
Infantile polycystic kidney disease (IPKD)	Autosomal recessive	Enlarged, cystic kidneys at birth	Hepatic fibrosis	Variable, death in infancy or childhood
Adult polycystic kidney disease (APKD)	Autosomal dominant	Large multicystic kidneys, liver cysts, flank pain	Hematuria, UTI, urolithiasis, hypertension	Chronic renal failure age 40-60 years
Simple cysts	None	Single or multiple cysts	Hematuria, pain	Benign
Peripelvic cyst	None	Cyst within the renal sinus, may be simple or lymphatic	May cause obstruction and hematuria	Benign
Uriniferous pseudocyst	None	Encapsulated urine in the renal sinus or retroperitoneum	May become infected	Benign
Aquired renal cystic disease	None	Cystic degeneration in end-stage kidney disease	Hemorrhage, erythrocytosis, malignancy	Dependence on dialysis

kidney may be demonstrated by ultrasound in the prenatal period.[80]

Nuclear medicine scintigraphy is employed to determine functional reserve of the affected kidney.[81] Tc-99m DMSA scan will determine the relative function value of the affected kidney compared with the normal side. Tc-99m DTPA slope will allow a relative estimate of blood flow. Radioiodinated ortho-iodohippurate (I-131-OIH, Hippuran) will allow determination of effective renal plasma flow, urine flow fractions, and tubular transport time. The drawback of this radiopharmaceutical is the relatively large dose to target organs, particularly in the presence of urinary tract obstruction.

SYNDROMES AND DISEASES ASSOCIATED WITH RENAL CYSTS

Bardet-Biedl Syndrome

A disorder characterized by obesity, mental retardation, retinitis pigmentosa, and hypogonadism.[82]

Tuberous Sclerosis

A condition in which mental retardation, adenoma sebaceum, renal angiomyolipomas, renal cysts, and hamartomas in different organs are present. (See Renal Angiomyolipoma in Chapter 9, "Renal Neoplasms").

von Hippel-Lindau Disease

Cerebellar hemangioblastoma and retinal angiomas are the central nervous system expression of the disease. Multifocal renal carcinoma and renal cysts with hyperplastic lining are present. Renal carcinoma is usually discovered early, since the patients are closely observed. Several partial nephrectomies may be performed in the patient's lifetime. Patients are followed either by CT or angiography every 1 or 2 years, searching for new renal carcinomas.[83] Diagnosis of a new carcinoma may be difficult, since the kidney is usually deformed from prior partial nephrectomies. Presence of multiple renal cysts makes the discovery of the malignant lesion that much more difficult. (See von Hippel-Lindau Disease in Chapter 9, "Renal Neoplasms").

Trisomy Syndrome

Multiple small cysts may be present in the subcapsular region and between the lobes.

REFERENCES

1. Potter EL. Bilateral renal agenesis. J Pediatr 1946; 24:68–76.
2. Leads from the MMWR. Renal agenesis surveillance-United States. JAMA 1988; 260:3114–3115.
3. Potter EL. Facial characteristics of infants with bilateral renal agenesis. Am J Obstet Gynecol 1946; 51:885–888.
4. Beeby DI. Seminal vesicle cysts associated with ipsilateral renal agenesis. Case report and review of the literature. J Urol 1974; 112:120–122.
5. Henay JA, Pfister RC, Meares EM Jr. Giant cyst of the seminal vesicle with renal agenesis. AJR 1987; 149:139.
6. Guys JM, Borella F, Panuel M, et al. The Mayer-Rokitansky syndrome. Report of 5 cases. Eur Urol 1988; 14:301–304.
7. Mascatello V, Liebowitz RL. Malposition of the colon in left renal agenesis and ectopia. Radiology 1976; 120:371–376.
8. Burgos FJ, Matorras R, Rivera M, et al. Double uterus associated with unilateral vaginal obstruction and ipsilateral renal agenesis: ultrasonographic diagnosis. JCU 1989; 17:296–298.
9. Wiersma AF, Peterson LF, Justema EJ. Arterial anomalies associated with unilateral renal agenesis. Obstet Gynecol 1976; 47:654–657.
10. Yoder IC, Pfister RC. Unilateral hematocolpos and ipsilateral renal agenesis: a report of two cases and review of the literature. Am J Roentgenol 1976; 127:303–308.
11. Macpherson RI. Supernumerary kidney: typical and atypical features. J Can Assoc Radiol 1987; 38:116–118.
12. Avni EF, Thoua Y, Van Gansbeke D, et al. Development of the hypodysplastic kidney: contribution of antenatal US diagnosis. Radiology 1987; 164:123–125.
13. Risdon RA, Young LW, Crispin AR. Renal hypoplasia and dysplasia: a radiological and pathological correlation. Pediatr Radiol 1975; 3:213–225.
14. Cha EM, Kanazari S, Khoury GH. Congenital renal hypoplasia: angiographic study. Am J Roentgenol 1972; 114:710–714.
15. Smith SJ, Cass AS, Hossein AH, et al. Unipapillary kidneys: a case report and literature review. Urol Radiol 1984; 6:43–47.
16. Peterson JE, Pinckney LE, Rutledge JC, et al. The solitary renal calyx and papilla in human kidneys. Radiology 1982; 144:525–527.
17. McMillan PJ, Gingell JC, Penry JB. Bilateral unipapillary kidneys and hematuria. J R Soc Med 1987; 80:456–457.
18. Cambell JE. Ureteral peristalsis in duplex renal collecting systems. Am J Roentgenol 1967; 99:577–584.
19. Bisset GS III, Strife JL. Duplex collecting system in girls with urinary tract infection: prevalence and significance. AJR 1987; 148:497–499.
20. Cronan JJ, Amis ES Jr, Zeman RK, Dorfman GS. Obstruction of the upper-pole moiety in renal duplication in adults. CT evaluation. Radiology 1986; 161:17–20.
21. Dietrich RB, Kangarloo H. Pelvic abnormalities in children: assessment with MR imaging. Radiology 1987; 163:367–369.
22. Culkin DJ, Wheeler JS Jr, Karasis M, et al. Treatment of renal calculus in inferior crossed renal ectopia. Urology 1988; 32:424–426.
23. Connor JM, Brautigan MW. The ectopic kidney in the emergency department. Ann Emerg Med 1987; 16:715–717.
24. Nussbaum AR, Hartman DS, Whitley N, et al. Multicystic dysplasia and crossed renal ectopia. AJR 1987; 149:407–410.
25. Milovic IS, Oluic DI. Thoracic renal ectopia. Br J Urol 1988; 62:183–184.

26. Goodman JD, Norton KI, Carr L, et al. Crossed fused renal ectopia: sonographic diagnosis. Urol Radiol 1986; 8:13–16.
27. Mellins HZ. Cystic dilatations of the upper urinary tract: a radiologist's developmental model. Radiology 1984; 153–159.
28. Griscom NT, Vawter GF, Fellers F. Pelvoinfundibular atresia: the usual form of multicystic kidney: 44 unilateral and two bilateral cases. Semin Roentgenol 1975; 10:125–131.
29. Felson B, Cussen LJ. Hydronephrotic type of unilateral congenital multicystic disease of the kidney. Semin Roentgenol 1975; 10:113–123.
30. Vinocur L, Slovis TL, Perlmutter AD, et al. Follow-up studies of multicystic dysplastic kidneys. Radiology 1988; 167:311–315.
31. Pedicelli G, Jequier S, Bowen AD, et al. Multicystic dysplastic kidneys: spontaneous regression demonstrated with US. Radiology 1986; 160:23–26.
32. Birken G, King D, Vane D, Lloyd T. Renal cell carcinoma arising in multicystic dysplastic kidney. J Pediatr Surg 1985; 20:619–621.
33. Stuck KJ, Koff SA, Silver TM. Ultrasonic features of multicystic dysplastic kidney: expanded diagnostic criteria. Radiology 1982; 143:217–221.
34. Sanders RC, Hartman DS. The sonographic distinction between neonatal multicystic kidney and hydronephrosis. Radiology 1984; 151:621–625.
35. Young LW, Wood BP, Spohr C, et al. Delayed excretory urographic opacification; a puddling effect in multicystic renal dysplasia. Ann Radiol (Paris) 1974; 17:391–396.
36. Kyaw MM. The radiological diagnosis of congenital multicystic kidney: "radiological triad." Clin Radiol 1974; 25:45–62.
37. Saxton HM, Golding SJ, Chantler C, Haycock GD. Diagnostic puncture in renal cystic dysplasia (multicystic kidney): evidence on the etiology of the cysts. Br J Radiol 1981; 54:555–561.
38. Diard F, Le Dosseur P, Cadier L, et al. Multicystic dysplasia in the upper component of the complete duplex kidney. Pediatr Radiol 1984; 14:310–313.
39. Nussbaum AR, Hartman DS, Whitley N, et al. Multicystic dysplasia and crossed renal ectopia. AJR 1987; 149:407–410.
40. Williams G, Blandy JP, Tresidder GC. Communicating cysts and diverticula of the renal pelvis. Br J Urol 1969; 16:163–170.
41. Timmons JW, Malek RS, Hattery RR, et al. Calyceal diverticulum. J Urol 1975; 114:6–9.
42. Hulbert JC, Reddy PK, Hunter DW, et al. Percutaneous techniques for management of calyceal diverticula containing calculi. J Urol 1986; 135:225–227.
43. Bronk JB, Parker BR. Pyelocalyceal diverticula in the Beckwith-Wiedemann syndrome. Pediatr Radiol 1987; 17:80–84.
44. Talner LB, Gittes RF. Megacalyces: further observation and differentiation from obstructive renal disease. Am J Roentgenol 1974; 121:473–486.
45. Kozakewich HPW, Lebowitz RL. Congenital megacalyces. Pediatr Radiol 1974; 2:251–258.
46. Garcia CJ, Taylor KJW, Weiss RM. Congenital megacalyces: ultrasound appearance. J Ultrasound Med 1987; 6:163–165.
47. Mandell GA, Snyder HM III, Heyman S, et al. Association of congenital megacalycosis and ipsilateral segmental megaureter. Pediatr Radiol 1987; 17:28–31.
48. Lenadruzzi G. Reporto pielografrio joco commune dilatazione delle vie urinarie intravensti. Radiol Med (Torino) 1939; 26:346–347.
49. Patriquin HB, O'Regan S. Medullary sponge kidney in childhood. AJR 1985; 145:315–317.
50. Afonso DN, Oliveira AG. Medullary sponge kidney and congenital hemi-hypertrophy. Br J Urol 1988; 62:187–188.
51. Eisenberg RL, Pfister RC. Medullary sponge kidney associated with congenital hemihypertrophy (asymmetry). A case report and survey of the literature. Am J Roentgenol 1972; 116:773–777.
52. Kerr DNS, Warrick CK, Hart-Mercer J. Lesions resembling medullary sponge kidney with congenital hepatic fibrosis. Clin Radiol 1962; 13:85–91.
53. Six R, Oliphant M, Grossman H. A spectrum of renal tubular ectasia and hepatic fibrosis. Radiology 1975; 117:117–122.
54. Kelly CJ, Neilson EG. Medullary cystic disease: an inherited form of autoimmune interstitial nephritis? Am J Kidney Dis 1987; 10:389–395.
55. Bodaghi E, Honarmand MT, Ahmadi M. Infantile nephronophthisis. Int J Pediatr Nephrol 1987; 8:207–210.
56. Kaplan BS, Milner LS, Jequier S, et al. Autosomal dominant inheritance of small kidneys. Am J Med Gen 1989; 32:120–126.
57. Olsen A, Hansen Hojhus J, Steffensen G. Renal medullary cystic disease. Findings at urography and ultrasonography. Acta Radiol 1988; 29:527–529.
58. Link DP, Hansen S, Palmer J. High dose excretory urography and medullary cystic disease of the kidney. AJR 1979; 133:303–305.
59. Boal DK, Teele RL. Sonography of infantile polycystic renal disease. AJR 1980; 135:575–580.
60. Stapelton FB, Magill HL, Kelly DR. Infantile polycystic kidney disease: an imaging dilemma. Urol Radiol 1983; 5:89–94.
61. Metreweli C, Garel L. The echographic diagnosis of infantile renal polycystic disease. Ann Radiol 1980; 23:103–107.
62. Davies CH, Stringer DA, Whyte H, et al. Congenital hepatic fibrosis with saccular dilatation of intrahepatic bile ducts and infantile polycystic kidneys. Pediatr Radiol 1986; 16:302–304.
63. Sellers AL, Winfield A, Rosen V. Unilateral polycystic kidney disease. J Urol 1972; 107:572.
64. Simon HB, Thompson GJ. Congenital polycystic disease. A clinical and therapeutic study of three hundred sixty-six cases. JAMA 1955; 159:657–662.
65. Segal AJ, Spataro RF, Barbaric ZL. Adult polycystic kidney disease: a review of 100 cases. J Urol 1977; 118:711–713.
66. Roberts PF. Bilateral renal carcinoma associated with polycystic kidneys. Br Med J 1973; 3:273–274.
67. McFarland WL, Wallace S, Johnson DE. Renal carcinoma and polycystic disease. J Urol 1972; 107:530–532.
68. Barbaric ZL, Spataro RF, Segal AJ. Urinary tract obstruction in polycystic renal disease. Radiology 1977; 125:627–629.
69. Levine E, Grantham JJ. High-density renal cysts in autosomal dominant polycystic kidney disease demonstrated by CT. Radiology 1985; 154:477–482.
70. Meziane MA, Fishman EK, Goldman SM, et al. Computed tomography of high density renal cysts in adult polycystic kidney disease. JCAT 1986; 10:767–770.

71. Hilpert PL, Friedman AC, Radecki PD, et al. MRI of hemorrhagic renal cysts in polycystic kidney disease. AJR 1986; 146:1167–1170.

72. Kutcher R, Schneider M, Gordon DH. Calcification in polycystic disease. Radiology 1977; 122:77.

73. Fortner A, Taylor A Jr, Alazraki NP, et al. Advantage of indium-111 leucocytes over ultrasound in imaging of an infected renal cyst. J Nucl Med 1986; 27:1147–1151.

74. McAfee JG, Samin A. In-111 labeled leucocytes: review of problems in image interpretation. Radiology 1985; 155:221–223.

75. Traisman ES, Conway JJ, Traisman ES, et al. Localization of urinary tract infection with Tc-99m glucoheptonate scintigraphy. Pediatr Radiol 1986; 16:403–407.

76. Schwab SJ, Bander SJ, Klahr S. Renal infection in autosomal dominant polycystic kidney disease. Am J Med 1987; 82:714–718.

77. Risdon RA. Renal dysplasia. J Clin Pathol 1971; 24:57–71.

78. Sanders RC, Nussbaum AR, Solez K. Renal dysplasia: Sonographic findings. Radiology 1988; 167:623–626.

79. Mahoney BS, Filly RA, Callen PW, et al. Fetal renal dysplasia: sonographic evaluation. Radiology 1984; 152:143–146.

80. Avoni EF, Thoua Y, Van Gansbeke F, et al. Development of hypodysplastic kidney: contribution of antenatal US diagnosis. Radiology 1987; 164:123–126.

81. Chachati A, Meyers A, Godon JP, et al. Rapid method for the measurement of differential renal function: validation. J Nucl Med 1987; 28:829–833.

82. Alton DJ, McDonald P. Urographic findings in the Bardet-Biedl syndrome. Radiology 1973; 109:659–663.

83. Malek RS, Omess PJ, Benson RC Jr, Zincke H. Renal cell carcinoma in von Hippel-Lindau syndrome. Am J Med 1987; 82:236–238.

6

Urolithiasis

UROLITHIASIS

Incidence.

- Renal stones: 5% of population
- Renal microliths: 20 to 100% on autopsy
- Recurrence: 40 to 70%
- Hospitalization: 14/10,000 population
- Medical intervention: needed in 20% of patients with stone disease

Composition.

- Calcium oxalate: 75%
- Calcium phosphate: 5%
- Uric acid: 8%
- Cystine, xanthine: 1%
- Struvite: 15%

Physical Properties.

- Radiopaque: 92%
   Calcium oxalate
   Calcium phosphate
   Struvite
- Radiolucent: 8%
   Uric acid
   Cystine, xanthine

Etiology.   Idiopathic, probably multifactorial, infection, hypercalcemia, renal tubular acidosis, hyperuricosuria, hyperoxaluria, cystinuria, and medullary sponge kidney.

Predisposing Conditions. Sarcoidosis, Cushing disease, outflow bladder obstruction, polycystic disease, calyceal diverticuli (Fig. 6–1), short bowel syndrome, Crohn's disease, some diversions, stents, indwelling catheters (Figs. 6–2, 6–3).

Risk Factors.   Dehydration, low urine volume, high concentration of minerals, presence of infection, lack of crystallization inhibitors, and abnormal urine pH.

Pathogenesis.   a) Nidus, such as a clump of epithelial cells, submucosal calcification (Randall's plaque) eroding into the collecting system, sloughed papilla, tubular cast, etc.; b) solute supersaturation; c) decreased levels of urinary organic or inorganic crystal-

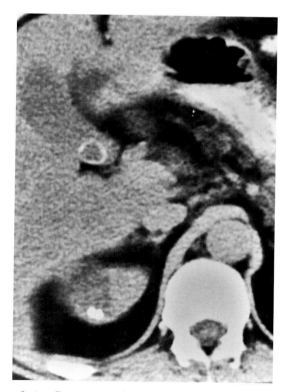

Figure 6–1.   Precontrast CT scan in the region of the upper pole of the right kidney and gallbladder. Radiopaque calculus is seen in the dependent part of the calyceal diverticulum. In the prone position the calculus would shift to the anterior wall of the diverticulum. Calcified gallstone is an incidental finding.

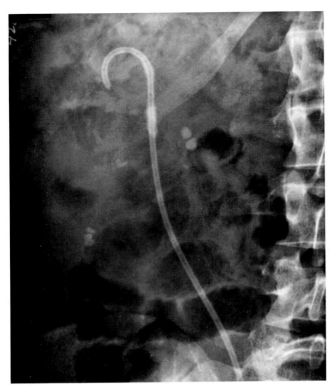

Figure 6–2. Plain radiograph of the right kidney. Several calcifications are seen in the area and they may or may not be in the kidney. Oblique view is needed for further delineation. The polyethylene stent is surrounded by encrusted calcific deposits. When the stent was removed calcific deposits were stripped and remained in the ureter. Retrograde endoscopy was required for complete removal.

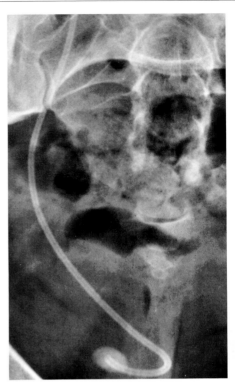

Figure 6–3. Plain radiograph of the right pelvis. Even silicon stents may form a nidus for calcific deposits, such as in this case. A large calcific encrustation is present at the tip of the catheter.

lization inhibitors (glycopeptides, chondroitin sulfate, citrate, ribonucleic acid, etc.).

Clinical Presentation. Renal colic, lumbar pain, hematuria, pyuria, crystaluria, urinary infection, renal failure, urgency, and frequency. Often asymptomatic.

Laboratory Findings. Urine crystals, hematuria.

Calcium Stones

Most stones contain calcium oxalate alone or in combination with hydroxyapatite (calcium phosphate). Most calcium oxalate stones are idiopathic, others result from metabolic, systemic, or inherited diseases. There is male preponderance and distinct geographic distribution in the "stone belts," such as the Southeast United States.

Hypercalciuria. There is a strong correlation between hypercalciuria and the number of stones formed.

Idiopathic hypercalciuria may be due to primary hyperabsorption of calcium from the intestine or impaired renal tubular calcium reabsorption (renal leak hypercalciuria).

Renal tubular acidosis (type I)[1] is a disorder of distal tubular cells where hydrogen ion gradient cannot be maintained. Urine pH is above 5.5 and there is renal leakage of calcium, phosphorus, sodium, and potassium. One of the inhibitors of stone formation (citrate) is absent.

Hyperoxaluria. Excessive urinary excretion of oxalate is also an important contributor toward calcium stone formation. This is usually an acquired disorder associated with small bowel inflammatory disease or resection, biliary, and pancreatic disease. In the presence of steatorrhea or altered enterohepatic circulation of bile salts, insufficient amounts of enteric calcium are available to complex with oxalate, allowing enhanced absorption.

High dietary intake of oxalate or substances metabolized to oxalate, such as vitamin C, may also lead to oxaluria.

Primary hyperoxaluria is a rare autosomal recessive inborn error of metabolism accompanied by excessive stone formation.

Hypercalcemia

Primary Hyperparathyroidism. Increased secretion of parathyroid hormone produces excessive reabsorption of calcium from bone, resulting in elevation of serum and urinary calcium levels. There is also increased absorption of calcium from the intestines.

Immobilization, Paget's disease, milk-alkali syndrome, Cushing disease, sarcoidosis, and hyperthyroidism are other examples.

Infectious Stones (Triple Phosphate or Struvite Stones)

Pseudomonas, Proteus, Klebsiella, and *Streptococcus* produce a urea-splitting enzyme by which there is an increase in urine pH and in concentration of ammonia and bicarbonate. Favorable conditions for precipitation of magnesium ammonium phosphate (struvite) and calcium phosphate (apatite) are thus formed (Fig. 6–4). Proteinaceous debris further augments stone growth.

Uric Acid Stones

Uric acid stones are relatively radiolucent, although larger stones may incorporate calcium and become somewhat radiopaque, or serve as a nidus for calcium oxalate stones. Most patients have low urine pH, which decreases uric acid solubility. Most patients with uric acid stones have normal uric acid metabolism. Forty percent of stones seen in patients with gout are uric acid. These stones are more common in rural farming communities than in industrialized centers and were also more common in the United States 100 years ago.

Cystine and Xanthine Stones

Cystinuria is an inherited error of the tubular transport system.[2] Cystine is poorly soluble in normal, somewhat acid urine. Cystine stones are relatively radiolucent.

Xanthinuria associated with stone formation is rare.

Milk of Calcium Urine

Milk of calcium urine is associated with obstruction (Fig. 6–5). Obstructed renal pelvis contains a particulate colloidal suspension of the various calcium salts. The particles tend to settle in the most dependent part of the cystic cavity. On the upright, cross-table supine projections, CT, and ultrasound, the layering of the colloidal suspension may be identified.[3]

Radiological Findings

Plain Radiograph. Most stones contain a proteinaceous matrix. Radiodensity of the calculus is directly proportional to the concentration of various calcium salts within the matrix. Most urinary tract calculi are *radiopaque* and are easily identified on a plain radiograph (Fig. 6–6).

Calculi composed of uric acid or cystine are frequently imperceptible on a plain radiograph and are referred to as *radiolucent.* Precipitation of calcium salts onto uric acid core occurs commonly, making these calculi somewhat radiopaque and frequently visible on plain radiographic examinations.

Plain radiograph is the most common imaging modality used for detection of urinary tract calculi. Inadequate exposure or inadvertent exclusion of the calculus from the field of view cannot be tolerated. Diagnosis may be difficult in the presence of calcifications outside of the urinary tract, such as gallstones, costochondral calcifications, phleboliths, calcified mesenteric lymph nodes (Fig. 6–7), and an endless variety of other calcifications occurring in the abdomen (Fig. 6–8).

When uncertain whether or not a suspicious radiodensity represents a calculus, an ipsilateral oblique projection will help determine if the density "moves"

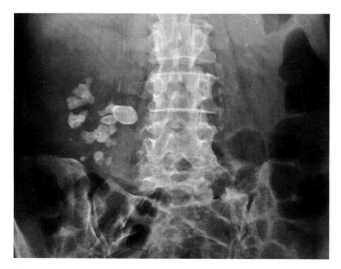

Figure 6–4. Plain radiograph of the abdomen. Multiple infectious renal calculi are present in the right kidney. The kidney is in low position and if percutaneous stone removal is planned, access to the kidney should be through the upper pole. Note aortic and iliac artery calcifications.

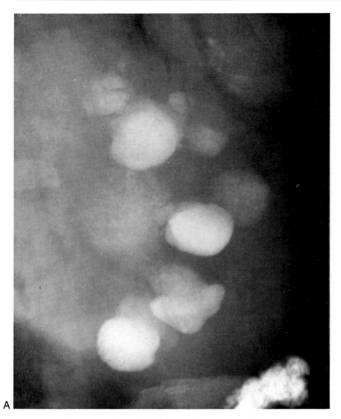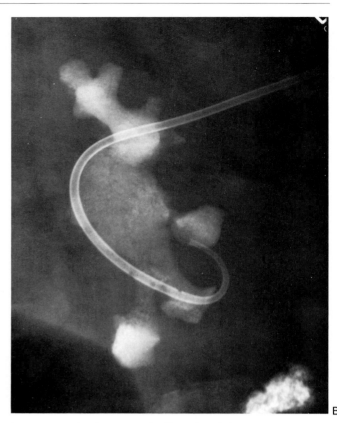

A   B

Figure 6–5. **(A)** Plain radiograph of the left kidney. Particulate suspension is present in dilated and obstructed collecting system. Layering was present on the upright projection. **(B)** Percutaneous nephrostomy was placed in the obstructed kidney. Mucinous fluid was obtained. Too big to be drained by such a small (8 F) catheter, the particles have coalesced. The nonfunctioning kidney was eventually removed.

as if it were in the urinary tract or not. Comparison with prior radiological examinations may show stone migration (Fig. 6–9).

The area where urinary calculi are the most difficult to detect is in the mid-ureteral segment in front of the sacroiliac joint. This area is known as the "graveyard of stones," since they are so easily overlooked because of overlying and confusing bone densities (Fig. 6–10A).

Tomography. Bowel gas is frequently present in quantities such that small urinary tract calculi may be easily overlooked. Under these circumstances simple plain tomography (no radiographic contrast administered) often reveals small unsuspected stones (Fig. 6–10B,C).

Radiation Dose. Since urolithiasis is a recurrent disease frequently requiring repeated radiographic examinations, cumulative radiation dose to the patient may be substantial over a period of years. One should be conservative and meticulous in obtaining technically superior radiographs and comparing current examination with the old. This will reduce the number of additional views or repeated exposures.

Sonography. Calculus appears as a markedly echogenic structure with prominent acoustical "shadowing" (Fig. 6–11). Sonography may be very useful in determining the character of a radiolucent intraluminal "filling defect." Uric acid stones will exhibit echogenicity and "shadowing" typical for a calculus, while transitional cell carcinoma, sloughed papilla, or a blood clot will not.

Unfortunately, marked echogenicity and acoustical "shadowing" may also be seen in the presence of gas, arterial calcification, clips, and tubes, and can occasionally be produced by cyst walls. False-positive diagnosis is therefore possible. Also, detection of small calculi is very much dependent on the examiner's expertise and is time consuming. Most ureteral calculi and renal calculi less than 3 mm in diameter are difficult or impossible to detect. Negative ultrasound examination does not exclude the presence of urolithiasis.

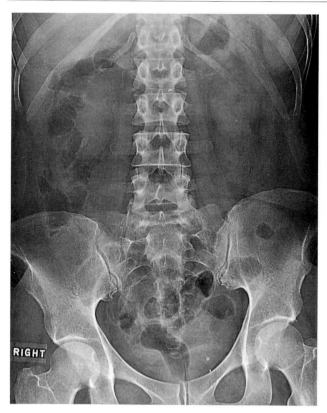

Figure 6–6.　Plain abdominal radiograph. Phlebolith in the true pelvis is clearly seen. On occasion, it may be misdiagnosed as a ureteral calculus. Distinguishing features are laminated appearance and position below the ischial spines. Less clearly visible is a small radiopaque calculus in the region of the left lower pole calyx. A cluster of small calculi in the lower pole calyx of the right kidney is easily overlooked.

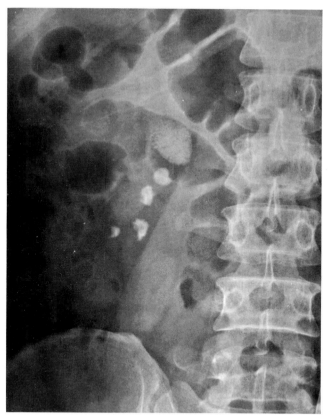

Figure 6–7.　Plain abdominal radiograph. A large renal calculus, almost stellate in appearance, is in the right renal pelvis. Several heavily calcified mesenteric lymph nodes are just inferior to the renal stone. On subsequent radiographs, they are seen to change position, influenced by bowel peristalsis.

CT.　Superior contrast discrimination of CT permits detection of most calculi, regardless of their calcium content (Fig. 6–12). The only drawbacks are the expense and the possibility of missing the stone between the slices. Therefore this imaging modality is reserved for occasions when other types of imaging are indeterminate. CT is particularly useful in differentiating soft tissue tumors from radiolucent calculi, both of which may present as an intraluminal filling defect on urography.[4]

Urolithiasis is commonly seen as a serendipitous finding on CT scans performed for evaluation of unrelated abdominal disease. Attempts to determine chemical composition by using CT numbers was not very successful or practical.

MR Imaging.　At the present time, MR imaging is not the modality of choice in evaluating urolithiasis. Motion artifacts and poor resolution in comparison with all other imaging techniques place MR at a distinct disadvantage. On T1- and T2-weighted images, calculi appear hypointense (dark) compared with the surrounding structures (Fig. 6–13).

Plain Radiographic Findings in Acute Renal Colic

Presence of Ureteral Calculus.　Curiously, in many patients presenting with renal colic, it is difficult to determine which among the many radiodense candidates on the plain radiograph is the offending calculus. Often it is difficult to determine if the calculus is present at all. The decision whether to proceed with ultrasound or an excretory urogram is dependent on the overall clinical picture. One may argue that if no large stone is visible, it must be small and likely to pass spontaneously. On the other hand, even a large radiolucent calculus with no chances of ever descending into the bladder may be overlooked.

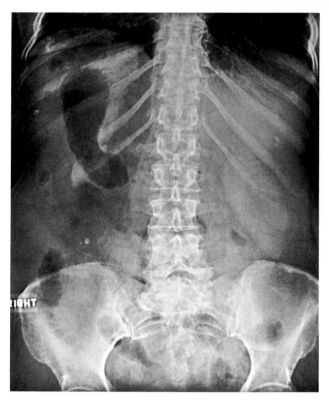

Figure 6–8. Plain abdominal radiograph. Faintly opaque right staghorn calculus is seen behind gastric gas shadow. Situs inversus is present, a finding that draws attention away from the stone.

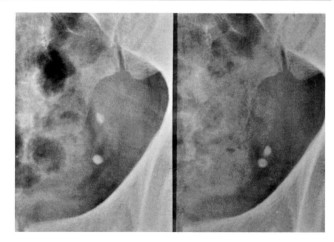

Figure 6–9. Plain radiographs of the pelvis obtained several days apart. Phlebolith is stationary while distal left ureteral stone is seen migrating distally. Patient is experiencing typical colicky pain.

One should always be looking for other possible causes for acute renal colic, such as sloughed papilla, blood clot, fungus ball, and congenital ureteropelvic junction obstruction (UPJ).

Scoliosis/splinting.   Mild splinting is a common occurrence but is not specific for urolithiasis.

Ileus.   Varying degrees of intestinal ileus may or may not accompany acute renal colic. Ileus is also not specific for urolithiasis.

Urinoma.   Rupture of the collecting system and extravasation of urine into the retroperitoneum may occur. Decompression into the retroperitoneum and perirenal space may ease acute colicky symptoms and give the false impression that the acute episode is over. Plain radiographic findings are:

1. Fluid in the perirenal space may obliterate perirenal fat and thus make the kidney invisible. Urine within the renal fascia (Gerota's) may be outlined by the fat in the paranephric space, just outside the fascia.
2. Fluid in the pararenal space may obliterate fat in

that space. From outside, fluid may outline the fat within the renal fascia, in the middle of which the kidney may be seen. This is known as *"renal halo sign."*
3. Fluid in retroperitoneum may obliterate the psoas margin. This sign is nonspecific, since psoas is not seen in 20% of normal individuals.

Diseases Mimicking Renal Colic

Acute pain mimicking renal colic may be associated with appendicitis, ruptured aortic aneurysm, dissecting aortic aneurysm, porphyruria, lumbar disc disease, etc.

Calculi and Contrast Studies

Acute, subacute, and chronic obstruction and the radiographic findings they effect on contrast examinations (Figs. 6–14, 6–15) are discussed in Chapter 7 ("Urinary Tract Obstruction"). Surrounded by radiographic contrast within the urinary tract system, the calculus may become invisible if no attenuation differences exist between two media (Fig. 6–16). Contrast may be denser than a moderately radiopaque stone, which is seen as a "filling defect" within the contrast (Fig. 6–17). Under such circumstances the stone is referred to as *relatively radiolucent* to radiographic contrast.

Radiolucent filling defects may represent air bubbles (introduced during a retrograde or antegrade examination), transitional cell carcinoma, blood clot, sloughed papilla, fungus ball, etc.

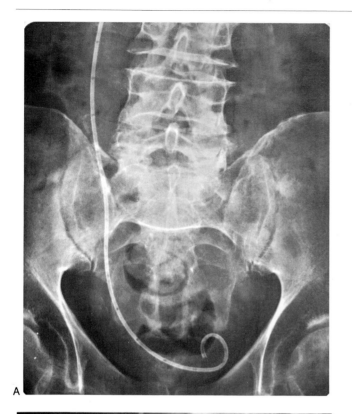

A

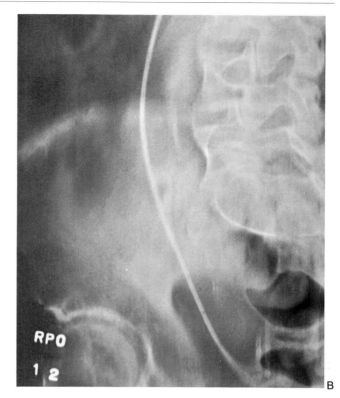

B

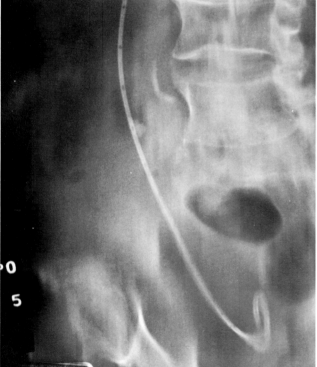

C

Figure 6–10.   (A) Plain radiograph. Presacral ureter is known as the "graveyard of stones." This is because so many are overlooked in this area. A right ureteral stent is in place, but one is uncertain whether a ureteral calculus is present or not. (B) The patient is positioned in ipsilateral posterior oblique position and several tomographic cuts are obtained. In this position the ureter is almost parallel with the film. No calculus is seen on this particular slice. (C) On the next anterior slice the ureteral calculus is in focus and is clearly visible.

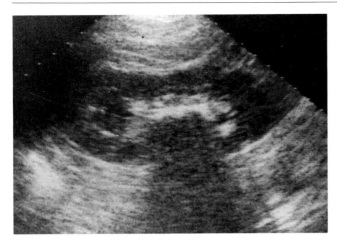

Figure 6–11. Acoustical "shadowing" behind a large hyperechoic renal stone.

Retrograde pyelography is occasionally necessary to determine whether a calcification in the lower pelvis is a phlebolith or a distal ureteral calculus. Since some phleboliths may be in close proximity to the ureter, this task may prove to be difficult.

On soft tissue window display on a contrast CT study, calcifications are obliterated by radiographic contrast. On the bone window, these calcifications may become readily visible.

RETROGRADE STONE REMOVAL

Basketing

The simplest retrograde stone removal technique involves placement of a caged wire basket into the ureter and alongside the stone. When opened and then closed in that location, the stone is trapped by the basket and retrieved using discretionary traction.

A variant of this technique employs an angioplasty-type balloon catheter, which is used to dilate the ureterovesical orifice and facilitate extraction.

Ureteropyeloscopy

Rigid or flexible ureteroscopes may be introduced in a retrograde manner all the way into the renal pelvis, usually requiring epidural anesthesia.[5] The ureteroscope is always passed over a guidewire (Fig. 6–18) and after dilatation of the ureterovesical orifice. Extraction of smaller calculi from the ureter and renal pelvis is possible (Fig. 6–19). Complications include ureteral perforation.

PERCUTANEOUS STONE REMOVAL

The first percutaneous extraction of urinary tract calculi was performed by Swedish radiologist Ingmar Fernström who published his results in 1976.[6] Remarkably, it took more than 20 years after the introduction of percutaneous nephrostomy for this breakthrough to occur. This, however, was a milestone in the evolving treatment of urolithiasis. Today, this procedure is preferred for treatment of large and very dense stones.

Procedure

The technique requires percutaneous placement of a working Teflon sheet into the kidney. The sheet must

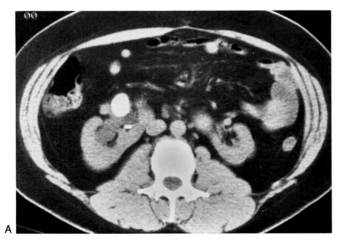

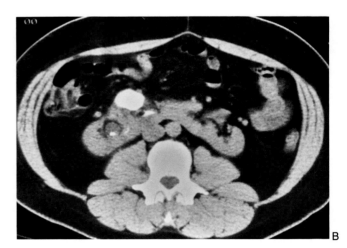

Figure 6–12. **(A)** Precontrast CT scan. A large radiodense calculus is present in the right renal pelvis and another smaller one just posterior to it. **(B)** More inferior slice in the same patient is diagnostic of a horseshoe kidney. The connecting isthmus is seen anterior to the great vessels. Inferior mesenteric artery is anterior and touching the isthmus. Another large radiodense right renal stone is present in the lower pole.

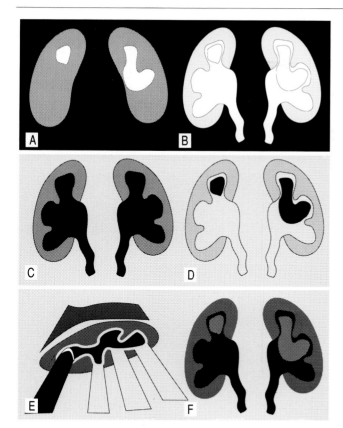

Figure 6–13. Schematic representation of calcified renal stones on different imaging modalities. **A:** plain radiograph or precontrast CT scan; **B:** intravenous or retrograde pyelogram or postcontrast CT scan; **C:** MR imaging, T1-weighted sequence; **D:** MR imaging, T2-weighted sequence; **E:** ultrasonography, **F:** Tc-99m DMSA scintigram.

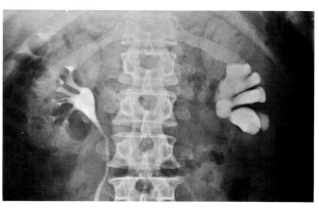

Figure 6–15. EXU. Many small calculi are scattered in the right kidney but are invisible in the presence of radiographic contrast. On the left there is a large calculus located in the renal pelvis causing moderate obstruction. Collecting system is dilated. A renal carcinoma measuring 3 cm in diameter is also present. The only telltale signs are flattening of the upper pole calyx on the very top and increased distance between the calyx and the top of the renal outline. Treatment was left partial nephrectomy and pyelolithotomy.

be of appropriate size to permit introduction of grasping instruments and rigid or flexible ureteroscope or pyeloscope. This usually requires 24, 26, 28, or 30 F size sheet. Placement of the sheet in an optimal position, so that it "looks" at the stone, markedly simplifies grasping and removal. To achieve optimal placement, puncture of the most appropriate calyx at an appropriate angle is mandatory.

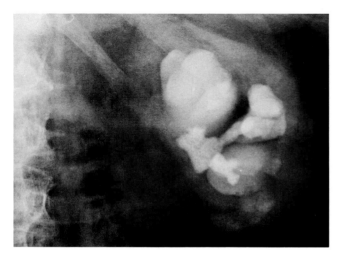

Figure 6–14. EXU. A large left renal stone is in the renal pelvis causing moderate partial obstruction to all calyces.

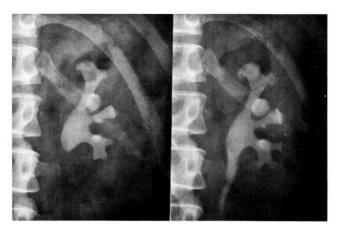

Figure 6–16. EXU. Staghorn is clearly seen on the scout radiograph (left). After injected contrast fills the renal pelvis, the calculus is almost impossible to recognize. This is one among many reasons why a preliminary radiograph is mandatory prior to injection of contrast material.

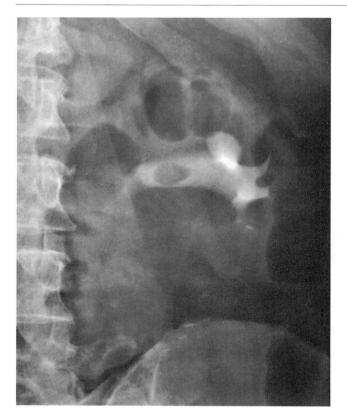

Figure 6–17. EXU. Uric acid stones are relatively radiolucent and may easily be missed on the preliminary radiograph. Since they displace contrast and themselves absorb very few x-rays, a "filling defect" is seen within the collecting system or ureter. Differential diagnosis includes sloughed papilla, blood clot, transitional cell carcinoma, arteriovenous malformation, fungus ball, etc.

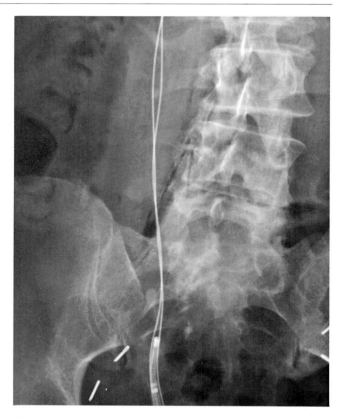

Figure 6–18. Retrograde ureteroscopy. A flexible ureteroscope is introduced into the right ureter over a guidewire. A second guidewire has also been introduced. This procedure is being done under epidural anesthesia. The telltale sign is the presence of air (streaking radiolucencies) in the soft tissues along the spine. Small amounts of air are introduced by the anesthesiologist during the spinal puncture until a "give" is felt, signaling entrance into the epidural space.

The procedure is usually performed under epidural or general anesthesia and under fluoroscopic control. Once the appropriate calyx is entered, the tract is enlarged by exchanging progressively larger dilators or a caged balloon catheter over a guidewire. Once dilatation is accomplished, the sheet is introduced over the last dilator (Fig. 6–20). After the stone is extracted, an appropriately large nephrostomy is left in place (Fig. 6–21).

Percutaneous Ultrasonic Lithotripsy

If the calculus is too large (Fig. 6–22) for simple percutaneous extraction, or too dense (Fig. 6–23), it may be fragmented and each fragment aspirated or extracted individually. Fragmentation is achieved with an ultrasonic lithotrite, an instrument with a probe which fits through the sheet and transmits focused acoustical energy to the stone when in contact with it.

In the presence of congenital anomalies percutaneous approach may be difficult and somewhat more hazardous (Fig. 6–24).

EXTRACORPOREAL LITHOTRIPSY

Electrohydraulic lithotripsy (EL) is currently the method of choice for initial management of most smaller renal calculi.[7-10] EL is a method that disintegrates renal calculi by means of a focused underwater shock wave that is created either by an underwater spark, a dish of piezoelectric crystals, or an acoustical membrane (Figs. 6–25, 6–26). The shock wave is focused by a hemiellipsoid cup, a dish, or an acoustical lens, and concentrated on the stone. After receiving a number of shock waves, the stone is shattered into small fragments. In some units the patient is positioned within a bathtub by a mobile

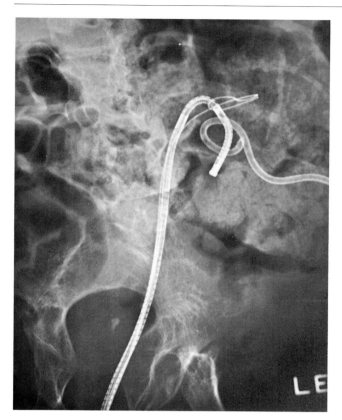

Figure 6–19. Retrograde pyeloscopy. Incredible flexibility of a fiberoptic pyeloscope is demonstrated here. The examiner is looking into the lower pole calyx. There is a percutaneous nephrostomy and a guidewire alongside the pyeloscope. Note also sacral agenesis, wide separation of the symphysis pubis, and a bladder calculus.

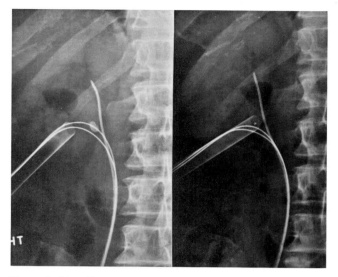

Figure 6–20. Percutaneous stone extraction. After percutaneous puncture, the tract to the renal pelvis is dilated to 28 F and a working sheath positioned so that it allows easy access to the stone. A safety wire is outside the sheath and a working wire is within the sheath. A retrograde catheter is also in place. The stone was easily removed under endoscopic control and no residual stones are seen on the postprocedural radiograph (right).

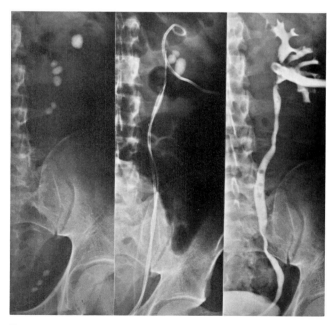

Figure 6–21. Sequence of images during percutaneous extraction of ureteral and renal calculi. Some nine calculi can be counted (left). After a percutaneous nephrostomy has been placed, all the calculi were pushed into the renal pelvis with retrograde catheters (middle). The tract was enlarged and all stones removed. Several air bubbles are seen in the mid-ureter during nephrostogram (right).

suspension mechanism, in others the patient is on top of a table. Centering is accomplished either by two fluoroscopes at 90° angles to each other, an ultrasound transducer, or a tilting C-arm.

The procedure is usually carried out under epidural anesthesia and, depending on the size of the stone, 800–2000 shock waves are administered. A vast majority of patients will spontaneously pass the stones within several days to a week. Larger calculi may require one or two additional treatments. Although the passage of small calculus fragments following therapy is usually associated with very minimal discomfort, the tendency is to place a ureteral stent prior to the procedure. This prevents ureteral obstruction and the passage of stone fragments is facilitated despite the presence of the stent within the ureteral lumen.

Staghorn and large pelvic calculi may be treated with a combination of percutaneous nephrolitho-

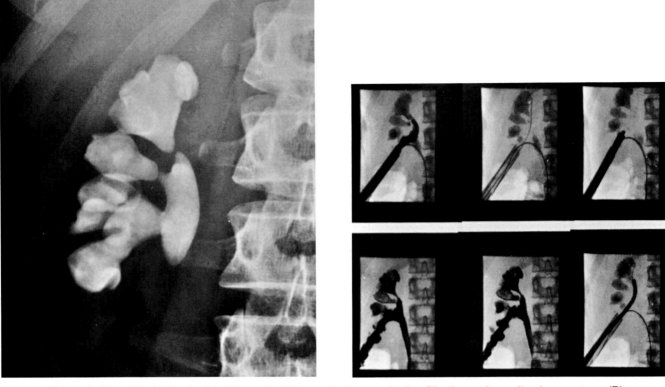

A   B

Figure 6–22. **(A)** Abdominal radiograph. A large staghorn calculus fills the entire collecting system. **(B)** Percutaneous nephrolithotripsy. Sequential spot films are obtained during percutaneous stone disintegration and complete removal.

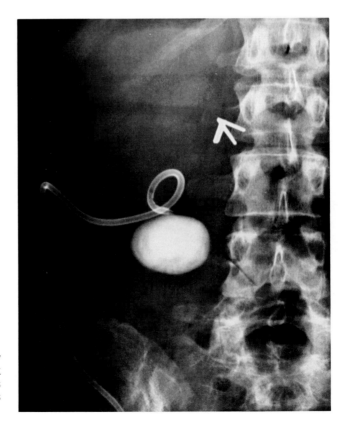

Figure 6–23. Abdominal radiograph. An example of a very dense stone. Successful treatment with extracorporeal shock wave therapy is very unlikely and percutaneous treatment is indicated. To that end a percutaneous nephrostomy has already been inserted.

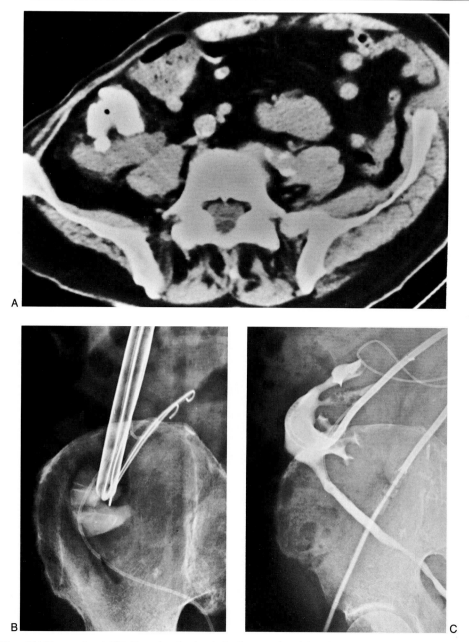

Figure 6–24. **(A)** Precontrast CT. Renal calculus is in the renal pelvis of a low-lying right kidney. Because of the reverse rotation of the kidney, percutaneous access to the kidney is very difficult. **(B)** A posterior outward oblique approach was used for percutaneous nephrolithotripsy. Sheath, working, and safety guidewires are in place. **(C)** Nephrostogram in the RPO projection. The approach through the middle calyx was the only way to gain access to the stone, which was completely removed.

tripsy and EL. Any smaller fragments that cannot be reached by percutaneous methods are subjected to EL therapy.

It is possible to treat a ureteral calculus if above the pelvic brim. However, to minimize possible ureteral injury, urologists prefer to manipulate the calculus in a retrograde fashion to either dislodge it backward into the renal pelvis or to place a stent alongside the calculus prior to treatment.

Congenital anomalies complicate the treatment, just as they do in percutaneous lithotripsy (Fig. 6–27).

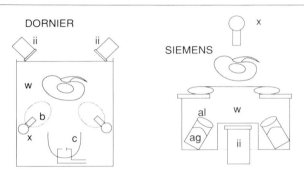

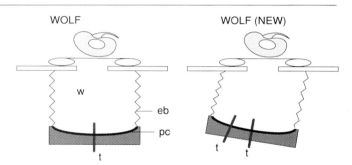

Figure 6–25. Schematic representation of Dornier and Siemens lithotriptors; al: acoustical lens; ag: acoustic generator; b: underwater balloon inflated during fluoroscopy to decrease tube load; c: hemiellipsoid cup with the electrode; ii: image intensifier; x: x-ray tube; w: water. The patient is submerged in water (Dornier) or on the top of the table dipping slightly into water well (Siemens).

Figure 6–26. Schematic representation of ultrasonic lithotriptor (Wolf). eb: expanding bellows; pc: piezoelectric crystals in a dish; t: localizing ultrasonic transducer. The new version allows the dish to be tilted for subcostal approach to the upper pole stones. Because the dish is larger than hemiellipsoid cup of the other units, the distribution of energy at the skin is larger so that the treatment is less painful and may be completed without epidural anesthesia.

Radiology Role

Excellent quality of abdominal radiographs is necessary for preprocedural evaluation and for follow-ups.[11] Because patients do not undergo bowel preparation for EL therapy, detection of small fragments may be somewhat difficult. A judicious use of plain film tomography may thus be indicated in some instances. Ultrasound is also helpful in the follow-up of larger fragments and in detecting hydronephrosis. In addition, perinephric hematoma or other renal anomalies, such as tumors and renal cysts, are every so often discovered by serendipity.

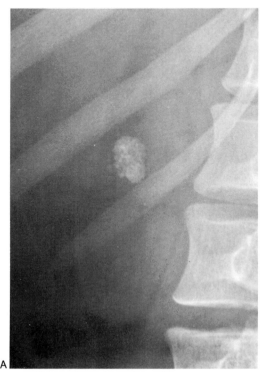
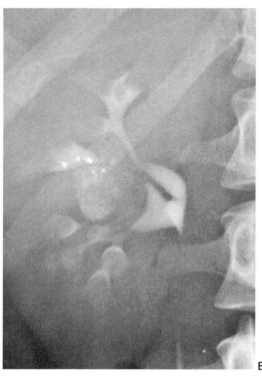

Figure 6–27. **(A)** Scout radiograph. Fragmented right renal calculus after EL treatment. **(B)** EXU. The fragments are in the narrow neck infundibular diverticulum and are retained for a long period of time. Retrograde endoscopic manipulation was necessary to evacuate the debris.

Percutaneous Nephrostomy

Some patients may need a percutaneous nephrostomy following EL treatment.[12] Obstruction (Fig. 6–28), fever, and increasing flank pain are indications for percutaneous nephrostomy tube placement in the post-treatment period (Fig. 6–29).[13] Small nephrostomy tubes under these circumstances are useless because they frequently occlude with debris. At least a 12 F nephrostomy tube or larger is desirable. Because the collecting system is frequently distorted or contracted by a fibrous process in patients with long-standing calculus disease, different types of nephrostomy tubes may have to be used, each tailored to the particular situation.

Percutaneous nephrostomy serves as the preamble to establishing a larger tract for percutaneous nephrolithotripsy in the case of a dense, big, or staghorn calculus.

Complications

Obstruction due to stone passage occurs in approximately 15% of the patients without the "double J"

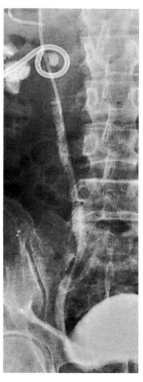

Figure 6–29. EXU. Calculous debris fills the entire ureter. Despite ureteral stent and percutaneous nephrostomy, the right kidney is obstructed (contrast in the bladder is from the left kidney). Both catheters are occluded and the nephrostomy has to be exchanged.

stent. Some centers have reported quite a high number of perinephric hematomas (Figs. 6–30, 6–31). Hematuria, hemorrhage, and cutaneous echymosis are seen.[14,15] Contusion of the bowel and lung are potential complications.

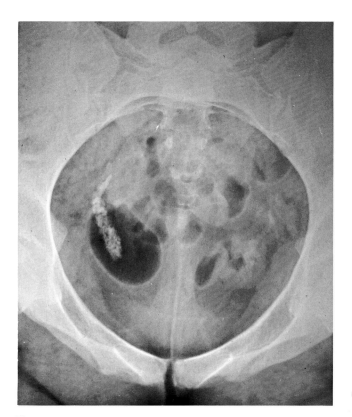

Figure 6–28. Plain radiograph. Accumulation of calculous debris in the ureter from a fragmented stone above may produce obstruction. This radiographic appearance is sometimes referred to as "Steinstrasse" (stone street), a term coined in Germany where EL was invented.

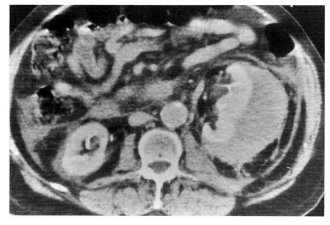

Figure 6–30. Contrast-enhanced CT. A large subcapsular hematoma is discovered after EL treatment of the left kidney. More surprising is a small spontaneous subcapsular hematoma of the right kidney, which was not treated by EL.

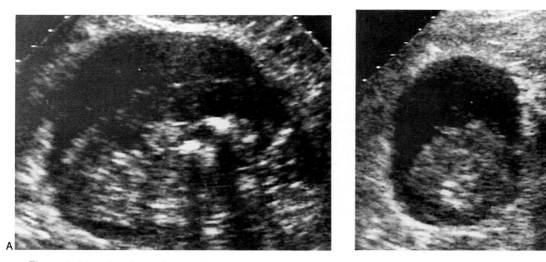

Figure 6–31.   Another subcapsular hematoma following EL treatment as seen on ultrasound in longitudinal (A) and transverse (B) planes.

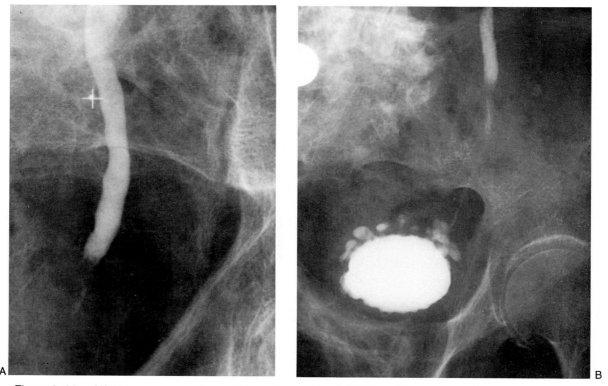

Figure 6–32.   (A) Nephrostogram in a patient with a solitary left kidney. There is complete distal left ureteral obstruction by a radiolucent uric acid stone. Oral and parenteral alkalinization could not be tolerated by the patient. A small catheter was placed through the nephrostomy tube close to the stone and alkaline perfusion started. Egress was through nephrostomy. (B) Within a few days there was complete dissolution of the uric acid stone and the obstruction is no longer present. Heavily trabeculated bladder is present, which makes retrograde ureteral catheterization and stone basketing almost impossible. Note Paget's disease in the right pubic bone. (From Barbaric ZL. Interventional uroradiology. Radiol Clin North Am 1979; 17:413–433. Reprinted with permission.)

Several recent reports raise the possibility that EL treatment may cause hypertension at some time interval after the procedure. Incidence may be as high as 8–10%. This new discovery may require some rethinking about the true usefulness of EL, particularly if prospective studies now being conducted confirm hypertension as a complication.

STONE DISSOLUTION

This is a rarely used method nowadays. By alkalinizing urine either by parenteral method or through the percutaneous nephrostomy, it is possible to dissolve the uric acid stone (Fig. 6–32).

REFERENCES

1. Buckalew VM Jr. Nephrolithiasis in renal tubular acidosis. J Urol 1989; 141:731–737.
2. Hernandez-Graulau JM, Castanega-Zuniga W, Hunter D, Hulbert JC. Management of cystine nephrolithiasis by endourologic methods and shock-wave lithotripsy. Urology 1989; 34:139–143.
3. Murray RL. Milk of calcium of the kidney: diagnostic features on vertical beam roentgenograms. Am J Roentgenol Radium Ther Nucl Med 1971; 113:455–459.
4. Parienty RA, Ducellier R, Pradel J, et al. Diagnostic value of CT numbers in pelvocalyceal filling defects. Radiology 1982; 145:743–747.
5. Roberts MC, Pollack HM, Banner MP, et al. Interstitial emphysema associated with epidural anesthesia for extracorporeal shock-wave lithotripsy. AJR 1987; 148:301–302.
6. Fernström I, Johannson B. Percutaneous pyelolithotomy: a new extraction technique. Scand J Urol Nephrol 1976; 10:257–260.
7. Chaussy C, Schmiedt E, Jocham D, et al. First clinical experience with extracorporeally induced destruction of kidney stones by shock-waves. J Urol 1981; 127:417–420.
8. Chaussy C, Schmiedt E, Jocham D, et al. Extracorporeal shock-wave lithotripsy (ESWL) for treatment of urolithiasis. Urology (Suppl) 1984; 23:59–66.
9. Drach GW, Dretler S, Fair W, et al. Report of the United States cooperative study of extracorporeal shock-wave lithotripsy. J Urol 1986; 135:1127–1133.
10. LeRoy AJ, Segura JW. Extracorporeal shock-wave lithotripsy. Radiol Clin North Am 1986; 24:623–631.
11. Bush WH, Gibbons RP, Lewis GP, Brannen GE. Impact of extracorporeal shock-wave lithotripsy on percutaneous stone procedures. AJR 1986; 147:89–93.
12. Tegtmeyer CJ, Kellum CD, Jenkins A, et al. Extracorporeal shock-wave lithotripsy: interventional radiologic solutions to associated problems. Radiology 1986; 161:587–592.
13. Cochran ST, Barbaric ZL, Mindell HJ, et al. Extracorporeal shock-wave lithotripsy: impact on the radiology department of a stone treatment center. Radiology 1987; 163:655–659.
14. Papanieoaou N, Stafford SA, Pfister RC, et al. Significant renal hemorrhage following extracorporeal shock-wave lithotripsy: imaging and clinical features. Radiology 1987; 163:661–664.
15. Rubin JI, Arger PH, Pollack HM, et al. Kidney changes after extracorporeal shock-wave lithotripsy: CT evaluation. Radiology 1987; 162:21–24.

7

Urinary Tract Obstruction

URINARY TRACT OBSTRUCTION

Etiology.   Calculi, clot, tumor, sloughed papilla, inadvertent ligation, congenital, extrinsic compression, retroperitoneal fibrosis, endometriosis.

Pathophysiology.   Tubular dilation, initial increase (in 1 hour) followed by decrease in renal blood flow, severalfold increase in renal lymphatic flow, initial increase in ureteral peristalsis followed by aperistalsis, dilatation, and parenchymal atrophy.

Clinical Presentation.   Acute colicky pain is due to stone transiting the ureter. Radiating pain, nausea, vomiting, gross hematuria. May be asymptomatic in chronic phase.

Laboratory Findings.   None, hematuria, pyuria, azotemia.

Acute Obstruction (Severe)

Radiological Findings.   Sonography may be normal in 50% of patients with acute obstruction. Therefore a normal sonogram does not exclude acute obstruction.[1-3] Grade I or II dilatation may be found in others but one has to keep in mind that presence of dilatation is not specific for obstruction and may be seen in other disorders. Only occasionally does sonography demonstrate a calculus at ureteropelvic junction (UPJ) or in the distal ureteral segment.

Several classic signs are seen on excretory urogram and CT:

1. *Dense nephrogram.* Early in the examination the obstructed kidney shows a faint nephrogram

which gradually, over a period of an hour, becomes very intense, much more so than the normal kidney (Fig. 7–1).[4] This increase in nephrogram intensity may persist for 24 hours and is due to the following: a) While sodium (Na) and water are reabsorbed from the tubules, molecules of the contrast material are not. The contrast becomes more concentrated compared with the normal kidney; b) Increase in tubular volume. Volume changes with the power of two of the radius; thus a small change in tubular radius will

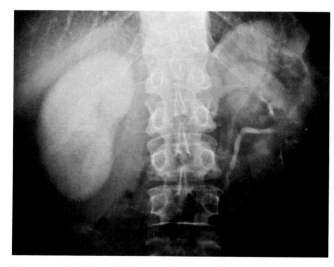

Figure 7–1.   Intensifying nephrogram in a patient with severe acute ureteral obstruction. At 1 hour after injection of contrast material, the nephrogram has reached its peak, but it will persist for several hours and gradually diminish over next 24 hours. Although other pathological conditions may produce persistent nephrogram, none attains so dense a nephrogram as does acute obstruction.

significantly increase tubular volume. The larger the volume, the more iodine atoms are in the path of the x-ray beam.

2. *Delayed appearance of contrast in the collecting system.* There still continues to be forward motion of urine through the collecting tubules, at least through the cortical nephrons (those with short loop of Henle) (Fig. 7–2). However, it may take a long time (sometimes 24 hours) for the contrast to faintly opacify the obstructed collecting system (Fig. 7–3).

3. *Poor concentration in the collecting system.* Despite the fact that the contrast is concentrated within the tubules, slow forward motion and dilution with urine already present in the collecting system are explanations for poor concentration in the collecting system. Poor concentration of the contrast in the collecting system may hamper diagnosis of the cause and the site of the ureteral obstruction.

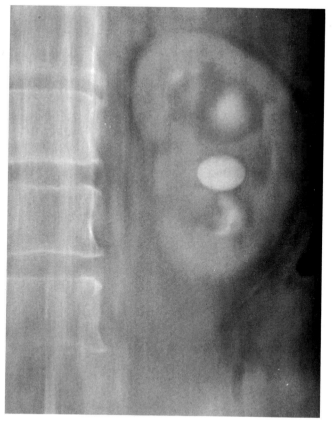

Figure 7–3. Acute obstruction. Dense nephrogram persists and the contrast is slowly excreted into the collecting system. Since the contrast is denser than urine, it tends to settle into the most dependent calyces. Even more time is needed for the contrast to accumulate and displace urine and enter into anteriorly located renal pelvis and ureter (patient supine).

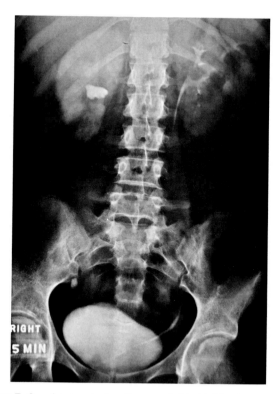

Figure 7–2. Acute obstruction on right. At 25 minutes after contrast injection, there is still no contrast present in the right collecting system. Only a delayed radiograph, perhaps even 12 or 24 hours after the injection, may faintly opacify the collecting system and ureter to the point of the obstruction. Here there are two calculi, one in the distal ureter and the other in the renal pelvis. Either might have caused obstruction and the diagnosis may be made on the delayed radiograph.

Acute Obstruction (Partial/Mild)

Radiological Findings. There are, of course, varying degrees of urinary tract obstruction, from complete to very mild. The less severe the obstruction, the less pronounced the radiographic findings. The most reliable diagnostic findings on an excretory urogram are:

1. *Delay in function.* This is the most valuable sign of obstruction if accompanied by mild dilation of the collecting system and the ureter.
2. *Standing column.* Mild dilation of the ureter seen throughout its entire length denotes lack of peristalsis (Figs. 7–4, 7–5, 7–6).

In a mild obstruction it is easier to determine size and cause of obstruction, since the contrast material is more concentrated and outlines the ureter much more distinctly than in a severe case of obstruction.

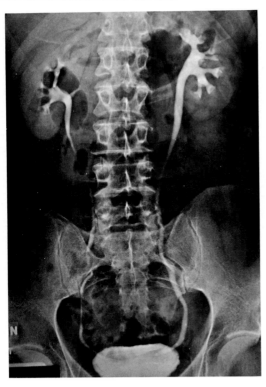

Figure 7–4. Standing column. Distal ureteral obstruction due to a small calculus. Dilatation of the left collecting system is obvious, as is the dilatation of the left ureter when compared with the opposite side.

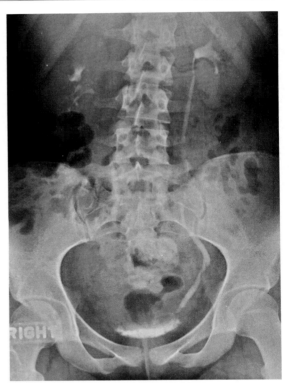

Figure 7–5. At times an upright postvoid radiograph may be the only one where difference in the caliber of two ureters is obvious. Small distal radiopaque calculus is causing mild obstruction. The collecting system is not dilated and the diagnosis of obstruction cannot be made by sonography.

Graphic description of an acute obstruction is presented in Figure 7–7.

Complicating Features of Acute Obstruction

There are several complicating features of acute obstruction that add to the spectrum of radiographic findings in this disease.

1. *Calyceal perforation* is seen in the presence of increased pelvic pressure due either to obstruction or retrograde pyelography. The fornix is the weakest point in the collecting system and a common site of rupture. Extravasated urine fills the renal sinus (*pyelosinus backflow*), perirenal space, and retroperitoneum (Fig. 7–8). Contrast assumes a characteristic "streaky" appearance as it descends between fascial planes and retroperitoneal fat. In the presence of extravasation, delay in excretion of the contrast material into the collecting system may not be readily apparent since the kidney has "decompressed" itself and need not be significantly obstructed because of retroperitoneal leak.

Urine outside the collecting system may be detected even without contrast administration on CT (Fig. 7–9), sonography (Fig. 7–10), and even on MR imaging (Fig. 7–11).

On rare occasions extravasated contrast in the renal sinus may be contained and may resemble a peripelvic cyst (Fig. 7–12).

2. *Renal sinus lymphocele.* This is a rare occurrence associated with acute obstruction where there is a localized collection of lymph in the renal sinus appearing as a cystlike structure on sonography or causing pelvicalyceal distortion on IVP and CT.

3. *Nondilated obstructive uropathy.* On rare occasions the upper urinary tract system need not be dilated even in the presence of severe obstruction.[5-8] This type of obstruction may be impossible to diagnose by such modalities as sonography and nonenhanced magnetic resonance imaging.

Chronic Obstruction (Complete)

Radiological Findings. When obstruction is complete, progressive dilation of the collecting system

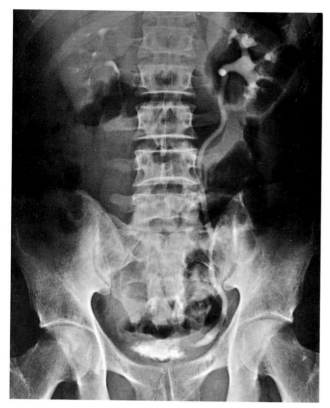

Figure 7–6. Standing column on the left in this patient is from residual edema induced by a calculus that has since passed.

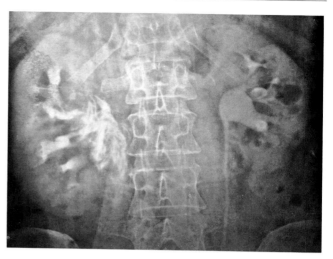

Figure 7–8. Acute obstruction and forniceal rupture. The kidney has "decompressed" into the renal sinus, perinephric space, and retroperitoneum. Because the pressure in the collecting system has diminished, antegrade flow of urine continues unabated. Ureter, however, did not fill with contrast and the site of obstruction remains elusive.

and ureters continues and the number of nephrons diminishes. After 6 to 12 weeks, loss of renal function is irreversible. At that time grade III or IV hydronephrosis is detected on sonography. One millimeter thick

remaining renal parenchyma may be opacified by intravenous or intra-arterial contrast injection. This is a specific radiographic sign pathognomonic for chronic obstruction and is known as *"shell nephrogram"* (Figs. 7–13–7–18).

Chronic Obstruction (Partial)

Radiological Findings

A. *Excretory urography and CT*
  1. *Delay in function* (Figs. 7–19, 7–20).
  2. *Dilatation.* Dilatation of the collecting system is usually detected on contrast examination (Figs. 7–21, 7–22) but may be identified on CT even without intravenous contrast (Fig. 7–23).
  3. *Negative pyelogram.* Contrast in the renal parenchyma may outline the dilated collecting system before being excreted into it (Figs. 7–24, 7–25).
  4. *Crescent sign of Dunbar.* When partial obstruction persists unchecked, dilation of the collecting system continues. The collecting tubules also dilate and gradually assume a position parallel to the renal outline. Concentrated radiographic contrast material in dilated tubules is seen as a crescent several millimeters long, a radiographic sign pathognomonic for chronic renal obstruction (Fig. 7–26).[9]

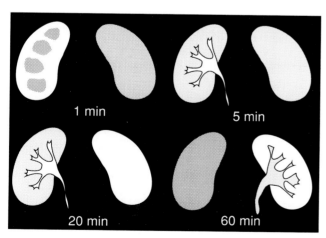

Figure 7–7. Schematic drawing of classic radiological findings on an excretory urogram in acute obstruction (in this case on the left). There is delayed function and slowly increasing nephrogram, which becomes intense. On delayed radiographs, sometimes even after several hours, the collecting system may become faintly opacified.

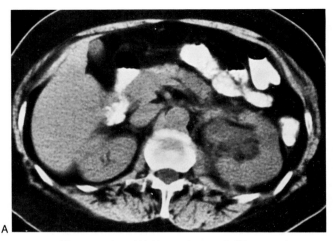

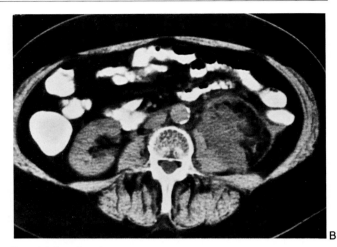

A   B

Figure 7–9. (A) Nonenhanced CT scan demonstrates dilated left collecting system in a patient with acute distal ureter obstruction. (B) A slice just inferior to the lower pole of the left kidney shows urine collecting alongside psoas and streaking within thickened renal fascia. Although not specific for urine, the fluid collection is most likely not an acute hematoma because acute hematoma attenuates more and would appear hyperdense compared with the psoas.

5. *Visualization of individual papillary ducts.* Similar to the crescent sign, if the collecting tubules are seen "en face," they may be seen as radiopaque dots on the excretory urogram.[10]

6. *Fluid-fluid interface sign.* Since specific gravity of excreted contrast is greater than that of urine, the contrast accumulates in the most dependent parts of the renal collecting system, gradually displacing urine (Figs. 7–27,

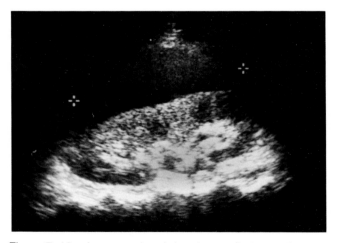

Figure 7–10. Large perinephric urinoma (between the cursors) is seen in a pregnant woman with acute ureteral obstruction due to urolithiasis. Despite advanced pregnancy, the collecting system is not significantly distended. Urinoma was drained percutaneously, followed by placement of a percutaneous nephrostomy that served during the rest of the pregnancy.

7–28). This, of course, is best seen on CT. On an excretory urogram, however, this contrast behavior may pose diagnostic difficulties early in the course of examination. On a radiograph taken with the patient in the upright position, fluid-fluid interface may be seen that is pathognomonic for urinary tract dilatation although not for urinary tract obstruction.

7. *Pelvocalyceal wall opacification.* In the presence of long-standing obstruction, pelvocalyceal wall becomes hyperemic, particularly in the presence of infection. Following an intravenous bolus of contrast, it is sometimes possible to observe a blush of the pelvocalyceal wall on urography. Hyperemic and thickened pelvocalyceal wall is best seen on CT (Fig. 7–27).

8. *Hold up of contrast on an upright radiograph.* Drainage by gravity or reflex contraction of the pelvocalyceal system while the patient is upright will eliminate any possibility of obstruction. Persistence of dilatation and contrast in such a position is very suggestive of obstruction.

B. *Sonography*

Dilatation of the collecting system and the ureter is evident, depending on the site, degree, and longevity of the obstruction (Fig. 7–29). Grades I, II, III, and IV are in common use (Fig. 7–30).

C. *Nuclear Medicine*

Tc-99m DTPA scan will show delayed appearance of the radionuclide, diminished uptake com-

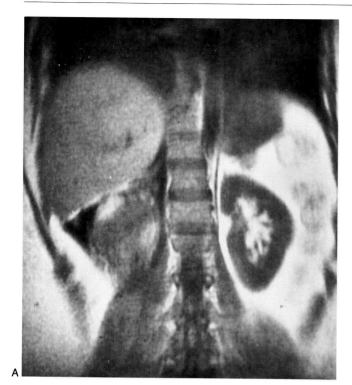
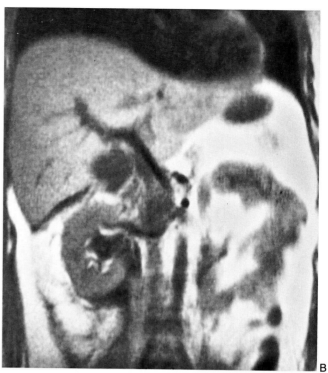

Figure 7–11. MR imaging is not the primary (or even secondary) method for determining the presence of acute urinary tract obstruction. In this patient in a more posterior coronal plane, a normal left kidney surrounded by perinephric fat is seen (**A**). On the right, hypointense fluid is present in the perinephric space (**A**). Dilated system and more perinephric fluid on the right is even more obvious on a more anterior slice (**B**). Obstruction is probably present and there has been a forniceal rupture. The site and cause of the obstruction, however, remain undetermined. Excretory urogram is the examination of choice.

pared with normal side, dilated collecting system, and, occasionally, dilated ureter to the point of the obstruction on delayed scans (Fig. 7–31).

D. *MR Imaging.*

Magnetic resonance imaging is not the primary method for evaluating urinary tract obstruction, but dilatation of the collecting system and the ureter is likely to be seen during evaluation of some other disease. Urine is of low signal intensity (dark) on T1-weighted sequences.

E. *Plain Radiography*

Plain radiography is an important means of detecting increasing dilatation in patients with calculous debris in the kidney after extracorporeal shock wave lithotripsy. Fluid-like debris in the kidney assumes the role of radiographic contrast. Milk of calcium urine may also show fluid-fluid levels in the upright position (Fig. 7–32).

Gas may also be detected and may serve as "negative" radiographic contrast. Beside infection, gas in the collecting system may be seen after

instrumentation, fistulas, and some types of urinary diversions (Fig. 7–33).

DILATED UPPER URINARY TRACT SYSTEM: OBSTRUCTED OR NOT?

Dilatation of the urinary tract system without obstruction may be seen in:

1. Vesicoureteral reflux.
2. Corrected long-standing obstruction with residual dilatation.
3. Chronic renal disease.
4. Prune belly syndrome.
5. Megacalycosis

Sometimes it is difficult to determine whether the dilated system is obstructed or not. The delay in function may not be perceivable and the collecting system may not empty that well on a radiograph

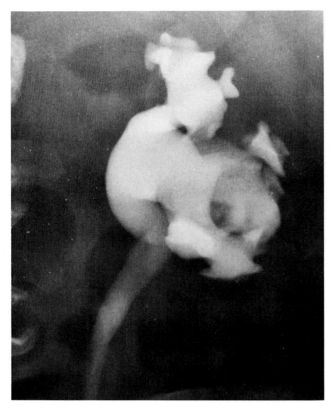

Figure 7–12. Localized pyelosinus backflow demonstrated on a retrograde pyelogram. Patient is acutely obstructed at mid-ureteral level and there is moderate dilatation of the collecting system.

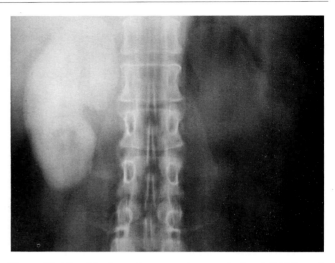

Figure 7–14. Shell nephrogram is seen in the left kidney in the early stage of an excretory urogram.

taken in an upright position. Diagnostic techniques have been devised to ascertain if dilatation of the upper system is due to obstruction or not.

Upright Postvoid Radiograph

This is probably the simplest and cheapest method by which obstruction can be excluded. Unobstructed system will empty by gravity, partially obstructed system will not (Fig. 7–34).

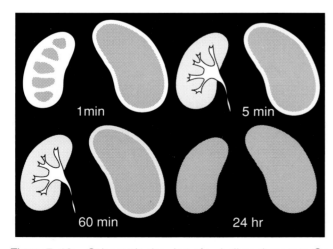

Figure 7–13. Schematic drawing of a shell nephrogram. On intravenous urography all that is left of renal parenchyma is opacified. This usually happens to be 1 to 2 mm thick and should not be confused with the subcapsular rim sign seen in renal infarction, renal vein thrombosis, or acute cortical necrosis.

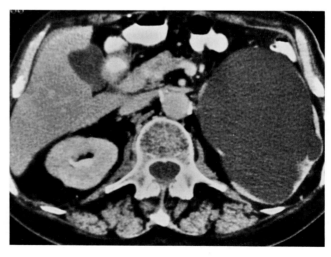

Figure 7–15. Contrast-enhanced CT scan demonstrates shell nephrogram in a massively enlarged and hydronephrotic kidney. The decision whether to treat the obstruction depends on the amount of functional reserve determined by nuclear medicine studies.

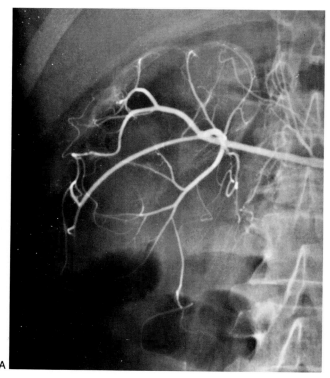
A

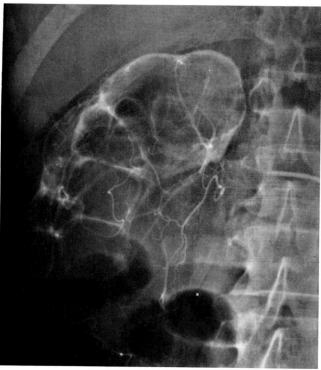
B

Figure 7–16. Selective right renal arteriogram in end-stage obstruction and hydronephrosis. Segmental and intralobar branches are splayed by hydronephrotic sac. Only 1 mm of parenchyma separates arcuate arteries from the renal outline **(A)**. Capsular, inferior adrenal, and pelvicalyceal arteries appear more prominent. Inside the shell nephrogram is a large nonopacified hydronephrotic sac **(B)**.

Furosemide (Lasix) Excretory Urogram

This study is usually reserved for intermittent ureteropelvic junction (UPJ) obstruction. Excretory urogram is performed and 5- and 10-minute radiographs are obtained. At that moment the patient is given

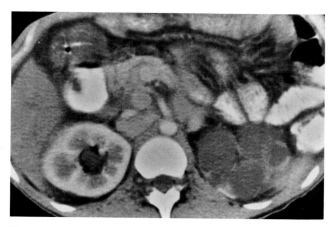

Figure 7–17. Contrast-enhanced CT. Nice example of early normal nephrogram on the right early after contrast injection. Cortex is clearly differentiated from the medulla. On the left a shell nephrogram is diagnostic of long-standing hydronephrosis with little, if any, parenchyma remaining.

intravenous fluids and a potent diuretic (furosemide 50 mg IV). As marked diuresis ensues, the ureteropelvic junction is challenged to permit increased flow of urine. The test is positive if during the functional challenge the patient experiences pain and if contrast is retained in the dilated collecting system while the normal side rapidly clears of contrast.[11]

Diuretic Renogram

This test is similar to the furosemide test except that a radionuclide is used instead of contrast. After challenge with diuretic, the washout rate of DTPA is observed.[12,13] Retention of the radionuclide over 10 minutes following furosemide infusion is considered diagnostic for obstruction (Fig. 7–35). Of the two tests just described, nuclear medicine is probably the more sensitive.

Double "J" Ureteral Stent

In a situation where the patient develops intermittent pain following a hydration challenge, it seems reasonable to place a ureteral stent for a period of a week

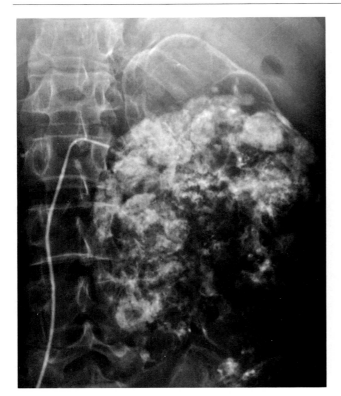

Figure 7–18. Late phase of a selective left renal arteriogram. A large hypervascular renal carcinoma replaces most of the mid and lower pole of the kidney. In the upper pole there is a distinct shell nephrogram indicating presence of long-standing hydronephrosis due to tumor obstruction.

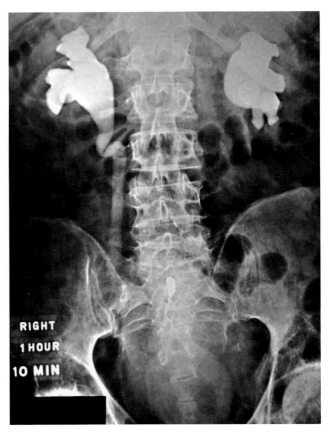

Figure 7–19. Marked bilateral delay in contrast excretion and dilatation of the collecting system. The degree of dilatation and particularly the tortuosity of the visualized right ureter suggest chronic obstruction. Obstructions need not be supravesical to cause these findings. In this patient there is marked outflow bladder obstruction due to prostatic enlargement. Continual high bladder pressures transmit to the ureters and kidneys and are as damaging as ureteral obstruction.

or two and repeat the challenge. Absence of pain under these circumstances would indicate the presence of obstruction, such as ureteropelvic junction obstruction. Such placement is relatively atraumatic, particularly in females.

Whitaker Test

When the above-mentioned tests are indeterminate and a decision regarding surgical correction must be made, a flow-pressure measurement study may provide the correct diagnosis.

Whitaker test is a mildly invasive study requiring a bladder catheter and a small percutaneous catheter (18 gauge or 5 F).[14–18] Bladder is kept empty by constant catheter drainage but intermittent empty bladder pressures are obtained and are assumed to represent intra-abdominal pressure (BP). Small percutaneous catheter is inserted into the kidney (Fig. 7–36). Contrast is constantly infused through the percutaneous catheter and the infusion rate is gradually increased over a period of time (Fig. 7–37).

During the infusion intrapelvic pressure (RP) is intermittently measured. The differential pressure (DP) between RP and BP represents true intrapelvic pressure. Infusion into the renal collecting system should continue for a period of time to overcome compliance of the dilated collecting system.[19,20]

At a flow rate of 10 ml/min, a DP below 10 to 12 cm H_2O excludes the presence of obstruction. A DP of 13 to 22 cm H_2O suggests mild or equivocal obstruction, while DP of 23 to 40 cm at the same flow rate indicates moderate obstruction. A DP above 41 cm indicates severe obstruction.[21–23]

Duplex Doppler Sonography

Resistive index is increased above 0.70 during obstruction and decreases after the obstruction has

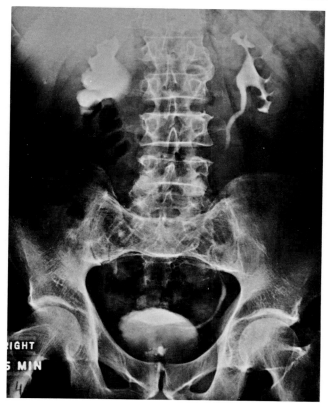

Figure 7–20. Fifteen minutes after administration of contrast material there is definite delay in contrast excretion and dilatation of the right collecting system. If immediate cause of obstruction is not evident right away, one should scrutinize the presacral areas for telltale signs of ureteral calculus. One, perhaps two, radiopaque right ureteral calculi are present. A radiograph obtained 15 minutes later (or an immediate prone radiograph) will confirm the diagnosis. Note prostatic calcifications.

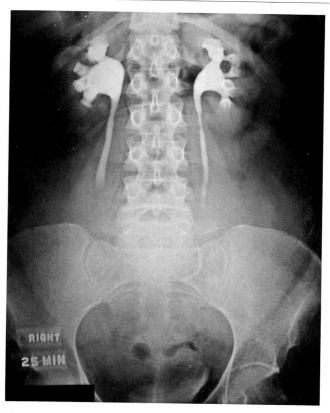

Figure 7–21. Bilateral dilatation of upper ureters and collecting system due to a large pelvic mass that is compressing ureters upon the pelvic brim, thus causing obstruction. Top of the mass extends to the level of L2 vertebral body. There is also functional delay, since at 25 minutes after contrast injection the bladder should be much fuller and more opacified.

been relieved.[24] Comparative studies are still needed to evaluate this novel approach.

False-positive diagnosis of grade I hydronephrosis can be lessened by using pulsed or color Doppler. Normal blood vessels may imitate dilatation and are easily separated from the collecting system.[25]

Minipercutaneous Nephrostomy

When all the above-mentioned tests fail to definitively confirm or exclude obstruction, a small 8 F or 10 F nephrostomy tube may be inserted and left in place for several weeks. Selective renal function studies at the time of nephrostomy insertion and several weeks later are compared. Interim improvement in renal function connotes the presence of obstruction.

PERCUTANEOUS NEPHROSTOMY

Percutaneous nephrostomy is a rapid, rather simple, and effective means of providing supravesical urinary diversion in the obstructed system of patients too ill to undergo corrective surgery for obstruction.[26,27] Examples are obstruction from any cause, with superimposed fulminating infection, severe electrolyte imbalance, severe renal failure, congestive heart failure, and bleeding disorders that would preclude surgery as a life-saving measure. Not all urinary obstructive processes need to be surgically corrected. For instance, a large obstructing neoplasm may well respond to chemotherapy or radiation therapy, or an obstructive calculus may be removed by retrograde endoscopic approach. Under the circumstances described above, percutaneous nephrostomy should be considered a life-saving pro-

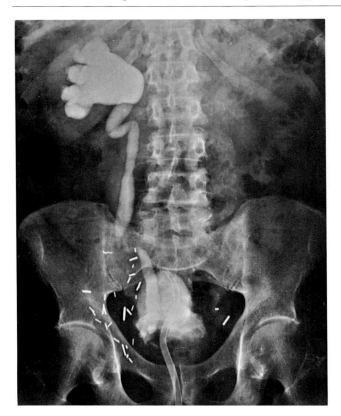

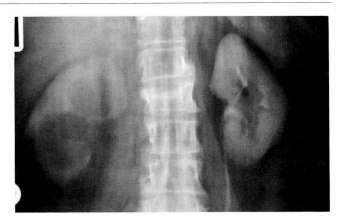

Figure 7–24. Negative pyelogram in a patient with distal ureteral obstruction. If given enough time, a follow-up radiograph several hours later is likely to show some contrast appearing in the collecting system. Thus, the obstruction site can be determined. This patient had a ureter partially clipped several years earlier during a transvaginal hysterectomy.

Figure 7–22. Right hydronephrosis and hydroureter in a patient with carcinoma of the bladder. Ureters dilate and also elongate with prolonged obstruction and thus become tortuous. Left kidney is not seen on this examination. Either it was removed or is nonfunctioning because of obstruction caused by the bladder tumor.

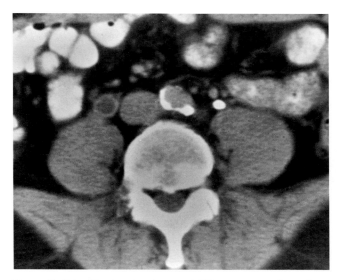

Figure 7–23. Contrast-enhanced CT scan several centimeters below the kidneys. Left ureter is densely opacified by contrast lying on top of the psoas and left of heavily calcified aorta. Dilated right ureter contains no contrast. Low attenuation within the ureter suggests presence of nonopacified urine. Therefore, dilatation as well as delay (or absence) of function may be implied from this single image without ever actually seeing the kidneys.

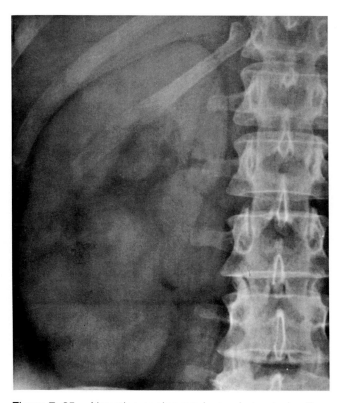

Figure 7–25. Negative pyelogram in an obstructed solitary right kidney 10 minutes after injection of contrast. Enlargement is probably due to combination of hypertrophy and obstruction.

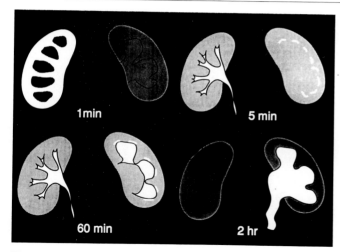

Figure 7–26. Schematic drawing of crescent sign of Dunbar. The crescents represent dilated and reoriented collecting tubules, which now lie parallel to the renal outline. If seen end-on, they will be seen as dots on the radiograph.

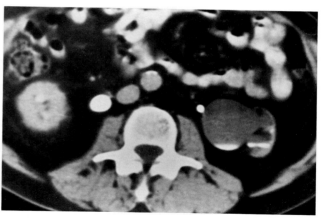

Figure 7–28. At first glance the diagnosis is obvious. Left hydronephrosis, fluid-fluid level, shell nephrogram, everything points to prolonged obstruction. The left kidney is small, but this "inappropriate" response to obstruction has been well documented. The bright dot at the medial aspect of the dilated left renal pelvis is not contrast but a ureteral catheter leading to the upper moiety, which is not obstructed. Also, there is a very dilated right ureter suggesting the presence of right obstruction.

cedure. Morbidity and mortality are far below those of operative nephrostomy. Most importantly, such simple percutaneous drainage buys precious time, during which many of the secondary problems described above may be brought under control (Figs. 7–38, 7–39, 7–40).[28,29]

Another indication for placing a percutaneous nephrostomy is to provide access to the upper urinary tract as a prelude to the numerous other radiological and endourological procedures discussed below.

Planning

The most important part is the preparatory stage. Consulting any prior radiological or ultrasound examinations, determining size, shape, and position of the collecting system, orientation of the pelvis and

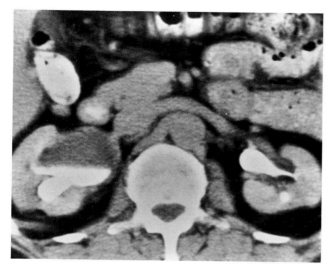

Figure 7–27. Fluid-fluid interface in a patient with distal ureteral obstruction. This is the same patient presented in Figure 7–23. It will take some time for the contrast level to rise and displace urine ahead of it. Since the ureteropelvic junction is anterior, it will take even longer for the ureter to opacify. Note thickened wall of the right renal pelvis.

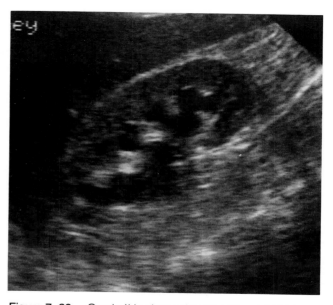

Figure 7–29. Grade II hydronephrosis of the right kidney.

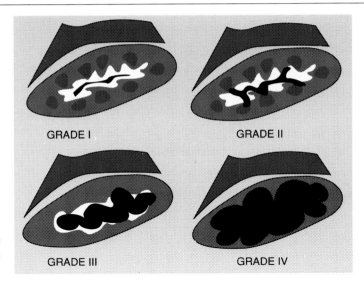

GRADE I GRADE II

GRADE III GRADE IV

Figure 7–30. Schematic drawing of four grades of hydronephrosis as seen on sonography.

infundibula and their relation to other major organ systems should never be overlooked. This is the time for planning the approach, the puncture site, the size and type of the catheter to be used, and for considering obstacles such as scoliosis, calculi, duplex system, high- or low-lying kidney, renal cysts, retrorenal liver (Fig. 7–41), spleen, and ascending and descending colon (Fig. 7–42). If at all possible, intravenous contrast should be given an hour or so before the procedure. Often, the collecting system will opacify sufficiently to greatly facilitate the puncture. If this is not feasible, ultrasound can be of great help, particularly if one is inexperienced. Having a biopsy transducer can also be very helpful.

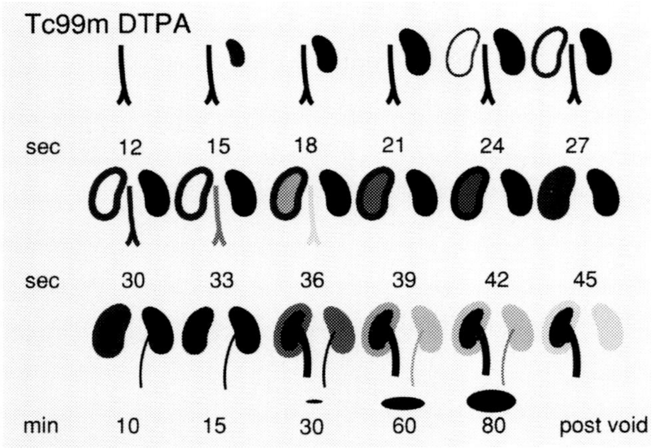

Positioning

The patient is positioned prone whenever possible (Fig. 7–43). This is not absolutely necessary, but such a position makes the interventional radiologist more comfortable. Sometimes the patient will not be able to tolerate the prone position and will have to be placed in the supine oblique position. In both positions the depth of field is impossible to determine and the position of the collecting system is determined almost by feel.

Procedure

As local anesthesia is given, we usually use a Lundequist needle catheter system to enter into the collecting system. As one approaches the renal outline under fluoroscopic control, the kidney and often the calyx will deflect slightly (Fig. 7–44). If they don't, the needle is out of the plane of the collecting system and puncture should not be attempted. Rather, the needle should be redirected either anteriorly or posteriorly and the procedure repeated. Once urine is aspirated, a 0.038 guidewire is introduced and positioned as deeply as possible within the collecting system or proximal ureter. This is accomplished with vascular dilators. The best type of nephrostomy tube is the Cope system. It has an inner stiffener so that it is easily introduced over the guidewire. A self-locking mechanism eliminates the need for skin suture, and it comes in a variety of sizes (8, 10, 12, and 14 F).

Tc99m DTPA

sec 12 15 18 21 24 27

sec 30 33 36 39 42 45

min 10 15 30 60 80 post void

Figure 7–31. Schematic drawing of appearance of urinary tract obstruction on Tc-99m DTPA scan. Scintigrams obtained after a bolus of the tracer demonstrate decreased excretion of the radionuclide in the right kidney and dilatation of the collecting system and ureter up to the point of obstruction.

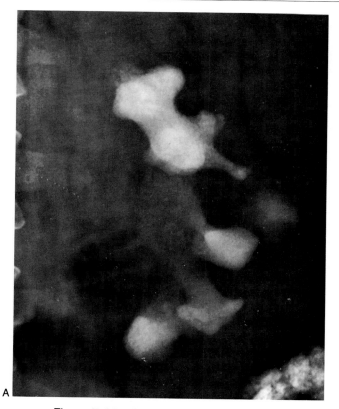
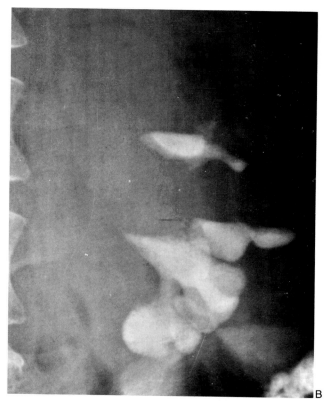

Figure 7–32. Milk of calcium urine in a completely obstructed and nonfunctioning kidney. In the supine position the appearance is that of a staghorn (**A**). In the upright position the small colloidal crystalline suspension layers in the dependent position (**B**).

Conversion to a Permanent Nephrostomy

Permanent percutaneous nephrostomy is the least desirable method of urinary tract diversion. Having to carry a bag and the social stigma associated with it are not the only problems. Frequent exchanges are necessary, urinary tract infections are common, and maintaining adequate hygiene may be difficult. Additionally, skin irritation and the usually inevitable progression of the primary disease, either malignancy or some other debilitating process, make it very difficult for many patients to deal with the permanent nephrostomy tube. Therefore it is only in very desperate situations that such a type of diversion should be considered.

The self-restraining Cope catheter system in a larger size (12 or 14 F) is an excellent choice for such a diversion. If, however, recurrent infections, particularly fungal infections, become a problem, the sinus tract needs to be enlarged to 20 or 24 F and a Foley or Mallecot catheter placed.

Internal Antegrade Ureteral Stenting

In many instances it is possible to negotiate a guidewire and a double pigtail catheter through an obstructed ureter in an antegrade fashion.[30] Two excellent stents are available with internal stiffeners. If anticipating antegrade stent placement during initial percutaneous nephrostomy placement, a more superior calyx should be chosen for initial entry into the collecting system. Such placement will greatly simplify stent placement, as at least one major curvature of the catheter has been eliminated and there are fewer vector lines to be concerned with. Choosing the proper length of the stent is important. Too long a stent will constantly irritate the bladder and make the patient miserable. Too short a stent may be lost within the upper urinary tract system without ever reaching the bladder, or it may retract from the bladder into the ureter. Such a stenting procedure may be used in patients with ileal loops, Kock's pouch, and other types of urinary diversion. One must understand the anatomical variance of these

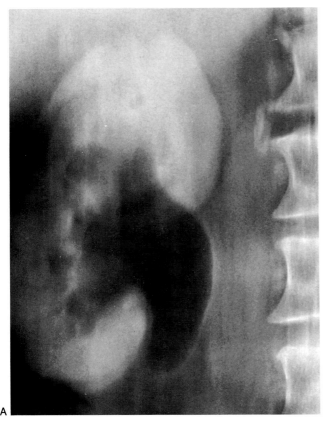
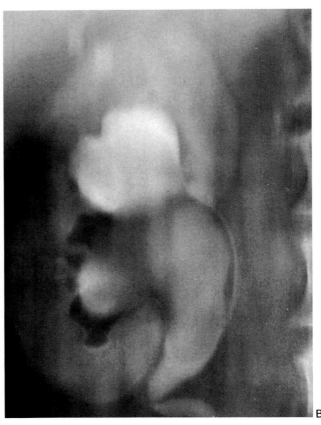

Figure 7–33.   Gas is present in the collecting system of the right kidney during an early nephrogram phase of an EXU (**A**). This is a solitary kidney in a patient with ureterosigmoidostomy, and gas most likely represents refluxing bowel gas. Dilatation of the collecting system suggests possible obstruction. Indeed, there was a mild mid-ureteral stricture (**B**).

operative procedures and make sure that the stents will be endoscopically retrievable at a future date (Fig. 7–45).

Besides providing for internal drainage in an obstruction, internal stenting may be successfully used in the management of iatrogenic ureteral fistulas. It is frequently possible to negotiate a ureteral lumen by using an antegrade approach, even if the retrograde approach proved impossible. Prolonged presence of the stent and adequate drainage are likely to result in complete healing without stricture formation (Fig. 7–46).

Percutaneous Endopyelotomy

Some types of urinary tract obstruction may be successfully treated using percutaneous approach. For example, percutaneous treatment of ureteropelvic junction obstruction is successful in over 85%.[31,32] The puncture site is usually through the posterior middle calyx with a posterolateral approach.[33–36] The tract is dilated to 28 or 30 F and

working sheet introduced. Under direct vision the entire thickness of the posterolateral wall (avoiding aberrant vessel if present) is divided, using either electrocautery or cold knife. The site may be enlarged with a balloon catheter. Finally, a universal 12 F stent is placed across the area of stenosis.

Percutaneous Removal of Lost Ureteral Stents

Lost ureteral stents may be removed percutaneously if endoscopic retrieval is impossible (Fig. 7–47).

URETEROPELVIC JUNCTION (UPJ) OBSTRUCTION

Congenital UPJ Obstruction

Incidence.   Most common abdominal mass during infancy and most common cause of urinary tract

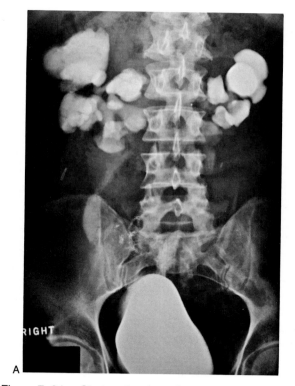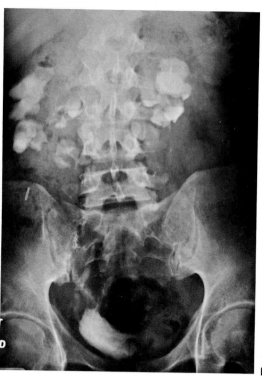

A   B

Figure 7–34. Obstruction or not? **(A)** EXU 30 minutes after contrast injection in a patient with prior history of obstruction, urolithiasis, and infection. Axes of both kidneys point inferomedially, characteristic for horseshoe kidneys. Dilated calyces are present bilaterally and could be due to current obstruction, effects of prior obstruction, urolithiasis, prior infections, etc. **(B)** In upright position the collecting system has appreciably emptied of contrast compared with first radiograph, thus excluding significant obstruction.

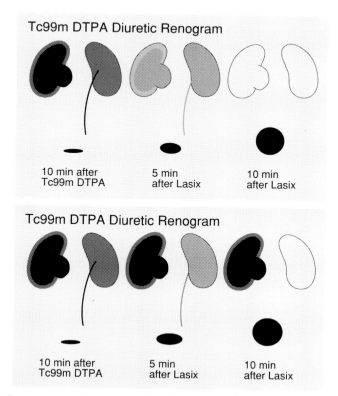

Figure 7–35. Schematic drawing of diuretic renogram. Ten minutes after challenge with diuretics, the normal side has cleared (top) while the radionuclide is still retained in the obstructed kidney (bottom).

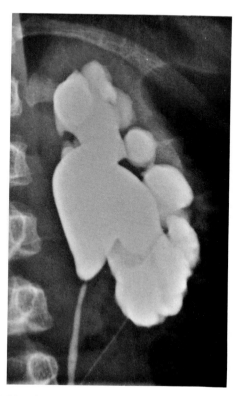

Figure 7–36. Ureteropelvic junction obstruction or no obstruction? Whitaker test discovers high intrapelvic pressures even with slow rate of antegrade perfusion.

125

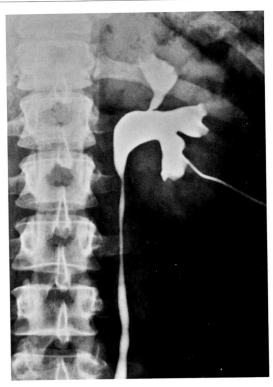

Figure 7–37. Whitaker test excludes presence of obstruction in a patient who had intermittent severe left flank pain and equivocal nuclear medicine challenge test.

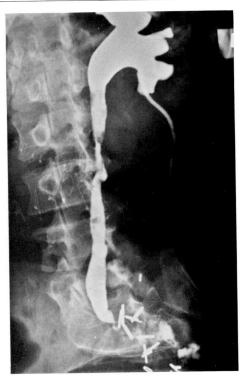

Figure 7–38. Several days after hemipelvectomy, the surgical wound is wet and infected. Urography demonstrates that the left ureter has been inadvertently clipped, resulting in obstruction, ureteral necrosis, urine leak, and sepsis. Percutaneous nephrostomy is placed to provide temporary drainage until infection is brought under control and a more opportune time is created for surgical correction.

obstruction in children. Frequently bilateral. More frequent in horseshoe and solitary kidney.

Pathology. Maloriented and attenuated smooth muscle with more than normal collagen between the muscle fibers resulting in afunctional and narrow segment. Varying degrees of hydronephrosis above the afunctional segment possible. May be considered the mildest expression of the hydronephrotic form of multicystic kidney disease.

Clinical Presentation. Intermittent acute flank pain, periodically provoked by massive diuresis (beer drinker's disease, Chilaiditi crisis, German disease). May be asymptomatic in the chronic stage. Palpable abdominal mass in infants. Prenatal diagnosis possible on sonography.

Radiological Findings. Varying degree of hydronephrosis and an extrarenal pelvis is present (Fig. 7–48). It is of some importance to visualize normal ureter distal to UPJ. This may be possible only on overhead lateral projection with the involved kidney away from the table. Frequently, there will be no evidence of obstruction at the time of examination and provocation tests (furosemide excretory urogra-

phy, Tc-99m DTPA scan, or Whitaker test) may be called for.

One should be aware that 15% of apparent obstructions are caused by an aberrant renal artery crossing the most proximal part of the ureter. This may have a characteristic appearance on an excretory urogram.[37,38] An angiogram should at least be considered in order to exclude or confirm the presence of the aberrant crossing vessel.

UPJ Obstruction Caused by Aberrant Renal Artery

Incidence. Fifteen percent of all patients with ureteropelvic junction obstruction.

Pathology. Extrinsic compression of the proximal ureter by a lower pole renal vessel. The vessel crosses the ureter anteriorly.

Clinical Presentation. Intermittent hydronephrosis is seen in most of the patients. Probably the most

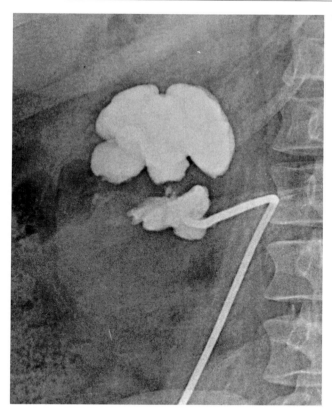

Figure 7–39. Patient with a solitary obstructed right kidney presents urosepsis. Percutaneous nephrostomy is placed that helps to eradicate infection and improve renal function. Nephrostogram demonstrates total ureteral obstruction, complete infundibular obstruction to the lower pole, and infundibular stenosis to the upper pole. Renal tuberculosis should be strongly suspected, but none was found.

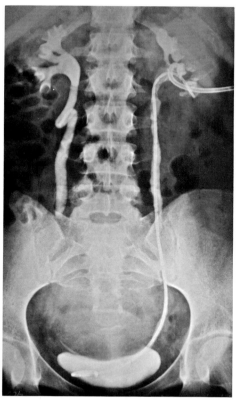

Figure 7–40. A 7-month pregnant woman had a percutaneous nephrostomy tube (PNT) placed because of urolithiasis and complete ureteral obstruction. Double "J" stents kept obstructing and kept compounding the problem. Patient carried the PNT until after delivery at which time this urogram was obtained. Note enlarged postpartum uterus. Urolithiasis was definitively treated at that time.

common cause of UPJ obstruction is a horseshoe kidney. Likely to present at a later age than congenital UPJ obstruction.

Treatment. Dismembered pyeloplasty, with anastomosis brought anteriorly to the aberrant obstructing lower pole vessel.

Radiological Findings. A small dilated proximal ureteral segment is almost diagnostic of the obstruction caused by the crossing vessel (Fig. 7–49). Since UPJ may be located anteriorly in an incompletely rotated kidney, an overhead contralateral projection or steep obliques may be needed to visualize these structures on an excretory urogram. Otherwise, the findings are identical to those in congenital UPJ obstruction.[39–42] Obstruction due to abberant vessels is common in horseshoe kidney (Fig. 7–50).

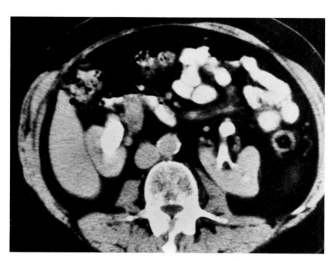

Figure 7–41. Retrorenal liver may present obstacles when upper pole approach is necessary, for instance in some types of percutaneous renal calculi removal or horseshoe kidney.

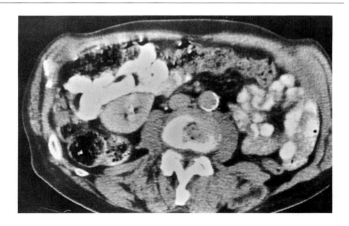

Figure 7–42.   Retrorenal colon is a normal positional variant. In this patient with solitary right kidney the colon is positioned in a way that virtually precludes percutaneous nephrostomy placement.

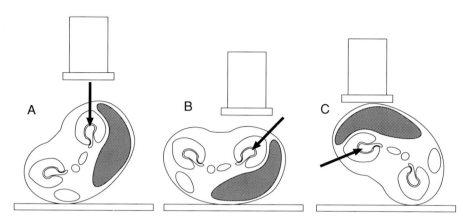

Figure 7–43.   Schematic drawing of different patient positions for percutaneous nephrostomy intended for the right kidney. **(A)** Prone oblique position is probably the easiest, although it forces the operator's hands into the primary x-ray beam. **(B)** Prone position is preferred by many as the operator's hands are out of the primary beam. Operator does not have depth of field perception. **(C)** Supine oblique position is necessary if for any reason the patient is unable to be placed prone.

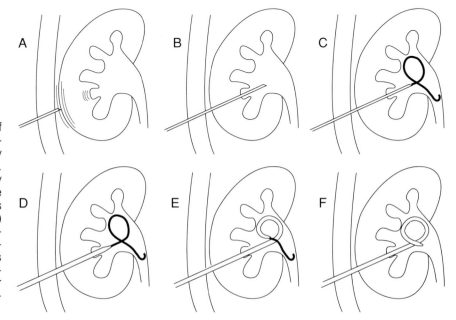

Figure 7–44.   Schematic drawing of PNT placement. **(A)** After local anesthesia is instilled, the introductory needle is directed toward the kidney. Slight deflecting motion of the kidney assures the operator that he is in the appropriate plane. **(B)** Puncture is made into the posterior calyx. **(C)** Proper position is confirmed by obtaining urine. Needle obturator is exchanged for a guidewire. **(D)** Tract is dilated using progressively larger dilators. **(E)** Finally PNT is placed over the guidewire, coiled in the collecting system, and **(F)** locked in place.

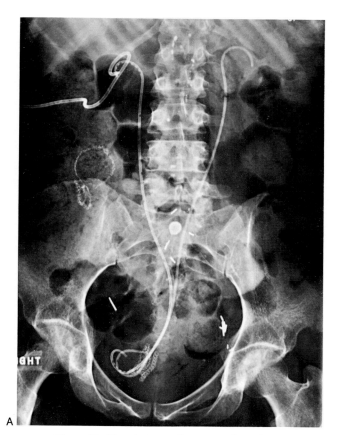
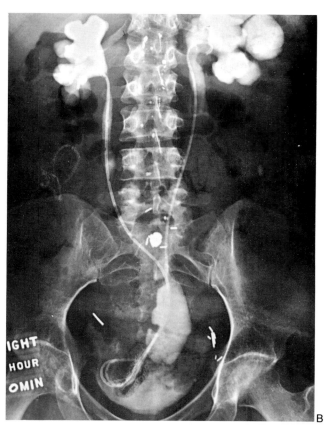

Figure 7–45. Antegrade stents placed in a patient with a Wallace loop, a type of continent diversion. **(A)** Note the bowel staples where the nipple has been created. **(B)** The antegrade stents are negotiated through the nipple and are easily retrievable endoscopically.

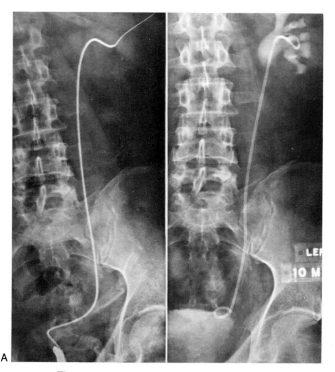
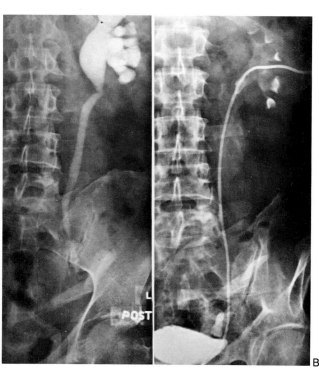

Figure 7–46. Sometimes it may be impossible to negotiate the catheter over the guidewire and endoscopic retrieval of the guidewire from the bladder is necessary. Having purchase from both sides of the wire, the stent is easier to place. **(A)** Obstruction and ureterocutaneous fistula are present after ureterolithotomy. Antegrade catheter is placed into the distal ureter but cannot be negotiated into the bladder. **(B)** Cystoscopically, the guidewire is retrieved from the bladder and antegrade stent is advanced. Stent is in good position on the follow-up EXU and was removed after several months.

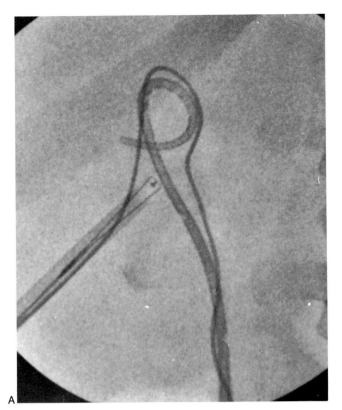

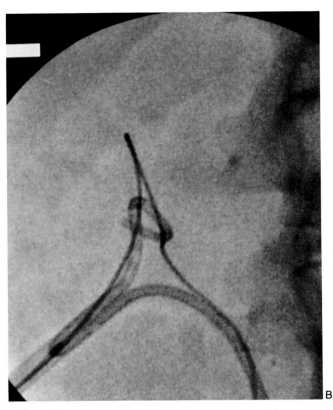

A

B

Figure 7–47. (A) A lost ureteral stent in the process of being percutaneously retrieved using a special grasper. (B) The jaws of the grasper are firmly locked around the stent, which is partially in the working sheet on its way out.

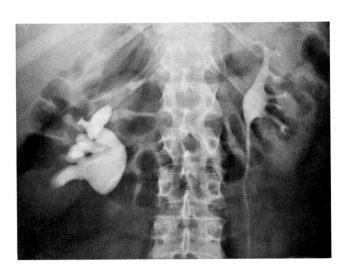

Figure 7–48. Mild ureteropelvic junction obstruction of the right kidney.

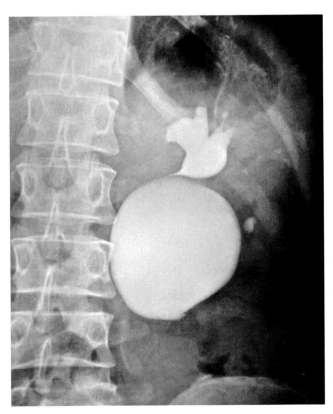

Figure 7–49. Proximal ureteral obstruction of the lower moiety in a duplex system close to UPJ is caused by a crossing vessel. The very proximal ureter can barely be visualized.

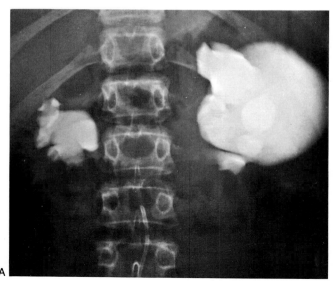

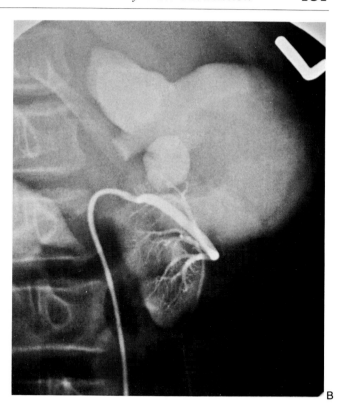

Figure 7–50. Proximal ureteral obstruction near or at UPJ in a patient with a horseshoe kidney. **(A)** EXU shows disproportionate dilatation of the renal pelvis compared with the calyces, particularly of the left kidney. Axes of both kidneys are oriented infereomedially, characteristic for horseshoe kidney. **(B)** Selective arteriogram of aberrant renal artery in the left posterior oblique projection demonstrates the vessel crossing the area of the obstruction.

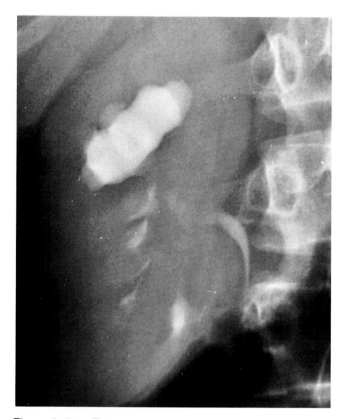

Figure 7–51. Fraley's syndrome caused by an upper pole crossing vessel. There is persistent dilatation of the upper pole calyx and retention of urine on the upright projection.

Simultaneous UPJ and UVJ Obstruction

Coexistence of UPJ and ureterovesical junction (UVJ) obstruction is a rare occurrence which makes the detection of either one of the two obstructions difficult.[43] Obstruction of the UVJ may be present even without ureteral dilatation and the obstruction may become evident only after UPJ has been surgically corrected.

FRALEY'S SYNDROME

Obstruction of the upper pole infundibulum may be caused by a crossing vessel (Fig. 7–51).[44,45] Pain and infection may be severe enough to require surgical management. On imaging studies, dilated upper pole calyx and varying degrees of parenchymal atrophy may be seen. Frequently an impression upon the upper infundibulum by the crossing vessel is seen on contrast studies.

REFERENCES

1. Laing FC, Jeffrey RB Jr, Wing VW. Ultrasound versus excretory urography in evaluating acute flank pain. Radiology 1985; 154:613–616.

2. Erwin BC, Carroll BA, Sommer FG. US in the evaluation of acute flank pain. Radiology 1985; 157:554.

3. Laing FC, Jeffrey RB Jr, Wing VW. US in the evaluation of acute flank pain: reply. Radiology 1985; 157:554.

4. Dyer RB, Munitz HA, Bechtold R, Choplin RH. Abnormal nephrogram. Radiographics 1986; 6:1039–1052.

5. Maillet PJ, Pelle-Francoz D, Laville M, et al. Nondilated obstructive acute renal failure: diagnostic procedures and therapeutic management. Radiology 1986; 160:659–662.

6. Goldfarb CR, Ongseng F, Chokshi V. Nondilated obstructive uropathy. Radiology 1987; 162:879–882.

7. Naidich JB, Rackson ME, Mossey RT, Stein HL. Nondilated obstructive uropathy: percutaneous nephrostomy performed to reverse renal failure. Radiology 1986; 160:653–656.

8. Naidich JB, Rackson ME, Mossey RT, Stein HL. Nondilated obstructive uropathy: reply. Radiology 1987; 162:879–882.

9. Dunbar JS, Nogrady MB. The calyceal crescent-roentgenographic sign of obstructive hydronephrosis. Am J Roentgenol 1970; 110:520–528.

10. Griscom NT, Kroeker MA. Visualization of individual papillary ducts (ducts of Bellini) by excretory urography in childhood hydronephrosis. Radiology 1973; 106:385–389.

11. Whitfield HN, Britton KE, Hendrey WF, Wickham JEA. Furosemide intravenous urography in the diagnosis of pelviureteric junction obstruction. Br J Urol 1979; 51:445–448.

12. Howman-Giles R, Uren R, Roy LP, et al. Volume expansion diuretic renal scan in urinary tract obstruction. J Nucl Med 1987; 28:824–828.

13. Bevis CRA, Shields RA, Lawson RS, et al. Comparison of technetium-99m-thiodiglycolic acid and iodine-123-hippuran in the evaluation of equivocal upper urinary tract obstruction. Br J Radiol 1987; 60:661–665.

14. Whitaker RH. Methods of assessing obstruction in dilated ureters. J Urol 1973; 45:15–22.

15. Marshal V. Whitaker RH. Ureteral pressure flow studies in difficult diagnostic problems. J Urol 1975; 114:201–207.

16. Whitaker RH. An evaluation of 170 diagnostic pressure flow studies of the upper urinary tract. J Urol 1979; 121:602–604.

17. Pfister RC, Newhouse JH. Interventional percutaneous pyeloureteral techniques: antegrade pyelography and ureteral perfusion. Radiol Clin North Am 1979; 17:341–350.

18. Pfister RC, Newhouse HJ, Hendren WH. Percutaneous pyeloureteral urodynamics. Urol Clin North Am 1982; 9:41–49.

19. Newhouse JH, Pfister RC, Hendren WH, et al. Whitaker test after pyeloplasty: establishment of normal ureteral perfusion pressures. AJR 1981; 137:223–226.

20. Hay AM, Norman WJ, Rich ML, et al. A comparison between diuresis renography and the Whitaker test in 64 kidneys. Br J Urol 1984; 56:561–564.

21. Senac MO, Miller JH, Stanley P. Evaluation of obstructive uropathy in children: Radionuclide renography vs. the Whitaker test. AJR 1984; 143:11–15.

22. Kass EJ, Majd M, Belman AB: Comparison of the diuretic renogram and the pressure perfusion study in children. J Urol 1985; 134:92–96.

23. Pfister RC, Papanicolay N, Yoder IC. Diagnostic morphologic and urodynamic antegrade pyelography. Radiol Clin North Am 1986; 24:561–570.

24. Platt JF, Rubin JM, Ellis JH, DiPietro MA. Duplex Doppler US of the kidney: differentiation of obstructive from nonobstructive dilatation. Radiology 1989; 171:515–517.

25. Scola FH, Cronan JJ, Schepps B. Grade I hydronephrosis: pulsed Doppler US evaluation. Radiology 1989; 171:519–520.

26. Goodwin WE, Casey WC, Woolf W. Percutaneous trocar (needle) nephrostomy in hydronephrosis. JAMA 1955; 157:891–894.

27. Barbaric ZL. Percutaneous nephrostomy for urinary tract obstruction. AJR 1984; 143:803–809.

28. Thompsen HS, Dorph S. Upper urinary tract: pyelography and interventional procedures. Acta Radiol (Stockh) 1987; 28:129–134.

29. Ball WS Jr, Towbin RB, Strife JL, et al. Interventional gentiourinary radiology in children: review of 61 procedures. AJR 1986; 147:791–796.

30. Mitty HA, Dan SJ, Train JS. Antegrade ureteral stents: technical and catheter-related problems with polyethylene and polyurethane. Radiology 1987; 165:439–442.

31. Lee WJ, Badlani GH, Karlin GS, Smith AD. Treatment of ureteropelvic strictures with percutaneous pyelotomy: experience with 62 patients. AJR 1988; 151:515–518.

32. Clayman RV, Hunter D, Surya V, et al. Percutaneous intrarenal electrosurgery. J Urol 1984; 131:866–867.

33. Whitfield HN, Mills V, Miller RA, Wickham JEA. Percutaneous pyelolysis: an alternative to pyeloplasty. Br J Urol 1983; 55 (suppl):93–96.

34. Bush WH, Brannen GE, Lewis GP. Ureteropelvic junction obstruction: treatment with percutaneous endopyelotomy. Radiology 1989; 171:535–538.

35. Korth K, Kuenkel M, Erschig M. Percutaneous pyeloplasty. Urology 1988; 31:503–509.

36. Cardella JF, Hunter DW, Castaneda-Zuniga WR, et al. Electrolysis for recanalization of urinary collecting system obstructions: a percutaneous approach. Radiology 1985; 155:87–90.

37. Snyder HM III, Lebowitz RL, Colodny AH, et al. Ureteropelvic junction obstruction in children. Urol Clin North Am 1980; 7:273–289.

38. Barry WF, Fetter BF, Glenn JF. The abnormal ureteropelvic junction: a muscle deficit. Radiology 1972; 104:43–44.

39. Stephens FD. Ureterovascular hydronephrosis and the "aberrant" renal vessels. J Urol 1982; 128:984–987.

40. Addonizio JC, Patel RC. Innocent aberrant renal vessels producing ureteropelvic junction obstruction. Urology 1980; 16:176–180.

41. Perlberg S, Pfau A. Management of ureteropelvic junction obstruction associated with lower polar vessels. Urology 1984; 23:13–18.

42. Hoffer FA, Lebowitz RL. Intermittent hydronephrosis: a unique feature of ureteropelvic junction obstruction caused by a crossing renal vessel. Radiology 1985; 156:655–658.

43. McGrath MA, Estroff J, Lebowitz RL. The coexistence of obstruction at the ureteropelvic and ureterovesical junctions. AJR 1987; 149:403–406.

44. Fraley EE. Vascular obstruction of superior infundibulum causing nephralgia. A new syndrome. N Engl J Med 1966; 275:1403–1409.

45. Fraley EE. Dismembered infundibulopyelostomy; improved technique for correcting vascular obstruction of the superior infundibulum. J Urol 1969; 101:144–148.

8

Urinary Tract Infection

RENAL BACTERIAL INFECTIONS

Acute Bacterial Pyelonephritis

Etiology. *E. coli, Proteus, Pseudomonas,* enterococ-cus, *or Klebsiella.*

Pathology. Acute interstitial inflammatory process of the renal parenchyma and renal pelvis with neu-trophilic leukocyte infiltration. Some tubular de-struction and microabscesses may be present. The process may be diffuse or focal. Unchecked inflam-mation may progress into a renal abscess or result in gradual atrophy by tubular destruction, glomerular hyalinization, and scarring.

Clinical Presentation. Abdominal and flank pain, costovertebral angle tenderness to percussion, fever, vomiting, frequency, oliguria. Asymptomatic in 50%.

Laboratory Findings. Bacteriuria, hematuria, py-uria, leukocyte casts, leukocytosis.

Radiological Findings. Pathological signs of any acute inflammatory process, including in the kidney, are: *rubor* (redness), *calor* (elevated temperature), *dolor* (pain), *tumor* (mass, enlargement), and *functio laesa* (impaired function).

Urographic, sonographic, or CT images cannot display redness or elevated temperature. A radiolo-gist can only occasionally suspect the presence of local pain, reflected in the curvature of the spine (splinting). What can be detected is mass effect and impaired function, but even these findings are seen in only 20% of all cases on excretory urography (Fig. 8–1). Thus, 80% of examinations in acute pyelone-phritis will be normal and are hardly worth the inconvenience for the average patient.

There are, however, more fulminating forms of pyelonephritis, with more pronounced symptoms, fever of unknown origin, or those that do not respond to antibiotic treatment within 48–72 hours.[1-3] These forms of pyelonephritis are commonly seen in pa-tients with urinary tract calculi, diabetes,[4] and neu-ropathic bladder. Regardless of severity, the fol-lowing are the positive findings encountered in this disease by imaging modalities using radiographic contrast:

1. *Renal enlargement.* Increase in size is due to in-flammatory edema, multiple microabscesses, and, at least in part, to tubular obstruction by purulent debris. Expansion is outward and also inward, toward the renal sinus, due to restriction imposed by the renal capsule. Elongation, nar-rowing, and splaying or "spidery" appearance of the collecting system may ensue. On rare occa-sions, the opposite kidney may enlarge, even with-out clinical signs of inflammation (Fig. 8–2).
2. *Diminished or absent function.* Contrast excretion into the collecting system may be diminished or completely absent.
3. *Inhomogeneous nephrogram.* Since some tubules (convoluted or collecting) are filled with inflam-matory debris, the nephrogram may appear quite bizarre. This can range from poorly defined areas of low attenuation ("patchy") nephrogram, in-creased[5] and decreased enhancement in wedge-shaped areas[3] (Fig. 8–3), to a very faint nephro-gram (Fig. 8–4).
4. *Thickening of the renal fascia.* This finding may indicate early perinephric extension of the inflam-matory process.

133

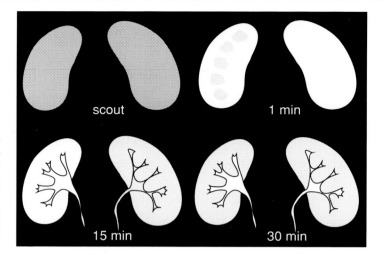

Figure 8–1. Schematic presentation of radiographic signs in acute pyelonephritis on urography. Renal enlargement of the affected kidney, rather poor nephrogram, and poor concentration of contrast in the collecting system. Spidery, elongated calyces are a reflection of inward renal expansion.

5. *Edema of the renal pelvis.* Striations and filling defects may be seen on excretory urography or pyelography (Fig. 8–5). Thickening of the pelvocalyceal wall has also been described.

Focal Acute Pyelonephritis (Acute Lobar Nephronia)

The term "acute lobar nephronia" was introduced to distinguish this localized disease from diffuse acute bacterial pyelonephritis.[6]

Mass effect may be seen on any one of imaging studies. On ultrasound there may be loss of corticomedullary junction and displacement of the central sinus complex by the mass, which in most instances is hypoechoic compared with normal renal parenchyma.[7]

On precontrast CT, the mass is of same radiodensity as the kidney. On contrast-enhanced CT, there is poor or absent nephrogram in the area (Fig. 8–6).[8] Renal sinus may be displaced (Fig. 8–7).

If urine cultures are negative, thin needle placement with irrigation utilizing a small amount of fluid may give the specific bacteriological diagnosis. Septic infarct enters into differential diagnosis under appropriate clinical setting (Fig. 8–8).

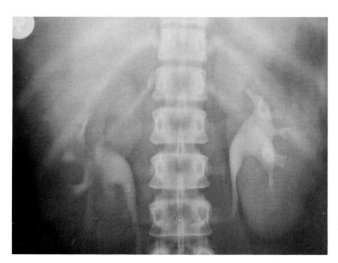

Figure 8–2. Bilateral renal enlargement in a patient with clinical right pyelonephritis. Concomitant diseases that may result in renal enlargement, such as early diabetes mellitus, were not present. Left renal enlargement was probably due to subclinical pyelonephritis.

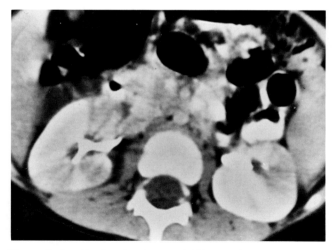

Figure 8–3. Contrast-enhanced CT scan in a patient with bilateral acute pyelonephritis. Wedge-shaped and patchy areas of decreased and somewhat striated nephrogram are the common finding on this examination. CT, with superior contrast resolution, outweighs other imaging modalities in determining the presence and the extent of the process.

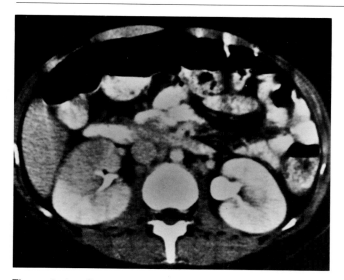

Figure 8–4. Contrast-enhanced CT in a patient with right acute pyelonephritis. Most of the kidney is involved with the inflammatory process. Poor nephrogram and renal enlargement are obvious when compared to the left kidney.

Renal and Perirenal Abscess

Etiology. *E. coli, Proteus, Staphylococcus, Pseudomonas,* enterococcus, *or Klebsiella.*

Pathology. Acute inflammatory process of the renal parenchyma with necrosis of the parenchyma and liquefaction. May extend into perinephric space. May contain gas.

Clinical Presentation. Fever, chills, abdominal and flank pain, nausea, vomiting, costovertebral angle tenderness. Urolithiasis, prior urological surgery, and diabetes mellitus are common predisposing factors. In 10% of patients fever and flank tenderness may be absent.

Laboratory Findings. Bacteriuria, hematuria, pyuria, leukocyte casts, leukocytosis. In some cases urine culture may be normal.

Radiological Findings. Renal abscess presents as a mass lesion in the kidney. Renal function may or may

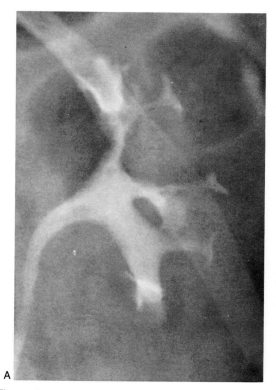

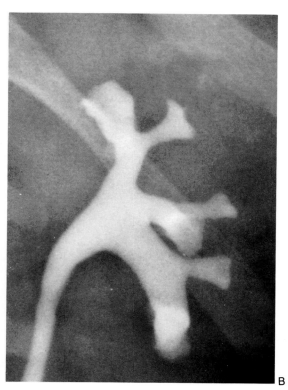

A

B

Figure 8–5. (A) Retrograde pyelogram in a patient with acute pyelonephritis. Mucosal irregularities are present and differential diagnosis includes mucosal edema, transitional cell carcinoma, and renal vein thrombosis. **(B)** Repeat retrograde pyelogram 2 weeks after appropriate antibiotic therapy shows resolution of mucosal irregularities. Mucosal edema due to inflammation has subsided.

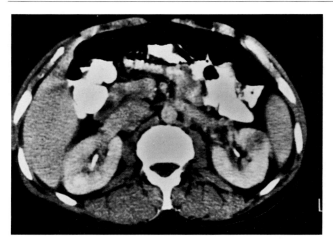

Figure 8–6. Focal acute pyelonephritis involves smaller area in the left kidney and also shows inhomogeneous nephrogram. Only local enlargement is present, mimicking a tumor mass.

not be affected. The mass is relatively hypovascular when seen on nephrotomography or dynamic CT scan. Thick wall, which may enhance, is the rule on both examinations (Figs. 8–9, 8–10). Ultrasound may also demonstrate a hypoechoic mass with internal echoes.

Larger renal abscesses should be drained percutaneously or otherwise (Fig. 8–11).[9,10] Small renal abscesses may be treated conservatively (Fig. 8–12).[11]

Large renal abscesses frequently perforate into the collecting system (Fig. 8–13). Perforation into other visceral organs is rare (Fig. 8–14).

Perirenal abscess presents as a fluid collection or low attenuation mass around the kidney; wall enhancement may be evident, and thickened renal fascia and septa are also seen within the perirenal space (Fig. 8–15). Gas formation is seen on occasion. Renal abscess and perinephric abscess may coincide (Fig. 8–16). Treatment should include drainage, preferably using percutaneous techniques.[12,13]

Emphysematous Pyelonephritis

Emphysematous pyelonephritis is a fulminating form of acute pyelonephritis seen mainly in diabetics and has a 50% mortality. Classic plain radiography or CT findings are diffuse radiolucencies throughout the kidney, minimal or no function, renal enlargement, and occasionally gas in the ureter and perinephric space (Fig. 8–17). The distribution of the gas throughout the kidney may also be localized. The term "emphysematous" relates to the crackling sounds the kidney emits when hand squeezed at autopsy, a sound similar to an emphysematous lung. CT is the best imaging modality. Ultrasound may demonstrate hyperechoic areas with intense acoustical shadowing.[14]

Following embolization of a renal carcinoma, gas may be seen in the infarcted tissues. Unless accompanied by signs of systemic infection, the presence of this gas is probably benign, similar to the gas seen in the soft tissues of a dead fetus.

Pyohydronephrosis

The concomitant presence of urinary tract obstruction and acute infection is a serious and, on occasion, life-threatening situation. The excretion of antibiotics into an obstructed system seriously diminishes.

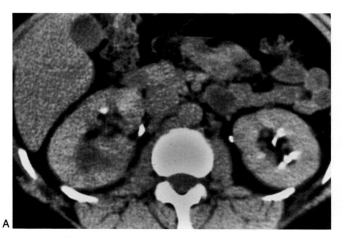

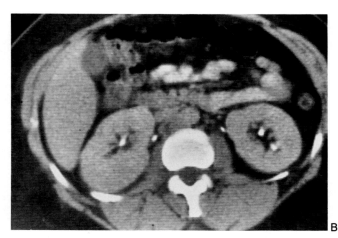

Figure 8–7. Focal acute pyelonephritis in the lower pole of the right kidney. The mass associated with the focal infection is impressing on the renal sinus and lower pole calyx resulting in incomplete filling (**A**). Moderate improvement is seen after 1 week of antibiotic therapy (**B**).

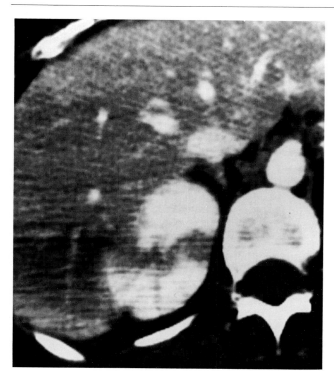

Figure 8–8. Contrast-enhanced CT scan in a patient believed to have had a septic renal infarct. Two triangular, wedge-shaped areas with absent nephrogram are present.

The presence of inflammatory cellular and bacterial debris further hampers any beneficial effect of the small quantities of antibiotic that may reach the renal collecting system. Lost or diminished function, renal enlargement, and the presence of dilatation strongly suggest the diagnosis. CT is the most convincing examination because it will show anatomical as well as functional status of the kidney. The diag-

nosis can be made as easily on ultrasound (Fig. 8–18) and IVP.

Treatment is urgent or otherwise a number of functioning nephrons will be irreversibly lost. The obstructed system must be decompressed as soon as possible, either by placement of retrograde stents or percutaneous nephrostomy. If nephrostomy is the method of decompression, antegrade nephrostogram should not be attempted until the infectious process is under control. Increased pressure in the collecting system could contribute to pyelointerstitial or pyelovenous backflow and sepsis.

Imaging Choices

Most patients with acute pyelonephritis are diagnosed on the basis of their clinical presentation. In most instances imaging contributes little to the diagnosis and in most cases the findings are normal. However, if a positive response to antibiotic therapy is not evident within 48 hours, an underlying complicating factor must be considered. Either there is obstruction, perinephric extension of the inflammatory process, abscess formation, or other complication. Most of the complicating features need specific treatment. The imaging study has to be the one that can evaluate parenchymal appearance, detect obstruction and its cause and level, and do it rapidly, reproducibly, and accurately. CT is the obvious method of choice in evaluating these patients as it most accurately defines the extent of the disease, guiding early and accurate therapy.[3,15,16]

Unusual Bacterial Infections

Urinary tract infection with nontyphi *Salmonella* is rare and almost always associated with a predispos-

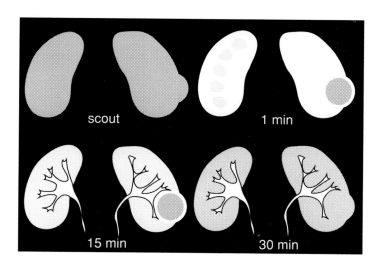

Figure 8–9. Schematic presentation of a renal abscess on contrast examination such as excretory urogram. A radiolucent mass, typically with thick enhancing wall, is present.

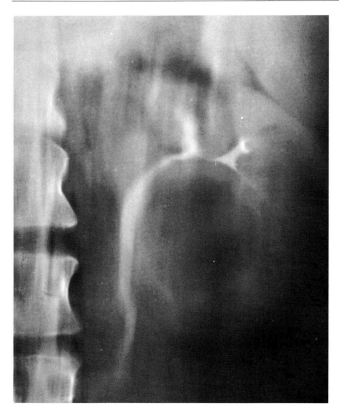

Figure 8–10. Renal abscess on excretory urography. Displacement of the collecting system, although obvious, is not specific. Radiolucency likewise may be seen in simple cysts. Enhancing wall, on the other hand, should suggest abscess as the diagnosis.

ing anomaly, such as ureteropelvic junction obstruction or urolithiasis.[17–19]

Urinary Tract Infection in Children

Etiology. *E. coli, Proteus* (associated with urolithiasis), *Staphylococcus* (in boys).

Incidence. Prevalence of asymptomatic bacteriuria in girls is 1.2 to 4% and practically nonexistent in boys in preschool and school-age groups.

Contributing Factors. *Vesicoureteral reflux* is commonly present. The reflux may be primary (maldevelopment of UPJ) or secondary (due to detrusor-sphincter dysenergia or Hutch diverticulum). Some bacterial endotoxins may paralyze the ureter so that reflux may appear worse in the presence of infection. *Aberrant micturition* (emptying the bladder into the ureter) results in residual and stagnant urine, promoting infection. Bacteria may be carried into the collecting tubules if *intrarenal reflux* is present.

Obstruction at any level, but more so outflow bladder obstruction, and obstruction at distal ureteral level, promote infection. This is probably because bacteria may not be as readily washed away in an impaired flow situation, and also because stagnant urine provides an opportunity for bacterial growth.

Bladder dysfunction may also be the cause for outflow bladder obstruction and excessive amount of residual urine.

Clinical Presentation. Lower urinary tract: dysuria, frequency, foul-smelling urine.

Upper urinary tract: flank pain, abdominal pain, fever.

Laboratory Findings. "Clean catch" bacteriuria greater than 100,000 colonies/ml, preferably in two consecutive specimens. Less than that if the specimen is collected by catheterization or suprapubic puncture.

Radiological Workup

1. Why? Imaging in children with documented urinary tract infection is geared to discover, exclude, or assess: a) vesicoureteral reflux; b) obstruction; c) bladder dysfunction; d) acute renal infection; e) chronic sequelae of infection (renal scars, calyceal clubbing); and f) monitor children at increased risk.[20,21]

 2. Who?[21]
   a. Children with well-documented urinary tract infection by culture.
   b. Children presenting with acute or critical illness, even without culture results.
   c. Children with bladder dysfunction.
   d. Children with renal failure and/or hypertension.
   e. Children at higher risk (siblings of patients with known reflux).

3. What age? Most renal scarring associated with infection and vesicoureteral reflux occurs early in life and the damage is done by the age of 5 and certainly by the age of 10 years.[21–22] Later than that, scarring is unusual unless there is massive reflux.

 4. What study?
   a. Infant or younger child presenting with well-documented urinary tract infection is examined by voiding cystourethrography (VCUG).[22] If reflex is discovered, an excretory urogram is done to critically assess the presence of renal scars.[21] If no reflux is detected, renal ultrasound is adequate to evaluate renal morphology.[21,23,24] Abnormal ultrasound findings may raise the need for an excretory urogram.

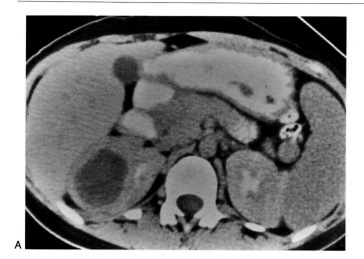

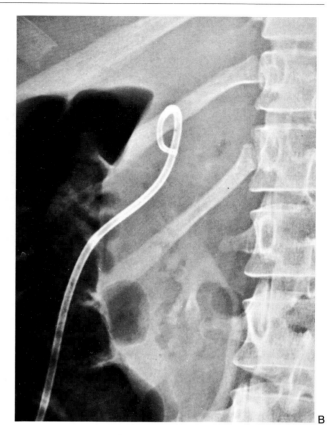

Figure 8–11. Upper pole abscess in the right kidney. Thick wall is present, although enhancement is not immediately obvious, probably because of inadequate bolus injection **(A)**. Percutaneous drainage in this high lesion was accomplished via the intercostal approach **(B)**.

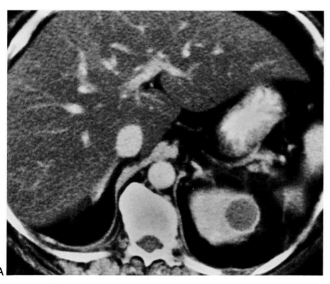

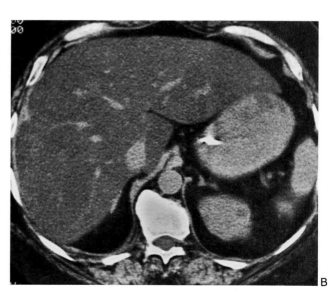

Figure 8–12. Smallish left upper pole abscess shows typical wall enhancement in addition to mass effect and radiolucent nonenhancing center. Aspiration under ultrasound was difficult and yielded only a few drops of purulent material which grew *E. coli* **(A)**. After a week of appropriate antibiotic therapy, the abscess is almost healed with marked diminution in size **(B)**. Note markedly radiolucent liver both on enhanced **(A)** and nonenhanced **(B)** scan due to fatty degeneration.

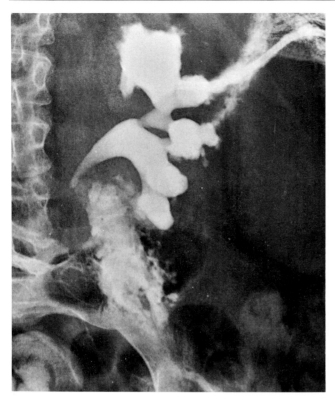

Figure 8–13. Large renal abscess was drained percutaneously. Communication with the collecting system was evident on the antegrade injection of contrast material. In addition, there is ureteral perforation and leakage of contrast material into the retroperitoneum where a retroperitoneal abscess is bound to form.

b. Afebrile child with lower urinary tract symptoms may be examined by nuclear cystogram and if reflux is detected it may be further characterized by a VCUG and excretory urogram. If nuclear cystogram is normal, ultrasound of the kidney is adequate to assess renal morphology and exclude obstruction.[21]

c. Older child or teenager whose kidneys are no longer in danger of scarring because of reflux, need only be examined by ultrasound,[25] or if unavailable, by excretory urography[26] or renal scintigram. VCUG is obtained if these are abnormal.

5. When in relation to infection? VCUG can be obtained any time after the acute episode is under control and over.[21] In an acutely ill child ultrasound may be obtained any time if obstruction is suspected.[24]

Radiological Findings. See "Refluxing Nephropathy" in Chapter 13.

TUBERCULOSIS

Incidence. Ten percent of patients with pulmonary TB.

Etiology. *Mycobacterium tuberculosis.*

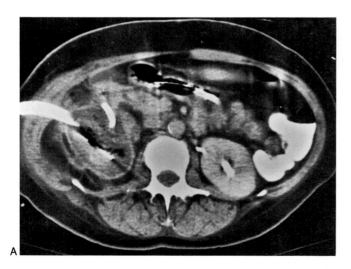

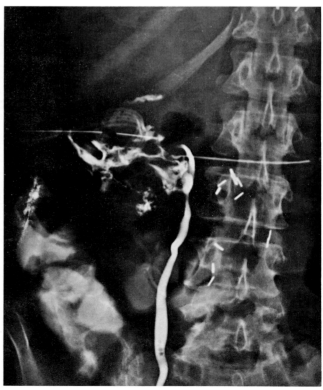

Figure 8–14. Contrast-enhanced CT scan in a patient who had surgical drainage of an "abscess in the gallbladder fossa" (elsewhere). Surgical drain is obviously transversing the nonfunctioning right kidney, which shows rim enhancement **(A)**. There is communication with the second part of duodenum on retrograde pyelogram **(B)**. Following right nephrectomy, the kidney was found to be necrosed.

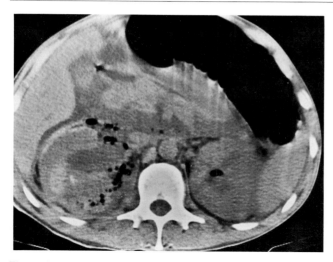

Figure 8–15. Right perirenal abscess in a patient with concomitant bilateral ureteral obstruction. Gas appears in the collecting system of the left kidney because a nephrostomy tube has been placed.

Pathology. Small tubercules in the renal cortex, and eventually in the medulla. Tubercles enlarge and undergo caseous necrosis. Spread is down the ureter. Fibrosis, scarring, and calcifications dominate in the healing stage. Genital organs may become involved.

Clinical Presentation. Pyuria, dysuria, hematuria, frequency, fatigue, malaise, cough.[27]

Laboratory Findings. A positive culture of tuberculous bacillus. Positive skin test and smear.

Radiological Findings.

1. *Papillary necrosis.* Bacillus is initially confined to the renal cortex and by tubular propagation spread occurs in the medulla where caseous ulcerative tubercle appears on a renal papilla. The earliest radiographic finding is a shaggy papilla leading to papillary necrosis (Fig. 8–19).[28] While other diseases associated with papillary necrosis cause occlusion of the vasa recta, the destruction of the papilla in tuberculosis is due to the specific type of necrotic, proteolytic process.

2. *Renal mass.* On occasion, the localized inflammatory process becomes bulky with subsequent development of a tuberculoma (Fig. 8–20). Caseous necrosis may eventually develop a cavity.[28–30]

3. *Mucosal irregularity.* As the bacilli seed down the urinary stream, foci of infection form in the pelvis (Fig. 8–21) and ureters with subsequent thickening and irregularity of the transitional epithelium.

4. *Infundibular stenosis.* Healing phase is characterized by stricture formation. Individual calyx may become obstructed and dilated *(hydrocalyx)* due to an infundibular stricture.[28] There may be no excretion of the contrast into the obstructed calyx *(amputated calyx)* (Fig. 8–22).

5. *Purse-string sign.* Retractable fibrosis of the pelvocalyceal system ensues in the healing stage. Pelvis assumes characteristic appearance when the cicatrized renal pelvis is retracted into the renal sinus (Figs. 8–23, 24).

6. *Ureteral strictures.* As the healing process continues, ureteral strictures, single or multiple (Fig. 8–25), and skipped areas of intact ureter may be seen *(corkscrew ureter)* (Fig. 8–21).[31] Eventually, the entire ureter may be involved and rigid in appearance *(pipe stem ureter)*.

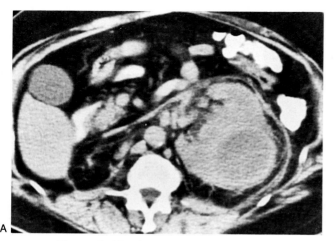
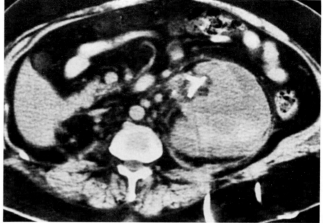

Figure 8–16. Large abscess in an obstructed solitary kidney **(A)**. During an attempted percutaneous nephrostomy tube placement, the abscess was transversed and perinephric hematoma and abscess eventually developed **(B)**. Acute hemorrhage appears radiodense. Note marked thickening of renal fascia associated with inflammatory process.

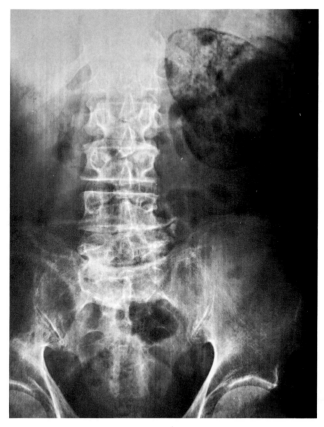

Figure 8–17. Plain radiograph in an elder diabetic presenting with emphysematous pyelonephritis and septic shock. Gas seen as radiolucencies permeates throughout the renal parenchyma and subcapsular areas. An associated renal mass is outlined by gas. Gas is also seen in the proximal ureter.

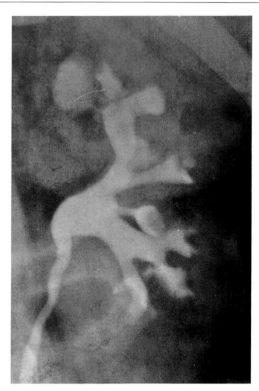

Figure 8–19. Varying stages of papillary necrosis in renal tuberculosis.

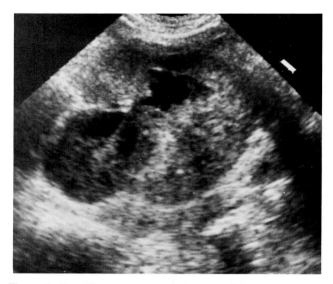

Figure 8–18. Transverse renal ultrasound demonstrates dilated collecting system and extrarenal pelvis. Cellular debris may be seen in the renal pelvis, forming a fluid-fluid level. The obstructed infected system was urgently drained by placing a percutaneous nephrostomy.

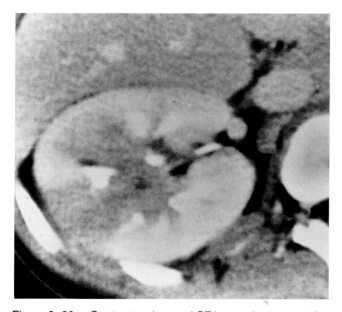

Figure 8–20. Contrast-enhanced CT in a patient presenting with fever of unknown origin. There was no hematuria and urine cultures were normal. The mass effect on the collecting system and patchy loss of nephrogram was an incidental finding. Eventually, open biopsy confirmed the diagnosis of renal tuberculosis.

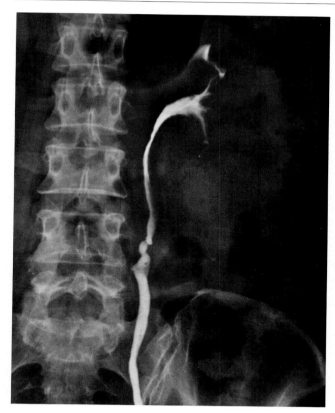

Figure 8–21. Subtle mucosal irregularity in the renal pelvis. Ureteral narrowing resembles a corkscrew.

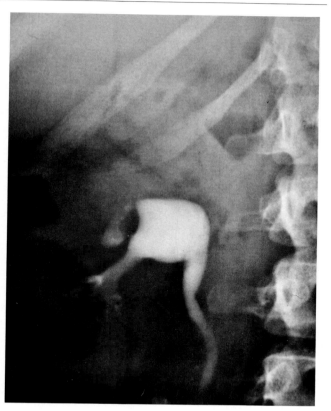

Figure 8–22. There is no filling of the upper pole calyx because the cicatrizing process has caused a stricture of the upper infundibulum. Hydronephrotic upper pole is not excreting contrast and there can be no reflux from the pelvis into the upper pole calyx. Also present are subtle changes involving the papillae in the mid and lower calyceal groups.

7. *Autonephrectomy.* Finally, the entire kidney is destroyed and replaced with a fibrotic process. Calcification eventually occurs throughout the shrunken kidney (Fig. 8–26).
8. Bladder eventually becomes involved. Small, *contracted, irregular bladder* of diminished capacity is demonstrated on contrast examination.
9. Tuberculous orchitis, epididymitis, and prostatitis are comparatively rare. Uterus, ovaries, and oviducts may also be affected.
10. Adrenal glands. It is rare to see adrenal gland involvement in the active stage of the disease. *Calcifications,* however, are seen in later stages of the disease.
11. *Psoas abscess.*
12. Renocolic fistula may be seen in extreme cases.
13. There may be increased incidence of renal carcinoma[32] and renovascular hypertension[33,34] in patients with end-stage renal tuberculosis.
14. Diagnosis of renal tuberculosis is easily made on excretory urogram or retrograde pyelogram when multiple radiographic findings, seemingly unrelated to each other, are present. Even if only one sign discussed above is present, tuberculosis

must be suggested in differential diagnosis (Fig. 8–27). Differential diagnosis includes papillary necrosis, infundibular stenosis of other origin (including neoplasm), and brucellosis.

URINARY BRUCELLOSIS

Etiology. *Brucella abortus* (cattle), *Brucella melitensis* (sheep), *Brucella suis* (pigs), *Brucella canis* (dogs). Gram-negative coccobacilli. Infection results from ingestion of raw milk or in slaughterhouse workers, farmers, and animal handlers.

Pathology. Penetration is through skin or mucous membranes and spread is via lymphatic system and hematogenously. Granulomas consisting of lymphocytes, epithelioid, plasma, and giant cells develop in many organs. Caseation necrosis may occur in severe cases. Many organ systems may be involved. In man

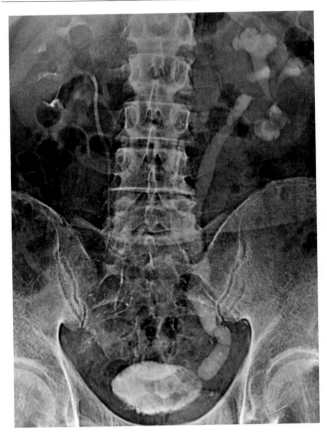

Figure 8–23. Purse-string sign in the left kidney. The renal pelvis is retracted into the renal sinus. Also present is distal left ureteral obstruction due to a stricture.

the testicle is the most common site in the genitourinary system, followed by the epididymis and prostate. Involvement of the bladder and upper urinary tract system is rare.

Clinical Presentation. Onset may be insidious with low-grade fever, weakness, sweat, or abrupt with high fever and chills. Chronic relapsing suppurative disease may also occur. Cystitis may be the only urinary tract symptom.

Radiological Findings. Brucellosis of the kidneys and ureter have striking similarity to renal tuberculosis.[35,36] Differentiating points described are insufficient for making specific diagnosis. Cicatrization, calcification, infundibular stenosis, and mass lesion simulating a tuberculoma may be seen. The only important differentiating finding from tuberculosis is that the ureter is usually uninvolved.

URINARY SCHISTOSOMIASIS (BILHARZIASIS)

Prevalence. Three hundred million worldwide, rare in the United States.

Etiology. *Schistoma haematobium.* Intermediate host is an aquatic snail of the genus *Bulinus.*

Pathology. Granulomatous inflammatory reaction to the eggs in the walls of the ureter and bladder (reversible by specific treatment), fibrosis and calcification in later stages, ureteral obstruction, small capacity bladder. Bladder carcinoma is common. Involvement of the spinal cord is rare.

Clinical Presentation. Chronic: terminal hematuria, urgency, frequency, blood clots in urine, pain, enuresis. Acute: Katayama fever (20–60 days after infection, rare with *S. hematobium*).

Laboratory Findings. Ova in the voided urine specimen. Complement fixation and fluorescent antibody tests positive.

Radiological Findings. Bladder *calcification* is readily identified on CT and plain radiograph (Fig. 8–28). Parallel calcification may be present in distal ureters *(railroad track)*.[37,38] In severe forms submucosal calcifications may be present even in the upper tract system. Rarely, calcification may be seen under the renal capsule (but not in the parenchyma), vas deferens, and seminal vesicles and even in appendix, colon, and rectum.

Contracted, small capacity bladder may be present. Granulomas are seen in an earlier stage of the disease and are seen as *intraluminal filling defects* on cystogram, urogram, CT, and ultrasound.[38–41] These cannot be differentiated radiologically from bladder carcinoma, which is associated with this disease. Carcinoma should be suspected if there is discontinuity of submucosal bladder calcification, which is frequently disrupted by tumor growth.

Ureteral strictures lead to upper tract obstruction and hydronephrosis[40] and hydroureter.[37] Vesicoureteral reflux may be present.

Prostate may enlarge in bilharzial prostatitis.

XANTHOGRANULOMATOUS PYELONEPHRITIS

Etiology. *Proteus mirabilis, E. coli.*

Pathology. Acute and chronic renal inflammatory process, may extend into perinephric space, many

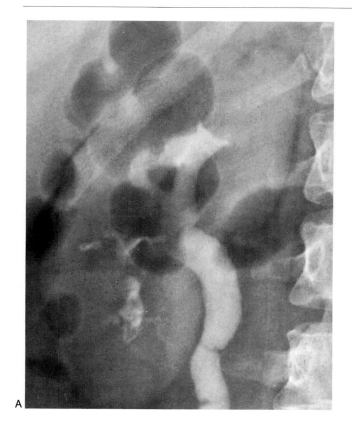

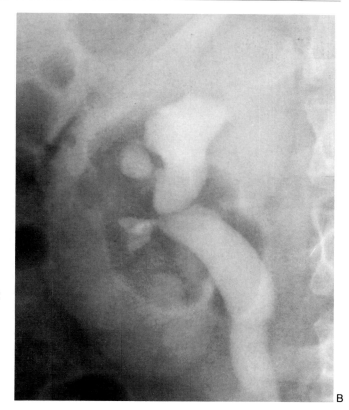

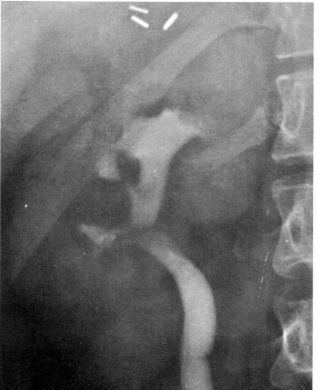

Figure 8–24. Renal tuberculosis was missed despite ureteral stricture causing dilatation and irregularities involving mid and lower calyceal groups **(A)**. Several months later, the renal pelvis is scarred and retracted into the renal sinus and there is amputation of the lower pole calyx and continued dilatation of the ureter **(B)**. The patient now has vesicocutaneous fistula following gynecological surgery and undergoes ureterovesical reimplantation. Diagnosis of renal tuberculosis is still not made. Two years later the purse-string sign is recognized, as is amputation of the lower pole calyx for what they really represent **(C)**.

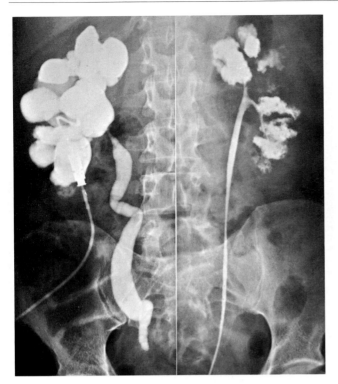

Figure 8–25.   Composite image of right nephrostogram and left retrograde pyelogram. Several tuberculous ureteral strictures produced hydronephrosis, which became secondarily infected and was treated with percutaneous drainage and appropriate antibiotics. On the left, rectractile fibrosis of the renal pelvis is apparent. Beyond, the contrast is admixed with caseous material replacing most of the kidney parenchyma. (From Barbaric ZL. Interventional uroradiology. Radiol Clin North Am 1979; 17:413–433. Reprinted with permission.)

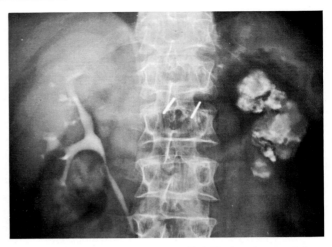

Figure 8–26.   Autonephrectomy. Calcified end-stage tuberculous kidney.

foam cells (histiocytes), fibrosis. Must be differentiated from fibrous histiocytoma.

Clinical Presentation.   Flank pain, low-grade fever, weight loss, malaise, urolithiasis. Mild hepatic dysfunction may be present.

Laboratory Findings.   *Proteus mirabilis* in the urine, typically low colony count, less than 1000/ml. Also frequently found is *E. coli.*

Radiographic Findings.   This inflammatory process is frequently associated with struvite (infectious,

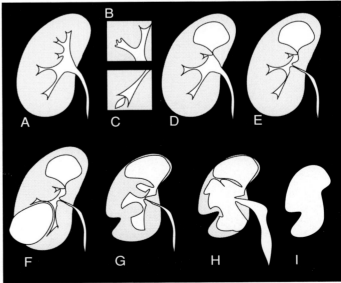

Figure 8–27.   Schematic presentation of progression and development of radiological signs in renal tuberculosis from normal (A), papillary irregularities (B), papillary necrosis (C), infundibular stenosis (D), pursestring sign (E), tuberculoma (F), parenchymal scarring (G), ureteral strictures and hydronephrosis (H), and autonephrectomy (I).

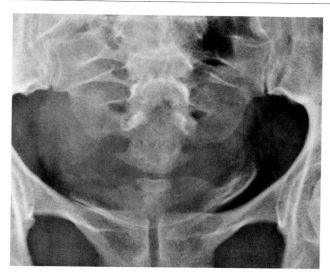

Figure 8–28. Bladder calcification in schistosomiasis.

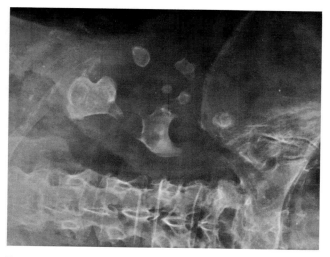

Figure 8–29. Xanthogranulomatous pyelonephritis. Non-functioning enlarged kidney is filled with infection stones. There was no appreciable hydronephrosis on pathological examination.

triple phosphate) stones. The kidney may be totally involved and nonfunctioning (Fig. 8–29).[42,43] Varying degrees of obstruction may be present and secondary infection by *E. coli* is not unusual.

Frequently, an inflammatory mass is formed (tumefactive form), which at times is difficult to differentiate from renal carcinoma.[42,44,45] Abnormal inflammatory vessels are apparent on angiography, which makes it indistinguishable from renal carcinoma. To make differentiation even more difficult, regional lymph nodes may be enlarged secondary to inflammation, which may simulate stage III renal carcinoma.

Marked thickening of the renal fascia and intrafascial septa may be observed (Fig. 8–30). Inflammatory

mass may extend into other retroperitoneal spaces and even involve adjacent organs.[42,45]

MALAKOPLAKIA

Etiology and Pathogenesis. Unknown. Probably acquired deficiency of the immune system. *E. coli* infection common.

Pathology. Umbilicated yellowish granulomas composed of periodic acid–Schiff (PAS)-positive histiocytes, which contain *Michaelis-Gutmann bodies*

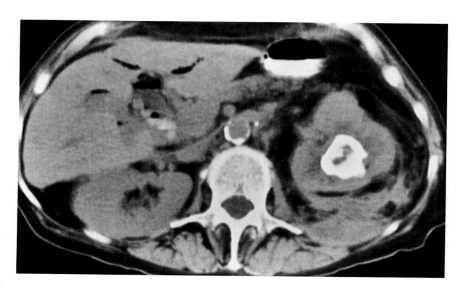

Figure 8–30. Xanthogranulomatous pyelonephritis. Inflammatory mass extends into the perinephric space and there is also an apparent process in the posterior pararenal space. Renal fascia is thickened. A large stone is present in the renal pelvis.

(small calculospherules, basophilic on PAS stain). Bladder is the most commonly involved organ. Prostate, testes, ureters, and the upper urinary system may also become involved.

Clinical Presentation.   Nonspecific. Urinary tract infection. Female predominance.

Radiological Findings.   Diagnosis is usually made during cystoscopy when yellowish patches 1 to 2 cm in diameter are found. These protrude above the mucosal surface and are characteristically umbilicated in the center.

On an excretory urogram there may be filling defects within the bladder or ureters.[46–49] Kidney involvement is rare. Granulomatous plaque may cause ureteropelvic junction obstruction, irregularities of the pelvocalyceal mucosa, or mimic a renal tumor.

FUNGAL INFECTIONS OF THE URINARY TRACT

Candidiasis (Monoliasis)

Etiology.   *Candida albicans.*

Pathology.   Acute suppurative process with abscess formation or chronic caseation of giant cell granulomas. Urinary tract may be involved in disseminated form of the disease, or the disease may be localized to the kidneys or bladder.

Clinical Presentation.   Unlike other fungal infections of the urinary tract that are comparatively rare, candidiasis is a relatively common urinary tract infection. Primary renal candidiasis presents a less serious clinical picture compared with systemic disseminated infection.

Radiological Findings.   Presence of nephrostomy catheters, patients receiving wide-spectrum antibiotics, steroids, and renal transplant and other immunosuppressed patients are at greater risk. Renal enlargement and poor function may be seen during an episode of pyelonephritis on an excretory urogram[50] or CT. Fungus balls may be present and cause obstruction (Fig. 8–31).[51,52] *Gas may be seen in the kidneys or the bladder* as the organism is gas-forming (Fig. 8–32). Ultrasound may also demonstrate intraluminal fungus balls.[53,54] In a later stage small contracted bladder and papillary necrosis may be seen.[55]

Percutaneous nephrostomy may be necessary to provide drainage.[56]

Rare Fungal Infections

Actinomycosis,[57,58] aspergillosis,[59–61] blastomycosis,[62] coccidioidomycosis,[63,64] cryptococcosis,[65] and histoplasmosis occur in patients who have disseminated disease or who are on immunosuppressive therapy. The radiological findings are mostly nonspecific. Abscesses, granulomatous reactions, fibrosis, and sinus tract formation constitute the pathological spectrum of varying fungal diseases.

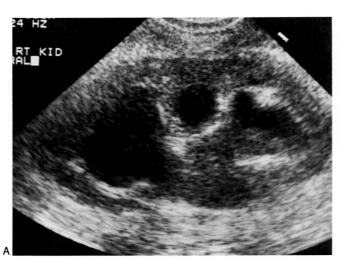
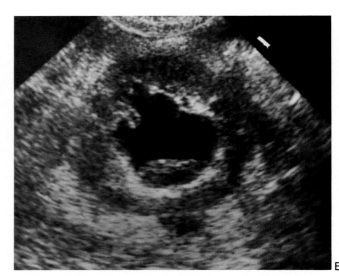

Figure 8–31.   Sonograms in longitudinal **(A)** and transverse **(B)** planes demonstrate hydronephrosis and intraluminal debris suggestive of a fungus ball. Patient was placed on appropriate antibiotic therapy and temporary drainage was established with percutaneous nephrostomy.

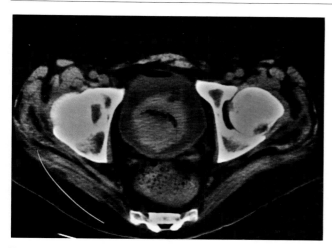

Figure 8–32. Bladder candidiasis. Fungus ball is present in the bladder in this immunosuppressed patient. Also, gas is seen within the fungus ball and at the top of the bladder. No bladder catheter was in place at the time.

Renal and perirenal abscess, inflammatory masses, and pyelonephritis have been described in actinomycosis, blastomycosis, and cryptococcosis.

Fungus balls causing ureteral obstruction were described with aspergillosis and are probably present in other fungal infections of the kidney as well.

Prostate, seminal vesicles, and scrotal contents are involved sometimes more frequently than the upper tract and have been described in actinomycosis, blastomycosis, cryptococcosis, and coccidioidomycosis. Enlarged and painful prostate, seminal vesicles, testicle, or epididymis may be present on physical examination.

ECHINOCOCCOSIS (HYDATID DISEASE)

Etiology. *E. granulosus, E. granulosus* var. *canadesins, E. multilocularis.*

Parasitology. Small, 3–9 mm tapeworm (cestodes). Definitive hosts are canines such as dogs, wolves, and foxes. Intermediate hosts harboring larval form (hydatid cyst) are sheep, cattle, deer, man, and others. Man is infected through contact with dog feces. Ingested oncosphere passes into portal circulation and is filtered through the liver and then lungs before 15% of surviving infective embryos reach systemic circulation. Hydatid cysts may develop in any tissues, including kidneys. Growth rate is 0.25–1 cm per year.

Pathology. Hydatid cyst is a fluid-filled structure containing infective larval forms. Thick germinal layer buds daughter cysts into the lumen. Outer wall is encapsulated fibrous tissue that may calcify. Multilocular, honeycomb cysts are seen associated with *E. multilocularis.*

Clinical Presentation. Pain, hematuria, anaphylactic shock if ruptured.

Laboratory Findings. Scolices in urine are very rare, hematuria.

Radiographic Findings. Mass lesion in the kidney is present, possibly with rim calcification.[66] Thick capsule and internal echoes separate this lesion from a simple cyst.[67,68] Daughter cysts may be visible. Hydatid cyst is almost impossible to differentiate from renal carcinoma or other necrotizing mass lesions in the kidney. Angiographic examination may demonstrate blush in the wall, which in the presence of calcification is very suggestive of the diagnosis.[66]

Calcification is best seen on CT scan but is not pathognomonic. On MR imaging hydatid cyst is hypoechoic on T1-weighted image and hyperechoic on T2-weighted images, again not very specific. The presence of multiple lesions, such as in the liver, lungs, and brain, facilitates the diagnosis,[68] but this presentation is seen in comparatively few patients.

Since spill of a ruptured hydatid cyst may cause anaphylactic shock, percutaneous cyst puncture is considered a contraindication. Recently, there has been a case report of an uneventful percutaneous hydatid cyst puncture in the liver.

REFERENCES

1. Silver TM, Kass EJ, Thornbury JR, et al. The radiological spectrum of acute pyelonephritis in adults and adolescents. Radiology 1976; 118:65–71.
2. Fierer J. Acute pyelonephritis. Urol Clin North Am 1987; 14:251–256.
3. Soulen MC, Fishman EK, Goldman SM, Gatewood OMB. Bacterial renal infection: role of CT. Radiology 1989; 171:703–707.
4. Gold RP, McClennan BL, Rottenberg RR. CT appearance of acute inflammatory abscess and the renal interstitium. AJR 1983; 141:343–349.
5. Ishikawa I, Saito Y, Onouchi Z, et al. Delayed contrast enhancement in acute focal bacterial nephritis: CT features. J Comput Assist Tomogr 1985; 9:894–897.
6. Rosenfield AT, Glickman MG, Taylor KJW, et al. Acute focal bacterial nephritis. Radiology 1979; 132:553–561.
7. Lee JKT, McClennan BL, Melson GL. Acute focal bacterial nephritis: emphasis on gray scale sonography and computed tomography. AJR 1980; 135:87–92.
8. Rigsby CM, Rosenfield AT, Glickman MG, et al. Hemorrhagic focal bacterial nephritis: findings on gray-scale sonography and CT. AJR 1986; 146:1173–1176.

9. Sacks D, Banner MP, Meranze SG, et al. Renal and related retroperitoneal abscesses: percutaneous drainage. Radiology 1988; 167:447–451.

10. Lang EK, Springer RM, Glorioso LW III. Abdominal abscess drainage under radiologic guidance: causes of failure. Radiology 1986; 159:329–332.

11. Whitfield JD, Noe HN. Conservative management of renal carbuncles in children. Urology 1989; 34:89–92.

12. Bernardino ME, Baumgartner BR. Abscess drainage in the genitourinary tract. Radiol Clin North Am 1986; 24:539–545.

13. Edelstein H, McCabe RE. Perinephric abscess. Modern diagnosis and treatment in 47 cases. Medicine (Baltimore) 1988; 67:118–131.

14. Allen HA, Walsh JW, Brewer WH, et al. Sonography of emphysematous pyelonephritis. J Ultrasound Med 1984; 3:533–537.

15. Piccirillo M, Rigsby CM, Rosenfield AT. Sonography of renal inflammatory disease. Urol Radiol 1987; 9:66–78.

16. Hoddick W, Jeffrey RB, Goldberg HI, et al. CT and sonography of severe renal and perirenal infections. AJR 1983; 140:517–520.

17. Ross SA, Towness PL, Hopkins TB. Salmonella enteritidis: a rare cause of pyelonephritis in children. Clin Pediatr 1986; 25:325.

18. Hagood PG, Steinhardt GF. Salmonella urinary tract infection associated with ureteropelvic junction obstruction. J Urol 1988; 140:351–352.

19. Borrero GO, Jafri SZH, Vazquez PM, et al. Computed tomography of acute renal abscess due to salmonella chester. Comput Radiol 1986; 10:41–42.

20. Hayden CK Jr, Swischuk LE, Fawcett HD, et al. Urinary tract infections in childhood: current imaging approach. Radiographics 1986; 6:1023–1034.

21. Lebowitz RL, Mandell J. Urinary tract infection in children: putting radiology in its place. Radiology 1987; 165:1–4.

22. Blickman JG, Taylor GA, Lebowitz RL. Voiding cystourethrography: initial radiological study in children with urinary tract infections. Radiology 1985; 156: 659–662.

23. Sty JR, Wells RG, Starshak RJ, et al. Imaging in acute renal infection in children. AJR 1987; 148:471–476.

24. Kangarloo H, Gold RH, Fine RN, et al. Urinary tract infection in infants and children evaluated by ultrasound. Radiology 1985; 154:367–370.

25. Leonidas JC, McCauley RGK, Klauber GC, et al. Sonography as a substitute for excretory urography in children with urinary tract infection. AJR 1985; 144:815–818.

26. Bisset GS III, Strife JL, Dunbar JS. Urography and voiding cystourethrography: findings in girls with urinary tract infection. AJR 1987; 148:479–484.

27. Gow JG. Genitourinary tuberculosis: a study of 700 cases. Lancet 1963; 2:261–265.

28. Kollins SA, Hartman GW, Carr DT, et al. Roentgenologic findings in urinary tract tuberculosis: a 10 year investigation. Am J Roentgenol 1974; 121:487–500.

29. Permkumar A, Lattimer J, Newhouse JH. CT and sonography of advanced urinary tract tuberculosis. AJR 1987; 148:65–68.

30. Goldman SM, Fishman EK, Hartman DS, et al. Computed tomography of renal tuberculosis and its pathological correlates. Comput Assist Tomogr 1985; 9:771–776.

31. Friedenberg RM, Nay C, Stachenfeld RA. Roentgenologic manifestations of the tuberculosis of the ureter. J Urol 1968; 99:25–29.

32. Niebling HA, Walters W. Adenocarcinoma and tuberculosis of the same kidney: review of the literature and report of the 7 cases. J Urol 1948; 59:1022–1035.

33. Marks LS, Poutasse EF. Hypertension from renal tuberculosis. operative case. Predicted by renal vein renin. J Urol 1973; 109:149–151.

34. Kaufman JJ, Goodwin WE. Renal hypertension secondary to renal tuberculosis. Am J Med 1965; 38:337–344.

35. Abernathy RS, Price WE, Spink WW. Chronic brucellar pyelonephritis simulating tuberculosis. JAMA 1955; 159:1534–1537.

36. Ibrahim AIA, Shetty SD, Saad M, Bilal NE. Genitourinary complications of Brucellosis. Br J Urol 1988; 61:294–296.

37. Hanafy HM, Youssef TK, Saad SM. Radiological aspects of bilharzial (schistosomal) ureter. Urology 1975; 6:118–121.

38. Hugosson CO, Olsen P. Early ureteric changes in Schistosoma Haematobium infection. Clin Radiol 1986; 37:501–504.

39. Hugosson C. Striation of the renal pelvis and ureter in bilharziasis. Clin Radiol 1987; 38:116–118.

40. Dittrich M, Doehring E. Ultrasonographical aspects of urinary schistosomiasis: assessment of morphological lesions in the upper and lower urinary tract. Pediatr Radiol 1986; 16:225–228.

41. Jorulf H, Lindstedt E. Urogenital schistosomiasis: CT evaluation. Radiology 1985; 157:745–747.

42. Beachley MC, Ranniger K, Roth FJ. Xantogranulomatous pyelonephritis. Am J Roentgenol 1974; 121:500–507.

43. Shanser RB, Herzog KA, Palubinskas AJ. Xantogranulomatous pyelonephritis in children. Pediatr Radiol 1975; 3:12–15.

44. Malek RS, Elder JS. Xantogranulomatous pyelonephritis: a critical analysis of 26 cases and the literature. J Urol 1978; 119:589–595.

45. Hartman DS, Davis CJ Jr, Goldman SM, et al. Xantogranulomatous pyelonephritis: sonographic pathologic correlation of 16 cases. J Ultrasound Med 1984; 3:481–488.

46. Sunshine B. Malakoplakia of the upper urinary tract. J Urol 1974; 112:362–365.

47. O'Dea MJ, Malek RS, Farorrow GM. Malakoplakia of the urinary tract. J Urol 1977; 118:739–742.

48. DeRidder PA, Koff SA, Gikas PW, et al. Renal malakoplakia. J Urol 1977; 117:428–431.

49. Puvaneswary M, Teong CC. Radiological, ultrasound and computed tomographic findings in a case of renal malakoplakia. Australas Radiol 1987; 31:192–194.

50. Clark RE, Minagi H, Palubinskas AJ. Renal candidiasis. Radiology 1971; 101:567–572.

51. Stuck KJ, Silver TM, Jaffe HM, Bowermam RA. Sonographic demonstration of renal fungus balls. Radiology 1982; 142:473.

52. Mazer MJ, Bartone FF. Percutaneous antegrade diagnosis and management of candidiasis of the upper urinary tract. Urol Clin North Am 1982; 9:157.

53. Kintanar C, Cramer BC, Reid WD, et al. Neonatal renal candidiasis: sonographic diagnosis. AJR 1986; 147: 801–803.

54. Cohen HL, Haller JO, Schechter S, et al. Renal candi-

diasis of the infant: ultrasound evaluation. Urol Radiol 1986; 8:17–18.

55. Knepshield JH, Feller HA, Leb DE. Papillary necrosis due to Candida albicans in a renal allograft. Arch Intern Med 1968; 122:441–444.

56. Bartone FF, Hurwitz RS, Rojas EL, et al. The role of percutaneous nephrostomy in the management of obstructing candidiasis of the urinary tract in infants. J Urol 1988; 140:338–341.

57. Ellis LR, Kenny GM, Nellans RE. Urogenital aspects of actinomycosis. J Urol 1979; 122:132.

58. Levine LA, Doyle CJ. Retroperitoneal actinomycosis: a case report and review of the literature. J Urol 1988; 140:367–369.

59. Melchoir J, Medust WK, Valk WL. Ureteral colic from a fungus ball: unusual presentation of systemic aspergillosis. J Urol 1972; 108:698–699.

60. Young RC, Bennett JE, Vogel CL, et al. Aspergillosis, the spectrum of the disease in 98 patients. Medicine (Baltimore) 1970; 49:147–173.

61. Zirinsky K, Auh YH, Hartman BJ, et al. Computed tomography of renal aspergillosis. J Comput Assist Tomogr 1987; 11:177–179.

62. Eickenberg HV, Amin M, Lich R Jr. Blastomycosis of the genitourinary tract. J Urol 1975; 113:650–652.

63. Kuntze JR, Herman MH, Evans SG. Genitourinary coccidioidomycosis. J Urol 1988; 140:370–374.

64. Huntington RW Jr, Waldman WJ, Sargent JA, et al. Pathological and clinical observation on 142 cases of fatal coccidioidomycosis with necropsy. In: Coccidioidomycosis. (Ajello L, ed). Tucson: University of Arizona Press, 1967.

65. Salyer WR, Salyer DC. Involvement of the kidney and prostate in cryptococcus. J Urol 1973; 16:139–143.

66. Baltaxe HA, Fleming RJ. The angiographic appearance of hydatid disease. Radiology 1970; 97:559–604.

67. Zuk JA. Renal hydatid disease. Importance of preoperative diagnosis. Br J Urol 1989; 63:100–101.

68. Gulati SM, Agarwal SB, Singh K, Pandey KK. Hydatid disease of kidney. Br J Clin Pract 1987; 41:798–801.

9

Renal Neoplasms

RENAL MASS

Detection

If a renal mass is what we are looking for, CT is the examination of choice. However, renal masses do not comprise the major component of uroradiological examinations. Different imaging modalities are employed in evaluating different urinary tract symptoms. Regardless of the imaging method used for initial examination of the kidney, certain radiological principles apply to all, and some apply only to certain types of examinations. However, every image obtained by any one of the available modalities must be scrutinized for telltale signs of a renal mass.

CHANGE IN SHAPE

A bulge in the renal outline may be seen on a plain radiograph, excretory urogram, angiogram, sonography, CT, and MR imaging. Frequently, such a change in shape may be the only radiographic sign suggesting the presence of the mass. Pseudotumors must be taken into account, since these normal variations in the renal contour may simulate true tumors.

DIFFERENT PHYSICAL PROPERTIES

Different x-ray attenuation values, enhancement (Fig. 9–1), texture, calcifications, echogenicity (Fig. 9–2), or MR signal characteristics (Fig. 9–3) may make a mass distinctively visible against the background of normal tissue or provide clues for a more definitive and, at times, specific diagnosis.

DISPLACEMENT

The mass must attain appreciable volume before displacement of adjacent structures becomes evident.

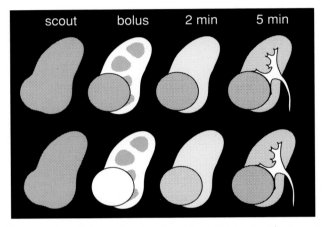

Figure 9–1. Schematic drawing of renal cyst or a hypovascular tumor (upper row) and hypervascular neoplasm (lower row) during an EXU. The hypervascular tumor enhances during the bolus phase.

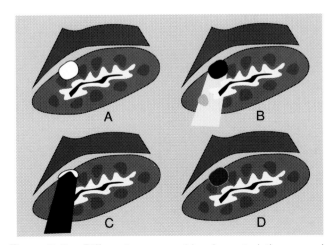

Figure 9–2. Different sonographic characteristics associated with renal masses of the same size. **(A)** Small echogenic angiomyolipoma. **(B)** Simple renal cyst with through transmission. **(C)** Heavily calcified renal mass with acoustical shadowing. **(D)** Solid renal mass, most likely renal carcinoma.

T1-weighted T2-weighted

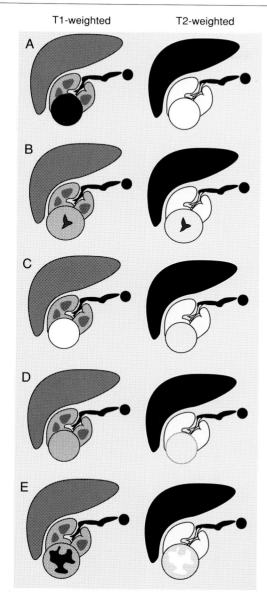

Figure 9–3. Schematic drawing of appearance of different mass lesions on MR imaging. (A) Simple cyst. (B) Oncocytoma. (C) Angiomyolipoma. (D) Renal carcinoma. (E) Necrotic renal carcinoma or metastasis.

1. Displacement of the adjacent calyx or calyceal group is likely to occur first. Slight elongation of the infundibulum may also be present (Fig. 9–4). If displacement is in an anteroposterior direction, it may be completely overlooked on an excretory urogram or retrograde pyelogram unless oblique projections are obtained.

2. Displacement of the renal pelvis and renal sinus fat occurs if the tumor is of appropriate size, or if a small tumor is located adjacent to these structures. Again, oblique projections on projectional examinations may be the only means of identifying the mass.

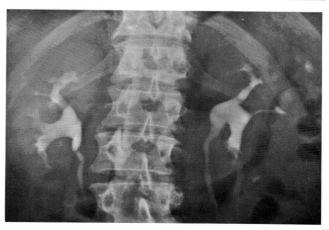

Figure 9–4. Calyceal displacement and splaying of the infundibula by a lower pole left renal mass.

The external impression upon a larger renal pelvis may imitate an intraluminal filling defect.

3. Displacement of the kidney may be present, but rarely before the renal mass becomes 4 cm in diameter. Change in renal axis is determined if the line connecting the uppermost and the lowermost calyces is no longer parallel to psoas outline. Lateral displacement of the lower pole places the mass at the medial aspect of the kidney. Renal displacement may be caused by an intrarenal mass expanding outward or by an extrarenal mass adjacent to the kidney. Mass posterior to the lower pole of the kidney may change the renal axis so that the axis extends in an anteroposterior direction (Fig. 9–5).

Anterior and posterior displacement may be completely missed, as may displacement of the collecting system, without oblique radiographs on projectional examinations. Large retrorenal masses are frequently overlooked by omitting these projections on EXU.

4. Displacement of other organs requires a mass of considerable size, which is unlikely to be overlooked on any examination.

Classification After Discovery

Discovering a mass is one thing. What to do with it is another. The following are well-established rules:

- **Rule 1:** *If the renal mass is solid, it must be considered malignant.*

  A solid mass has an 85% chance of being a renal cell carcinoma. Add to that another 10% for renal sarcomas, lymphoma, transitional cell carcinoma, or metastases. The odds are rather small that the solid mass lesion is a benign tumor, such as oncocytoma, angiomyolipoma, and fibroma.

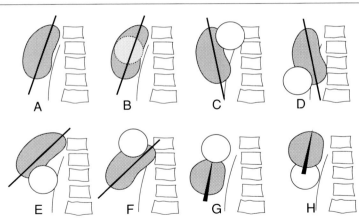

Figure 9–5. (A) Normal renal axis. (B) If the mass is posterior to the mid-kidney, there may be no change in axis. (C,D,E,F) Change in alignment of renal axis depends on the relative size and location of the tumor. If the mass arises from the anterior aspect of the upper pole (G) or posterior to the lower pole (H), the change in axis is in an anteroposterior direction and the kidney may appear shortened in AP projection.

- **Rule 2:** *The only exception to Rule 1 is the unquestionable presence of fat within the mass.*

  Discovery on CT of even small amounts of fat within what otherwise is a soft tissue tumor implies the presence of an angiomyolipoma. Lipoma and hibernoma are usually uniformly of fat density. Renal liposarcoma may contain elements of fat. This tumor originates in renal sinus, is seen in the elderly, and is rare. A large renal carcinoma, however, may encapsulate sinus fat and mimic an angiomyolipoma.

- **Rule 3:** *If a cystic renal mass does not meet the radiological criteria for a simple renal cyst, it must be considered malignant.*

  Cystic renal carcinomas do exist. Some types of malignant tumors are predominantly cystic: Wilms tumor, for example.

- **Rule 4:** *The presence of an oncocytoma (a benign tumor) may be suggested on radiological examination. However, the diagnosis is made only if on multiple histological sections (not aspiration biopsy) renal carcinoma cells are absent amid oncocytoma cells.*

  Considering the relative rarity of oncocytoma compared with renal cell carcinoma, committing to a diagnosis of oncocytoma solely on the basis of radiological findings is inappropriate. The diagnosis may be suggested prior to definitive therapy and may influence the surgeon to consider partial nephrectomy. A detailed histological examination of the *entire* specimen is necessary for exclusion of renal cell carcinoma.

- **Rule 5:** *Renal pseudotumor may be differentiated from a neoplasm in most instances.*

  Many normal kidneys have been removed because of incomplete understanding of congenital or developmental variances that can resemble a neoplasm.

- **Rule 6:** *Aspiration biopsy of an arteriovenous malformation or a renal artery aneurysm may result in major hemorrhage.*

Dynamic CT or color Doppler ultrasound should be sufficient to confirm the diagnosis should any doubt still remain.

- **Rule 7:** *There is no substitute for clinical judgment.*

  While most solid renal masses are indistinguishable from renal carcinoma, some may be differentiated on the basis of their clinical presentation. For example, focal acute bacterial pyelonephritis is likely to have presenting symptoms different from those of renal carcinoma. Reevaluation of the lesion after antibiotic therapy is a prudent approach.

Decision algorithm is provided for guidance (Fig. 9–6). The list of differential diagnoses of renal masses is lengthy (Tables 9–1, 9–2).

RENAL PSEUDOTUMORS

Pseudotumors are mass effects in the kidney produced by exaggerated normal tissue, abnormal development, or any other non-neoplastic process that may suggest the presence of a neoplasm.[1,2]

Hypertrophied Septum of Bertin

No hypertrophy is involved; rather, there is an exaggerated amount of normal cortical tissue, usually between the upper and middle calyceal groups (Figs. 9–7, 9–8). Distortion and elongation of adjacent calyces may be present so that the possibility of a renal carcinoma may be entertained. If there is uncertainty about the diagnosis, dynamic CT is diagnostic (Fig. 9–9). If there is still doubt about the diagnosis, Tc-99m DMSA scan is an appropriate examination. This radionuclide is bound by tubules so that there is a void in the suspected area in the presence of a tumor.

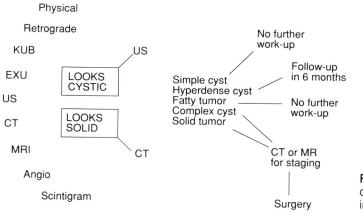

Physical
Retrograde
KUB   US
EXU   ┌─────────┐
US   │ LOOKS   │
CT   │ CYSTIC │
        └─────────┘
MRI   ┌─────────┐
        │ LOOKS   │
Angio   │ SOLID   │
        └─────────┘
Scintigram

No further work-up
Simple cyst
Hyperdense cyst
Fatty tumor ——— No further work-up
Complex cyst
Solid tumor

Follow-up in 6 months

CT or MR for staging

Surgery

Figure 9–6. Steps taken after discovery of a renal mass by any imaging modality.

Table 9-1. Renal Masses Classified by Pathology

MALIGNANT	BENIGN	INFLAMMATORY
Renal carcinoma	Simple cyst	Abscess
Lymphoma	Angiomyolipoma	Pyelonephritis
Leiomyosarcoma	Oncocytoma	Xanthogranulomatous-pyelonephritis
Hemangiopericytoma	Pseudotumor	Infected renal cyst
Liposarcoma	Reninoma	Tuberculosis
Rhabdomyosarcoma	Pheochromocytoma	Rheumatic granuloma
Shwannoma m.	Leiomyoma	
Osteosarcoma	Hemangioma	
Fibrous histiocytoma	Cystic nephroma	
Neurofibrosarcoma	Fibroma	
Metastases	AVM	
Invasion by adjacent neoplasm	Hemangiopericytoma	
Carcinoid	Hibernoma	
Adult Wilms	Renal artery aneurysm	
Wilms		
Mesoblastic nephroma		
Leukemia		

Table 9-2. Renal Masses Classified by Radiographic Appearance

SIMPLE CYSTS	COMPLEX CYSTS	FATTY TUMORS	ALL OTHERS
Cyst	Cystic nephroma	Angiomyolipoma	Renal carcinoma
Multiple cysts	Renal carcinoma	Lipoma	Metastases
Peripelvic cyst	Hemorrhagic cyst	Hibernoma	Lymphoma
Calyceal diverticulum	Metastases	Liposarcoma	Sarcomas
	Wilms		Lobar nephronia
	Infected cyst		Abscess
	Lymphoma		Tuberculosis
	Tuberculosis		Oncocytoma
	Septated cyst		Fibroma
	Renal artery aneurysm		Xanthogranulomatous-pyelonephritis
	AVM		Pheochromocytoma
	Hydrocalyx		Wilms
			Rheumatic granuloma
			Reninoma
			Leiomyoma
			Hemangioma
			Nephroblastomatosis
			Adenocarcinoma
			Transitional cell carcinoma
			Carcinoid

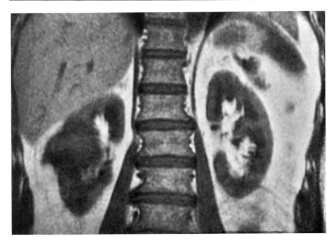

Figure 9–7. T1-weighted sequence in coronal plane. Right renal mass is isointense to the cortex and is deforming renal outline and distorting renal sinus fat. This represents a renal cell carcinoma. On the left a septum of Bertin is seen between two pyramids, almost dividing the renal sinus in two.

Lobar Dysmorphism

Abnormal orientation of a renal lobe between upper and middle calyceal groups closely resembles an exaggerated septum of Bertin. The dysmorphic lobe characteristically points to and drains into a posteriorly located calyx.[3] It may present as a renal mass, usually distorting middle and upper calyceal groups. The presence of a posterior calyx is the diagnostic feature on IVP or CT (Fig. 9–10). On nephrotomography or angiography *the doughnut sign* may be present. It is a cortical blush surrounding relatively radiolucent medulla in the capillary phase.[4] Tc-99m DMSA scan is rarely indicated, since urographic findings are usually so convincing.

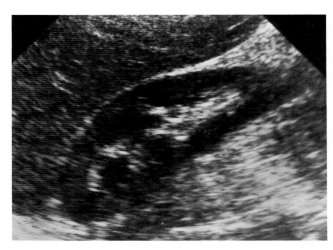

Figure 9–8. Septum of Bertin in the right kidney almost divides right renal sinus in two.

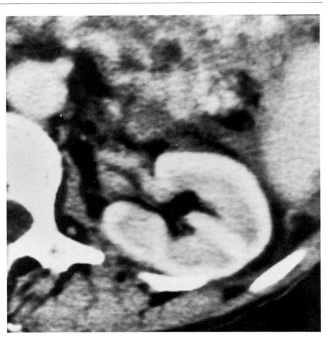

Figure 9–9. Septum of Bertin protruding into the renal sinus seen on a dynamic CT scan.

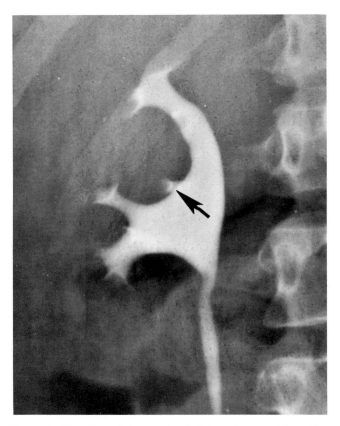

Figure 9–10. Pseudotumor due to lobar dysmorphism. The upper and middle infundibula are splayed apart by a maloriented renal lobe. The clue to its presence is a small, posteriorly located calyx (arrow).

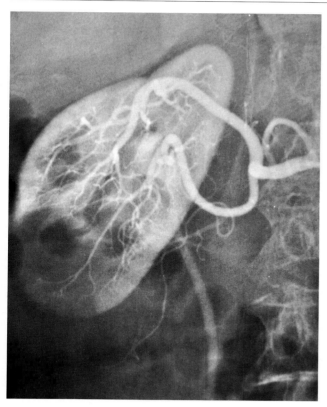

Figure 9–11. Accessory renal hilus extending along antero-superior area of the kidney. A superior polar vessel is seen entering the area.

Accessory Renal Hilus and Junctional Parenchymal Defect

Another anomaly that may mimic a mass lesion on ultrasound or excretory urography is extension of the renal sinus toward the anterosuperior surface of the right kidney (Fig. 9–11). The normal infolding of parenchyma may give a false impression of a tumor. Steep oblique projection during excretory urography and ultrasound may be necessary to make the diagnosis. Junctional parenchymal defect may be located posteriorly as well (Fig. 9–12).

Fetal Lobation

Separate renal lobes are fused at birth. Occasionally, a fissure separating two or more lobes may still be present on the renal surface and may sometimes be exaggerated, resembling a renal mass (Fig. 9–13). Fetal lobation and junctional parenchymal defect may be indistinguishable (Fig. 9–14).

Renal Infarct

Acute renal infarct may cause mass effect within the kidney with calyceal displacement seen on excretory urogram.[5] This may be exaggerated in the presence of fetal lobation or junctional parenchymal defect. A triangular or large irregular zone of nonenhanced renal parenchyma is detected on contrast CT scan (see Fig. 12–4).

Subcapsular cortical rim sign should always be looked for. This sign is pathognomonic for renal infarction and consists of a 1 or 2 mm thin enhancing rim of parenchyma along the outer renal margin. The outer rim is probably supplied via perforating capsular arteries.

Intrarenal Hematoma

Hemorrhage into the renal parenchyma may also simulate renal neoplasm.[6] Small renal neoplasms

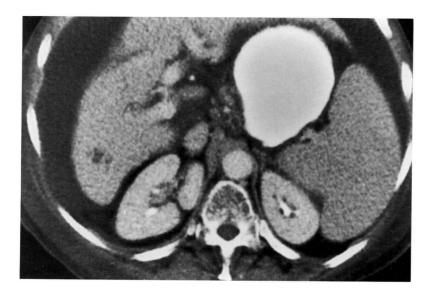

Figure 9–12. Contrast-enhanced CT demonstrates a deep fissure in the posterior surface of the kidney, representing junctional parenchymal defect. Note also a metastasis in the liver and ascites.

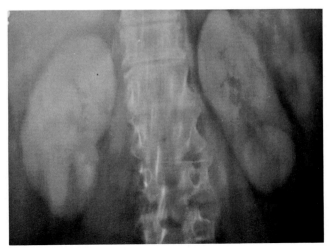

Figure 9–13. Fetal lobation in the lower pole mimicking a renal tumor.

may cause intrarenal or subcapsular hemorrhage. Therefore, CT examination is indicated, even if the patient was on anticoagulants during the acute episode.[7]

Peripelvic Lipomatosis

An abundance of fat in the renal sinus occurs with age and gradual renal parenchymal atrophy. As the number of functioning nephrons hyalinize and disappear, parenchyma regresses both centrifugally and centripetally. Sinus fat fills the vacated area.

Sometimes there is an abundance of fat even without renal atrophy, possibly caused by intermittent

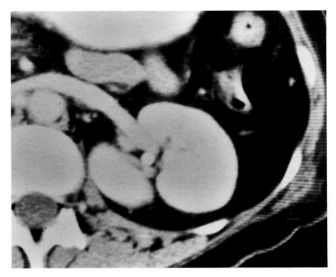

Figure 9–14. Posterior fetal lobation or junctional parenchymal defect.

urinary extravasation into the sinus, for instance in patients with prostatic enlargement and outflow bladder obstruction.[8] A higher than normal concentration of uric acid is detected in the fat. An element of fibrosis (fibrolipomatosis) may also be present.

Calyceal displacement and elongation are common (Fig. 9–15). Radiolucencies in the renal sinus are seen on CT,[9] MR images, and nephrotomograms. On occasion, a fatty mass is localized on only one area *(lipomatosis circumscripta)*.

Renal Scarring

Renal scarring associated with chronic refluxing nephropathy may exaggerate the appearance of intact and perhaps somewhat hypertrophied normal parenchyma. Other pseudotumors in the affected kidney may exaggerate these differences even more, making differentiation from a true malignancy that much more difficult.

Dromedary Hump

The spleen influences the shape of the lateral renal margin.[2] Occasionally, a very prominent hump along this margin may resemble a renal neoplasm or a renal cyst (Fig. 9–16). On excretory urogram or CT, an undisturbed calyx may be seen draining that area (Fig. 9–17). If in doubt, Tc-99m DMSA scan is indicated (Fig. 9–18).

Vascular Impressions

Vascular impressions on the pelvocalyceal system may simulate a neoplasm. Ureteral compression during urography usually resolves the dilemma (Fig. 9–19).

BENIGN RENAL NEOPLASMS

Renal Angiomyolipoma

Incidence. In patients with tuberous sclerosis, 80%. Fifty percent of all renal angiomyolipomas are seen in tuberous sclerosis. However, small angiomyolipomas are seen more commonly in asymptomatic patients.

Pathology. Variable amounts of fat, muscle, and vascular tissues (benign hamartoma), hypervascular, simultaneous presence in the liver and regional lymph nodes possible.

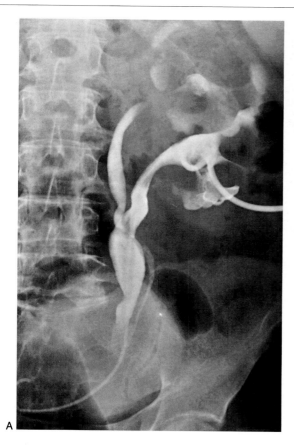

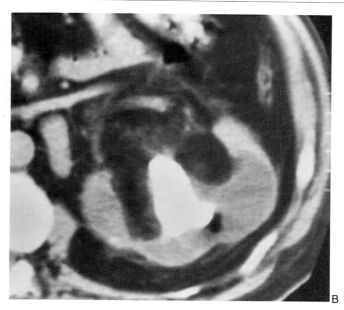

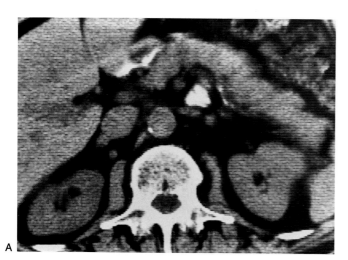

Figure 9–15. Peripelvic lipomatosis in a patient with a bifid collecting system and urolithiasis. **(A)** Nephrostogram shows displacement of the pelvocalyceal system. **(B)** Low attenuation renal sinus masses are present. Differential diagnosis includes peripelvic cysts.

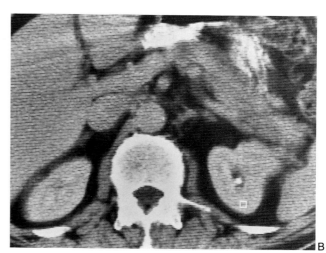

Figure 9–16. Renal pseudotumor. **(A)** Precontrast CT scan demonstrates a "lump" along the anterior superior left renal outline. **(B)** The "mass" enhances uniformly and with the same intensity as the surrounding parenchyma. Unfortunately, this normal kidney was removed for fear of malignancy.

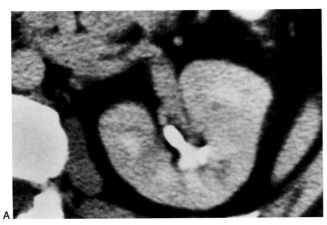
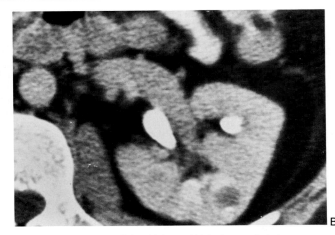

Figure 9–17. Left renal pseudotumor. The "mass" along the anterior part of the kidney **(A)** is immediately adjacent to the calyx seen on the next cut caudad **(B)**. A small renal cyst is seen posteriorly.

Clinical Presentation. Acute retroperitoneal hemorrhage, palpable mass, gastrointestinal symptoms due to mass compression, incidental finding in young women (4–40 mm).

Treatment. Small tumors—none; hemorrhage—transcatheter embolization; very large tumors—nephrectomy or partial nephrectomy.

Radiological Findings. The presence of fat in a tumor is the characteristic signature of an angiomyolipoma. Therefore the preferred imaging modality is CT.[10] Radiolucent mass of any size may be seen (Fig. 9–20). Recent hemorrhage may be identified in the perinephric space. In small tumors even meager amounts of fat may be detected on 5 mm cuts.

On ultrasound, angiomyolipomas have a highly echogenic appearance without through transmission. Small angiomyolipomas are a common finding on sonography in younger women (Fig. 9–21).[11]

On MR imaging, the fat as well as the rich vascular elements are also evident. Enlarged renal vein may be seen to traverse the lipomatous tumor.

On angiography, the tumor is very vascular.[12] This differs from renal liposarcoma, which is seen in older patients and is hypovascular.

Fatty, muscular, and vascular components vary from tumor to tumor. In rare instances there may be no fat detectable even on thin cuts, and differentiation from malignant tumors is not possible.

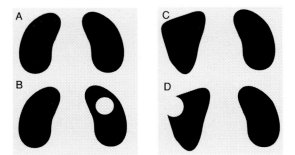

Figure 9–18. Schematic drawing of Tc-99m DMSA scintigram in **(A)** septum of Bertin. **(B)** Cyst or tumor in that area. **(C)** Dromedary hump. **(D)** Tumor mimicking a dromedary hump.

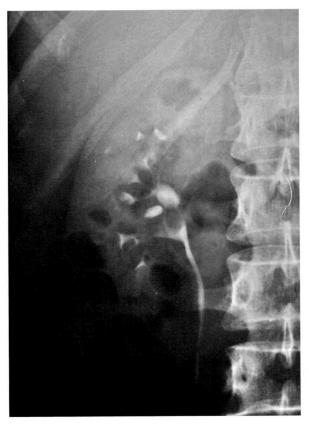

Figure 9–19. Vascular impression upon the renal pelvis.

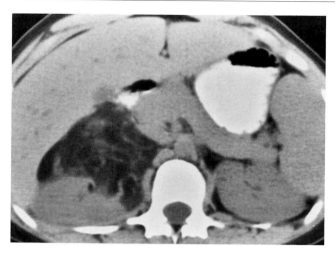

Figure 9–20. Precontrast CT scan demonstrates low attenuation renal mass with definite fatty component.

Cysts may occasionally be seen together with angiomyolipomas in patients with tuberous sclerosis (Fig. 9–22).[13]

There have been several isolated case reports of concurrent renal carcinoma.[14–16] Malignancy should be suspected in the presence of calcification within the tumor, or when the margin between the tumor and the kidney is irregular and indistinct.

An angiomyolipoma may be discovered in the regional lymph nodes[17] or liver, but this is not considered a manifestation of malignancy.

Transcatheter embolization may be considered for ablation of a tumor, particularly if well circumscribed, or for control of hemorrhage (Fig. 9–23).[18]

Lipoma and Hibernoma

Lipoma is a rare benign tumor of the kidney and most probably originates from the renal sinus fat. Diagnostic feature is radiolucent appearance on CT[19] or the tumor is isointense to the retroperitoneal fat on MR sequences. Radiolucency may be detectable on an excretory urogram, and pelvocalyceal distortion due to mass effect may be evident. Differential diagnosis includes other fatty renal tumors and localized peripelvic lipomatosis *(lipomatosis circumscripta).*

Hibernoma is a benign tumor arising from metabolically active brown fat (commonly found in hibernating animals).[20] On CT and MR imaging, it should resemble a lipoma. There may be a higher association of these tumors with pheochromocytoma.[21]

In some mammals brown fat is found in the forniceal areas of the renal pelvis. It is suspected that clumps of brown fat serve a yet undetermined regulatory renal function, since their vascular supply resembles that of the pituitary gland.

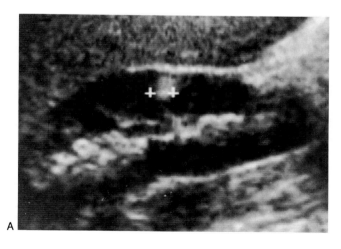

A

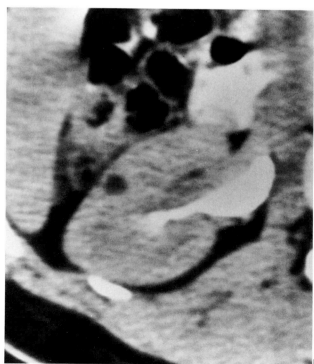

B

Figure 9–21. (A) Typical small angiomyolipoma presents as an echogenic mass without through transmission on sonography. (B) Thin CT cuts allow more precise measurement of the attenuation values in such small lesions.

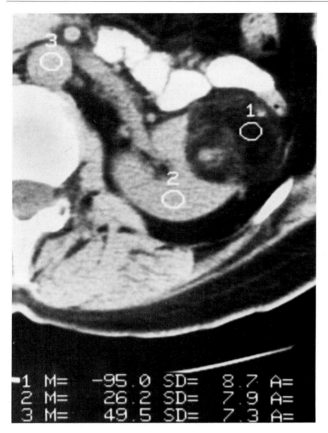

Figure 9–22. Renal angiomyolipoma. Cursors are placed over the tumor, normal kidney, and aorta. Attenuation values expressed in Hounsfield units show without a doubt that the mass has large areas of fat.

Oncocytoma

Incidence and Pathology. Proximal tubular cell adenoma (oxyphilic adenoma). Pathological diagnosis is made when *multiple sections* of the specimen show no evidence for clear cell carcinoma.

Clinical Presentation. Usually silent, hematuria, tumor mass effect.

Radiological Findings. Nonspecific findings of a solid renal mass are seen on excretory urogram, ultrasound, or retrograde examination.

In most patients CT examination is likewise nonspecific, demonstrating a solid renal mass indistinguishable from renal carcinoma (Fig. 9–24). In some instances, however, a *central scar* can be identified and is suggestive for diagnosis, providing that a *homogeneous pattern* is present on US.[22]

Two very suggestive signs have been described on angiographic examination:

1. *Spoke wheel* sign where arterial supply enters the tumor in a concentric fashion from periphery inward and resembles a wheel with spokes (Fig. 9–25). This sign is usually seen in larger tumors.[23,24]
2. *Homogeneous blush* in capillary phase.

One must remember that identical signs may be seen in renal carcinoma and at best are suggestive but not diagnostic of oncocytoma. These criteria are reliable only if the mass is 3 cm or larger.

MR imaging cannot differentiate this tumor from renal carcinoma (Fig. 9–26).[25,26]

Thin needle aspiration biopsy of suspected oncocytoma has been suggested by some as a means of differentiating this tumor from renal carcinoma. The presence of benign cells in the aspirate *does not* exclude malignancy, however, since pathological criteria for diagnosing this tumor are not only the presence of oncocytes, but also the *absence of malignant cells on multiple sections.* We have yet to see a case where even in the presence of suggestive radiologic signs, surgery was cancelled. On the other hand, the presence of these signs may influence the urologic surgeon to consider partial nephrectomy instead of radical nephrectomy.

Multilocular Cystic Nephroma (MLCN)

Etiology. Unclear. Possibly Wilms tumor which has undergone benign differentiation or, more likely, a variant of multicystic dysplastic kidney (MDK).

Incidence. In children 50% of tumors occur before age 5 years (female to male ratio, 1 to 1). In adults usually found between ages 40 to 70 years (female to male ratio, 2 to 1).

Pathology. Unilateral septated, compartmentalized cystic renal mass. Individual cysts not communicating. Fibroblastic connective tissue septa, columnar epithelial lining.

Clinical Presentation. Palpable abdominal mass (children). Hematuria.

Treatment. Partial nephrectomy if radiological findings strongly favor MLCN. However, the diagnosis is difficult, since differential diagnosis includes complex cyst and cystic renal cell carcinoma. Many patients will therefore have an operation appropriate for cancer.

Radiological Findings. Cystic nephroma tends to be large when discovered in adults as well as children. A cystic mass with low Hounsfield number values is seen on CT. Multiple septa are usually also visible and may enhance with contrast (Fig. 9–27).

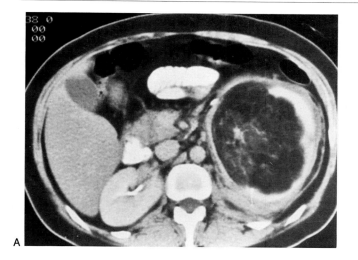

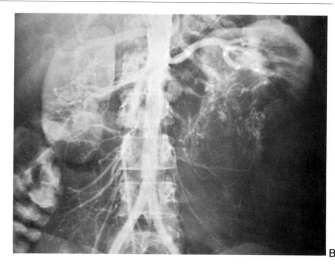

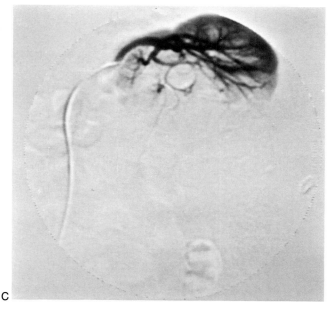

Figure 9–23. (A) Large angiomyolipoma presenting with an episode of acute hemorrhage. (B) Aortogram demonstrates neovascularity and renal displacement by the tumor mass and hematoma. (C) Subtraction selective renal arteriogram after successful supraselective embolization of the tumor, sparing the remainder ot the kidney.

Calcifications may be present in the septa and less commonly at the periphery.[27] Similar findings are seen on ultrasound and MR imaging.[28]

Cysts do not communicate. Needle aspiration with contrast instillation fills only an individual cyst and is noncontributory to the diagnosis. Fluid is clear and acellular.

As expected, tumor is hypovascular on angiographic study. Differential diagnosis includes cystic Wilms tumor and renal carcinoma. Malignancy is suspected if the septa are thickened and calcified.[29] Cystic compartments in cystic renal carcinoma are usually smaller than in MLCN and in the former may be associated with areas of hemorrhage.

Renal Adenoma

One to 2 cm adenomas are a very common finding at autopsy. Recently, they have been considered to represent renal cell carcinomas rather than benign tumors. Radiographically, they are indistinguishable from renal carcinoma (Fig. 9–28).

Rare Benign Renal Tumors

RENINOMA

Reninoma is one of the few surgically curable causes of hypertension. It is a benign tumor originating

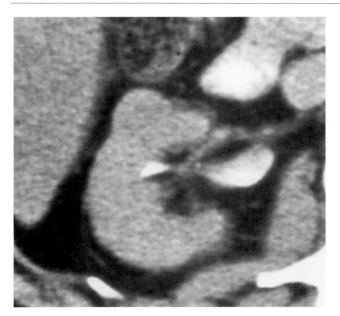

Figure 9–24. Small oncocytoma is indistinguishable from renal carcinoma and most other solid renal tumors.

from renin-producing cells within the juxtaglomerular apparatus. Reninoma is relatively hypovascular on angiographic examination. High ipsilateral renins from renal vein samples are diagnostic.[30]

FIBROMA

Fibroma is a benign tumor originating from the renal sinus or renal capsule. The tumor may calcify and is usually small (Fig. 9–29). CT cannot differentiate this benign tumor from renal carcinoma. Because of high connective tissue component, the tumor may appear hypointense (dark) on T2-weighted and isointense to the liver on T1-weighted sequences.

RENAL MEDULLARY FIBROMA

These are small, whitish tumors within the medulla that rarely attain a sufficiently large size to be detected on any imaging modality (Fig. 9–30).[31] On T2-weighted sequences, the tumor is hypointense (dark).[32]

LEIOMYOMA

Leiomyoma of the renal pelvis may present as an intraluminal filling defect and cause displacement of the collecting system.[33,34]

NEUROLEMMOMA

Rare benign parenchymal renal tumor, hypovascular, without distinguishing radiographic features.

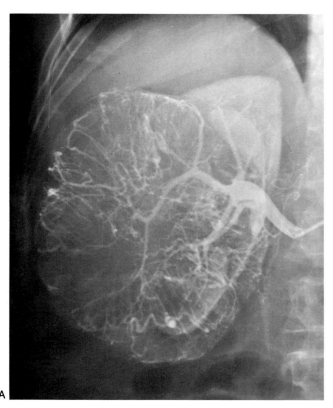
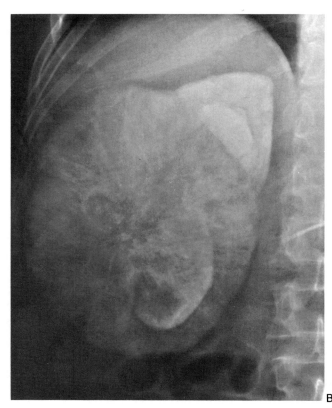

A

B

Figure 9–25. Spoke-wheel appearance **(A)** with relatively homogeneous capillary blush **(B)**.

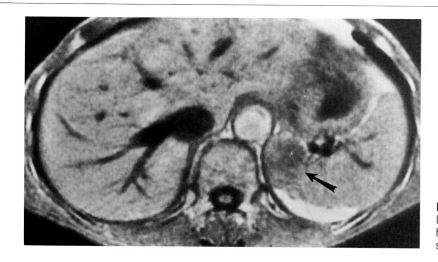

Figure 9–26. Oncocytoma of the left upper pole seen as a relatively hypointense area between aorta and spleen on T1-weighted sequence.

HEMANGIOMA

Intermittent hematuria over a number of years is suggestive of the diagnosis. The tumor is usually small *(capillary hemangioma)* and medullary in location. Large tumors *(cavernous hemangioma)* may be detected on angiography (hypervascular), CT, and MR imaging where the tumor is hyperintense to the kidney on T2-weighted sequence.

HEMANGIOPERICYTOMA

Rare neoplasm without distinguishing features occasionally associated with *hypoglycemia.*[35]

EXTRAMEDULLARY HEMATOPOIESIS

Intrarenal agnogenic myeloid metaplasia is a rare cause of intrarenal mass lesion.[36]

LYMPHANGIOMA

Rare benign neoplasm presenting as a multiloculated renal mass.[37]

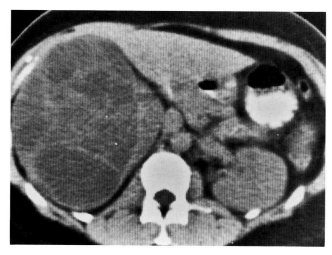

Figure 9–27. Cystic nephroma. Multiloculated cystic renal mass with large compartments is seen on nonenhanced CT. Compartments in cystic renal carcinoma are usually smaller.

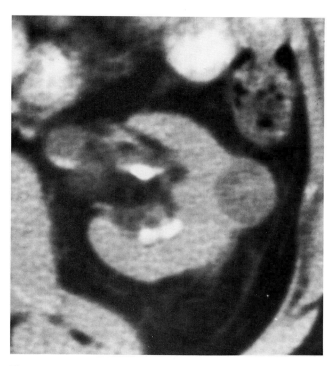

Figure 9–28. Benign renal adenoma growing within a renal cyst. Although at first glance the lesion resembles a cyst, it becomes obvious that there are internal inhomogeneities.

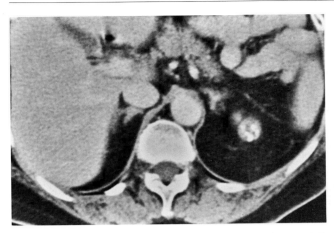

Figure 9–29. Small and calcified left upper pole renal fibroma.

MALIGNANT TUMORS OF THE KIDNEY

Renal Carcinoma

Incidence. One in 13,000 population, male preponderance, 50% mortality, peak incidence 45 to 60 years of age. Small 1–2 cm tumors are common at autopsy, perhaps 1/300.

Etiology. Idiopathic, hereditary HLA-BW17 chromosome, von Hippel-Lindau disease, smoking, fatty diet, end-stage renal disease, and dialysis.

Pathology. Proximal tubular cell neoplasm, clear and granular cell type, yellowish (high lipid content), hemorrhage, central necrosis, cystic component

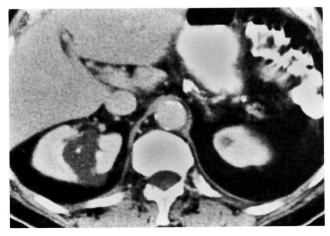

Figure 9–30. Noncalcified renal medullary fibroma in the right upper pole.

15%, venous invasion 40%, calcification 13%, arteriovenous shunts in the tumor are present in 5%.

Metastases. Hematogenous and lymphatic route. Lung, liver, skeleton, brain, adrenal.

Clinical Presentation. Weight loss, painless hematuria, fatigue, palpable mass, flank pain, fever, anemia, hypertension, spermatic varicocele, leg edema, renal colic, high output cardiac failure due to arterovenous shunting, and symptoms attributable to distant metastasis. Asymptomatic 30%, perhaps more. Many small renal cell carcinomas are discovered serendipitously or incidently at CT or ultrasound examination performed for indications unrelated to the urinary tract.[38,39] Occasional spontaneous regression.

Laboratory Findings. Hematuria, ESR, hypercalcemia, polycythemia, anemia.

Staging. The system commonly used is that developed by Robson et al.[40] (Fig. 9–31).

Radiological Findings

Excretory Urography. EXU still remains the examination of choice for evaluating hematuria. The mass may be obvious or its presence may be suspected because of a bulge of the renal outline, renal sinus, or pelvocalyceal system displacement (Fig. 9–32). Occasionally, it can be determined if the mass is hypovascular or hypervascular (Fig. 9–1). Presence of a hypervascular mass with evidence of invasion into the collecting system makes the diagnosis of renal carcinoma almost certain.

CT. CT is the method of choice for detection and staging of renal carcinoma. On nonenhanced scan, renal carcinoma has similar attenuation value to the kidney (Figs. 9–33, 9–34). Carcinoma usually enhances less than the kidney on contrast study (Fig. 9–35). Larger carcinomas may have an inhomogeneous appearance due to areas of necrosis or hemorrhage (Figs. 9–36, 9–37, 9–38).[41,42] CT is particularly well suited for detecting calcification within the mass.

Because of frequent use of CT and sonography, renal carcinoma is detected earlier and staged more accurately than ever before.[38,41–44]

Sonography. Ultrasound detects a solid mass that is usually isoechoic to the renal parenchyma without through transmission (Fig. 9–39). The main purpose of this examination is to separate benign renal cysts from solid tumors (Fig. 9–40). Superior extension of the tumor in the intrahepatic portion of the inferior vena cava and the right atrium is usually well demon-

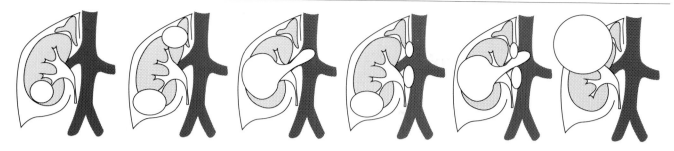

Stage I	Stage II	Stage III A	Stage III B	Stage III C	Stage IV A

Figure 9–31. Stage I: Tumor confined within the renal capsule. Stage II: Capsular penetration, adrenal involvement. Stage IIIA: Venous involvement. Stage IIIB: Regional lymph node involvement. Stage IIIC: Venous *and* regional lymph node involvement. Stage IVA: Direct extension to adjacent organs. Stage IVB (not shown): Distant metastases.

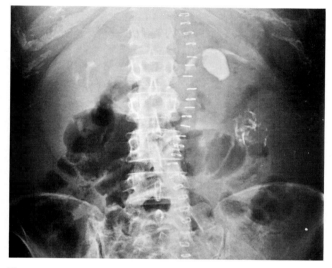

Figure 9–32. Large left renal mass with dystrophic calcifications. Collecting system is distorted and displaced cephalad by what proved to be renal carcinoma. The tumor was a surprise finding during a laparotomy performed to remove "enlarged spleen."

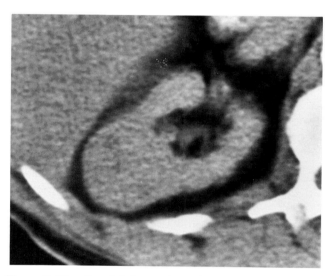

Figure 9–33. Small right renal carcinoma has similar attenuation to the kidney on precontrast scan. For this reason, a small tumor that does not alter the renal outline or displace the collecting system may go unrecognized unless a contrast study is also performed.

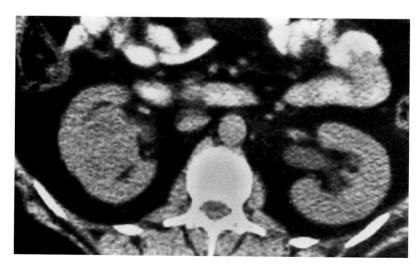

Figure 9–34. Renal carcinoma on a precontrast scan is recognized as a mass extending into renal sinus and displacing renal sinus fat.

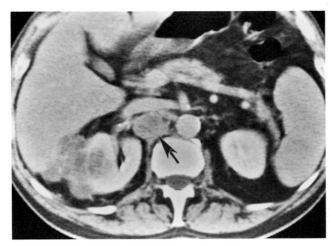

Figure 9–35. Most carcinomas enhance somewhat after a bolus of contrast material is delivered. The enhancement is usually less than that of the normal surrounding renal parenchyma, as in this case. Lobulated renal carcinoma has extended through the renal capsule. An enlarged retrocaval lymph node (arrow) enhances less than the great vessels.

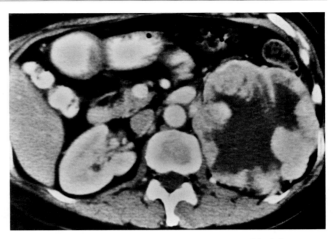

Figure 9–37. Huge left renal carcinoma with inhomogeneous enhancement. The low attenuation areas represent areas of necrosis. Enlarged venous channels usually surround a large tumor such as this, even when the renal vein is not involved and is seen enhancing posterior to the tumor in this case.

strated using this technique. The disadvantage of sonography is its inability to accurately assess regional lymph node involvement.

MR Imaging. At the present time, MR imaging is at a disadvantage regarding detection and classification of a mass lesion as cystic or solid. On T1-weighted sequences, most renal carcinomas tend to be iso- or somewhat hyperintense compared to the renal cortex (Fig. 9–7). On T2-weighted sequences, the tumor usually exhibits a strong signal, but so does the renal cortex (Fig. 9–41).[45,46] A smaller tumor may be invisible because on both sequences it may be

indistinguishable from the surrounding parenchyma. Therefore in many instances the presence of the tumor may be suspected only if deformity of the renal outline or renal sinus is produced by the mass.

One of the drawbacks of MR imaging is its inability to display discrete calcifications. This, of course, is one of the major differentiating features between malignant and benign renal masses. Add to that the inevitable image degradation due to respiratory, intestinal, vascular, and involuntary motion, and the impracticality of this examination for detection of smaller renal carcinomas becomes obvious (Fig. 9–42). Hemorrhage and necrosis within the tumor may be detected (Fig. 9–43).

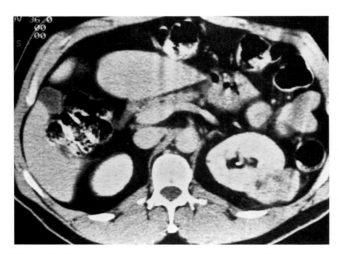

Figure 9–36. Inhomogeneous enhancement of a left renal carcinoma.

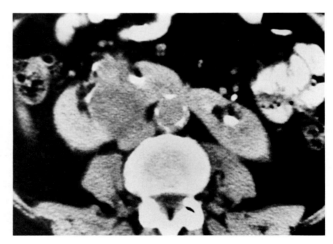

Figure 9–38. Inhomogeneous enhancement of a renal carcinoma in a horseshoe kidney.

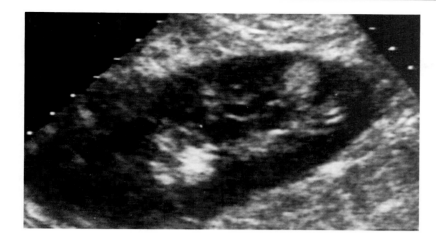

Figure 9–39. A small renal carcinoma in the lower pole is somewhat more hyperechoic than usual, but not as hyperechoic as the renal sinus fat.

An advantage of MR imaging over other modalities is in detection of venous propagation of the tumor and in those instances where the patient is allergic to radiographic contrast materials.[45–47]

Angiography. All questions regarding staging can usually be answered by CT. Angiography is seldom used for diagnostic purposes. If rich vascularity is seen on an angiogram, a diagnosis of renal carcinoma is almost a certainty, in contrast to lymphoma or metastases, which are hypovascular (Fig. 9–44). Papillary or spindle renal carcinomas may be hypovascular, however, and the trend to aspiration biopsy regardless of vascularity is rendering diagnostic angiography almost obsolete.

Arteriovenous fistular shunts are found in 5% of larger renal carcinomas (Fig. 9–45). Shunts may be very large and cause high-output cardiac failure (Fig. 9–46).

Palliative or preoperative embolization of cancerous tumors may be employed primarily to control bleeding (Fig. 47). One should expect postinfarction syndrome to develop with symptoms that are proportional to the volume of the infarcted cancer and normal renal parenchyma. The symptoms are pain, fever, and leukocytosis.

The detection rate of different imaging modalities in depicting renal carcinoma 3 cm or smaller is presented in Table 9–3.[41,45] It appears that CT is currently still the imaging modality of choice, although fast developments in MR technology may reverse the trend (Fig. 9–48 A,B).

Staging. Both CT and MR are well suited for estimating local extension. At the present time, CT has a slight edge in detecting smaller tumors (contralateral lesion, for instance), lymph node involvement (Fig. 9–49), and extension through renal fascia. MR has a slight edge in detection of venous tumor extension (Fig. 9–50), involvement of the adjacent musculature, and differentiating lymph nodes from vessels in patients allergic to contrast material. If venous extension is detected, cephalad extension must be determined, and in particular, its relation to the hepatic veins and right atrium. Tumor in the left renal vein may cause venous outflow obstruction and development of collaterals, including spermatic varicocele (Fig. 9–51 A,B).

Metastases. Skeletal metastases are osteolytic and radiolucent on radiography and CT imaging. There may be bone expansion, scalloping of the inner margins, and break through the bony cortex (Fig. 9–52). Metastases are usually hypervascular if the primary tumor is hypervascular. Pathologic fracture may be the initial presenting symptom. On MR imaging, the usual medium signal intensity (gray) of the bone marrow is replaced by hypointense (dark) area on T1-weighted image. On T2-weighted image, me-

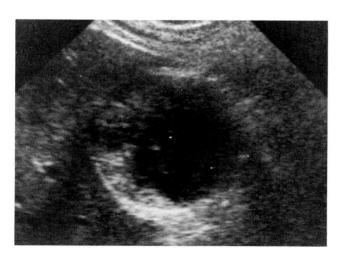

Figure 9–40. Renal carcinoma growing within a renal cyst.

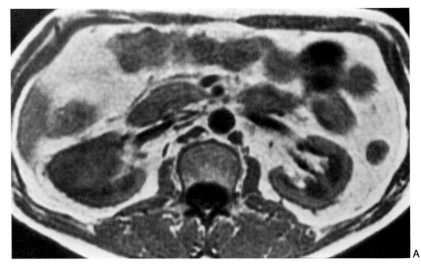

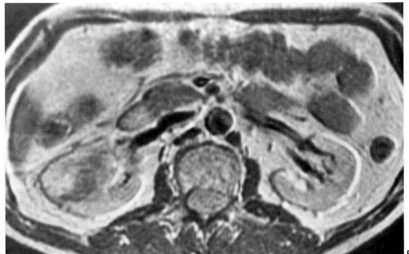

Figure 9–41. (A) Right renal carcinoma on T1-weighted sequence is isointense to the renal cortex. (B) On T2-weighted sequence the tumor remains mostly isointense to the renal cortex, but both have stronger signal intensity and are brighter.

tastases are usually isointense to the marrow and difficult to spot.

Liver metastases are relatively radiolucent on a precontrast scan and may be invisible after contrast infusion. Cavernous hemangioma is the most important differential diagnosis. Tc-99m red blood cell scan or MR imaging of the liver may help establish the diagnosis. On MR imaging, hemangioma is intensely bright and well circumscribed on T2-weighted sequence, metastasis usually less so.

Direct extension into the ipsilateral adrenal is common and so are hematogenous adrenal metastases (Fig. 9–53).

Thoracic metastases are usually nodular, "cannon ball" type lung lesions. Hilar and mediastinal adenopathy are grave prognostic signs. Ribs should be carefully scrutinized for the presence of lytic metastases.

Brain metastases are usually multiple and diagnosed as mass lesions on CT or MR.

Metastases to the Kidney (Renal Metastases)

Incidence. Twelve percent on autopsy of cancer patients.

Pathology. Hypovascular, seldom large, seldom necrotic. Primary sites are lung, breast, and gastrointestinal tract. Lymphoma and melanoma also commonly metastasize to the kidney.

Clinical Presentation. Usually asymptomatic. Sometimes pain and gross hematuria.

Laboratory Findings. Hematuria, proteinuria.

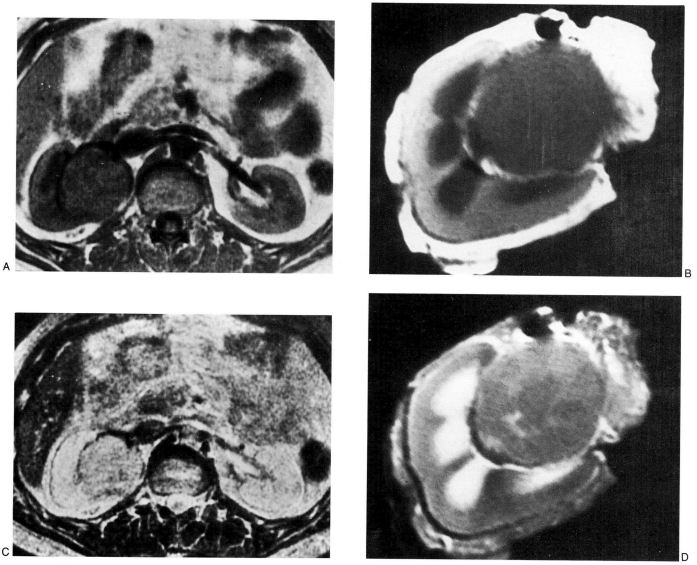

Figure 9–42. Example of image degradation due to motion. **(A)** T1-weighted sequence showing a renal carcinoma in the right kidney in a live patient. **(B)** T1-weighted sequence of the specimen immediately after surgery. **(C)** T2-weighted sequence in a live patient. **(D)** T2-weighted sequence of the specimen. The specimen, of course, is stationary and the anatomical detail is exquisite.

Radiological Findings. Renal metastases are usually small, multiple, clinically silent, and are associated with widespread metastatic disease elsewhere.[48,49] Principal method of detection is CT. The mass on the precontrast scan is almost isodense to the kidney and enhances only slightly on the postcontrast scan (Fig. 9–54). Acute hemorrhage within the mass may appear hyperdense (Fig. 9–55 A,B). Nonspecific appearance of a solid renal mass is present on sonography and urography. Most metastases are hypovascular on angiographic examination, with the notable exceptions of carcinoid, choriocarcinoma, and melanoma.

Renal metastases present a management problem when the primary malignant process is in remission, since concomitant renal cell carcinoma cannot be excluded without aspiration biopsy (Fig. 9–56).[50]

Renal Lymphoma

Incidence. Five percent of patients have renal involvement when first staged, 33% at autopsy. Primary renal lymphoma is rare.

Pathology. Multiple or solitary nodular lesions, diffuse lymphomatous infiltrates within interstitial

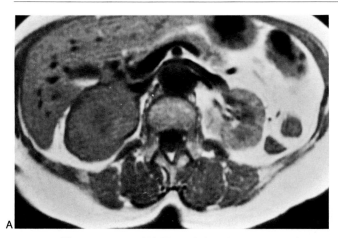

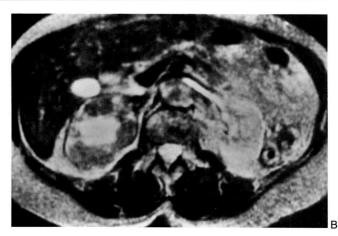

Figure 9–43.   (A) T1-weighted sequence demonstrates a renal carcinoma isointense to the renal parenchyma. (B) On T2-weighted sequence there are areas within the tumor that become markedly hyperintense and represent either necrosis or hemorrhage.

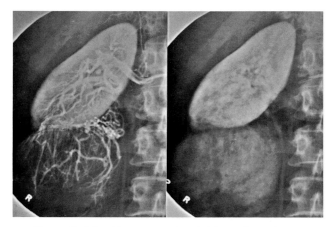

Figure 9–44.   Hypervascular right renal carcinoma.

spaces, renal or ureteral invasion from adjacent lymphomatous masses.

Clinical Presentation.   Usually asymptomatic. Some patients present in renal failure and ureteral obstruction.

Laboratory Findings.   Azotemia, hypercalciuria, proteinuria.

Radiological Findings.   Well over half of the kidneys affected have multiple or solitary lymphoma nodules or masses. These enhance slightly on the contrast CT scan, but much less than the adjacent normal renal parenchyma. Masses are hypoechoic or anechoic, but unlike renal cysts there is no through

Figure 9–45.   Sequence of radiographs from a selective left renal arteriogram demonstrating arteriovenous shunting. The renal vein (arrows) becomes opacified during the arterial phase.

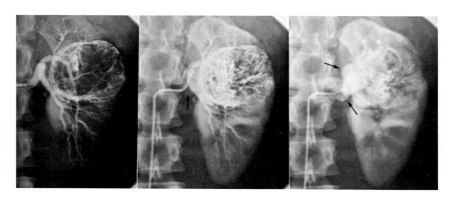

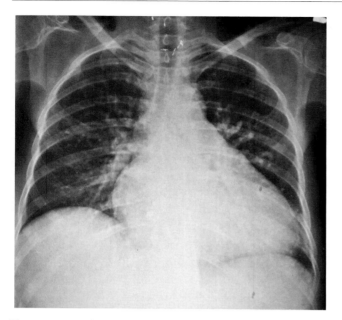

Figure 9–46. Cardiomegaly in a patient with a renal cancer with a large arteriovenous shunt.

transmission.[51,52] Angiography may demonstrate hypovascular masses and a fuzzy renal outline (Fig. 9–57).[53]

A less common mode of presentation is diffuse renal involvement resulting in global renal enlargement. Invasion of the renal sinus from the adjacent involved lymph nodes in a retrograde fashion may also be seen (Fig. 9–58). At times, perinephric spaces may also contain lymphomatous masses (Figs. 9–59, 9–60).

The major diagnostic problem is differentiating a renal lymphoma mass from a renal carcinoma. In many instances the radiographic findings are atypical. There may also be coincidental presence of both malignancies. Aspiration biopsy is the next logical step in arriving at a histological diagnosis. Radiological findings are summarized in Table 9–4.

MR is nonspecific and resembles renal carcinoma. T1-weighted sequences demonstrate a lesion isointense to the kidney (Fig. 61). T2-weighted sequences show the lesion to be of high signal intensity (bright).

Ureteral obstruction by enlarged lymph nodes may be seen.

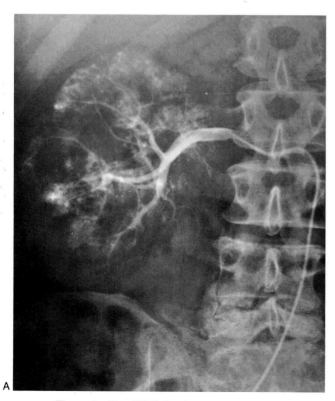

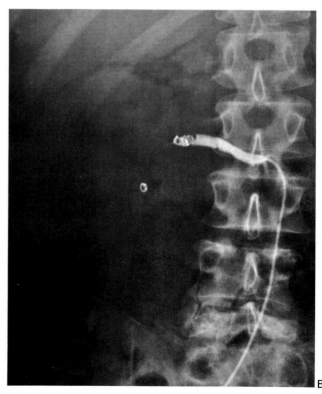

A B

Figure 9–47. (A) Selective renal arteriogram prior to renal artery embolization. (B) Selective renal arteriogram after embolization with wire coils showing complete obstruction.

Table 9-3.   Detection Rates in Depicting Renal Carcinoma 3 cm or Smaller[41,45]

MODALITY	%
CT	94
US	79
Angiography	74
IVP	67
MRI	62

Renal Leukemia

Incidence.   Fifty percent at autopsy of patients with leukemia.

Pathology.   Interstitial foci or infiltrates of leukemia cells, occasionally forming masses.

Clinical Presentation.   Usually silent. Enlarged kidneys may be palpable. Ureteral obstruction and renal failure are rare.

Laboratory Findings.   Hyperuricemia, uremia (rare).

Radiological Findings.   Bilateral symmetrical renal enlargement is present in most patients. In children renal enlargement may be the only presenting clinical finding.[54,55] Occasionally, one kidney may be more involved and larger than the other. Rarely, a renal mass is present. Hydronephrosis due to ureteral obstruction is rare. As the kidneys enlarge, calyceal splaying and narrowing may become apparent. The examination of choice is ultrasound, which will demonstrate enlarged kidneys and, possibly, presence of hypoechoic infiltrates. Mass lesions and hydronephrosis may also be evident.

Renal Sarcoma

Incidence.   Rare.

Pathology.   Leiomyosarcoma, hemangiopericytoma, liposarcoma, rhabdomyosarcoma, malignant schwannoma, neurofibrosarcoma, osteosarcoma, malignant fibrous histiocytoma (fibroxanthosarcoma).

Clinical Presentation.   Large abdominal masses, abdominal pain, discomfort, metastasizes readily.

Laboratory Findings.   Occasional hematuria, hypoglycemia (hemangiopericytoma).

Radiological Findings.   Usually a large hypovascular mass displaces the kidney rather than invading it.[56] The lack of renal parenchymal invasion and absence of lymphadenopathy are major differentiating radiographic signs to renal carcinoma (Fig. 9–62).

Ossification may occur in primary renal osteosarcoma and small specks of calcification may be seen in others.

Since the detected mass is solid, precise preoperative diagnosis is rarely possible. Efforts should be focused on determining local extension and detection of distant metastases.

On rare occasions, the differential diagnosis between benign angiomyolipoma and renal liposarcoma may be brought into question. The latter may exhibit spotty radiolucencies due to presence of fatty tissues within the tumor. Angiographic examination may sometimes be indicated. A hypervascular lesion with venous lakes and a swirled appearance favors an angiomyolipoma, while a hypovascular tumor is

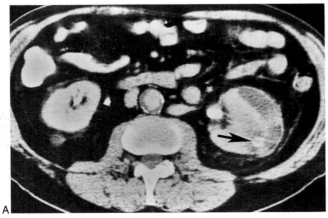
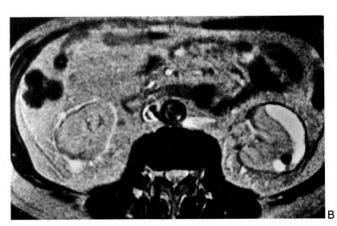

Figure 9–48.   (A) A subcapsular hematoma and an underlying small renal mass with areas of calcification (arrow) are detected on CT in a patient with left flank pain. (B) Hematoma is clearly visible on MR imaging (T2-weighted sequence) and the tumor, including calcification (low signal), is recognizable. Spontaneous subcapsular hemorrhage should spur the search for an underlying renal cancer or angiomyolipoma.

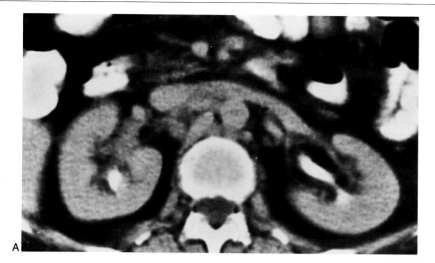

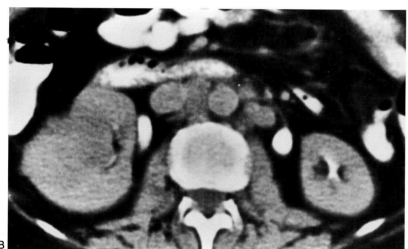

Figure 9–49. While searching for lymph nodes, it is useful to identify left renal vein and follow it to the vena cava. Retrocaval nodes are then detected without difficulty **(A)**. By following the inferior vena cava (and aorta) cephalad and caudad, it is easy to spot extraneous soft tissue densities in the retroperitoneum. **(B)** Right renal cancer is present with metastatic lymph nodes interposed between inferior vena cava and aorta, and in the left para-aortic region.

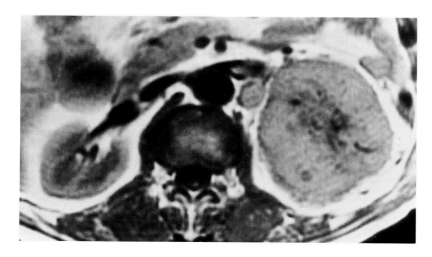

Figure 9–50. Left renal carcinoma propagating within the lumen of the left renal vein and extending posteriorly into the lumbar vein. Extension into the lumbar vein may be misinterpreted as regional lymph node metastasis.

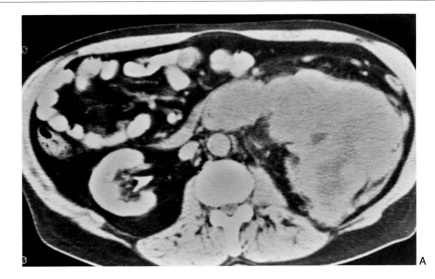

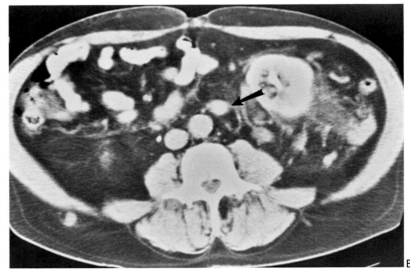

Figure 9–51. (A) Large upper pole left renal carcinoma propagates within the lumen of the left renal vein. (B) On a more caudal cut, a larger spermatic vein is visualized (arrow), as well as many dilated collateral vessels posterior to the lower pole of the kidney.

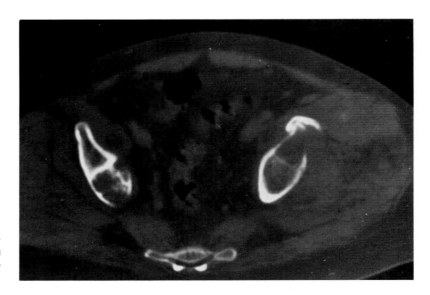

Figure 9–52. Osteolytic metastases from renal carcinoma with scalloping and a break-through cortex.

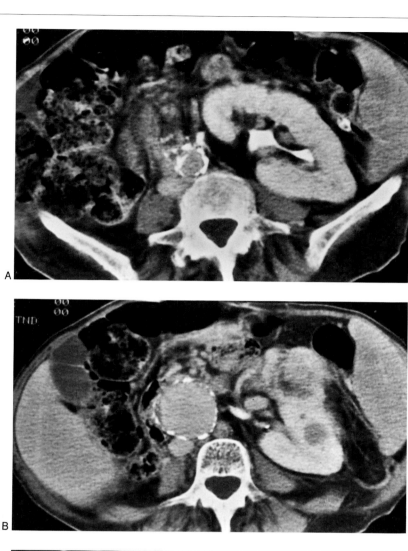

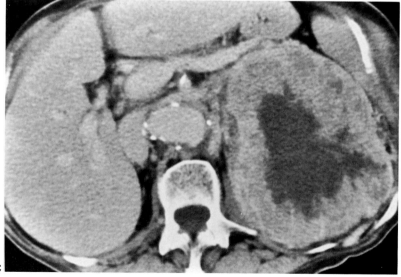

Figure 9–53. (A) Inferior displacement and change in axis of the solitary left kidney is caused by a renal carcinoma **(B)** originating from the posterior cortical area. **(C)** More cephalad cut shows the true size of the necrotic tumor. A small right adrenal metastasis is present although indistinguishable from inferior vena cava.

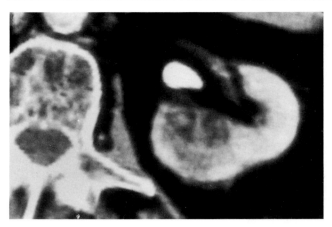

Figure 9–54. Renal metastasis from carcinoma of the colon. There are no distinguishing features from renal carcinoma.

likely a liposarcoma. Renal liposarcoma is a rare lesion seen predominantly in elderly patients.

Adult Wilms Tumor (Nephroblastoma)

Wilms tumor is rarely found in adults and is mostly seen before 35 years of age. There are no radiographic findings that can differentiate this tumor from most renal tumors, including renal cell carcinoma. Complex mass may be present, frequently with areas of necrosis, hemorrhage, and cystic components.[57–59] The tumor is hypovascular, although very fine zigzag or creeping vine neovascularity may be seen on angiography. Fine calcifications within the tumor may be seen on CT.

Transitional Cell Carcinoma (TCC) of the Renal Pelvis

Etiology. Infection, hydrocarbons, smoking, calculi, cyclophosphamide,[60] analgesic abuse, thorium deposition in the kidney.[61] Smoking and phenacetin abuse increase risk synergistically.[62,63]

Incidence. Five to 10% of all renal neoplasms.

Pathology. Multicentric, hypovascular, metastases to bone (lytic and mixed), lung and local invasion. Calcification is extremely rare. Polychronotopic, tends to have multiple recurrences in different areas and at different times. Forty to 80% of patients with upper tract tumor develop TCC elsewhere in the urinary tract. Three percent of patients with bladder TCC develop upper tract tumor.

Clinical Presentation. Hematuria, ureteral obstruction, weight loss.

Laboratory Findings. Hematuria, positive urine cytology.

Radiological Findings. The classic descriptive differential diagnosis of "filling defect" on excretory urography includes the common three: TCC, blood clot, and radiolucent calculus. Less common are fungus ball, sloughed papilla, fibroepithelial polyp, malakoplakia, vessel impression, metastases, invasion by hypernephroma, arteriovenous malformation, etc. The filling defect is usually first detected on an excretory urogram (Fig. 9–63) or retrograde pyelogram (Fig. 9–64). The diagnosis is confirmed by a

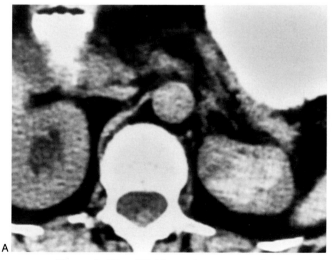
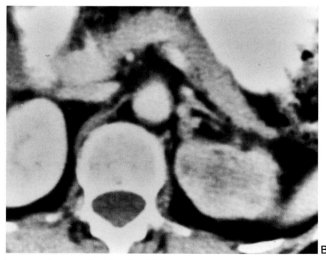

A   B

Figure 9–55. **(A)** Hyperdense areas in metastatic carcinoma of the colon in the kidney represent acute hemorrhage. **(B)** On postcontrast scan, the mass is relatively radiolucent.

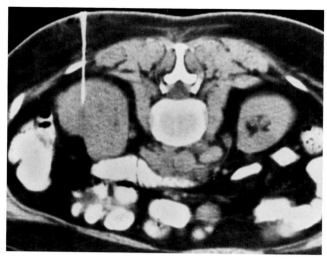

Figure 9–56. Aspiration biopsy of a renal mass in a patient with a breast carcinoma. Note regional lymph node enlargement.

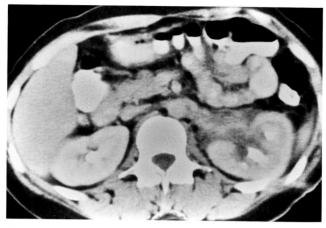

Figure 9–58. Infiltration of the renal sinus, as seen here in the left kidney, is usually by extension from adjacent lymph nodes.

positive urinalysis for TCC and/or selective retrograde washings and brush biopsy (Fig. 9–65).

Depending on the pattern of growth, the tumor may obstruct a major infundibulum and produce a hydrocalyx (Fig. 9–66). The result is an "amputated calyx," a finding that is highly suggestive of TCC, tuberculosis, or an inflammatory stricture (Fig. 9–67).

A very small tumor may be invisible to all types of imaging. This may be very disconcerting when, in the presence of hematuria, TCC cells are found in the urine on multiple occasions and yet no lesion can be identified on radiographic examinations. Coarse punctate calcifications may be seen on rare occasions.[64]

As the tumor grows, the renal sinus fat is invaded and eventually the renal parenchyma becomes invaded as well. Consequently, ill-defined soft tissue mass is seen on CT and ultrasound, obliterating the pelvic wall, and renal sinus fat is seen growing within the kidney (Fig. 9–68).[65,66] The tumor has low attenuation value on contrast-enhanced scan. No acoustical shadowing is present on ultrasound. Renal angiogram will demonstrate a hypovascular mass without any specific findings.

Because TCC tends to be multicentric, the entire transitional epithelium surface throughout the urinary tract must be carefully scrutinized for additional lesions (Fig. 9–69).

Renal Squamous Cell Carcinoma and Adenocarcinoma of the Renal Pelvis

Etiology. Infection, calculi, bladder schistosomiasis with reflux (squamous cell).

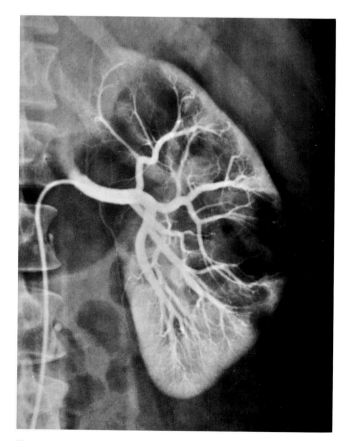

Figure 9–57. Multiple hypovascular renal masses in renal lymphoma.

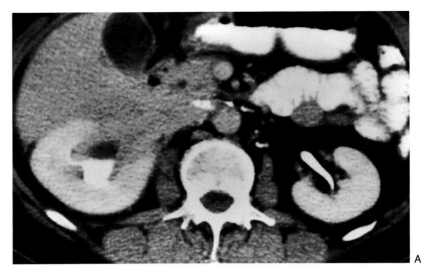

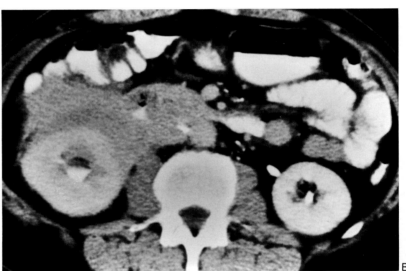

Figure 9–59. Lymphoma invading renal sinus **(A)** and perinephric space anterior to the right kidney **(B)**.

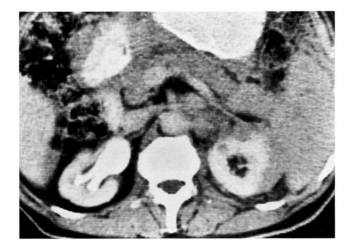

Figure 9–60. Histiocytic lymphoma extending into the left perinephric space. Note enlarged lymph nodes.

Incidence.   Rare.

Pathology.   Infiltrative.

Clinical Presentation.   Chronic urinary tract infection, recurrent renal calculous disease.

Radiological Findings.   These tumors originate from the collecting system epithelium and infiltrate the kidney from within. Partially functioning or completely afunctional but enlarged kidney is the usual finding on any radiographic examinations. CT is the examination of choice, since the local extension of the tumor is well depicted.

von Hippel-Lindau Disease

Etiology.   Rare familial disease, inherited as an autosomal dominant trait with incomplete penetrance.

Table 9–4. Radiological Findings in Renal Lymphoma

CT	SONOGRAPHY	ANGIOGRAPHY
Multiple renal masses 45% Solitary mass 15% Invasion from outside 25% Diffuse infiltration 10% Perinephric involvement 5%	Hypoechoic Anechoic No through transmission Diminished central sinus echoes	Hypovascular Capsular artery displacement Fuzzy renal outline

Pathology. Cerebellar hemangioblastoma, retinal angiomas. Multiple renal carcinomas are seen in 40% of patients. There are also multiple renal cysts resembling cysts in polycystic renal disease. Pheochromocytoma is present in 10%. Pancreatic tumors or cysts may also be present.

Clinical Presentation. Onset is in third decade of life. Symptoms are usually related to cerebellar or retinal involvement. Renal carcinomas, when diagnosed, are usually removed, employing partial nephrectomy in an attempt to preserve renal function.[67–69] Yearly follow-up imaging of the kid-

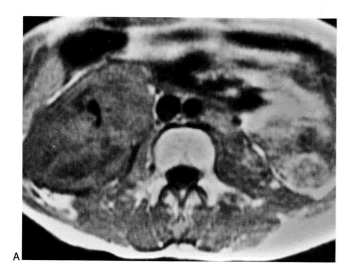

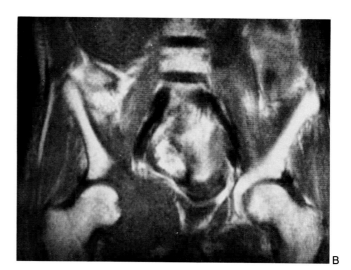

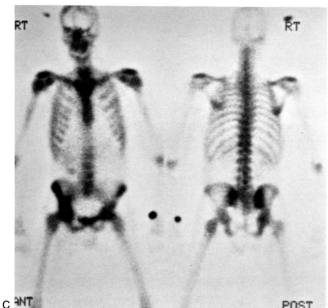

Figure 9–61. **(A)** Renal lymphoma is isointense to the renal cortex on T1-weighted sequence, as seen in the right kidney. **(B)** Metastases to the bone are hypointense (dark) compared to relatively hyperintense (bright) bone marrow. In this patient the right acetabulum is completely replaced by lymphoma. **(C)** Bone scan shows increased uptake in the area.

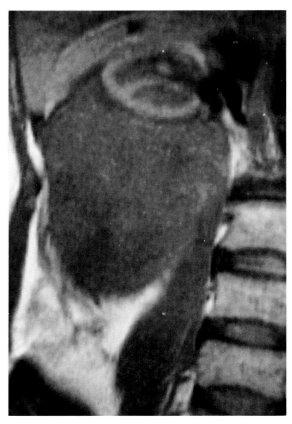

Figure 9–62. Renal fibrosarcoma. The tumor clearly does not originate from the renal cortex, which is seen undisturbed on this T1-weighted coronal sequence.

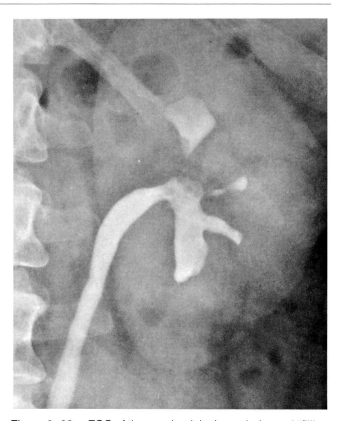

Figure 9–63. TCC of the renal pelvis. Irregularity and "filling defect" are seen in the renal pelvis. There is also narrowing of the upper pole infundibulum.

neys by CT or angiography searching for renal carcinoma is recommended. Cause of death is usually intracranial hemorrhage but death from metastatic renal carcinoma is also frequent.

Radiological Findings. Solid renal tumors are found on CT. Renal and pancreatic cysts may also be present. The diagnosis of recurrent carcinoma is difficult following one or several partial nephrectomies (Fig. 9–70). Following partial nephrectomy, the kidney remnant may assume bizarre shapes, sometimes mimicking a tumor.

RENAL NEOPLASMS IN CHILDREN

Mesoblastic Nephroma (Fetal Renal Hamartoma)

Etiology. Unknown.

Incidence. Most common renal neoplasm in infants. Male to female ratio, 2:1.

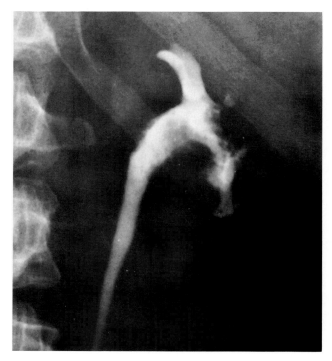

Figure 9–64. TCC of the renal pelvis.

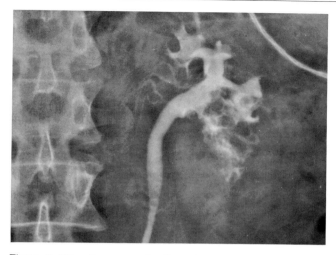

Figure 9–65. One complication of retrograde pyelography is pyelolymphatic backflow as seen in this study. Unfortunately, there is also a large irregular "filling defect" occupying most of the mid and lower collecting system. There is a danger of forcing the malignant cells into the lymphatic circulation if pressures during retrograde injection are too high.

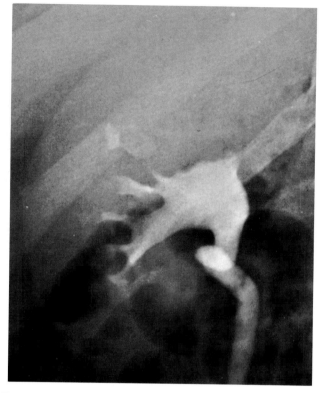

Figure 9–67. "Amputated" upper pole calyx by infiltrating TCC causing obstruction of the upper infundibulum.

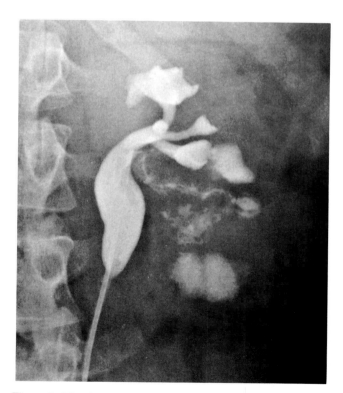

Figure 9–66. Lower pole hydrocalyx caused by an expanding TCC in the major infundibulum.

Pathology. Benign, yellowish medullary renal mass lacking capsule, composed of spindle cells. Cystic changes possible. May penetrate renal capsule. Entrapment of tubular structures.

Clinical Presentation. Abdominal mass, usually seen in first 4 months of life.[70,71] May be diagnosed in utero.

Treatment. Nephrectomy.

Radiological Findings. Focal, usually large solid renal mass is identified on ultrasound. Some internal echoes are present. Functioning renal parenchyma may be demonstrated within the tumor.[72] Differential diagnosis includes Wilms tumor and nephroblastomatosis.

Nephroblastomatosis

Incidence. Rare.

Pathology. Pathologic persistence of metanephric blastema in the renal parenchyma. Could be consid-

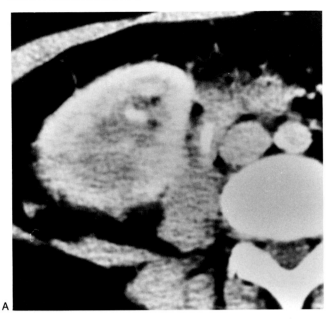
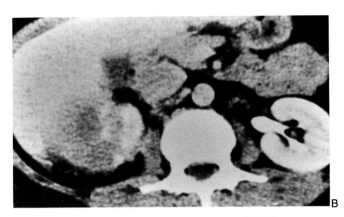

Figure 9–68. **(A)** Infiltrating TCC has replaced renal sinus fat and is invading renal parenchyma. **(B)** The inferior vena cava is expanded and an intraluminal filling defect may be recognized (compare with vena cava on A). Unlike renal carcinoma, TCC rarely propagates via veins, although this proved to be such a case.

ered malformation or neoplasm. Deep cortical and multifocal nephroblastomatosis is precursor of Wilms tumor. No mitotic figures.

Radiological Findings. Subcapsular tumor nodules are seen on ultrasound as mass lesion isoechoic or hyperechoic to the kidney. Isoechoic lesions may be missed and contrast-enhanced CT is the examination of choice.[73–75] On CT, nephroblastomatosis presents as low attenuation, nonenhancing masses. Since these may develop into Wilms tumor, follow-up is recommended.[76]

Wilms Tumor (Nephroblastoma)

Incidence. Most common abdominal malignancy in children. Incidence is 7.8 per 1,000,000 children (under age of 15 years) per year. Peak incidence is 2.5 to 3 years of age. Male to female ratio, 1.2:1. Bilateral in 5%; familial in 1%. If parent or sibling has bilateral Wilms, incidence is 30%. Congenital anomalies are present in 15% (genitourinary, hemihypertrophy, aniridia, neurofibromatosis, Drash's syndrome, Beckwith-Wiedemann syndrome, chromosomal abnormalities).

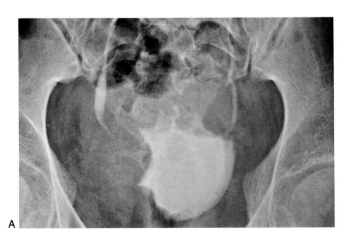
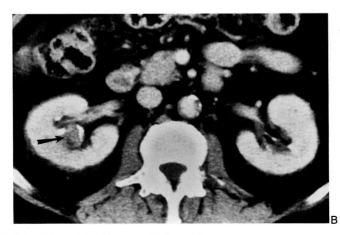

Figure 9–69. Synchronous TCC in the bladder **(A)** and right kidney **(B)** (arrow).

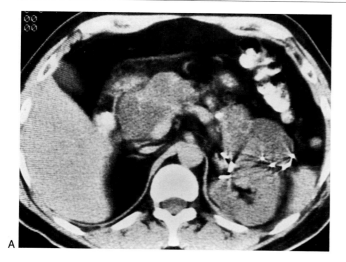

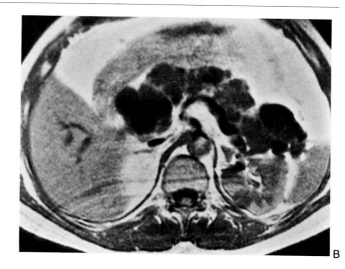

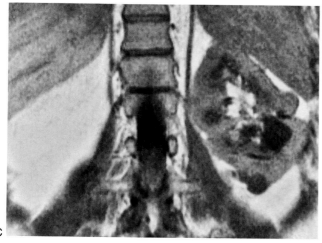

Figure 9–70. **(A)** CT and **(B)** MR T1-weighted sequence in a patient with von Hippel-Lindau disease showing multiple pancreatic cysts and one or two ill-defined renal cysts. **(C)** Coronal T1-weighted sequence demonstrates several low-intensity lesions, probably renal cysts, and a small mass, isointense to the cortex, along the lateral renal outline. The kidney is misshapen after several wedge resections of small renal carcinomas. The right kidney has been removed because of renal carcinoma.

Wilms tumor is two to eight times more common in patients with horseshoe kidney than in the general population.[77,78]

Pathology. Malignant embryonic neoplasm containing blastemal, embryonic, and stromal tissues. Mass with pseudocapsule, may be cystic. Calcifications in 15%. Renal vein, caval, and atrial extension are possible. Metastases are to lymph nodes, lungs, liver, skeleton, and central nervous system.

Histologic types are: a) favorable, 90% (lack of anaplastic and sarcomatous elements); and b) unfavorable, 10% (presence of anaplastic and sarcomatous elements).

Clinical Presentation. Common presentation is a symptomatic abdominal mass.[79] Uncommon presentation is fever, pain, hematuria, anorexia, hypertension. Extension into the vena cava is present in 6%.

Treatment. Surgery and multiagent chemotherapy. Radiation therapy is added in more advanced stages.

Radiological Findings. Sonography is the screening examination of choice to determine whether the mass is cystic or solid and to confirm if it is renal in origin. Vascular extension may be detected and particular attention is directed to clear the vena cava and right atrium of any possible tumor involvement. Liver metastases are also looked for.

MR imaging is the method of choice in further evaluation and staging of the disease.[80] Variable signal intensities are seen on T1- and T2-weighted sequences, depending on the presence of cystic components and hemorrhage. Great vessels are usually well depicted and abnormal lymph nodes detected.

CT is almost as good as MR imaging except for the necessity of intravenous contrast.[81] Since lung metastases are present in 10% of patients at the time of diagnosis, CT of the thorax is usually part of imaging workup.

It is of importance to exclude involvement of the renal pelvis or ureter because the presence of tumor in these areas is an indication for nephro-ureterectomy.[77] Thus, some recommend urography[82] or retrograde pyelography in case of non-visualization.

REFERENCES

1. King MC, Fridenberg RM, Tena LB. Normal renal parenchyma simulating tumor. Radiology 1968; 91:217–222.
2. Felson B, Moskowitz M. Renal pseudotumors: The degenerated nodule and other lumps, bumps, and dromedary humps. Am J Roentgenol 1969; 107:720–729.
3. Charghi A, Dessureault P, Drouin G, et al. Malposition of a renal lobe (lobar dysmorphism): a condition simulating renal tumor. J Urol 1971; 105:326–329.
4. Dacie JE. The "central lucency" sign of lobar dysmorphism (pseudotumor of the kidney). Br J Radiol 1976; 49:39–42.
5. Ranninger K, Abrams E, Bordent A. Pseudotumor resulting from a fresh renal infarct. Radiology 1969; 92:343–344.
6. Sukthomya C, Levin B. Pseudotumors of the kidney secondary to anticoagulant therapy. Radiology 1967; 88:701–703.
7. Sussman SK, Baker ME, Saeed M, et al. Polar infarct in a transplanted kidney: cause of a pseudomass. Urol Radiol 1987; 9:42–43.
8. Olsson O, Weiland PO. Renal fibrolipomatosis. Acta Radiol [Diagn (Stockh)] 1963; 1:1061–1070.
9. Simpson EL, Mintz MC, Pollack HM, et al. Computed tomography in the diagnosis of renal pseudotumors. CT 1986; 10:341–344.
10. Bosniak MA, Megibow AJ, Hulnick DH, et al. CT diagnosis of renal angiomyolipoma: the importance of detecting small amounts of fat. AJR 1988; 151:497–501.
11. Bret PM, Bretagnolle M, Gaillard D, et al. Small, asymptomatic angiomyolipomas of the kidney. Radiology 1985; 154:7–11.
12. Love L, Frank SJ. Angiographic features of angiomyolipoma of the kidney. Am J Roentgenol 1965; 95:406–408.
13. Mitnick JS, Bosniak MA, Hilton S, et al. Cystic renal disease in tuberous sclerosis. Radiology 1983; 147:85–87.
14. Gutierrez OH, Burgener FA, Schwartz S. Coincident renal cell cancer and renal angiomyolipoma in tuberous sclerosis. AJR 1979; 132:848.
15. Honey KJ, Honey RM. Tuberous sclerosis and bilateral renal carcinoma. Br J Urol 1977; 49:441–446.
16. Suslavich F, Older RA, Hinman CG. Calcified renal carcinoma in a patient with tuberous sclerosis. AJR 1979; 133:524–526.
17. Sant GR, Ucci AA, Meares EM. Multicentric angiomyolipoma: Renal and lymph node involvement. Urology 1986; 28:111–113.
18. Earthman WJ, Mazer MJ, Winfield AC. Angiomyolipo-
mas in tuberous sclerosis: subselective embolotherapy with alcohol, with long-term follow-up study. Radiology 1986; 160:437–441.
19. Dineen MK, Venable DD, Misra RP. Pure intrarenal lipoma: report of a case and review of the literature. J Urol 1984; 132:104–107.
20. Leiphart CJ, Nudelman EJ. Hibernoma masquerading as a pheochromocytoma. Radiology 1970; 95:659–660.
21. English JT, Patel SK, Flanagan MJ. Association of pheochromocytomas with brown fat tumors. Radiology 1973; 107:279–281.
22. Quinn MJ, Hartman DS, Friedman AC, et al. Renal oncocytoma: new observations. Radiology 1984; 153:49–53.
23. Sos TA, Gray GF Jr, Baltaxe HA. The angiographic appearance of benign renal oxyphilic adenoma. Am J Roentgenol 1976; 127:717–722.
24. Neisius D, Braedel HU, Schindler E, et al. Computed tomographic and angiographic findings in renal oncocytoma. Br J Radiol 1988; 61:1019–1025.
25. Remark RR, Berquist TH, Lieber MM, et al. Magnetic resonance imaging of renal oncocytoma. Urology 1988; 31:176–179.
26. Ball DS, Friedman AC, Hartman DS, et al. Scar sign of renal oncocytoma: Magnetic resonance imaging appearance and lack of specificity. Urol Radiol 1986; 8:46–48.
27. Madewell JE, Goldman SM, Davis CJ, et al. Multilocular cystic nephroma: a radiographic-pathologic correlation of 58 patients. Radiology 1983; 146:309–321.
28. Dikengil A, Benson M, Sanders L, Newhouse JH. MRI of multilocular cystic nephroma. Urol Radiol 1988; 10:95–99.
29. Hartman DS, Davis CJ Jr, Sanders RC, et al. Multiloculated renal mass: considerations and differential features. Radiographics 1987; 7:29–42.
30. Dunnick NR, Hartman DS, Ford KK, et al. The radiology of juxtaglomerular tumors. Radiology 1983; 147:321–326.
31. Glover CD, Buck AC. Renal medullary fibroma. A case report. J Urol 1982; 127:758–760.
32. Cormier P, Patel SK, Turner DA, Hoeksema J. MR imaging findings in renal medullary fibroma. AJR 1989; 153:83–84.
33. Zolickofer C, Castaneda-Zuniga W, Nath HP, et al. The angiographic appearance of intrarenal leiomyoma. Radiology 1980; 136:47–49.
34. Uchida M, Watanabe H, Mishina T, et al. Leiomyoma of the renal pelvis. J Urol 1981; 125:572–574.
35. Asa SL, Bedard YC, Buckspan MB, et al. Spontaneous hypoglycemia associated with hemangiopericytoma of the kidney. J Urol 1981; 125:864–867.
36. Redlin L, Francis RS, Orlando MM. Renal abnormalities in agnogenic myeloid metaplasia. Radiology 1976; 121:605–608.
37. Jacobs JE, Sussman SK, Glickstein MF. Renal lymphangioma—a rare cause of a multiloculated renal mass. AJR 1989; 152:307–308.
38. Smith SJ, Bosniak MA, Megibow AJ, et al. Renal carcinoma: earlier discovery and increased detection. Radiology 1989; 170:699–703.
39. Levine E, Huntrakoon M, Wetzel LH. Small renal neoplasms: clinical, pathologic, and imaging features. AJR 1989; 153:69–73.
40. Robson CJ, Churchill BM, Anderson W. The results of radical nephrectomy for renal cell carcinoma. J Urol 1969; 101:297–301.

41. Amendola MA, Bree RL, Pollack HM, et al. Small renal carcinomas: resolving a diagnostic dilemma. Radiology 1988; 166:637–641.
42. Zeman RK, Cronan JJ, Rosenfield AT, et al. Renal cell carcinoma: dynamic thin-section CT assessment of vascular invasion and tumor vascularity. Radiology 1988; 167:393–396.
43. Johnson CD, Dunnick NR, Cohan RH, et al. CT staging of 100 tumors. AJR 1987; 148:59–64.
44. Lang EK: Angio-computed tomography and dynamic computed tomography in staging of renal cell carcinoma. Radiology 1984; 151:149–155.
45. Hricak H, Theoni RF, Carroll PR, et al. Detection and staging of renal neoplasms: a reassessment of MR imaging. Radiology 1988; 166:643–649.
46. Fein AB, Lee JKT, Balfe DM, et al: Diagnosis and staging of renal cell carcinoma: a comparison of MR imaging and CT. AJR 1987; 148:749–753.
47. Patel SK, Stack CM, Taner DA. Magnetic resonance imaging in staging of renal cell carcinoma. Radiographics 1987; 7:703–716.
48. Choyke PL, White EM, Zeman RK, et al. Renal metastases: Clinicopathologic and radiologic correlation. Radiology 1987; 162:359–363.
49. Mitnick JS, Bosniak MA, Rothberg M, et al. Metastatic neoplasm to the kidney studied by computed tomography and sonography. J Comput Assist Tomogr 1985; 9:43–49.
50. Kutcher R, Greenbaum E, Rosenblatt R, et al. Prostatic carcinoma metastatic to the kidney: diagnosis by thin needle aspiration biopsy. Urol Radiol 1986; 8:98–99.
51. Horii SC, Bosniak MA, Megibow AJ, et al. Correlation of CT and ultrasound in evaluation of renal lymphoma. Urol Radiol 1983; 5:69–76.
52. Jafri SZH, Bree RL, Amendola MA, et al. CT of renal and perirenal non-Hodgkin's lymphoma. AJR 1982; 138:1101–1105.
53. Pick RA, Castellino RA, Seltzer RA. Arteriographic findings in renal lymphoma. Am J Roentgenol 1971; 111:530–534.
54. Gore RM, Skolnik A. Abdominal manifestation of pediatric leukemias: sonographic assessment. Radiology 1982; 143:207–210.
55. Araki T. Leukemic involvement of the kidney in children: CT features. J Comput Assist Tomogr 1982; 6:781–784.
56. Shirkhoda A, Lewis E. Renal sarcoma and sarcomatoid renal cell carcinoma: CT and angiographic features. Radiology 1987; 162:353–356.
57. Hartman DS, Davis CJ Jr, Madewell JE, et al. Primary malignant renal tumors in the second decade of life: Wilms' tumor vs renal cell carcinoma. J Urol 1982; 127:888–891.
58. Kumar R, Amparo EG, David R, et al. Adult Wilms tumor: clinical and radiographic features. Urol Radiol 1984; 6:164–169.
59. Kioumehr F, Cochran ST, Layfield L, et al. Wilms tumor (nephroblastoma) in the adult patient: clinical and radiological manifestations. AJR 1989; 152:299–302.
60. Brenner DW, Schellhammer PF. Upper tract urothelial malignancy after cyclophosphamide therapy: a case report and literature review. J Urol 1987; 137:1226–1227.
61. Oyen RH, Gielen JL, Van Poppel HP, et al. Renal thorium deposition associated with transitional cell carcinoma: radiologic demonstration in two patients. Radiology 1988; 169:705–707.
62. McCredie M, Steward JH, Jord JM. Analgesic and tobacco as risk factors for ureter and renal pelvis. J Urol 1983; 130:28–30.
63. McCredie M, Steward JH, Carter JJ, et al. Phenacetin papillary necrosis: independent risk factors for renal pelvic cancer. Kidney Int 1986; 30:81–84.
64. Dinsmore BJ, Pollack HM, Banner MP. Calcified transitional cell carcinoma of the renal pelvis. Radiology 1988; 167:401–404.
65. Gatewood OMB, Goldman SM, Marshal FF, et al. Computed tomography in the diagnosis of transitional cell carcinoma of the kidney. J Urol 1982; 127:876–887.
66. Baron RL, McClennan BL, Lee JTK, Lausan TL. Computed tomography of transitional cell carcinoma of the renal pelvis and ureter. Radiology 1982; 144:125–130.
67. Spencer WF, Novick AC, Montie JE, et al. Surgical treatment of localized renal cell carcinoma in von Hippel-Lindau's disease. J Urol 1988; 139:507–509.
68. Malek RS, Omess PJ, Benson RC Jr, Zincke H. Renal cell carcinoma in von Hippel-Lindau syndrome. Am J Med 1987; 82:236–238.
69. Loughlin KR, Gittes RF. Urological management of patients with von Hippel-Lindau's disease. J Urol 1986; 136:789–791.
70. Walker RD. New concepts in the treatment of genitourinary cancer in childhood. Semin Surg Oncol 1989; 5:227–234.
71. Chan HS, Cheng MY, Mancer K, et al. Congenital mesoblastic nephroma: a clinicoradiologic study of 17 cases representing the pathologic spectrum of the disease. J Pediatr 1987; 111:64–70.
72. Kirks DR, Kaufman RA. Function within mesoblastic nephroma: imaging—pathologic correlation. Pediatr Radiol 1989; 19:136–139.
73. Cormier PJ, Donaldson JS, Gonzales-Crussi F. Nephroblastomatosis: missed diagnosis. Radiology 1988; 169:737–738.
74. Fernbach SK, Feinstein KA, Donaldson JS, Baum ES. Nephroblastomatosis: comparison of CT with US and urography. Radiology 1988; 166:153–156.
75. Montgomery P, Kuhn JP, Berger PE, Fisher J. Multifocal nephroblastomatosis: clinical significance and imaging. Pediatr Radiol 1984; 14:392–395.
76. Rosenfield NS, Shimkin P, Berdon W, et al. Wilms tumor arising from spontaneously regressing nephroblastomatosis. AJR 1980; 135:381.
77. Mesrobian HGJ. Wilms tumor: past present, future. J Urol 1988; 140:231–238.
78. Mesrobian HGJ, Kelalis PP, Harabovsky E, et al. Wilms tumor in horseshoe kidneys: a report from the National Wilms Tumor Study. J Urol 1985; 133:1002.
79. Siegel MJ, Shackelford GD. Wilms tumor in children: abdominal CT and ultrasound evaluation. Radiology 1986; 160:501–506.
80. Kangarloo H, Dietrich RB, Erlich RM, et al. Magnetic resonance imaging of Wilms tumor. Radiology 1987; 163:291–294.
81. Peretz GS, Lam AH. Distinguishing neuroblastoma from Wilms tumor by computed tomography. J Comput Assist Tomogr 1985; 9:889–894.
82. Nakayama DK, Ortega GJ, D'Angio, O'Neill JA Jr. The nonopacified kidney with Wilms tumor. J Pediatr Surg 1988; 23:152–155.

10

Renal Cysts

SIMPLE RENAL CYSTS

Incidence. Found in 50% of the population over 50 years of age. Rarely seen in young adults and children.[1] There is no male/female preponderance.

Etiology. Probably secondary to tubular obstruction.

Pathology. Expansion of the distal tubules and collecting ducts. Contain clear or straw-colored fluid. Flattened epithelial or fibrous lining. Calcification in the wall possible. One percent of cysts may contain neoplasm at the base.

Clinical Presentation. In most cases cysts are asymptomatic and an incidental finding on radiologic examinations performed for other reasons. Symptoms are related to:

1. Mass effect such as compression of other organs, obstruction of the ureteropelvic junction, dull pain, or discomfort.
2. Hematuria.
3. Acute pain due to acute hemorrhage into the cyst or cyst rupture.
4. Hypertension. Hypoperfusion caused by parenchymal compression (as the cyst is expanding) may induce hyperreninemia.

Radiological Findings

EXU. Mass may be detected on plain radiograph. Excretory urography and tomography will demonstrate relatively radiolucent mass (Fig. 10–1). The outer cyst wall is either "pencil thin" or invisible. The expanding cystic mass may deform the renal parenchyma, resulting in *"claw"* or *"beak"* sign. Excretory urography, however, is much too insensitive to classify a newly discovered mass as cystic or solid.

188

To accomplish this, other imaging modalities are called for.

Sonography. Ultrasound will demonstrate a hypoechoic mass with through transmission (Fig. 10–2). The posterior wall of the mass is sharply demarcated. The wall must be thin. There should be no internal echoes, intraluminal filling defects, or floating debris. Ultrasound examination of the cyst is very much operator-dependent and is not as simple as it sounds. Some parts of the kidneys, the left upper pole, for example, are more difficult to examine than the right kidney where the liver provides an acoustical "window" for easier examination. Although ultrasonographic examination is 95% accurate, any deviation from strict ultrasonographic criteria for the simple cyst enumerated above should raise the possibility of the presence of renal carcinoma and call for a more definitive study, such as CT.

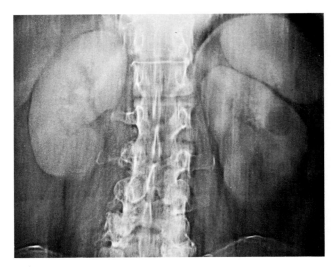

Figure 10–1. Radiolucent left renal cyst detected on tomography during early nephrogram phase.

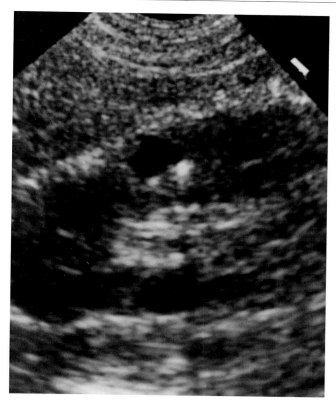

Figure 10–2. Small right renal cyst is sonolucent, which on this particular display is represented as dark. Through transmission is seen in the parenchyma extending beyond the cyst, seen here as brighter echoes. A small calculus in the adjacent calyx is hyperechoic (bright in this display) and exhibits intense acoustical shadowing distally.

CT. CT is the examination of choice if sonographic findings are questionable. Cysts are commonly discovered during CT examination of other organs and no other examination is usually necessary if the findings meet the criteria for benignity. Pencil-thin walls with smooth inner margins, without septations, without calcifications, lack of enhancement, and attenuation value from 0 to 20 HU constitute the signs of benignity (Fig. 10–3).

MR Imaging. Simple renal cyst is hypointense (black) compared with all parenchymal organs on T1-weighted sequences and hyperintense on T2-weighted sequences. It has the same signal characteristics as urine. Any deviation from this appearance suggests either the presence of a hemorrhagic cyst or a tumor.

Angiography. Angiography has no active role in distinguishing benign simple renal cyst from malignancy. During angiographic examinations for other indications, renal cysts may be discovered and it is prudent to familiarize oneself with their appearance on this examination.

The cyst is completely avascular. The base of the cyst should be smooth. Cyst wall must be paper thin. No vessel should transverse the cyst. There should be no calcifications (Fig. 10–4).

Even using these criteria, a hypovascular solid tumor such as lymphoma or papillary cell renal carcinoma may be overlooked. It is prudent to confirm the presence of the cyst by ultrasound.

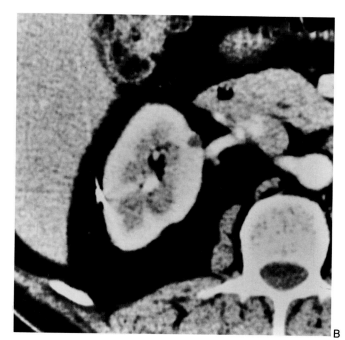

Figure 10–3. Small simple renal cyst in a patient who has undergone partial nephrectomy for renal carcinoma in the same kidney. **(A)** Precontrast scan. **(B)** Postcontrast scan.

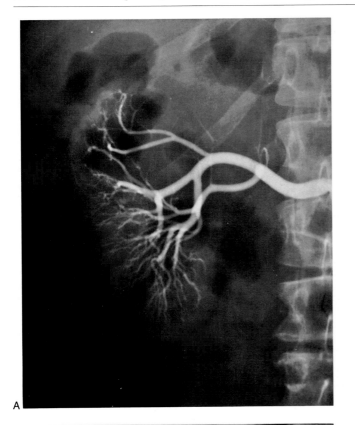

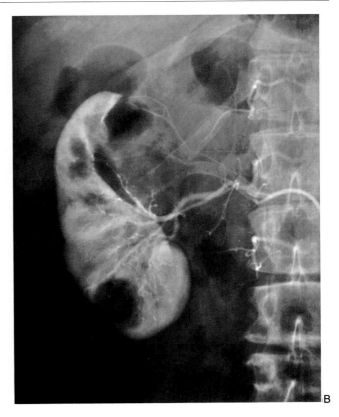

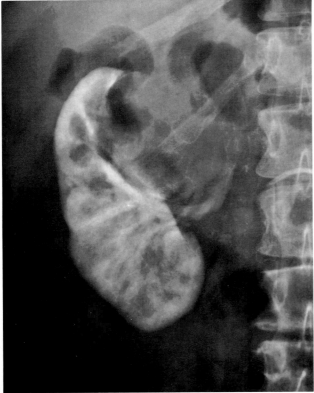

Figure 10–4.   Two simple renal cysts are present. **(A)** The upper cyst is big and displaces the upper pole away from midline, while the lower cyst is still not seen. **(B)** During the early nephrogram phase both cysts are readily visible. Several capsular vessels cross the upper cyst anteriorly or posteriorly to it. **(C)** The small lower cyst again becomes invisible, obscured by dense nephrogram in the normal parenchyma in front and behind it.

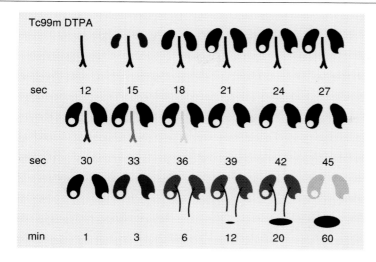

Figure 10–5. Schematic drawing of intraparenchymal and peripheral simple renal cysts as they may appear on Tc-99m DTPA scintigraphy.

Nuclear Medicine. On Tc-99m DMSA scintigram, the cyst and solid tumor appear as a cold defect (Fig. 10–5). There is no particular value in this modality for separating simple cyst from a malignant process.

COMPLEX CYSTS

If renal cystic lesion does not meet the criteria for a simple cyst, particularly on CT and ultrasound, it must be considered malignant. It is often up to the radiologist to recommend further management of such lesions, since the decision whether the cyst should be neglected, followed, aspirated, or operated on so heavily depends on radiological criteria. To facilitate this task, classification into four categories is proposed.[2]

Radiological Findings. Presence of one or more of the following radiological findings is diagnostic of a complex cyst (Fig. 10–6):

1. *Thick wall.* Anything thicker than pencil thin is considered abnormal (Fig. 10–7). Cystic renal carcinoma or necrotic tumor often present in this manner. Surgery is inevitable. Very small intraparenchymal cysts may appear to have a thick wall, which in reality represents normal surrounding parenchyma (Fig. 10–8).
2. *Irregularity at the base of the cyst.* Any irregularity at the base of the cyst should be considered a

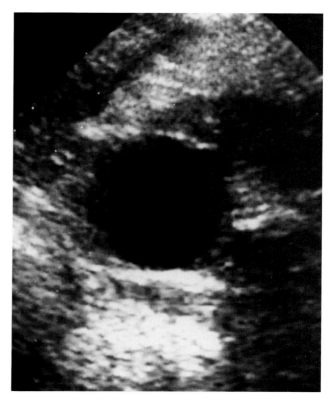

Figure 10–7. Thick wall renal mass with through transmission. This is a complex cyst and is considered malignant.

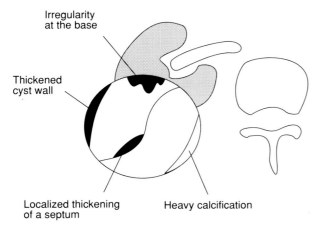

Figure 10–6. Schematic drawing of a complex cyst.

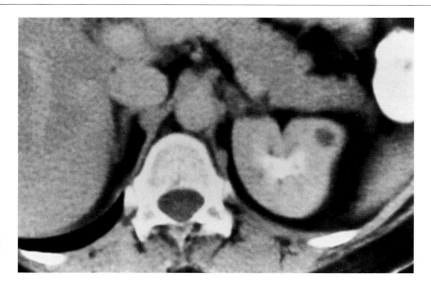

Figure 10–8. Small simple intra-parenchymal cyst appearing to have a thick wall. Several thin CT cuts will allow more precise acquisition of CT numbers from the lesion.

malignant growth (Fig. 10–9). A major problem is in instances where the cyst is molded by obstacles during its expansion. For example, a vessel or an infundibulum may cause an impression on the base of the cyst to suggest an irregularity (Fig. 10–10).

3. *Septations.* a) A thin septum may be ignored. Even a few thin septa pose no concern (Fig. 10–11). However, if there are many septa, partial nephrectomy is considered. Just how many are "many" still remains a judgment call; b) if the septum or septa are thicker than pencil thin or if there is localized thickening, presence of malignancy is strongly suspected.

4. *Calcifications.* Before the era of CT, calcifications were considered pathognomonic for malignancy. Now, however, small amounts of calcifications are made readily visible by modern imaging techniques (Fig. 10–12). Miniscule crescent or linear calcifications contained in the cyst wall (not in the middle of the mass) can be neglected. Of course, all other criteria for a benign cyst, such as lack of septa, thin wall, and low attenuation value must be met. More pronounced and heavier calcifications, even though still contained in the cyst wall, are suspicious for malignancy (Fig. 10–13). If calcification is within the middle of the "cystic" mass, and if it is not shifting as sometimes seen in calyceal diverticuli, there is not much doubt regarding diagnosis.[3] The mass is most likely malignant.

5. *High attenuation values.* In a well-calibrated CT imager, the measured attenuation values of a simple cyst should be between 0 and 20 HU.

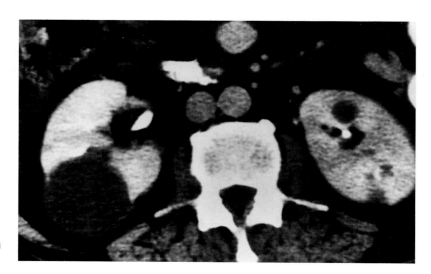

Figure 10–9. Right renal cyst with ill-defined irregularities at the base.

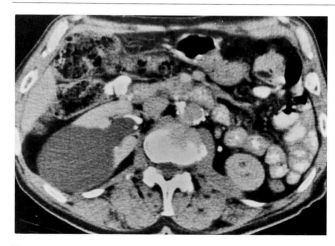

Figure 10–10. An expanding right renal cyst is extending into the renal sinus as well as perinephric space. The appearance of irregularity at the base was suggested on sonography.

Values higher than that imply the presence of a cyst high in protein content, a hemorrhagic cyst (see below), or a solid tumor.

6. *Contrast enhancement.* Cysts do not enhance following contrast injection. Any enhancement from the precontrast scan is diagnostic of a solid tumor (Fig. 14). Of course, arteriovenous malformations, renal artery aneurysms, etc., are considered, but usually there is no difficulty in separating these from a solid tumor. Because of volume averaging, it may be difficult to measure CT numbers from very small cysts. MR imaging is of little practical value.[4]

HEMORRHAGIC CYSTS

It is unclear why some cysts contain blood. It is a very common occurrence in patients with polycystic renal disease, where many benign cysts are seen to contain old or fresh blood. Bleeding into the cysts may be insidious and unnoticeable, or it may be acute and associated with severe flank pain (Fig. 10–15).[5] Most smaller hemorrhagic cysts are benign. The incidence of carcinoma in hemorrhagic cysts has not been established. Older literature (before the era of ultrasound and CT) suggests 30% of hemorrhagic cysts larger than 3 cm in diameter are malignant. However, since necrotic renal carcinomas were included in the count, this often quoted number is invalid.

Radiological Findings

1. *Hyperdense cyst.* On precontrast CT scan, hemorrhagic cysts are usually denser than the surrounding renal parenchyma (Fig. 10–16).[6] This is not always necessarily true, as hemorrhagic cysts may be isodense or even radiolucent on precontrast CT scan. On postcontrast scan the nephrogram is usually more radiopaque, so that the hemorrhagic cyst appears relatively radiolucent. Differential diagnosis of hyperdense cyst includes a cyst containing a higher than usual concentration of protein.[7] Isodense cysts must be differentiated from renal carcinoma. Both are considered complex cysts. Sonography is usually required to establish the cystic nature of either a hyperdense or isodense lesion, although it may prove to be unreliable in cysts smaller than 1 or 2 cm (Fig. 10–17).

2. *Settling debris.* On sonography, minute echogenic foci may be detected within the cyst immediately

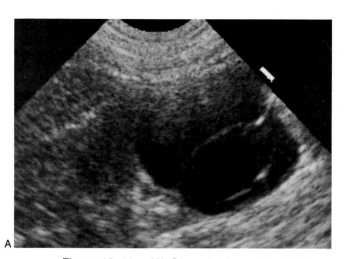
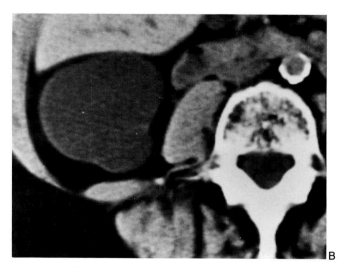

Figure 10–11. (A) Several thin septa with two specks of calcification are detected in a renal cyst on sonography. (B) Septa are barely visible on thick sections of the CT scan.

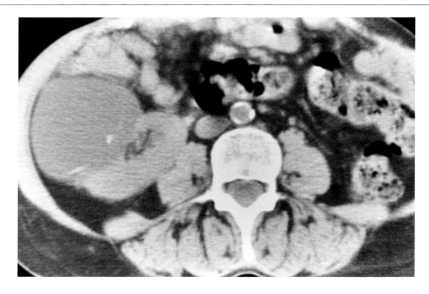

Figure 10–12. Heavier septal calcifications such as these may still be of no concern, but anything heavier should be considered a sign of malignancy.

after the patient is shifted into another position. These represent cellular debris settling into a dependent position and are more easily seen on real-time compared with the film record.[8]

3. MR imaging of hemorrhagic cysts may be very confusing. Different possible combinations have been observed and are clearly influenced by age.

The most common pattern is where the hemorrhagic cyst is hyperintense on T1- and T2-weighted sequences. However, a cyst pattern in which it is isointense to the cortex on T1-weighted sequence and hyperintense to the cortex on T2-weighted sequence (Fig. 10–18), or hypointense on both sequences (Fig. 10–19), has also been

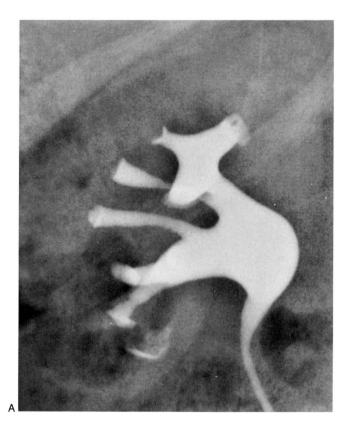

A

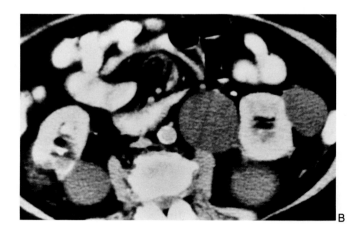

B

Figure 10–13. (A) Heavy calcification is clearly visible inferior to the lower pole calyx on retrograde pyelography. (B) CT scan in the same patient demonstrates numerous simple cysts in both kidneys. Calcification is located between two cysts without evidence of a solid component (arrow). In this situation a follow-up rather than surgery is a prudent approach.

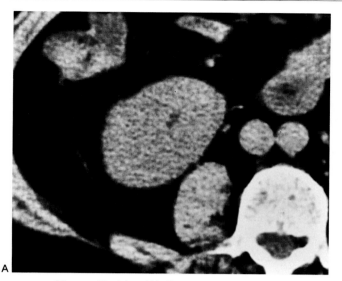
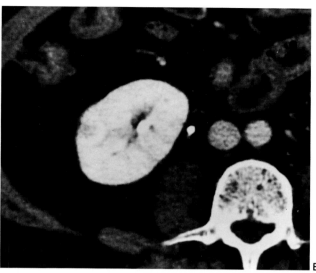

Figure 10–14. **(A)** Precontrast scan in the patient presented in Figure 10–3. **(B)** Postcontrast scan demonstrates inhomogeneous area of enhancement in the part of the kidney that was not subject to surgery. This lesion is a cancer until proved otherwise.

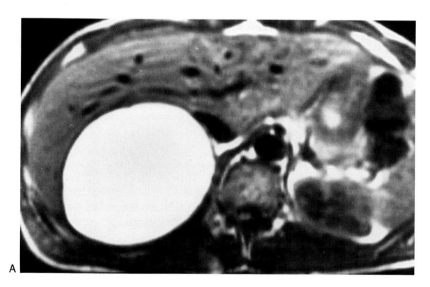

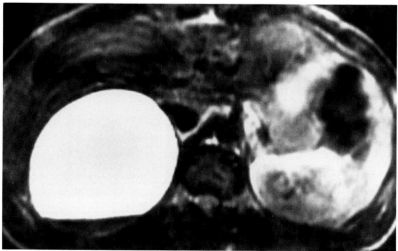

Figure 10–15. Hemorrhagic renal cyst associated with sudden onset of flank pain. **(A)** T1-weighted sequence 1 month after onset of symptoms shows the entire cyst to be hyperdense. **(B)** On T2-weighted sequence most of the cyst remains hyperdense with the exception of settling debris forming a fluid-fluid interphase. (Figures courtesy of R. Sukov, M.D.)

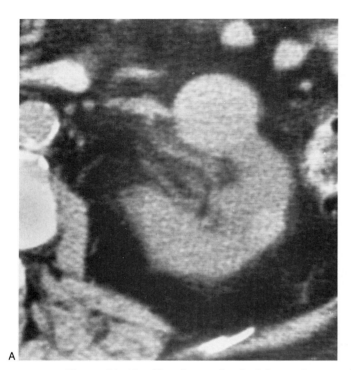
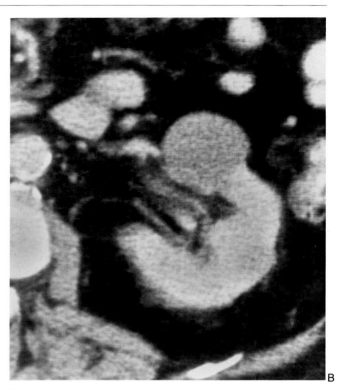

Figure 10–16. Two hemorrhagic left renal cysts. (A) On precontrast scan, the cysts are hyperdense compared with the surrounding parenchyma and (B) relatively radiolucent on postcontrast scan.

observed (Fig. 10–20). Unfortunately, renal carcinoma also exhibits this combination of signal intensities. Either way, sonography or CT is necessary when a new mass is discovered on MR imaging. The only exception is when a fluid-fluid interphase is discovered, confirming the cystic nature of the lesion (Fig. 10–15).

Disposition

If a hyperdense cyst is less than 3 cm, peripheral in location, smooth, round, does not contain calcifications or septations, and is nonenhancing, it is probably benign and it should be followed either by CT or ultrasound 6 months after discovery.

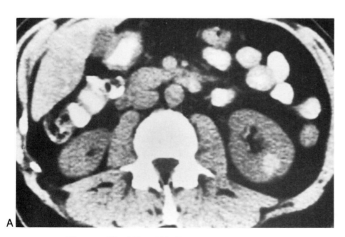
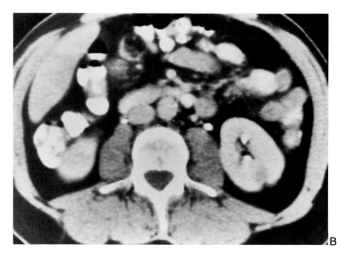

Figure 10–17. (A) Precontrast scan shows a hyperdense small renal mass. (B) The lesion is relatively radiolucent compared to the surrounding normal nephrogram on the postcontrast scan. A "solid" mass was found on sonography. A hemorrhagic cyst without evidence of malignancy was discovered at surgery.

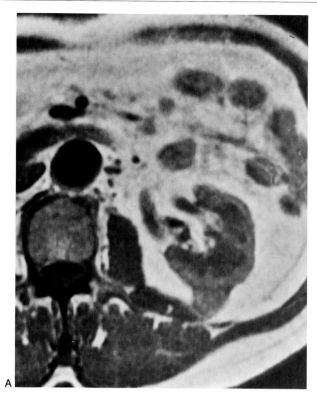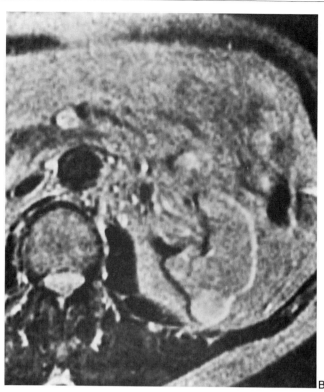

Figure 10–18. (A) Mass lesion isointense to the cortex on T1-weighted sequence. (B) The lesion is hyperintense on T2-weighted sequences. There is an irregularity at the cyst base which proved to be a small carcinoma at the base of a hemorrhagic cyst.

If the cyst is larger than 3 cm but otherwise has all the hallmarks of a benign cyst, it should probably be aspirated and its content examined for malignant cells. Many surgeons feel uncomfortable with such a lesion and may consider partial nephrectomy.

If any radiological findings suggestive of a complex cyst are found in addition to hemorrhage, the cyst is considered malignant.

Summary of possible findings and action to be taken is presented in Figure 10–21.

RENAL CYST PUNCTURE AND ASPIRATION

Renal cyst puncture was the precursor of interventional radiology. Many radiologists became proficient in placing needles into cysts, and other percutaneous applications followed.

Renal cyst puncture is seldom performed now for the purpose of differentiating benign from malignant processes. Clear fluid may be found in cystic renal neoplasms and cytology need not be positive for malignant cells.[9] Therefore the final arbiter as to

whether the cyst is malignant or benign is CT followed closely by renal ultrasound.

Rare indications for cyst puncture and fluid aspiration are in those instances where the cyst may cause mild impairment to the pelvocalyceal urine flow (Fig. 10–22) and hamper clearing of calculous debris after extracorporeal shock wave lithotripsy. Also, in some patients undergoing percutaneous nephrolithotripsy, the need may arise to decompress a renal cyst to provide better access to a renal calculus.

Shifting of renal calculi following cyst aspiration may cause ureteral obstruction and acute renal colic.[10]

Finally, a renal cyst may cause hypertension by compressing adjacent renal parenchyma, thus inducing ischemia and increased renin production. Aspiration may confirm the diagnosis.

The procedure may be done under ultrasound, fluoroscopic, or CT guidance. A 20 or 22 gauge needle is used and aspirate sent for cytology. If the fluid is cloudy, it is also sent for culture and sensitivity. The inside of the cyst may be examined by instilling diluted radiographic contrast (Fig. 10–23). Any irregularity is indicative of a tumor within the cyst.

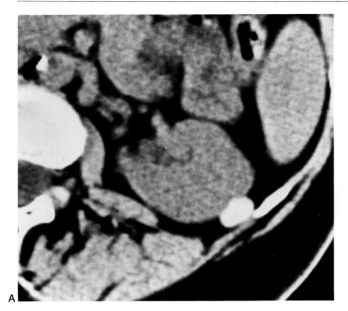

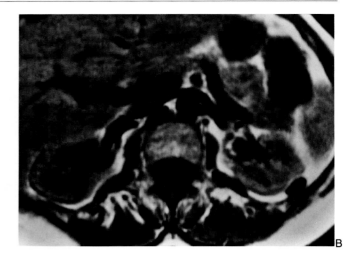

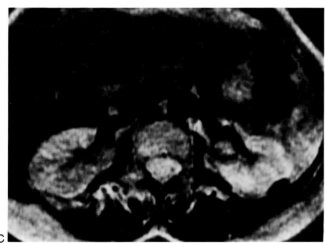

Figure 10–19. **(A)** Hyperdense small renal mass on precontrast scan. **(B)** The mass is low signal intensity (dark) on both T1- and T2-weighted sequences **(C)**. Only a hemorrhagic cyst or a heavily calcified lesion can produce this set of findings. Because the lesion was so small sonography failed to confirm it as a cyst but unequivocally showed lack of acoustical shadowing, which one would expect if calcification were present.

Complications include hemorrhage, pneumothorax, and infection.[11,12]

Renal Cyst Ablation

On rare occasions, renal cysts may cause symptoms, such as dull pain, abdominal discomfort, or vague gastrointestinal symptoms. In rare instances, a renal cyst may cause increased renin production by compressing adjacent renal parenchyma, making it hypoxic.[13] Aspiration of cyst fluid and concomitant disappearance of symptoms confirm the diagnosis.[14] However, the majority of renal cysts reaccumulate fluid over a period of time and relief of symptoms

may be transient. If diagnosis of a symptomatic renal cyst is certain, ablation may be considered instead of surgery.

A small 5 F pigtail catheter is introduced percutaneously into the cyst. All fluid is removed and 98% ethanol is instilled through the catheter. The volume of ethanol introduced should be 20% of the cyst fluid volume removed. Ethanol is left in place for 15 to 20 minutes, keeping in mind that it should be in contact with all surfaces of the cyst and particularly with the surface facing the renal parenchyma. For this reason, the patient or the table may have to be turned or tilted. After 20 minutes, the ethanol is withdrawn (Fig. 10–24).[15]

T1-weighted   T2-weighted

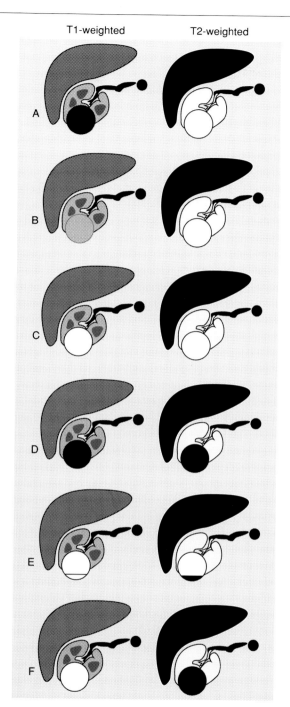

Figure 10–20. Varying appearances of hemorrhagic renal cysts on MR imaging. **(A)** Simple cyst; **(B,C,D,E)** pathologically proved hemorrhagic cysts; **(F)** possible hemorrhagic cyst.

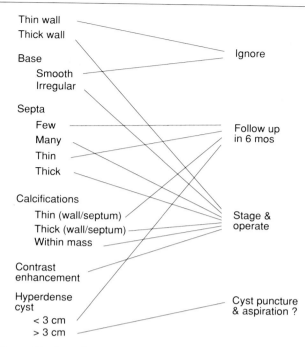

Figure 10–21. Suggested course of action to be taken upon discovering a complex renal cyst.

MILK OF CALCIUM RENAL CYST

"Milk of calcium renal cyst" is not a true cyst, but rather a communicating or a closed-off calyceal diverticulum. The cavity is lined with transitional epithelium and contains a particulate colloidal suspension of various calcium salts. The particles tend to settle in the most dependent part of the cystic cavity. With the patient in the supine position, plain radiography usually demonstrates a rounded "full moon" appearance. On the upright or cross-table supine projections, the horizontal beam is parallel with the layered surface and the "full moon" becomes a "half moon" (Fig. 10–26).[17]

The layering of the colloidal suspension may also be identified on CT, ultrasound,[18] and MR imaging.[19] Changing a patient's position from supine to prone during cross-sectional studies will demonstrate "half moon" shift into a different plane.[20]

RENAL SINUS CYSTS

Parapelvic cysts are simple renal cysts originating from the renal parenchyma, which are primarily expanding within the renal sinus.[21]

Peripelvic cysts are cysts originating from the sinus

Formerly Pantopaque®, an oily myelographic contrast, was used instead of ethanol.[16] One can still encounter very dense contrast in the cysts of these patients (Fig. 10–25).

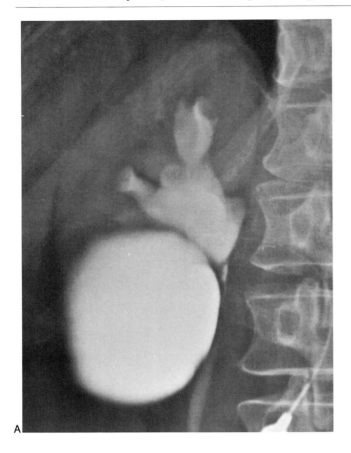

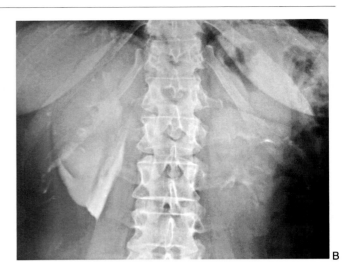

Figure 10–22. **(A)** Right renal cyst has been punctured and filled with contrast material. The cyst is causing partial obstruction by compressing upon the upper ureter in a patient complaining of intermittent flank pain. **(B)** Because of close proximity to the ureter, no sclerosing agents were installed. Instead, the cyst was punctured multiple times causing some extravasation. The pain disappeared after cyst decompression.

structures. These cysts are most likely lymphatic in origin.

Differential diagnosis includes peripelvic lipomatosis, infundibular diverticulum, loculated urinoma, renal artery aneurysm, renal vein varix, arteriovenous malformation (AVM), and pancreatic pseudocyst extending into the renal sinus.[22] Solid tumors, such as renal sinus angiomyolipoma, hibernoma (brown fat tumor), and renal carcinoma also enter differential diagnosis.

The collecting system is usually moderately affected, usually displaced (Fig. 10–27), and occasionally obstructed. On sonography, these cysts are difficult to classify as benign, since their expansion is hampered by the vessels and collecting system. Therefore they are seldom perfectly round. On sonography, replacement lipomatosis is echogenic while peripelvic cysts are hypoechoic. MR imaging (Fig. 10–28) and CT (Fig. 10–29) can easily be used to distinguish replacement lipomatosis from cysts. Dynamic CT scan is usually sufficient to determine if the lesion is enhancing, or whether it represents a major vascular problem such as AVM.

Sonography may be useless in detecting concomi-

tant hydronephrosis and obstruction, making a contrast study necessary (Fig. 10–30).

ACQUIRED CYSTIC DISEASE OF THE KIDNEYS (ACDK)

Etiology. Unknown.

Incidence. Up to 80% of patients on chronic hemodialysis or peritoneal dialysis develop renal cysts. Of these, between 8 and 16% will develop renal neoplasms.[23,24]

Clinical Presentation. Usually asymptomatic. Hematuria. Presenting symptoms may be caused by distant metastases.[25–27] Yearly follow-up by CT or ultrasound is generally recommended.

Radiological Findings. The best imaging modality is CT. Multiple small or moderate-sized cysts develop over a period of time, usually after 3 years of dialysis (Fig. 10–31). While small initially, the cysts may

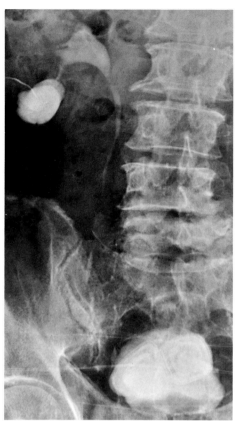

Figure 10–23. Renal cyst aspiration and "cystogram" were performed because of several septa found on sonography. Clear fluid with no malignant cells was obtained. Incidental discovery is bladder urolithiasis.

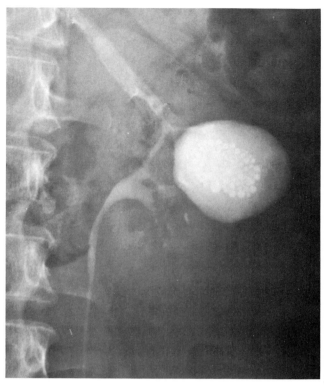

Figure 10–25. Pantopaque was introduced into this cyst many years ago without apparent success. A second cyst puncture was performed and iodinated contrast introduced that uniformly fills the cyst. Globules of oily contrast are seen at the bottom and the center of the cyst.

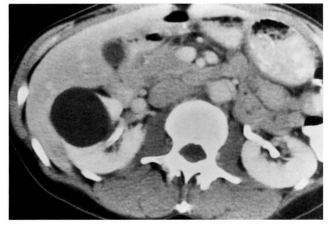

Figure 10–24. This patient presents with dull pain that could be attributed to the cyst. Note relative position of the cyst to the liver and potential difficulties that may be encountered during cyst puncture. The pain disappeared after puncture and aspiration but slowly reappeared after several weeks. Ethanol ablation was performed at that time.

become quite large. Carcinoma is detected, since it is more radiodense than cysts (Fig. 10–32, 10–33).

Sonography is somewhat more difficult to perform on what are usually small kidneys and small cysts. A solid mass in the presence of surrounding cysts is very suggestive of carcinoma.

MR imaging is unlikely to replace CT in evaluating these patients, since hemorrhagic renal cysts cannot be differentiated from solid tumors.

PSEUDOCYSTS

Uriniferous Perirenal Pseudocyst (Urinoma)

Chronically encapsulated urinoma within the layers of renal fascia may present as a tumor mass displacing the kidney on excretory urography.[28] The wall of the pseudocyst is a newly formed fibrous capsule derived from the reaction of surrounding tissues or

A

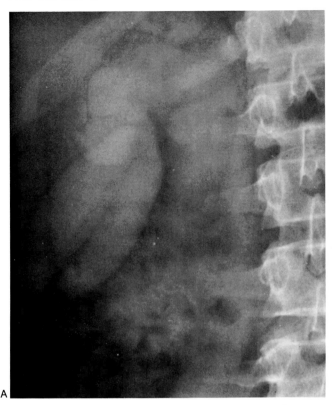

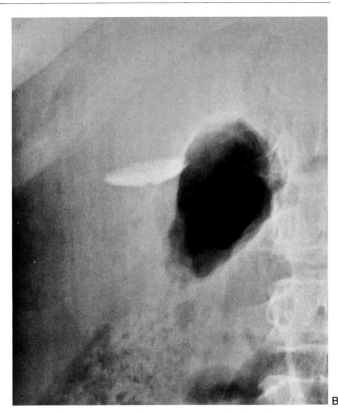

B

Figure 10–26. **(A)** Round faint density ("full moon") in the right upper quadrant may be mistaken for gallstones. **(B)** In the upright AP projection calcified particles shift in the most dependent part of the cavity ("half moon"). This still could represent "milk of calcium bile" and only an oblique or lateral projection in this case confirmed the presence of a "milk of calcium renal cyst."

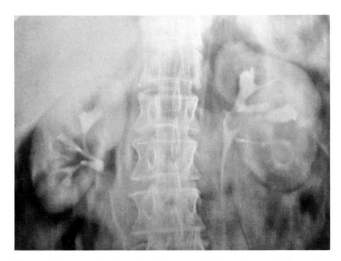

Figure 10–27. Left peripelvic cyst displacing and distorting left pelvocalyceal system.

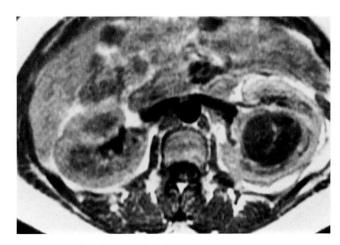

Figure 10–28. T1-weighted sequence demonstrates several hypointense left peripelvic cysts.

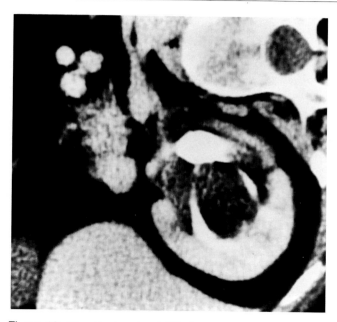

thickened renal fascia. Obstruction may or may not be present at the time of discovery. Any obstructive process may cause urine extravasation into the perirenal spaces, although that process might have happened some time ago. A pseudocyst by virtue of displacement and mass effect may cause secondary ureteral obstruction. Occasionally, contrast will be seen entering the pseudocyst. Diagnosis is confirmed by ultrasound and/or CT scan.[29] Retrograde pyelogram may be necessary to delineate obstruction.

Figure 10–29. Postcontrast CT demonstrates nonenhancing peripelvic masses. On thin sections, CT numbers may differentiate cysts from replacement lipomatosis.

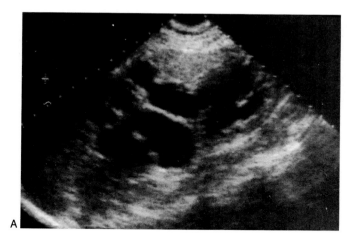

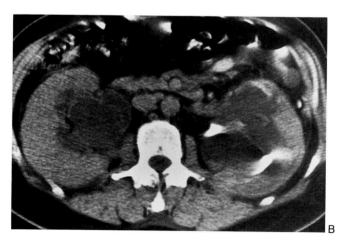

A

B

Figure 10–30. **(A)** Right renal sonogram fails to detect hydronephrosis in a patient with concomitant right obstruction and bilateral peripelvic cysts. **(B)** Right obstruction is suspected on CT because of delay in function on that side. Left collecting system is distorted by peripelvic cysts. Right percutaneous nephrostomy was placed and yielded purulent urine in a system completely obstructed by a ureteral calculus.

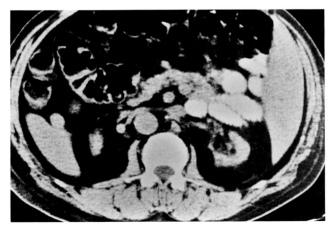

Figure 10–31. Small cyst heralds the development of acquired cystic renal disease in a small kidney. Also present is situs inversus.

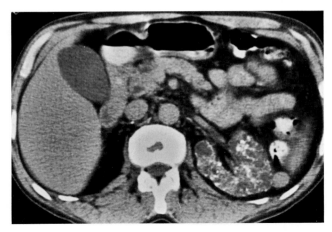

Figure 10–32. Acquired cystic renal disease in a patient with solitary kidney and nephrocalcinosis. The small mass arising from the lateral aspect of the kidney is denser compared with comparably sized cysts and most likely represents a solid tumor.

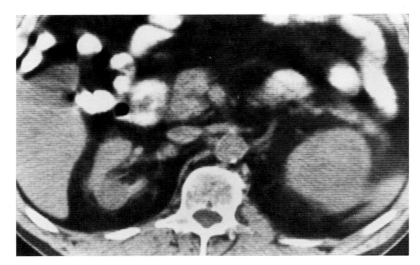

Figure 10–33. Large renal carcinoma in the left lower pole in a patient with acquired cystic renal disease. Note small right kidney with a small cyst.

REFERENCES

1. Steinhardt GF, Slovis TL, Perlmutter AD. Simple renal cysts in infants. Radiology 1985; 155:349–350.
2. Bosniak MA. The current radiological approach to renal cysts. Radiology 1986; 158:1–10.
3. Wayman PJ, McClennan BL, Lee JKT, et al. CT of calcified renal masses. AJR 1982; 138:1095–1099.
4. Marotti M, Hricak H, Fritzsche P, et al. Complex and simple renal cysts: comparative evaluation with MR imaging. Radiology 1987; 162:679–684.
5. Thompson KR, Lipchik EO, Frank IN. Hemorrhagic tension cyst of the kidney. J Urol 1977; 117:120–121.
6. Sussman S, Cochran ST, Pagani JJ, et al. Hyperdense renal masses: a CT manifestation of hemorrhagic renal cyst. Radiology 1984; 150:207–211.
7. Fishman MC, Pollack HM, Arger PH, Banner MP. High protein content: another cause of CT hyperdense renal cyst. J Comput Assist Tomogr 1983; 1103–1106.
8. Gooding GAW. Sonography of hemorrhagic cysts with computed tomographic correlation. J Ultrasound Med 1986; 5:699–702.
9. Amis ES, Cronan JJ, Pfister RC. Needle puncture of cystic renal masses: a survey of the Society of Uroradiology. AJR 1987; 148:297–299.
10. Cronan JJ, Messersmith RN, Amis ES Jr, Kidd DD. Obstructive migration of renal calculi following cyst aspiration. Radiology 1984; 152:317–319.
11. Branitz BH, Schlossberg IR, Freed SZ. Complications of renal cyst puncture. Urology 1976; 7:578–580.
12. Lang EK. Renal cyst puncture and aspiration: a survey of complications. AJR 1977; 128:723–727.
13. Hoard TD, O'Brien DP III. Simple renal cyst and high

renin hypertension cured by cyst decompression. J Urol 1976; 115:326–327.

14. Dean AL: Treatment of solitary cyst of kidney by aspiration. Trans Am Assoc Genitourin Surg 1939; 32:91.

15. Bean WJ: Renal cysts: treatment with alcohol. Radiology 1981; 138:329–331.

16. Raskin MM, Roen SA, Viamonte M Jr. Effect of intracystic Pantopaque on renal cysts. J Urol 1975; 114:678–679.

17. Murray RL. Milk of calcium of the kidney: diagnostic features on vertical beam roentgenograms. Am J Roentgenol Radium Ther Nucl Med 1971; 113:455–459.

18. Widder DJ, Newhouse JH. The sonographic appearance of milk of calcium in renal caliceal diverticuli. J Clin Ultrasound 1982; 10:448–450.

19. Kinard RE, Orrison WW, Brogdon BG, et al. MR imaging of milk of calcium renal cyst. J Comput Assist Tomogr 1986;10:1057–1058.

20. Yashiro N, Yoshida H, Araki T. Bilateral "milk of calcium" renal cysts: CT findings. J Comput Assist Tomogr 1985; 9:199–201.

21. Amis ES Jr, Cronan JJ. The renal sinus: an imaging review and proposed nomenclature for sinus cysts. J Urol 1988; 139:1151–1159.

22. Lilienfeld RM, Lande A. Pancreatic pseudocysts presenting as thick-walled renal and perinephric cysts. J Urol 1976; 115:123–125.

23. Dunnill MS, Millard PR, Oliver D. Acquired cystic disease of the kidneys: a hazard of long-term intermittent maintenance hemodialysis. J Clin Pathol 1977; 30:868–877.

24. Jabour BA, Ralls PW, Tang WW, et al. Acquired cystic disease of the kidneys. Computed tomography and ultrasonography appraisal in patients on peritoneal and hemodialysis. Invest Radiol 1987; 9:729–732.

25. Editorial review. Acquired cystic disease: replacing one kidney disease with another. Kidney Int 1985; 28:99–105.

26. Cho C, Friedland GW, Swenson RS. Acquired cystic disease and renal neoplasms in hemodialysis patients. Urol Radiol 1984; 6:153–157.

27. Scanlon MH, Karasick SR: Acquired renal cystic disease and neoplasia: complications of chronic hemodialysis. Radiology 1983; 147:837–838.

28. Myers M. Uriniferous perirenal pseudocyst. New observations. Radiology 1975; 117:539–545.

29. Healy ME, Teng SS, Moss AA. Uriniferous pseudocyst: computed tomographic findings. Radiology 1984; 153:757–762.

11

Adrenal Disorders

NORMAL ANATOMY

Adrenal glands are seen on 99% of CT and MRI examinations. Usually two limbs are seen in the shape of an inverted "V." Right adrenal is located in the superior portion of the perirenal space and posterior to the inferior vena cava (IVC). The left adrenal gland is somewhat anterior and medial to the upper pole of the left kidney. Arterial supply to the adrenal glands is from: a) Inferior adrenal arteries (branch of renal end capsular arteries); b) middle adrenal artery (branching from aorta); and c) superior adrenal arteries (branches from hepatic, splenic, phrenic, etc., arteries).

Venous drainage is via the central vein which drains in the IVC in the right and left renal vein. Left inferior adrenal vein and left inferior phrenic vein usually join into a common trunk before emptying into left renal vein (Fig. 11–1).

In cases of renal ptosis where the kidney descends when upright, adrenal gland remains in its normal position within the perirenal space.

ADRENAL MASS

1. *Indirect evidence.* On plain radiography or urography, the presence of the mass may be suspected even without visualizing the adrenal mass per se. Its presence may be suggested by inferior or lateral displacement of the kidney (Fig. 11–2) and by flattening the top of the renal outline.

2. *Direct evidence.* Mass is seen on any of the cross-sectional imaging methods (Fig. 11–3) (CT, MR, US, or scintigraphy), on angiography or plain film radiography if calcified.

Size

1. *Adrenal mass less than 3.5 cm in diameter.* Because nonfunctioning adrenal adenomas are so common, a newly found mass smaller than 3.5 cm in diameter in a patient without known malignancy elsewhere is assumed benign if:[1–4]
   a. No known malignancy is present elsewhere.
   b. There is no evidence of a functioning adrenal tumor.
   c. The mass is homogeneous in appearance.
   d. There is no enhancement on CT scan.
   e. The mass is unilateral.
Follow-up scan is needed from 4 to 6 months after the discovery. If there is no interval change in size, the mass is considered benign. Laboratory workup to exclude functioning cortical neoplasm or pheochromocytoma may be obtained.

Any enlargement in this span of time is strongly suggestive of malignancy, such as adenocarcinoma, and adrenalectomy is indicated.[1]

2. *Adrenal masses larger than 3.5 cm in diameter.* In the absence of primary malignancy elsewhere the tumor is considered a primary malignant neoplasm of the adrenal gland and adrenalectomy is indicated.

Texture

1. *Homogeneous mass.* Homogeneous appearance favors benign disease while inhomogeneous pattern is more readily associated with malignancy.[5]

2. *Inhomogeneous mass.* Inhomogeneity on CT within the mass may represent a necrotic tumor or hemorrhage into the tumor or into the adrenal gland. On MR imaging necrotic tumor is partially iso- or hypointense on T1-weighted image and hyperintense on T2.[6–8] Hemorrhage may have varying intensities,

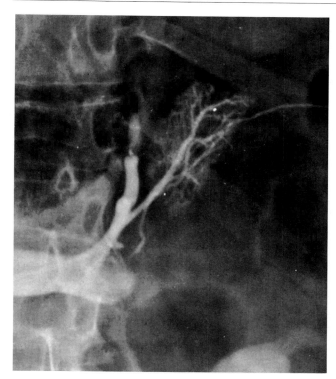

Figure 11–1. Retrograde left adrenal vein venogram demonstrates anatomical relation of left inferior adrenal vein to left inferior phrenic vein. Dilution of the blood specimen from the latter during selective blood sampling may yield erroneous results.

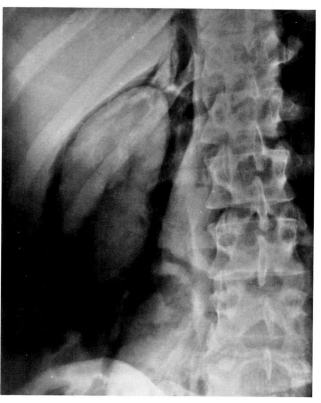

Figure 11–3. In the pre-CT era the radiologist had to employ desperate measures to visualize the adrenal gland directly. Retroperitoneal gas insufflation was the only method available for detecting small adrenal tumors and deciding on which side to operate.

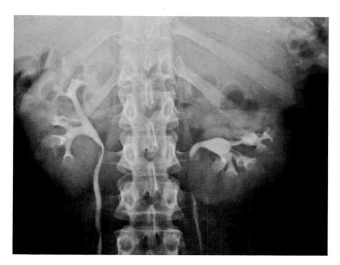

Figure 11–2. Although the outlines of a suprarenal mass may be faintly visualized on this excretory urogram, it is the inferior displacement of the kidney and change of its axis that draws attention to the tumor.

depending on the time of occurrence, but in general it is hyperintense on both T1- and T2-weighted images (Fig. 11–4).

3. *Fluid.* Adrenal cysts are an uncommon adrenal mass. HU value is low and ultrasound demonstrates hypoechoic smooth wall cystic structure with through transmission, just as in renal cysts. Occasionally, rim calcification is seen in the cyst wall.

4. *Calcifications.* Calcifications in normal or enlarged adrenal are common and nonspecific (Fig. 11–5). Calcifications may be seen in malignant and nonmalignant entities so that their presence (or absence) rarely contributes to a specific diagnosis. Calcification is seen in adenoma, adenocarcinoma, metastases, tuberculosis, neuroblastoma, old hemorrhage, Wolman disease, adrenal cysts, etc. As is always the case, calcification is seen much more readily on CT examinations than on plain radiographs. Small amounts of calcifications are difficult to see on MR imaging, but larger amounts are detect-

Spin-Echo, T1-weighted   Spin-Echo, T2-weighted

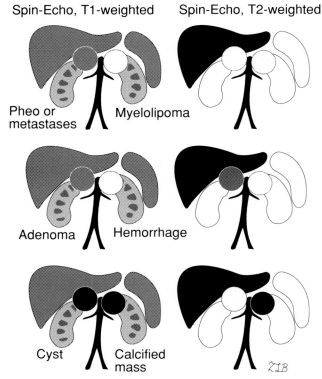

Pheo or metastases   Myelolipoma

Adenoma   Hemorrhage

Cyst   Calcified mass

Figure 11–4. Schematic drawing of MR signal intensities of different adrenal masses on T1- and T2-weighted sequences.

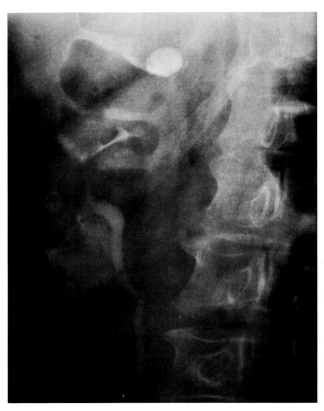

Figure 11–5. Small heavy round calcification of unknown etiology in the right adrenal gland. Because of its small size, only a follow-up may be required after 6 months.

able. Calcification is of low signal intensity (dark) on both T1- and T2-weighted images.

5. *Radiolucent masses.* Low attenuation value (−50 HU) indicates presence of fat within the tumor. The only tumor that exhibits this characteristic is a myelolipoma, which originates from extraosseous, myeloprolific, blood-forming remnants. Benign adenomas also have a relatively low attenuation value.

6. *Hyperdense masses.* Adrenal hemorrhage in acute stages is hyperdense on CT.

7. *Enhancement.* Contrast enhancement on CT also favors malignancy,[4] and so does enhancement on MR imaging after intravenous administration of Gd-DTPA.[9]

Renal Vein or IVC Extension

This finding is diagnostic for malignancy. Neoplasms that may propagate in this manner are adrenal adenocarcinoma, neuroblastoma, and some adrenal metastases, such as renal carcinoma and lymphoma.

ADRENAL SIZE

Size ranges for adrenal glands have not been firmly established. In general, the limb thickness approximates that of the diaphragmatic crura. Bilateral enlargement is seen in adrenal hyperplasia. Atrophy may be detected in association with functioning adrenal adenoma, either in the same gland or on the opposite side.

TWO MOST COMMON ADRENAL TUMORS

The two most common adrenal masses are *nonfunctioning adenoma* and *adrenal metastases*. Indeed, these two entities comprise about 90% of all adrenal tumors. Differentiating these tumors is of great importance when a primary malignancy is present elsewhere because it may significantly influence the choice of treatment.

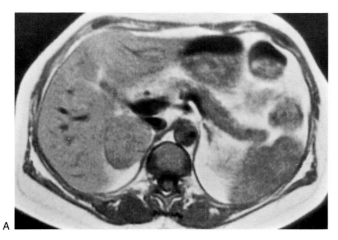

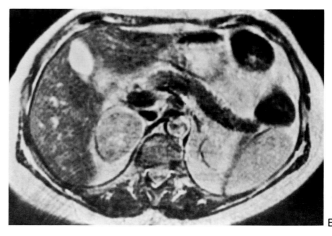

A   B

Figure 11–6. (A) MR image. Of course, not all adenomas will appear homogeneous. Here, the right adrenal mass appears homogeneous on T1-weighted sequence. (B) On T2-weighted sequence some inhomogeneity is detected. Note change in signal intensity of the liver, gallbladder, pancreas, great vessels, and the opposite normal adrenal.

Nonfunctioning Adrenal Adenoma

Benign nonfunctioning adenoma is the most common primary adrenal tumor. Adenomas are usually small, and they may occasionally calcify. They tend to appear homogeneous (Fig. 11–6) on cross-sectional imaging modalities, may have low attenuation values (Fig. 11–7), and enhance very little (Fig. 11–8). Adenomas may become large over a period of time (Fig. 11–9).

Adrenal Metastases

Metastasis is the most common adrenal mass in patients with primary malignancy. It may require a thin needle aspiration biopsy to confirm the diagnosis and differentiate from nonfunctioning adenoma. Presence of bilateral mass lesions favors malignancy.[3]

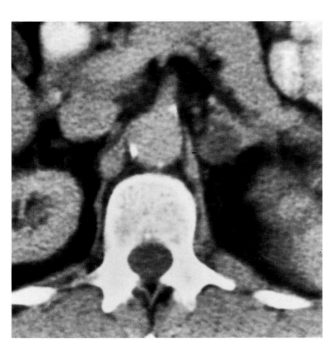

Figure 11–7. Small low-density nonfunctioning adenoma in left adrenal gland.

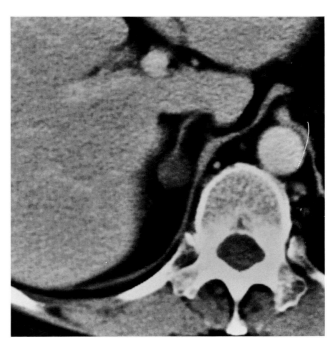

Figure 11–8. Nonfunctioning adenomas usually do not significantly enhance either on CT or MR imaging. This differs from metastasis or other malignant tumors, which often reveal inhomogeneous enhancement.

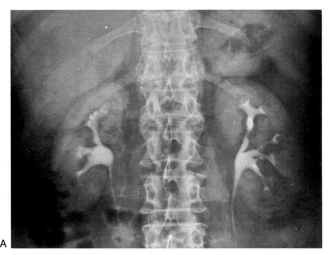
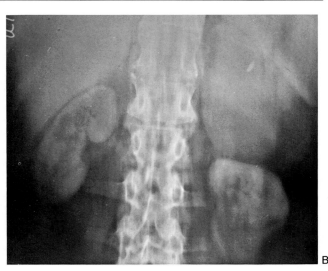

A   B

Figure 11–9. **(A)** A left adrenal nonfunctioning adenoma measuring about 4 cm in diameter is overlooked on an intravenous urogram. **(B)** Nine years later the mass had grown substantially when it was incidentally discovered on another intravenous urogram.

In the presence of primary malignancy elsewhere, deciding whether an adrenal mass is an insignificant nonfunctioning adenoma or a metastasis (lung, kidney, melanoma, colon) is quite difficult without adrenal biopsy.

After biopsy, CT is the most reliable method of determining whether a lesion is malignant or benign. A mass that demonstrates an inhomogeneous enhancement following contrast administration is most likely a metastasis (Fig. 11–10).[4,5] However, when a metastasis is small, these features may not be as readily apparent and differentiation from an adenoma may be impossible.

MR imaging is the next most sensitive method of discriminating adenoma from a metastasis. In general, both lesions will have similar appearance in T1-weighted images, but on T2-weighted images metastases tend to become bright (hyperintense) while adenoma remains isointense to the kidney.[6–8]

Dynamic fast gradient-echo imaging with Gd-DTPA appears even more reliable and may become the method of choice in differentiating these two entities. Adenomas show only mild enhancement and quick washout, while metastases show strong enhancement and prolonged washout.[9]

Differentiating features are summarized in Table 11–1.

OVERPRODUCTION OF CORTICOSTEROIDS

Clinical Presentation. Moon facies, truncal obesity, hypertension, hirsutism, diabetes, buffalo hump, osteoporosis, purplish abdominal striae, muscle wasting, weakness, amenorrhea, acne, fungal infections, emotional lability, polyuria, urolithiasis.

Laboratory Findings. Elevated plasma cortisol, elevated urinary steroids, loss of diurnal variation in steroid production, leukocytosis, eosinopenia, lymphopenia, impaired glucose tolerance test.

Cushing's Disease

Etiology. Pituitary adenoma causing secondary adrenal hyperplasia and overproduction of corticosteroids.

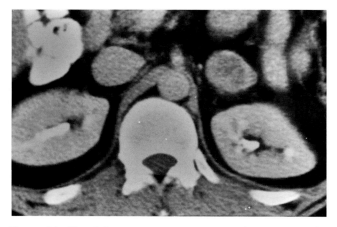

Figure 11–10. Inhomogeneous contrast enhancement of a left adrenal mass that proved to be a metastatic malignant melanoma.

Table 11–1. Differential Diagnostic Features Between Adenoma and Metastases

IMAGING	ADENOMA	METASTASES
Size	Any size	Any size
Bilateral	Usually not	More likely
Texture	Homogeneous	Inhomogeneous
Enhancement	Homogeneous	Inhomogeneous
MR T$_1$-weighted	Medium intensity	Medium intensity
MR T$_2$-weighted	Medium intensity	High intensity
Dynamic Gd-DTPA	Mild enhancement	Strong enhancement

Radiological Findings (Table 11–2)

Secondary Adrenal Hyperplasia. ACTH-producing pituitary chromophobe adenoma is the most common cause of overproduction of adrenocorticosteroids. The overproduction of ACTH causes adrenal hyperplasia. Adrenal hyperplasia may be diffuse or nodular.

1. Diffuse hyperplasia. Mild bilateral adrenal enlargement is seen on CT scan in as many as 50% of cases (Fig. 11–11). Other patients will have normal-sized glands, but never atrophy of the normal glandular tissue.

2. Macronodular hyperplasia. Adrenal hyperplasia in this disease may present as small nodules that mimic an adrenal tumor. These are usually less than 2 cm in diameter. A solitary nodule may be misdiagnosed as a functional adrenal adenoma and unnecessarily surgically removed. Macronodular hyperplasia should be suspected if there is enlargement of the opposite gland, enlargement of the remainder of the ipsilateral gland, or if there are several identifiable nodules.[10]

Pituitary Tumor. Inferior petrosal venous sampling may confirm the diagnosis and lateralize the tumor. High ACTH levels are present compared with the peripheral venous specimen.[11]

High resolution MR imaging of pituitary microadenomas (1.5 T) appears to be the imaging method of choice. Focal glandular hypointensity on T1-weighted sequences is the most useful finding.[12] Gd-DTPA-enhanced high resolution MR imaging is even more promising.[13]

Ectopic Adrenocorticotropic Hormone (ACTH) Syndrome

Etiology. Bronchial carcinoid (most common), thymic and gut carcinoid, oat-cell carcinoma, islet-cell carcinoma, medullary thyroid carcinoma, pheochromocytoma, and rarely other neoplasms.

Clinical Presentation. There is increased production of ACTH by the neoplasm. It may be difficult to differentiate from Cushing disease. ACTH levels are equal in petrosal vein and peripheral vein samples.

Radiological Findings. Secondary adrenal hyperplasia is more pronounced compared with the patients with pituitary microadenoma. The glands tend to be bigger and are only occasionally normal in size (Fig. 11–12).[14] On MR imaging, the enlarged adrenal glands are usually of low signal intensity on T1-weighted sequences and are isointense to the liver on T2-weighted sequences. Pheochromocytoma may be suspected if a high signal intensity adrenal mass is present on T2-weighted sequences.

CT is the method of choice for detection of the primary ACTH-secreting tumor. Slice thickness through the chest should be 5 mm, since the bronchial carcinoid is usually small and difficult to detect.

Table 11–2. Spectrum of Findings in Adrenal Cortical Hyperfunction

	MASS	NODULES	ADRENAL SIZE	SERUM ACTH	PETROSAL VEIN ACTH
Pituitary adenoma	±	+	++	++	++++
Ectopic ACTH	±	+	+++	++	++
Adrenal adenoma	+++	+	−		
PPNAD*	±	++	−		
Adrenal carcinoma	++++		±−		
Aldosteronoma	+++	+			

*PPNAD: primary pigmented nodular adrenocortical disease.

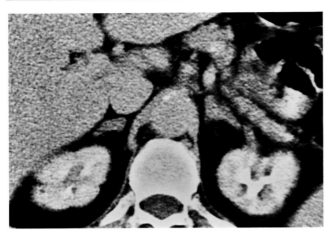

Figure 11–11. Mild bilateral adrenal hyperplasia in a patient with Cushing's disease. The size in absolute numbers is difficult to obtain. A more useful method is to compare adrenal size relative to the adjacent crus of the diaphragm.

Increased ACTH levels may be found in targeted venous samples, but only after the primary neoplasm is demonstrated on CT.[10] "Blind" sampling along the inferior or superior vena cava is usually not contributory.

Hyperfunctional Adrenal Adenoma (Cushing Syndrome)

Etiology. Functional benign cortical adenoma is the second most common cause of hyperadrenocorticism and Cushing syndrome.

Radiological Findings. The tumor is usually 2 cm or larger and homogeneous. Central necrosis is rarely if ever found in this tumor on cross-sectional imaging. The tumor may be relatively hypolucent on CT. Recognizable atrophy of ipsilateral or contralateral normal adrenal tissue is frequent. Practically every adenoma producing Cushing syndrome is detected on 5 mm thick CT scans of the adrenal glands.[10] Arteriography has no place in evaluating this disease, but for the sake of completeness, tumor may be hypo or hypervascular. Treatment is surgical.

Primary Pigmented Nodular Adrenocortical Disease

Incidence and Etiology. Rare disease affecting mainly infants and adolescents. May be familial. Possibly an autoimmune disease.

Pathology. Dark nodules containing lipofuscin and composed of polyhedral cells are present in otherwise hypoplastic adrenal gland. The nodules are typically very small.

Clinical Presentation. The symptoms of hypercortisolism are less pronounced than in more common Cushing syndrome caused by a hyperfunctioning adenoma. Severe osteoporosis is common.

Treatment. Bilateral adrenalectomy.

Radiological Findings. Irregular, "lumpy," or "knobby" gland or small nodules may be identified on high resolution CT scan, depending on their

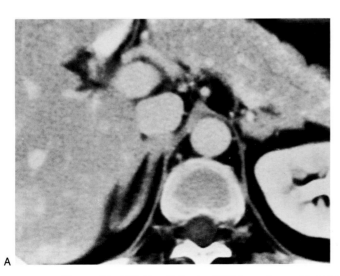

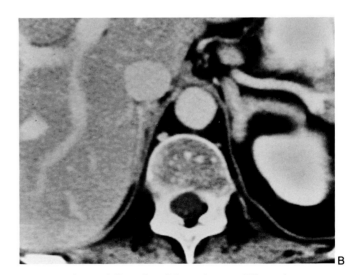

A   B

Figure 11–12A,B. Ectopic ACTH syndrome in patient with metastatic medullary thyroid carcinoma. Bilateral adrenal hyperplasia is present.

size,[14] and are suggestive of diagnosis in the appropriate clinical setting. The nodules may appear hypolucent on CT scan and hypointense on MR imaging. Osteoporosis and collapse of the vertebral bodies are commonly seen on plain radiography.

Adrenal Carcinoma

Adrenal carcinoma may (Cushing syndrome) or may not be hormonally active. Functional tumors are more common and account for about 80% of all adrenal carcinoma. Nonactive tumors may be clinically silent and become symptomatic due to their large size. There are two peaks in the second and fifth decades of life. There is slight female preponderance. Males tend to have higher incidence of nonfunctioning tumors.[15]

Clinical Presentation.   Symptoms are pain, weakness, anorexia, and fever.

Physical examination: abdominal mass, 50%; Cushing syndrome, 20%; Cushing syndrome and virilization, 15%; virilization, 15%; feminization, 6%.

Staging.

- Stage I: Tumor less than 5 cm, negative nodes, no local invasion.

- Stage II: Tumor larger than 5 cm, negative nodes, no local invasion.
- Stage III: Positive nodes or local invasion.
- Stage IV: Positive nodes and local invasion or distant metastases.

Radiological Findings.   Adenocarcinoma of the adrenal gland is usually large and is best examined by CT (Fig. 11–13). Calcification is present in 50% of all cases and is usually scattered within the tumor mass (Fig. 11–14). Occasionally, calcification can be peripheral. Areas of necrosis are present and the tumor is usually inhomogeneous (Fig. 11–15). The tumor may be hypo or hypervascular on arteriography. Extension and involvement of adjacent organs is possible. Extension into the renal vein (Fig. 11–16), inferior vena cava and even the right atrium is common and MR imaging may be useful (Fig. 11–17).

On occasion, a very large adrenal tumor may be difficult to differentiate from renal carcinoma. MR imaging or CT reconstruction in the sagittal plane may be very useful in such circumstances.

Embolization of the adrenal carcinoma may be done to reduce hormone overproduction and for palliation.[16]

Metastases are to the lung (Fig. 11–18) and bones, usually lytic.

PRIMARY ALDOSTERONISM

Incidence.   Occurs in 0.5% of patients with sustained hypertension.

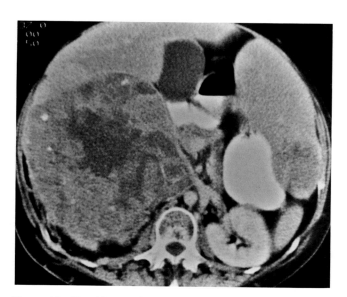

Figure 11–13.   Huge adrenal carcinoma exhibits inhomogeneous contrast enhancement on CT scan. Several areas of dystrophic calcifications are seen. Stomach, pancreas, and superior mesenteric vein are displaced to the left. The tumor extends into the inferior vena cava and partially occludes the left renal vein. A large collateral lumbar vein connects left renal vein to the left ascending lumbar vein (just left of the aorta) and provides for the venous outflow from the left kidney. There is also a hypolucent metastasis to the posterior aspect of the spleen.

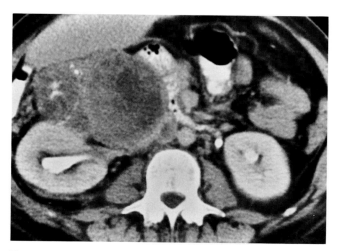

Figure 11–14.   Dystrophic calcification is seen in this adrenal carcinoma, localized more to one side. Extension into the inferior vena cava is apparent. Duodenum is displaced to the left.

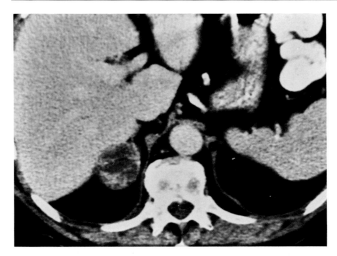

Figure 11–15. Inhomogeneous enhancement strongly suggests the presence of a malignant lesion. Not all adrenal carcinomas are large when first detected. Hormonal overproduction may focus attention on the adrenal gland, such as in this patient with an adrenal carcinoma measuring 3.9 cm.

Pathology. Functioning cortical adenoma (aldosteronoma) is present in 85% of the patients with primary aldosteronism. Bilateral or extra-adrenal tumors are extremely rare. A small proportion of patients has bilateral adrenal hyperplasia, which may be micro or macronodular.

Clinical Presentation. Hypertension.

Laboratory Findings. Hypokalemia, hyperkaluria, suppressed plasma renin activity, elevation of 24-hour urinary aldosterone, hypokalemic alkalosis, abnormal glucose tolerance test.

Radiological Findings. Localization of the tumor is of primary importance, since the surgical approach is not transabdominal (as in pheochromocytoma) but posterior 11th rib incision. Since the tumor is small and hypovascular, the examination of choice is thin-section CT. Most tumors are visualized on 5 mm thin sections (Fig. 11–19).

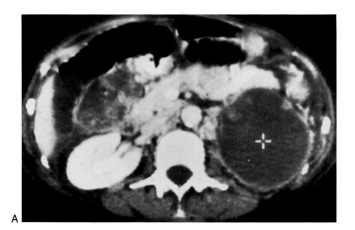

A

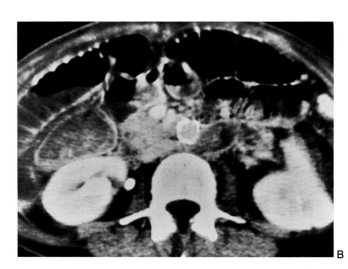

B

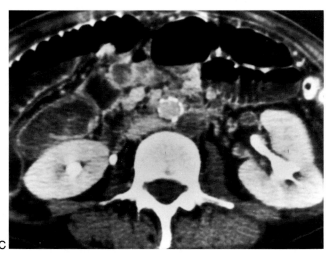

C

Figure 11–16 (A). Relatively low-density adrenal carcinoma did not enhance much on contrast CT scan. The walls of the lesion are thick and somewhat irregular and in the anteromedial part of the mass there are small areas of different texture. In trying to establish whether the tumor has extended into the left renal vein, it becomes apparent that this vessel is absent. (B) More inferior slice demonstrates the tumor, still somewhat radiolucent, propagating within the retroaortic left renal vein. (C) The most inferior slice where the retroaortic left renal vein (filled with tumor) is seen, confirming that the tumor did not extend into the inferior vena cava. The tumor may be seen in a segmental renal vein, just anterior to the renal pelvis.

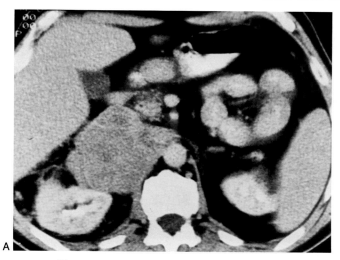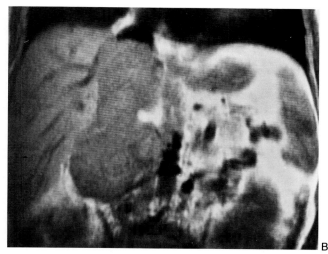

Figure 11–17. **(A)** Moderate sized adrenal carcinoma with a well-defined plane between the kidney. Extension into the inferior vena cava is present. **(B)** MR imaging on the same patient defines the upper extension of the tumor and in particular the relation with the hepatic veins (T1-weighted sequence).

A problem arises when the functioning tumor is only a few millimeters across. In the presence of clinical symptoms and normal-appearing CT, nuclear medicine scan using I-131-6-iodomethyl-19-norcholesterol (NP-59) has been useful in determining the presence of a functioning tumor.[17] The accuracy increases with dexamethasone suppression of the normal functioning adrenal tissues.

When these diagnostic procedures fail to localize the tumor, selective adrenal vein sampling for serum aldosterone levels is performed (Fig. 11–20). Retrograde adrenal venography may also be considered; however, adrenal gland hemorrhage and infarction following such retrograde contrast injection have been described. Sampling on the right side may be

difficult, since small adrenal vein orifice may be difficult to identify. On the left side, care must be taken not to selectively sample left inferior phrenic vein or to allow dilution of the specimen from this vessel.

MRI shows a mass isointense with the liver both in T1- and T2-weighted sequences.

PHEOCHROMOCYTOMA

Incidence. Bilateral, 10%. Extra-adrenal, 10–15% (sympathetic chain, organ of Zuckerkandl). Occurs in 0.6% of all hypertensive patients.

Pathology. Functional benign tumor of the adrenal medulla. Occasionally malignant. Metastases in liver, lungs, lymph nodes, and bones may be functional. May calcify.

Clinical Presentation. Paroxysmal or sustained hypertension, flushing, sweating, fainting, precordial pain, palpitations. May produce ectopic ACTH syndrome.

Laboratory Findings. Elevated serum catecholamines, elevated urinary metanephrines and vanillylmandelic acid (VMA). Hyperglycemia. Positive glucagon test (5 minutes after injection of 1 mg glucagon there is a rise in serum catecholamines above 2000 pg/ml).

Radiological Findings. This tumor is isointense to the kidney on T1-weighted and hyperintense on T2-

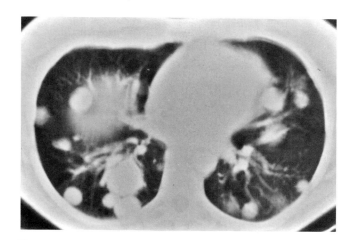

Figure 11–18. Multiple lung metastases from an adrenal carcinoma.

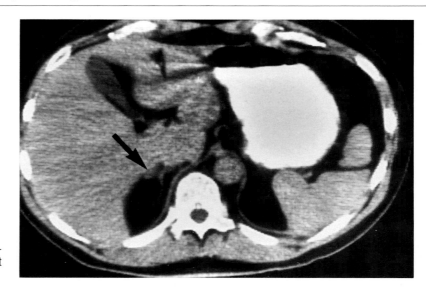

Figure 11–19. Miniscule aldosteronoma in the lateral limb of the right adrenal gland (arrow).

weighted sequences.[18,19] Therefore the tumor, particularly extra-adrenal tumors, is contrasted against the background. Since 15% of pheochromocytomas are extra-adrenal, MR is the imaging method of choice.[19,20] In addition, a degree of specificity is extracted from this imaging technique. Besides suprarenal areas, the sympathetic chain, the pelvis, and the thorax should be examined.

CT is almost as good as MR imaging, offering somewhat better resolution and less dependency on patient cooperation. The tumor may be homogeneous or inhomogeneous, and may have lesser attenuation values than the kidney. Calcifications are nonspecific.

On arteriography, pheochromocytoma is hypervascular. Angiography, however, is no longer routinely performed in search of pheochromocytoma. A note of caution is appropriate should such an examination be performed. Intra-aortic and selective intra-arterial contrast may cause sudden release of catecholamines and malignant hypertensive crises. To prevent such a hypertensive episode, two methods are practiced: 1) Phenoxybenzamine is administered to the patient prior to angiography. The critics of this method point out that irreversible hypotensive reaction may ensue.

2) Anesthesiologist monitors blood pressure and controls hypertensive episode if it does occur with nitroprusside drip.

Malignant Pheochromocytoma

Up to 10% of all pheochromocytomas may be malignant. Metastases to lymph nodes and skeletal system are common (Fig. 11–21). Skeletal metastases may be osteoblastic.

Sipple's Syndrome

Multiple endocrine adenomatoses are present, consisting of medullary thyroid carcinoma with amyloid stroma and pheochromocytoma. Pheochromocyto-

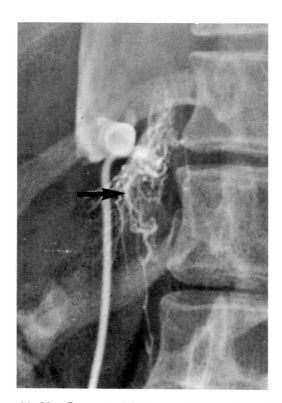

Figure 11–20. Because aldosteronomas may be small, adrenal vein sampling may rarely be needed. Retrograde venography may be hazardous because acute hemorrhage into the adrenal gland may be induced. On this old example of right retrograde adrenal vein venogram, a small mass is identified because of displacement of small intra-adrenal veins (arrow).

mas are bilateral in this disease 63 to 84% of the time. Parathyroid adenomas may also occur. Autosomal dominant inheritance.

Nuclear Medicine

New medullary agent I-131 MIBG (methyodobenzyl-guadinine) is specific for detecting primary and metastatic pheochromocytoma and neuroblastoma.

Pheochromocytoma and Renal Artery Stenosis

Several cases of renal artery narrowing in the close proximity of a pheochromocytoma have been described.[21] Narrowing may disappear spontaneously after adrenalectomy.

OTHER ADRENAL TUMORS

Adrenal Cyst

Adrenal cyst is a relatively uncommon adrenal mass (Fig. 11–22). Congenital, lymphatic obstruction and old hemorrhage are implicated as causes. Cysts may calcify (Fig. 11–23). Protein content in the fluid makes it appear hypointense (dark) on T1-weighted and hyperintense (bright) on T2-weighted images. If large (Fig. 11–24), cyst may be aspirated and emptied.

Myelolipoma

As previously mentioned, this unique tumor originates from the myeloproliferative, blood-forming remnants within the adrenal gland. Just like bone marrow, it contains an abundant amount of fat and therefore it is usually isointense to retroperitoneal fat on both T1- and T2-weighted sequences (Fig. 11–25), radiolucent on projectional radiography, and exhibits low attenuation value or Hounsfield number on CT.[22,23]

Myelolipomas may contain different proportions of fat and myeloid tissues, in which case the diagnosis may be difficult.[24] Calcification and hemorrhage may also be present.

Tuberculosis

Tuberculoma, caseous necrosis, scarring, and calcification is the mode of progression of this disease. Hemorrhage in the adrenal gland is possible.

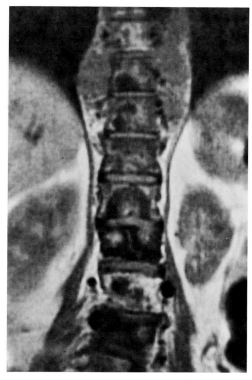

Figure 11–21. Metastatic malignant pheochromocytoma originating from organ of Zuckerkandl has metastasized into the paraspinal lymph nodes in the thorax as well as in the retroperitoneal nodes. In many areas in the spine whitish bone marrow is replaced by hypointense metastases (T1-weighted sequence).

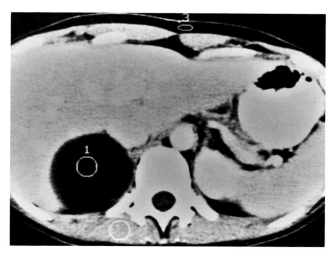

Figure 11–22. Simple adrenal cyst. CT values are between 0 and 20 HU. The walls should be thin and no internal echoes should be present.

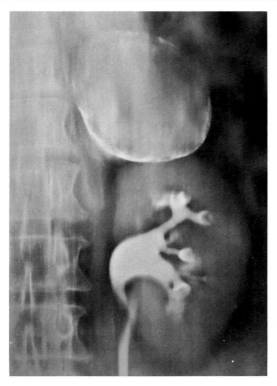

Figure 11–23. Calcified left adrenal cyst. Note flattening of the upper pole and mild inferior displacement of the left kidney.

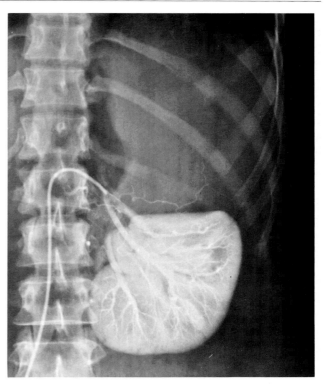

Figure 11–24. A large adrenal cyst was followed for 8 years without intervention. As expected, the cyst is hypovascular on angiography and this study is no longer indicated.

Hemorrhage

Acute bleeding in the adrenal gland may be seen postpartum in neonates, meningococcemia (Waterhouse-Friderichsen syndrome), acute trauma, adrenal carcinoma, pheochromocytoma, tuberculosis, metastases, during acute stress, and spontaneously.

It presents as a mass lesion on cross-sectional imaging (Fig. 11–26) and in later stages calcification is common (Fig. 11–27).[25,26] The mass may become cystic on follow-up examinations.

Adrenal hematoma is usually hyperintense both on T1- and T2-weighted images, but this obviously depends on the acuteness of the process.

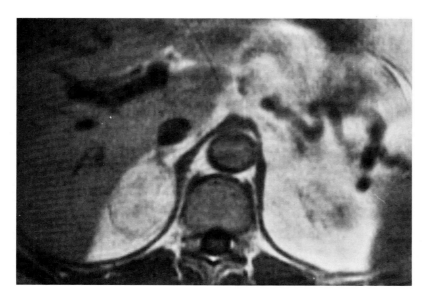

Figure 11–25. Presumed right adrenal myelolipoma followed for 2 years without change in size (T1-weighted sequence). The signal intensity is similar to that of the surrounding fat.

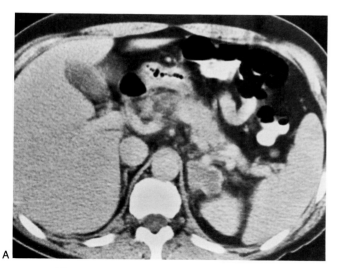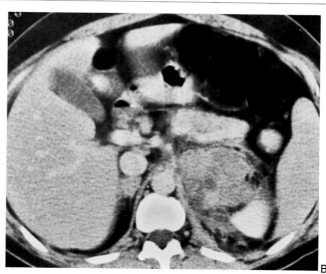

A B

Figure 11–26. **(A)** Relatively hypolucent left adrenal mass in a patient with lymphoma is most likely an old hematoma from previous adrenal hemorrhage. **(B)** One week later, patient developed acute flank pain due to spontaneous hemorrhage into the left adrenal gland. The left gland is now markedly enlarged with hyperdense areas of fresh hemorrhage. Since the last CT scan, there was also an acute hemorrhage into the previously normal right adrenal gland, although much smaller compared with the left.

Lymphoma

Most adrenal lymphomas are secondary non-Hodgkin's lymphomas and may be seen in one-third of patients with this disease.[27] Frequently, there is simultaneous renal involvement. Primary adrenal lymphoma is rare.[28]

Wolman's Disease

A rare fatal autosomal recessive disease seen in the first few months of life. Abnormal fatty metabolism is expressed in excessive storage of triglycerides and cholesterol in body organs. There is hepatosplenomegaly. Both adrenal glands are markedly enlarged and calcified.[29]

Pseudotumors

Normal tissues such as retroperitoneal fat (Fig. 11–28) and fluid-filled gastric fundus may mimic an adrenal mass. A radiograph taken with the patient in the prone position may allow air to fill the fundus, establishing the diagnosis. Pancreatic pseudocysts

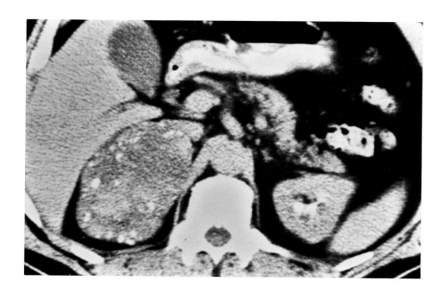

Figure 11–27. Old calcified adrenal hematoma. This case is a good example of the difficulty at times in differentiating a benign from a malignant lesion. Calcifications and inhomogeneous pattern are present and adrenal carcinoma may be considered.

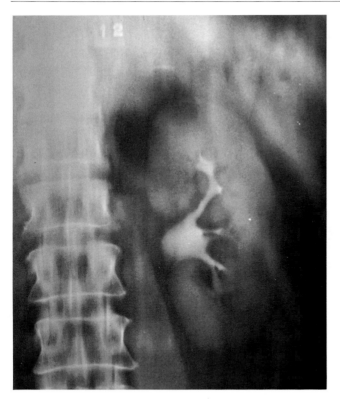

Figure 11–28. A radiolucent, well-circumscribed mass is seen on a tomographic cut along the medial aspect of the upper pole of the left kidney. Both the mass and the kidney are in focus (or in the imaging plane). CT showed only normal retroperitoneal fat and normal undisturbed adrenal gland.

and splenic artery aneurysm may also be misconstrued as an adrenal mass (Fig. 29).

NEUROBLASTOMA

Incidence.   Most common solid malignant tumor in childhood.

Pathology.   Neural crest tumor originating from adrenal (50%) or sympathetic chain. Venous inva-

sion common. Extension into spinal canal. Ganglioneurinoma is a matured form of neuroblastoma.

Clinical Presentation.   Large palpable abdominal mass. Distant metastases present in 66% of patients at the time of diagnosis.

Laboratory Findings.   Vanillylmandelic acid (VMA) test positive in 80%.

Radiological Findings.   Ultrasound is the first examination of choice. Determination is made very rapidly if the palpable mass is solid or cystic (hydronephrosis, multicystic kidney, renal cyst).

In the presence of a solid abdominal mass and positive VMA test, imaging efforts are directed toward proper staging of the disease. Since vascular encasement and spinal cord involvement are crucial in determining surgical resectibility, MR imaging is the examination of choice.[30]

The tumor is of high intensity on T2-weighted images and about same intensity as the liver on T1-weighted sequence. Internal architecture may be uniform or showing areas of hemorrhage and necrosis. Common low-intensity calcifications are usually not detected by this imaging technique.

Renal involvement, secondary hydronephrosis, lymph node enlargement, and bone metastases may all be identified. Occasionally, the tumor may appear to be arising from the kidney, simulating Wilms tumor.[31]

Encasement of the great vessels is seen to a greater advantage than on CT, since vessels are so well depicted. Encasement of renal, celiac, and splenic veins as well that of the inferior vena cava has been documented.

Finally, MR is an excellent imaging modality for monitoring effectiveness of therapy in regard to change in tumor size.

CT is very close to MR imaging, although it requires intravenous contrast to visualize major abdominal vessels and their relation to the tumor.[32,33]

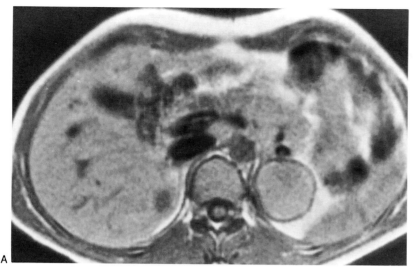

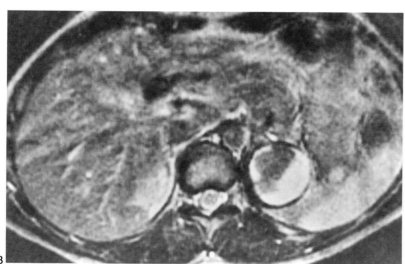

Figure 11–29. (A) Pancreatic pseudocyst masquerading as an adrenal tumor. Thick wall and relatively homogeneous appearance are seen on T1-weighted sequence. (B) On T2-weighted sequence, most of the cyst is hyperintense with intraluminal defects. The cyst was percutaneously aspirated elsewhere with what is now most likely a hemorrhagic component.

REFERENCES

1. Copeland PM. The incidentally discovered adrenal mass. Ann Intern Med 1983; 98:940–945.
2. Bernardino ME. Management of the asymptomatic patient with unilateral adrenal mass. Radiology 1988; 166:121–123.
3. Belldergun A, Hussain S, Seltzer SE, et al. Incidentally discovered mass of the adrenal gland. Surg Gynecol Obst 1986; 163:203–208.
4. Hussain S, Belldergun A, Seltzer SE, et al. Differentiation of malignant from benign adrenal masses: predictive indices on computed tomography. AJR 1985; 144:61–65.
5. Berland LL, Koslin DB, Kenney PJ, et al. Differentiation between small benign and malignant adrenal masses with dynamic incremented CT. AJR 1988; 151:95–101.
6. Reining JW, Doppman JL, Dwyaer AJ, et al. Adrenal masses differentiated by MR. Radiology 1986; 158:81–84.
7. Chang A, Glazer HS, Lee JKT, et al. Adrenal gland: MR imaging. Radiology 1987; 163:123–128.
8. Glazer GM, Woolsey EJ, Borrello J, et al. Adrenal tissue characterization using MR imaging. Radiology 1986; 158:73–79.
9. Krestin GP, Steinbrich W, Friedmann G. Adrenal masses: evaluation with fast gradient-echo MR imaging and Gd-DTPA-enhanced dynamic studies. Radiology 1989; 171:675–680.
10. Doppman JL, Miller DL, Dwyer AJ, et al. Macronodular adrenal hyperplasia in Cushing disease. Radiology 1988; 166:347–352.
11. Oldfield EH, Chrousos GP, Schulte HL, et al. Preoperative lateralization of ACTH-secreting pituitary microadenomas by bilateral and simultaneous inferior petrosal venous sampling. N Engl J Med 1985; 312:100–103.
12. Peck WW, Dillon WP, Normam D, et al. High-resolu-

tion MR imaging of pituitary microadenomas at 1.5 T: Experience with Cushing disease. AJR 1989; 152:145–151.

13. Steiner E, Imhof H, Knosp E. Gd-DTPA enhanced high resolution MR imaging of pituitary adenomas. Radiographics 1989; 9:587–598.

14. Doppman JL, Travis WD, Nieman L, et al. Cushing syndrome due to primary pigmented nodular adrenocortical disease: findings at CT and MR imaging. Radiology 1989; 172:415–420.

15. Nader S, Hickey RC, Selin RV, Samaan NA. Adrenal cortical carcinoma: a study of 77 cases. Cancer 1983; 52:707–711.

16. O'Keeffe FN, Carrasco CH, Charnsangavej C, et al. Arterial embolization of adrenal tumors: results in nine cases. AJR 1988; 151:819–822.

17. Ikeda DM, Francis IR, Glazer GM, et al. The detection of adrenal tumors and hyperplasia in patients with primary aldosteronism: comparison of scintigraphy, CT, and MR imaging. AJR 1989; 153:301–306.

18. Fink IJ, Reining JW, Dwyer AJ, et al. MR imaging of pheochromocytomas. J Comput Assist Tomogr 1985; 9:454–458.

19. Quint EL, Glazer GM, Francis IR, et al. Pheochromocytoma and paraganglioma: comparison of MR imaging with CT and I-131 MIBG scintigraphy. Radiology 1987; 165:89–93.

20. Grenberg M, Moawad AH, Wieties BM, et al. Extraadrenal pheochromocytoma: detection during pregnancy using MR imaging. Radiology 1986; 161:475–476.

21. Bezirdjian DR, Tegtmyer CJ, Leef JL. Intrarenal pheochromocytoma and renal artery stenosis. Urol Radiol 1984; 3:121–122.

22. Vick CW, Zeman RK, Mannes E, et al. Adrenal myelolipoma: CT and ultrasonographic findings. Urol Radiol 1984; 6:7–13.

23. Musante F, Derchi LE, Zappasodi F, et al. Myelolipoma of the adrenal gland: sonographic and CT features. AJR 1988; 151:961–964.

24. Gould JD, Mitty HA, Pertsemlidis D, Szporn AH. Adrenal myelolipoma: diagnosis by fine needle aspiration. AJR 1987; 148:921–922.

25. Murphy BJ, Casillas J, Yrizarry JM. Traumatic adrenal hemorrhage: radiologic findings. Radiology 1988; 169:701–703.

26. Baker ME, Spritzer C, Blinder R, et al. Benign adrenal lesions mimicking malignancy on MR imaging: report of two cases. Radiology 1987; 163:669–671.

27. Miyake O, Namiki M, Sonoda T, Kitamura H. Secondary involvement of genitourinary organs in malignant lymphoma. Urol Int 1987; 42:360–362.

28. Shea TC, Spark R, Kane B, Lange RF. Non-Hodgkin's lymphoma limited to the adrenal gland with adrenal insufficiency. Am J Med 1985; 78:711–714.

29. Harrison RB, Francke P Jr. Radiographic findings in Wolman's disease. Radiology 1977; 124:188.

30. Fletcher BD, Kopiwoda SY, Strandjord SE, et al. Abdominal neuroblastoma: magnetic resonance imaging and tissue characterization. Radiology 1985; 155:699–703.

31. Rosenfield NS, Leonidas JC, Barwick KW. Aggressive neuroblastoma simulating Wilms tumor. Radiology 1988; 166:165–167.

32. Lowe RE, Cohen MD. Computed tomographic evaluation of Wilms tumor and neuroblastoma. Radiographics 1984; 4:915–928.

33. Peretz GS, Lam AH. Distinguishing neuroblastoma from Wilms tumor by computed tomography. J Comput Assist Tomogr 1985; 9:889–894.

12

Renal Vascular Disorders

RENAL EMBOLISM AND INFARCTION

Etiology. Embolus, trauma, transcatheter embolization, renal artery dissection, inadvertent renal artery ligation.

Clinical Presentation. Acute flank pain, hematuria. Symptoms are related to the volume of infarcted tissue and may be mild in small infarcts and very pronounced in large. Occlusion of the main renal artery of a solitary kidney, renal allograft, or bilateral occlusion is complicated by renal failure. Hematuria and blood clots may cause temporary ureteral obstruction.

Radiological Findings. Contrast-enhanced CT is the examination of choice. Triangular or wedge-shaped nonperfused area is seen in segmental infarction (Fig. 12–1). *Cortical subcapsular rim sign* represents 2 to 3 mm thick dense outer nephrogram overlying the infarcted segment (Figs. 12–2, 12–3).[1,2] This sign is almost pathognomonic for infarction, although it has been described in renal vein thrombosis, acute cortical necrosis, and acute tubular necrosis. Presumably the outer 3 mm of cortex have dual blood supply, from renal arteries and from small capsular perforators.[3] Associated subcapsular hematoma may be present at times.

Partially perfused adjacent areas, associated intraparenchymal hemorrhage, and edema may mimic a mass and suggest a neoplastic process.[4,5] Surgery or angiography can be delayed, since such a pseudotumor is likely to disappear within several weeks, at which time loss of parenchyma will be evident on follow-up CT (Fig. 12–4 A,B,C).

Angiography may disclose an intra-arterial filling defect, a cutoff vessel (Fig. 12–5), and lack of perfusion of the infarcted segment (Figs. 12–6, 12–7, and 12–8). Capsular arteries within perinephric space and adjacent to the infarct frequently become prominent within days after the event and may be mistaken for neoplastic vessels. After several weeks, a scar forms (Fig. 12–9).

SUBCAPSULAR AND PERINEPHRIC HEMATOMA

Etiology

1. *Spontaneous.* Malignant tumors are probably the most common cause, followed by benign tumors such as angiomyolipoma. Less common are vas-

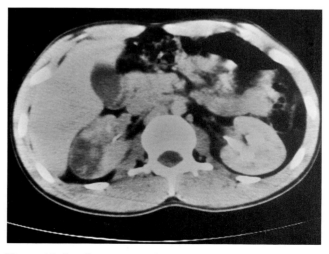

Figure 12–1. Segmental infarct involving lateral part of the right kidney. Triangular nonperfused area with the apex pointing toward renal hilum is seen on contrast-enhanced CT scan.

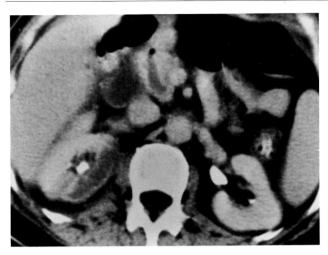

Figure 12–2. Here the infarcted segment is quite large, probably due to occlusion of the posterior ramus. Cortical subcapsular rim sign is seen, representing the outer 2–3 mm of cortex perfused by small perforating capsular arteries.

cular diseases, such as polyarteritis nodosa and arteriovenous malformations (AVM), hemorrhagic cysts, infection, and infarction. On occasion, no underlying causes have been found.[6]

2. *Traumatic and iatrogenic.* Blunt or penetrating trauma, ESWL, percutaneous nephrostomy, biopsy, surgery, and anticoagulation.

Clinical Presentation. Acute flank pain. Hematuria may or may not be present.

Radiological Findings. CT is the examination of choice. Acute subcapsular hematoma is denser than the kidney on CT (Fig. 12–10). Within days it becomes relatively radiolucent (Fig. 12–11). Adjacent parenchyma may be displaced tangentially to the unyielding renal capsule. Perinephric hematoma dissects between the lamelar septa and fat within the perinephric space (see Fig. 6–30).

Because of high association of spontaneous subcapsular hematoma with an underlying malignant (or benign) tumor, the kidney must be carefully examined (Fig. 12–12). The neoplasm may be small, therefore contrast enhancement and 5 mm thin slices should be obtained, looking for telltale signs of renal carcinoma or angiomyolipoma.[7–9]

Subcapsular and perinephric hematoma may be identified on ultrasound as hypoechoic (see Fig. 6–31). Angiography is rarely needed and may be considered for embolization and to establish diagnosis of polyarteritis nodosa. In the presence of hemorrhage, smaller tumors are detected with difficulty on angiography.

RENAL ARTERY ANEURYSM

Etiology. Congenital, atherosclerosis, hypertension.

Pathology. Degeneration of media (atherosclerotic aneurysms). Intimal dissection (dissecting aneurysms).

Clinical Presentation. Usually asymptomatic. Hypertension, acute pain, retroperitoneal hemorrhage are all rare.

Treatment. Small, less than 2 cm, calcified renal artery aneurysms are ignored unless contributing to renal vascular hypertension. Larger aneurysms, particularly those that are not calcified, are surgically removed or can be embolized.

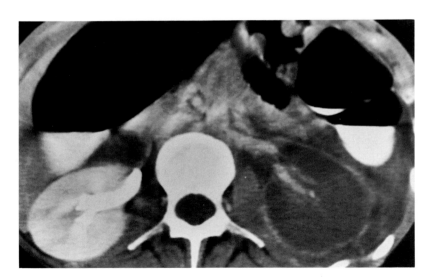

Figure 12–3. Infarction of the entire left kidney. Left kidney is not enhancing except for the outer subcortical area. Patient presents with acute flank pain while being treated for subacute bacterial endocarditis. Differential diagnosis includes renal vein thrombosis.

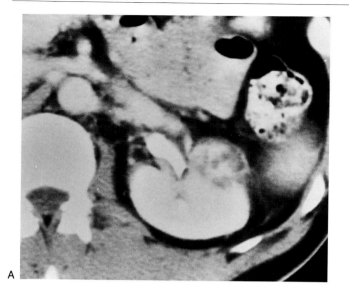

A

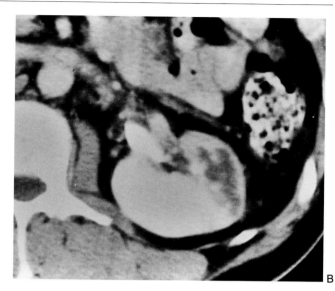

B

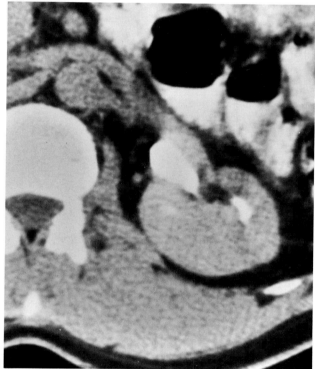

C

Figure 12–4. (A) Left renal pseudotumor due to acute renal infarction. Mass at the anterior aspect of the left kidney appears inhomogeneous and could very well represent a malignant tumor. (B) One slice caudad demonstrates classic cortical subcapsular enhancement and underperfused area, signs typical for infarction. (C) One month later a repeated CT scan demonstrates atrophy of the renal parenchyma in the area of infarct.

Radiological Findings. An aneurysm may be detected on a plain radiograph if calcified (Fig. 12–13). More likely, it is a serendipitous discovery during a CT scan or sonography (Fig. 12–14). Angiography is necessary to judge resectability (Fig. 12–15). Embolization may be accomplished by depositing detachable balloons within the aneurysm.

Dissecting aneurysms are similar to aortic dissections. Indeed, many aortic dissections extend into the renal artery. Spontaneous renal artery dissection without aortic involvement is rare. Narrowing of the renal artery, filling of the false channel, and visualization of the intimal flap on angiography are the principal findings (Figs. 12–16, 12–17).

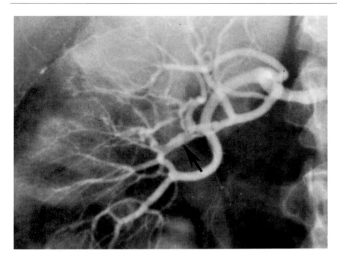

Figure 12–5. Right renal arteriogram. Intraluminal "filling defect" representing embolus is seen in the segmental artery (arrow).

RENAL VASCULAR HYPERTENSION

Incidence. Five percent of all hypertensive patients.

Etiology. Atherosclerosis, fibromuscular dysplasia, renal artery dissection, thrombosis, neurofibromatosis, midaortic syndrome, renal artery aneurysm, tumor encasement, AV fistulas, extrinsic compression (Page kidney, renal cyst, obstruction), radiation-induced stenosis.[10]

Pathophysiology. Renin is produced in the juxtraglomerular cells in the macula densa and its secretion is increased in the presence of significant renal artery stenosis. Renin acts on circulating angiotensinogen to produce angiotensin I (A I). Angiotensin-converting enzyme acts on A I to produce angiotensin II (A II), a very potent vasoconstrictor (Fig. 12–18).

Saralasin is A II antagonist and partial agonist. Captopril is an inhibitor of angiotensin-converting enzyme. Both blunt A II response.

Clinical Presentation. Sudden onset of hypertension, abdominal bruit, "inappropriate hypertension." Efforts by the medical community to diagnose the presence of renal artery stenosis have significantly decreased. This is largely due to the expense of relatively insensitive radiological procedures and because of the liberal use of new and very effective antihypertensive medications. However, renal vascular hypertension is one of the curable types of hypertension (other than aldosteronoma and pheochromocytoma). Thus, successful treatment of renal vascular hypertension can eliminate a life-long dependence on antihypertensive medication.

Laboratory Findings. A rise in peripheral vein renins is detected in 50%, and a rise in renin levels in renal vein of the affected kidneys is detectable in 80%.

Radiological Findings. The basic design of nonangiographic radiological diagnostic procedures is based on: a) Increased amount of time for intrave-

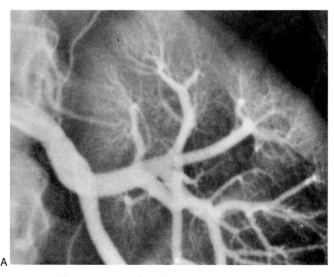

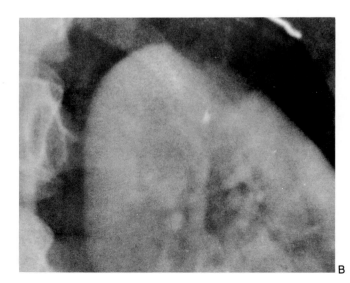

Figure 12–6. Small embolus due to improper catheter technique is almost unnoticed **(A)**. Several seconds later a small triangular nephrogram defect and lingering contrast in the acutely occluded artery are diagnostic **(B)**.

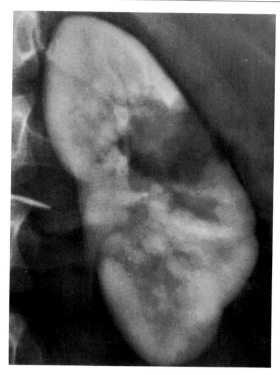

Figure 12–7. Typical segmental infarct seen in the nephrogram phase on the left renal arteriogram.

nously injected contrast (or radionuclides) to reach the affected kidney; b) presence of collateral arterial supply; c) increased reabsorption of sodium and water from the tubules by the affected kidney; and d) parenchymal atrophy.

Urography. Rapid sequence urogram (or hypertensive IVP) differs from regular excretory urogram in that during the first 5 minutes radiographs of the kidneys are obtained at 1 minute intervals (Fig. 12–19).[11] The positive signs are:

1. *Smaller size:* Affected kidney is 1.5 cm smaller in the longest diameter compared with the normal kidney. Atrophy occurs after prolonged renal hypoxia.
2. *Delay in the appearance of the nephrogram* on the affected side.
3. *Delay in appearance of the contrast in the pelvocalyceal system* (Fig. 12–20). This delay occurs because contrast takes longer to transit the area of obstruction and to negotiate the newly developed collaterals.
4. *Ureteral or pelvocalyceal notching:* Periureteral collaterals develop gradually and may indent both ureters and pelvocalyceal walls (Fig. 12–21).

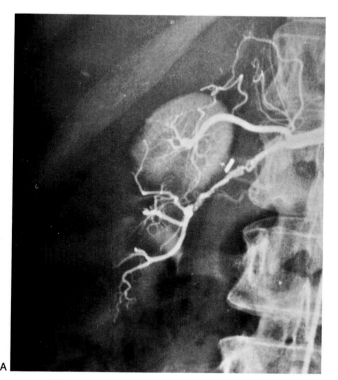

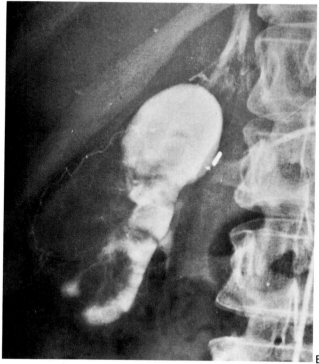

A

B

Figure 12–8. Selective right renal arteriogram. Large segmental infarction is present in a patient who has recently undergone surgical repair of fibrodysplastic renal artery. Main branch, as well as the upper pole segmental branch are normal. The main segmental branch is irregular, and another main branch is occluded, explaining the paucity of smaller branches (**A**). In the nephrogram phase large anterolateral segment is not perfused (**B**). Note filling of the capsular branches and inferior adrenal arteries on the top of the kidney and adrenal blush in the later phase.

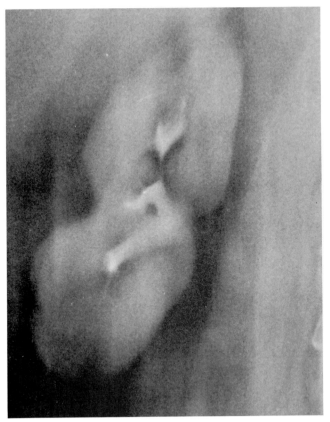

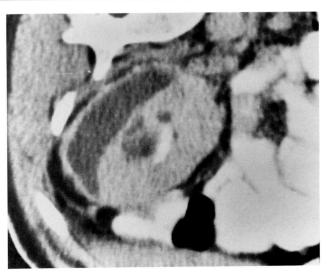

Figure 12–11. Contrast-enhanced CT. Subacute subcapsular hematoma several weeks old is relatively radiolucent. A small radiolucent mass measuring 2 cm in diameter is in the renal parenchyma immediately adjacent to a hematoma and most likely represents an angiomyolipoma (which has a tendency to bleed).

Figure 12–9. Renal scar several months after an acute renal infarct.

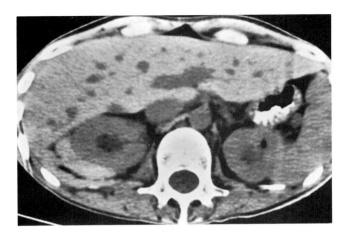

Figure 12–10. Nonenhanced CT. Acute subcapsular and perinephric hematoma immediately after an attempted right percutaneous nephrostomy. Fresh blood clot is hyperdense compared with the renal parenchyma.

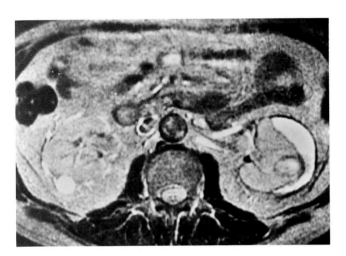

Figure 12–12. MR image, T2-weighted sequence. Hyperintense left subcapsular hematoma is present. A small tumor measuring 2–3 cm in diameter is adjacent and immediately under the hematoma. Here it is unclear if the tumor is a benign angiomyolipoma, renal carcinoma, or something else. Thin CT sections with and without contrast will yield more information. Unless distinct areas of fat are found within the tumor, it is presumed to be malignant. Note small cyst in the right kidney.

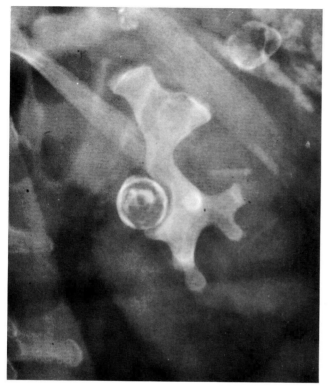

Figure 12–13. Plain radiograph. Calcified left renal artery aneurysm in a solitary kidney with staghorn calculus. Note how the growth of the staghorn has been influenced by the aneurysm. (Photograph courtesy of Dr. Shlomo Raz.)

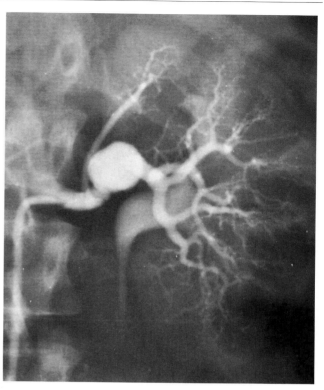

Figure 12–15. Selective left renal arteriogram is done to judge resectability of a noncalcified aneurysm.

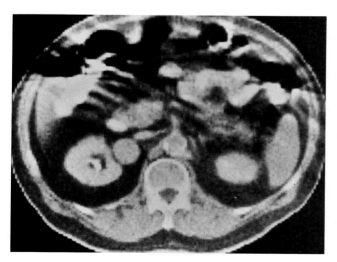

Figure 12–14. Right renal artery aneurysm discovered serendipitously on contrast-enhanced CT scan performed for other reasons.

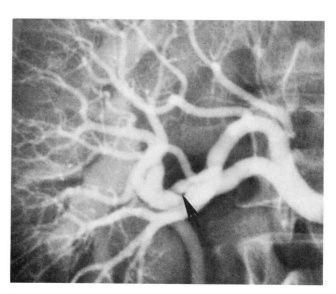

Figure 12–16. Spontaneous dissection of the right renal artery. Intimal flap is seen as a thin strip, almost resembling a cardiac valve (arrow).

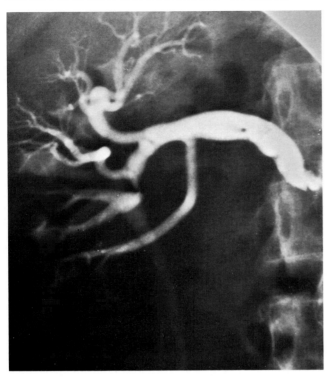

Figure 12–17. Spontaneous dissection of the right renal artery. Several small radiolucencies are present in the main renal artery. The dissection extends distally into the lower branch, at which point the segmental branch becomes narrow.

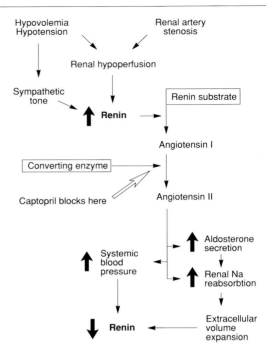

Figure 12–18.   Renin-angiotensin axis.

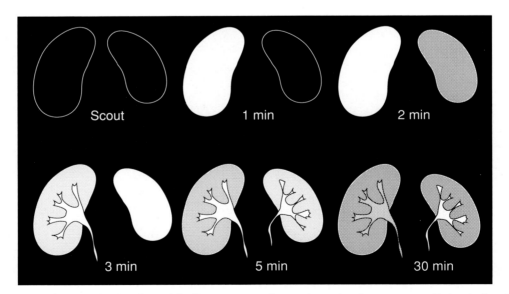

Figure 12–19.   Schematic drawing of findings expected on a hypertensive urogram. Delay in function is detected on early radiographs within 1 to 5 minutes following injection of contrast. Hyperconcentration in the affected kidney is rarely seen and may be somewhat more obvious on later radiographs.

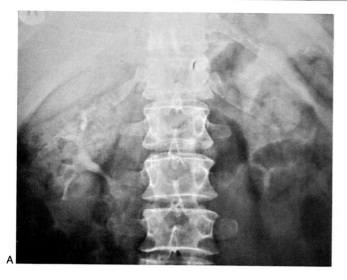

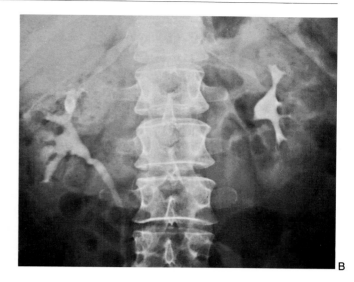

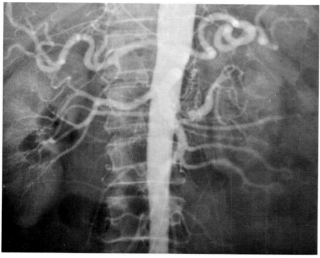

Figure 12–20. (A) Four minutes after a bolus of contrast was injected, the collecting system of normal right kidney is already opacified. The smallish left kidney is not. (B) At 15 minutes, it becomes obvious the delay in function on the left is not because of obstruction, renal vein thrombosis, or pyelonephritis. Hyperconcentration of the contrast, as seen in the left kidney of this patient, is not seen in conditions other than renal vascular hypertension. (C) Severe left renal artery stenosis is confirmed on angiography.

5. *Hyperconcentration on delayed films:* This finding is difficult to perceive and is due to increased sodium and water reabsorption in the affected kidney.

Excretory urography is no longer the primary method for screening patients with suspected renal vascular hypertension because the false-negative rate is 20%. However, radiologists must be familiar with these signs, since functionally significant renal artery stenosis may be detected during the course of an excretory urogram performed for other purposes (Fig. 12–22).

Tc-99m DTPA Scintigraphy. Without captopril. The procedure and findings are analogous to the rapid sequence urogram (Fig. 12–23). After an intravenous bolus of radionuclide, scintigrams are obtained 5–15 seconds apart, which is several times more frequent than rapid sequence urogram (Fig. 12–24). For this reason, the delay in function may be detected somewhat more readily.

With captopril. Renal uptake is recorded quantitatively before and 1 hour after oral administration of 25–50 mg of captopril. The test is positive if there is a decline in Tc-99m DTPA uptake after captopril.[12] Captopril dramatically reduces blood pressure in patients with functionally significant renal artery stenosis, more so than in patients with essential hypertension. There is also more pronounced vasodilatation of efferent arterioles compared with afferent arterioles. This results in a significant decrease in glomerular capillary pressure and glomerular filtration rate and explains the difference in uptake before and after captopril.

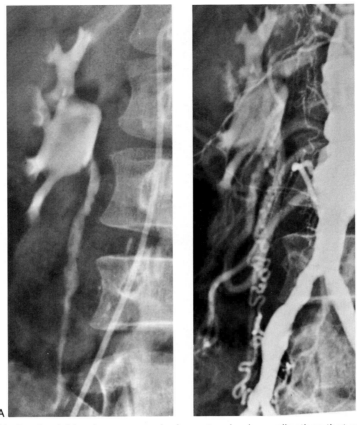

A   B

Figure 12–21. **(A)** Ureteral notching in renovascular hypertension is smaller than that caused by periureteral venous or lymph node enlargement. **(B)** Serpiginous periureteral collaterals that caused the notching arise from lumbar or internal iliac branches and deliver blood to the arterial system of the kidney distal to stenosis.

Intravenous Digital Subtraction Angiography (DSA-IV). Injection of contrast material through a centrally placed venous catheter allows for a more compact bolus of contrast material to reach the abdominal aorta. Electronic digital temporal subtraction eliminates spurious shadows so that the renal arteries usually become visible. The disadvantage of this particular examination is that several injections usually have to be made, resulting in a substantial dose of contrast material. Examinations are often unsuccessful due to respiratory motion and peristaltic activity. Others report a very high success rate.[13]

Arteriography. Arteriography is the examination of choice for determining the presence of renal artery stenosis.[14] This examination may be performed on an outpatient basis, significantly decreasing the cost. It should therefore precede every other test, including renal vein renin sampling. If stenosis is not present, there is no longer doubt of false-negative rates associated with other examinations. In most instances a significant unilateral stenosis will be treated even if ipsilateral renins are not found to be elevated. Before the study is begun, the decision may be made whether to immediately proceed with balloon angioplasty at the time of diagnosis. A surgeon familiar with the case should be available in the hospital.

Angiographic findings accurately reflect various diseases:

1. *Atherosclerosis* is the most common cause of renal stenosis in male patients over the age of 50 years. Renal artery orifice is usually involved and the atheroma may be calcified. The aorta may also be heavily involved (Fig. 12–25).
2. *Fibromuscular dysplasia* is the most common cause of renal artery stenosis in female patients under the age of 40 years. The process appears to be self-limiting at age 40. There are several subtypes (Fig. 12–26):[15] a) Intimal, a weblike obstruction composed only of intima; b) medial hyperplasia involving the inner media; c) medial fibroplasia, typical beady appearance involving midarterial segment (Fig. 12–27). This type is

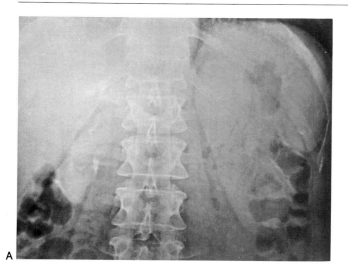

A

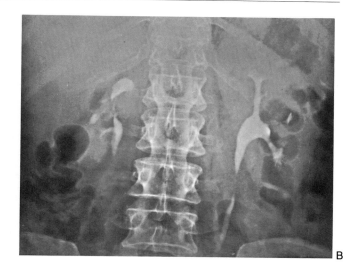

B

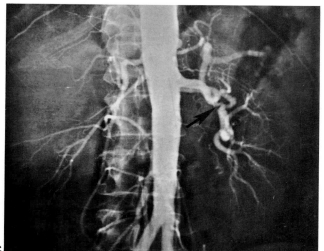

C

Figure 12–22. An example of unsuspected renovascular hypertension detected on urography. **(A)** Five minutes after injection, the contrast is excreted in the right collecting system, while none is seen on the left. Although the right kidney is small, there is calyceal clubbing in the upper pole and focal scarring typical for reflux nephropathy. **(B)** At 10 minutes, contrast appears in what otherwise looks like a normal left kidney. Any delay in excretion when compared to the opposite kidney is highly significant. **(C)** Renal artery stenosis is present on the left (arrow) with poststenotic dilatation. Right renal artery, although small, has no areas of narrowing.

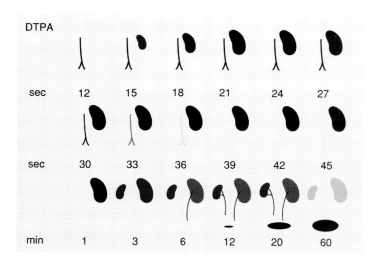

Figure 12–23. Schematic drawing of sequence of events in renovascular hypertension produced by right kidney artery stenosis. There is delay in appearance of the radionuclide in the renal vascular bed, tubules, and collecting system.

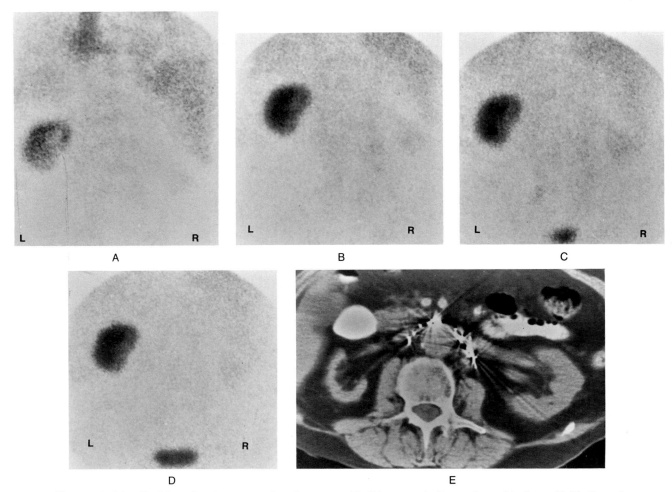

Figure 12–24. Tc-99m glucoheptonate has been used in this case. In the early rapid phase **(A,B)**, there is rapid appearance and accumulation of radionuclide in the left kidney (remember scintigrams are read "backwards"). On later scintigrams **(C,D)**, there is still no evidence of renal perfusion or function. The right kidney, if it exists at all, has complete renal artery occlusion and is not functioning. **(E)** CT scan done for other reasons demonstrates a small right kidney.

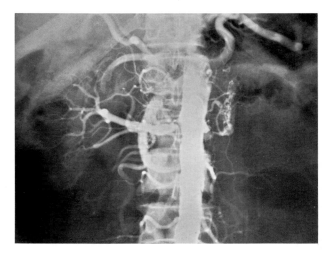

Figure 12–25. An example of atherosclerotic bilateral renal artery stenosis. These lesions are typically seen at the ostium. Poststenotic dilatation is seen on the right but not on the left.

frequently associated with small, noncalcified renal artery aneurysm involving segmental branches (Fig. 12–28); d) perimedial fibroplasia involving the outer media; and e) adventitial, usually involving a longer, smooth segment (Fig. 12–29).

3. *Neurofibromatosis.* Prolific fibrotic changes occur in the media. Stenosis is not caused by a neurofibroma.

4. *Arteritides.* These include *Takayasu's aortitis, moya-moya disease,* etc. (Fig. 12–30).

5. *Midaortic syndrome.* This is an unusual cause of renovascular hypertension in children. There is a narrowing of the infrarenal abdominal aorta, which may involve renal arteries (Fig. 12–31). The disease is self-limiting by the age of 15 years, but if left untreated it is ultimately fatal.[16]

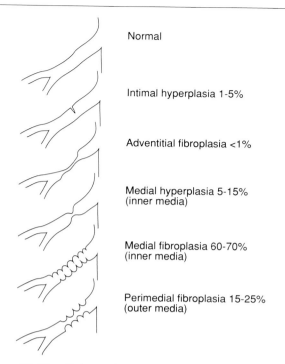

Normal

Intimal hyperplasia 1-5%

Adventitial fibroplasia <1%

Medial hyperplasia 5-15%
(inner media)

Medial fibroplasia 60-70%
(inner media)

Perimedial fibroplasia 15-25%
(outer media)

Figure 12–26. Schematic drawing and frequency of different types of fibromuscular dysplasia.

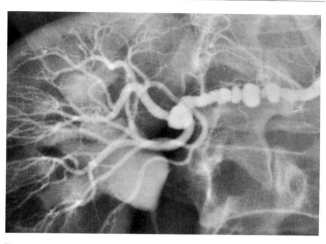

Figure 12–28. Medial fibroplasia and a small aneurysm at the bifurcation into anterior and posterior rami.

6. *Spontaneous renal artery dissection.* This disease has a quite characteristic appearance on selective renal angiography. It is rare and associated with essential hypertension and atherosclerotic disease. (Fig. 12–32).[17] Renal artery dissection may also complicate dissecting aneurysm of the abdominal aorta.

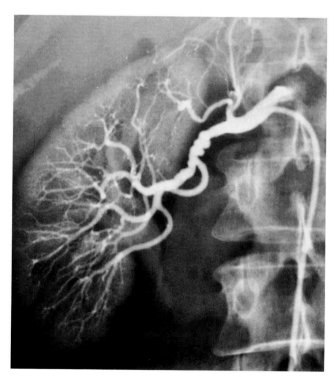

Figure 12–27. Medial fibroplasia with beady appearance of the middle arterial segment.

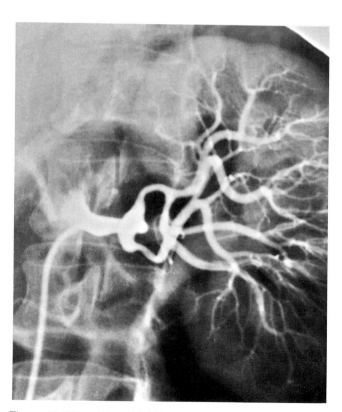

Figure 12–29. Adventitial fibroplasia. There is no beading. Smooth narrowing involves anterior and posterior rami and extends into segmental branches.

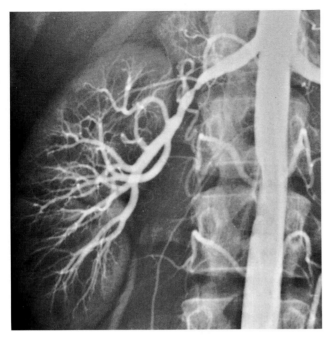

Figure 12–30.   Right renal artery stenosis involving the middle arterial segment. There is also localized narrowing of the infrarenal abdominal aorta. The two processes are probably related.

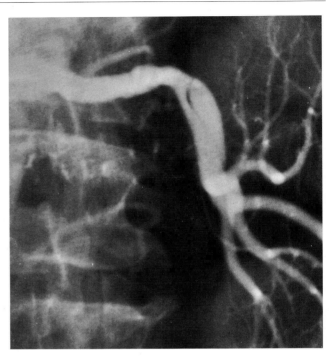

Figure 12–32.   Spontaneous dissection of left renal artery. Intimal flap is seen as a radiolucent line.

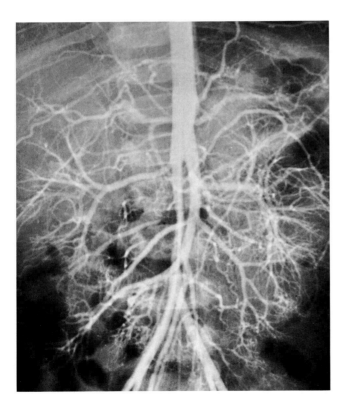

Figure 12–31.   Middle aortic syndrome in a child. Infrarenal aorta is narrower than the superior mesenteric artery, which is slightly to the left. One way to identify the aorta is to identify common iliac arteries and trace them back to the bifurcation.

7. *Renal artery aneurysm.* Aneurysm may cause renal vascular hypertension because of extensive compression on the segmental branches of the renal artery and occasionally to the distal embolic phenomena from the thrombi forming within the aneurysm (Fig. 12–15).
8. *Renal transplant arterial anastomosis.* About 5% of renal allografts may develop stenosis at the arterial anastomotic site.
9. *Graft stenosis.* Patients with renal artery bypass graft (Fig. 12–33, 12–34).
10. *Tumor encasement or displacement* (Fig. 12–35).
11. *Radiation injury* is a rare cause of arterial narrowing (Fig. 12–36).
12. *Inadvertent ligation or clipping.*

Percutaneous Transluminal Angioplasty of the Renal Arteries (PTA).   Renal artery stenosis is crossed with an appropriate angiographic catheter. Intra-arterial heparin and antispasmodics are administered to prevent renal artery spasm and thrombosis. The stenosis is crossed with a guidewire over which the balloon-carrying catheter is positioned (Fig. 12–37). The balloon diameter (when inflated) should be 1 to 2 mm wider than the lumen of the normal renal artery segment adjusted to stenosis. The balloon is inflated several times for 15 seconds at a time, until "sausaging" has completely disappeared. The process distends and overstretches the media. Postprocedural

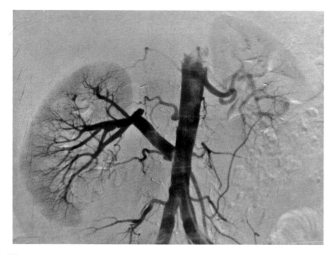

Figure 12–33. Renal artery graft (end-to-side aorta, end-to-end distal renal artery). One segmental branch to the lower pole of the right kidney is occluded but is reconstituted (seen on a later film) via the capsular collaterals.

medications are administered to lower clotting factors. Complications include intimal tear, thrombosis of the renal artery, and renal artery rupture.[18,19]

Technically successful angioplasty ranges from 90% in patients with fibromuscular dysplasia (FMD) (Fig. 12–38) to 25% or less in patients with bilateral ostial atherosclerotic lesion. Cured (or significantly improved) range from 90% for FMD, 82% for nonostial atherosclerosis (Fig. 12–39), 50% for renal allografts, to very poor in patients with bilateral ostial atherosclerosis.[19–21]

Transcatheter Renal Artery Embolization and Ablation. In some instances small hyperreninemic kidney may be too small to contribute useful renal function or to justify percutaneous transluminal angioplasty, nephrostomy, or bypass graft.[22–25] Ablation of such a kidney may be possible if a catheter can be wedged through the stenotic segment. Small amounts of alcohol or other embolic material are

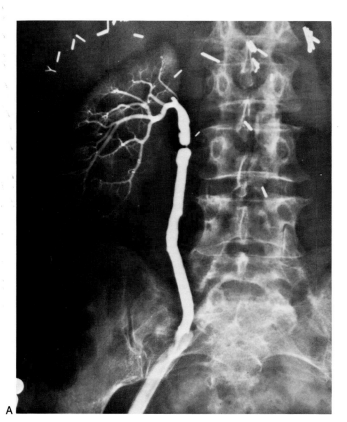

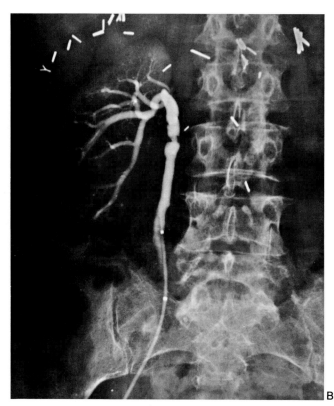

A

B

Figure 12–34. A complicated saphenous graft between right common iliac artery and right renal artery. A significant stricture is present at the anastomotic site between the graft and distal renal artery (**A**). Only partial success is achieved with balloon angioplasty (**B**).

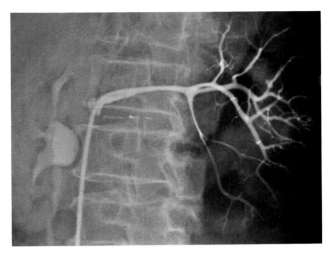

Figure 12–35. Renal artery encasement with liposarcoma originating from left renal pelvis. The main renal artery and several segmental branches are elongated and narrow.

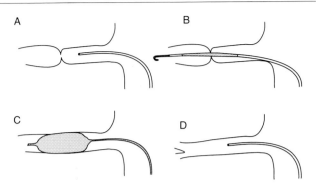

Figure 12–37. Schematic drawing of balloon angioplasty technique. **(A)** Artery is selectively catheterized. **(B)** The narrow segment is crossed with a guidewire and the angioplasty balloon catheter. **(C)** Dilatation is accomplished in several 10- to 15-second attempts. **(D)** Postangioplasty angiogram is performed.

needed to completely ablate the renal vascular bed of the affected kidney and eliminate renin production (Fig. 12–40).

Other Causes for Hyperreninemia

1. *Page kidney* is a kidney with a normal renal artery where renal parenchyma is constricted by a cicatrizing hematoma. This hampers free perfusion of the kidney and induces increased renin production. CT scan and MRI show thickened fibrotic mass surrounding the kidney.

2. *Renal cyst or tumor* may compress adjacent renal parenchyma, rendering it hypoxic.[26]

3. *Arteriovenous fistula* causes hyperreninemia by virtue of blood "steal" from the normal renal parenchyma, since the perfusion pressure in such a renal arterial system is low.

4. *Hydronephrosis* may on occasion produce high renin output, which is corrected after decompression.

5. *Nephrosclerosis.* Obstructive small vessel disease may also be responsible for relative hypoxia and resultant increase in renin production.

6. *Chronic pyelonephritis* is rarely associated with hyperreninemia.

7. *Abdominal aorta aneurysm.*

Comments

Prior to proceeding with work-up for suspected renovascular hypertension, these points should be considered:

1. There is no reason to subject the patient to the inconvenience and expense of various diagnostic

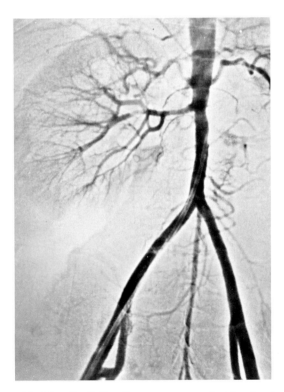

Figure 12–36. Radiation therapy was part of the treatment for left Wilms tumor when this patient was a child. This has resulted in radiation injury and arrest in the growth of the aorta. The infrarenal aortic segment is short and narrower than the external iliac artery. Also, the very proximal right renal artery is somewhat narrow.

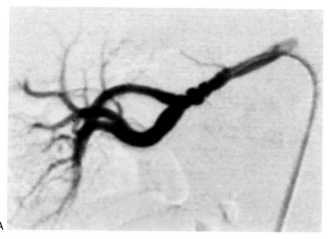

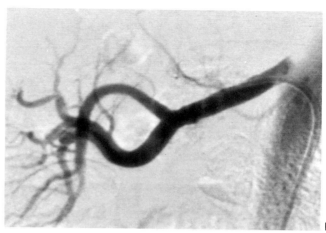

Figure 12–38. Pre **(A)** and post **(B)** renal artery angioplasty in a patient with FMD.

procedures if medical treatment will only be instituted anyway.

2. In the presence of significant renal artery stenosis normal renin values from ipsilateral renal vein should not be trusted. If renins do not "lateralize" one has two choices: Repeat selective renal vein renin test at a later date or proceed with angioplasty, dismiss-

ing selective renin test with 20% false-negative rate. The problem with repeating the test is that if it is normal again, one would still proceed with angioplasty, if the angiographic findings are convincing. If one cannot rely on a negative renin test in an angiographically convincing case, why should one in a marginal situation? The answer is that the decision

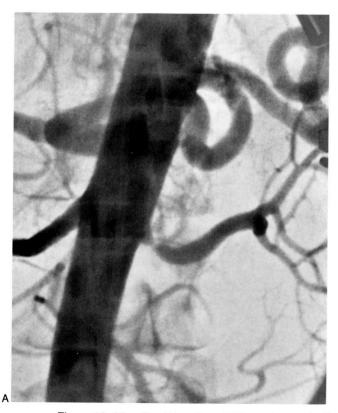

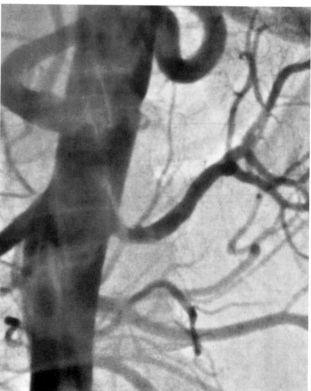

Figure 12–39. Pre **(A)** and post **(B)** renal artery balloon angioplasty in a fairly simple nonostial atherosclerotic lesion.

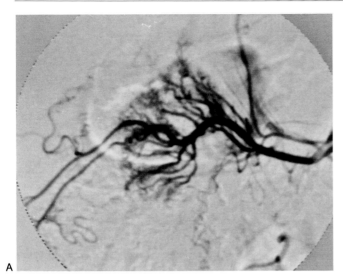
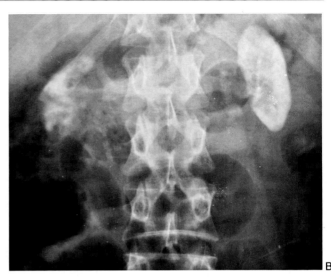

A   B

Figure 12–40. Ablation of small nonfunctioning kidneys in a patient with a successful renal transplant. **(A)** Catheter is positioned beyond the takeoff of the adrenal and first capsular branch. Nonetheless, reflux into these vessels and the presence of large perforating capsular arteries necessitated the use of a supraselective small catheter wedged into smaller arterial branches to avoid embolization of organs other than kidneys. **(B)** Postembolization radiograph demonstrates persistent dense nephrogram in both embolized kidneys. On the right, patchy areas that have escaped infarction are supplied by the perforating capsulars and do not show appreciable nephrogram.

regarding treatment may be made with greater confidence if the test is positive.

3. The decline in number of patients undergoing investigation for renovascular hypertension and PTA is the result of better medical therapy and expensive screening. Unfortunately, the disease is progressive, and if this trend continues, there may be many small useless kidneys around in the future, many of which could have been saved.

4. Of children with sustained hypertension, 50% are likely to have renovascular hypertension. Mid-aortic syndrome and neurofibromatosis are more common in the pediatric age group.[27]

ARTERIOVENOUS MALFORMATION AND FISTULA

Congenital arteriovenous malformation (AVM) is a rare cause of hematuria. The lesion may simulate a large renal mass,[28] intraluminal renal filling defects (Fig. 12–41, 12–42), or may be so small as to be undetectable on most radiographic studies (Fig. 12–43) including angiography. Color Doppler may suggest the presence of the AVM. Angiography can aid in making final diagnosis and determine if the lesion is resectable or whether transcatheter embolization is the preferred method of treatment (Fig. 12–44).[29]

Two types have been described: cirsoid and aneurysmal. Both are more common in women, the cirsoid type in younger adults, aneurysmal type in the elderly. Arteriographic findings range from a cluster of small vessels to large vascular conduits (Fig. 12–45). An early draining vein is pathognomonic and should be looked for diligently.

Arteriovenous fistulas are the product of trauma, usually penetrating trauma from biopsy, bullet, or knife wound (Fig. 12–46).

By diverting blood away from the kidney, an AVM or arteriovenous fistula may create a condition of relative hypoperfusion of the normal renal parenchyma, the so-called "steal" phenomenon. Hyperreninemia and hypertension may result. Selective renins are useless because of the dilutional effect of large blood volume flowing through the fistula.

Color Doppler may demonstrate pulsation, which likely represents perivascular tissue movement.[30–32] Arteriovenous fistulas are a common complication of renal biopsy. Many such fistulas spontaneously close. Some will require transcatheter embolization for control of either hemorrhage or hypertension.

Arteriovenous shunting occurs in 5% of renal carcinomas. Shunting may be so severe as to result in cardiac failure. A case of arteriovenous shunting has been described in an angiomyolipoma, although this is considered rare.[33]

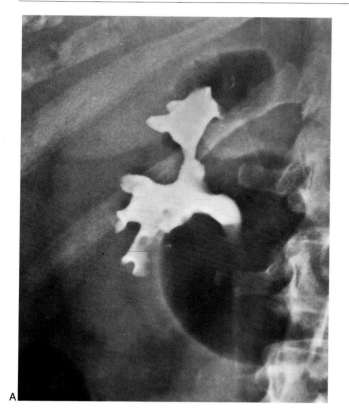

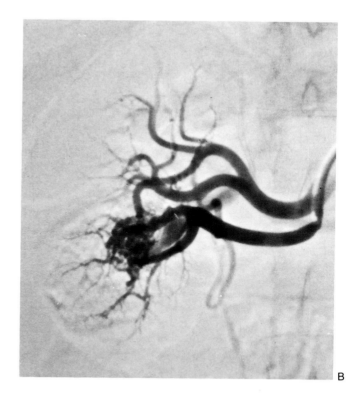

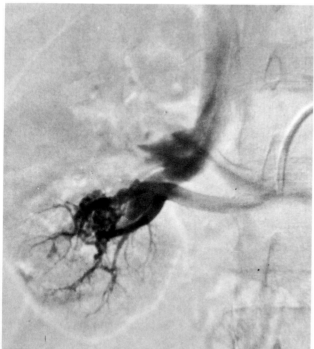

Figure 12–41.   AVM in the lower pole of the right kidney. **(A)** Irregular filling defect in the renal pelvis, particularly in the lower pole calyx, could represent transitional cell carcinoma or several other entities. **(B)** During the arterial phase, there is a cluster of vessels from which an early-filling draining vein emanates. **(C)** In the late arterial phase even the inferior vena cava is densely opacified with contrast. (From Po JB et al. Arteriovenous malformation: the value of renal angiography for a filling defect in the renal pelvis. J Urol 1975; 114:607–609. Reprinted with permission.)

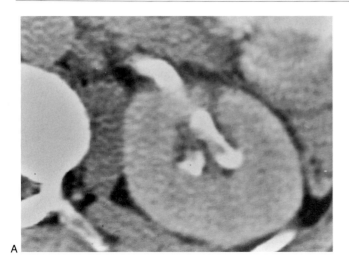

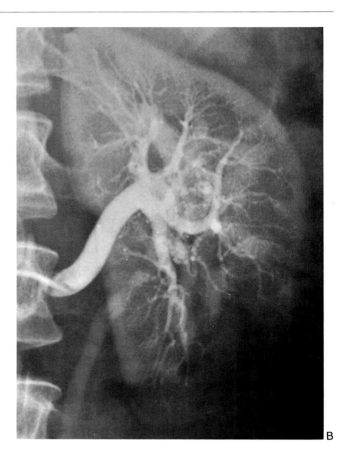

Figure 12–42. AVM in a patient with intermittent gross hematuria. **(A)** CT demonstrates irregular filling defects in the renal pelvis. **(B)** On selective renal angiogram, the AVM is less well defined compared with the previous case. Small irregular tortuous vessels are seen in the area of the renal hilus. There is no distinct feeder branch that could be selectively embolized. (Photograph courtesy of Dr. Luff).

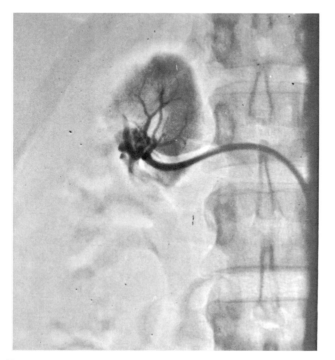

Figure 12–43. Small AVM in the upper pole of the right kidney. Although the lesion seen here is a very small cluster of rounded vessels feeding a small early-draining vein, intermittent hematuria resulted in dangerously low hematocrit.

RENAL VEINS

Anatomy

The right renal vein is several centimeters long, inserts into the inferior vena cava at a level L1-L2, and is angulated cephalad. Twenty percent of the population have two right renal veins, the inferior usually smaller in caliber (Fig. 12–47).

The left renal vein is longer than the right, has a more horizontal pathway, and inserts into the inferior vena cava in the region of L2, almost at 90° (Fig. 12–48, 12–49). Before entering into the vena cava, it crosses the abdominal aorta anteriorly in the space between the aorta and superior mesenteric vessels. Left renal vein receives tributaries from a left gonadal vein and inferior adrenal vein. Inferior adrenal vein also receives the inferior phrenic vein, which usually has a valve 1 to 2 cm above its confluence with the inferior adrenal vein. Both right and left renal veins have communicating veins connecting them with the ascending lumbar veins (Fig. 12–50). These communicating channels can enlarge considerably during the presence of renal vein thrombosis or other distal obstructive lesions.

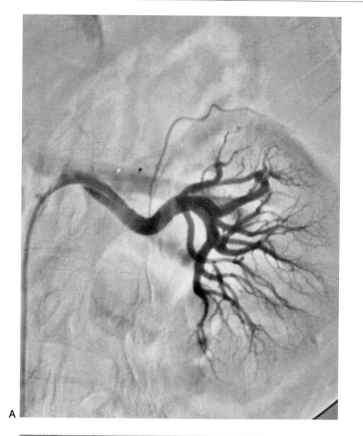

A

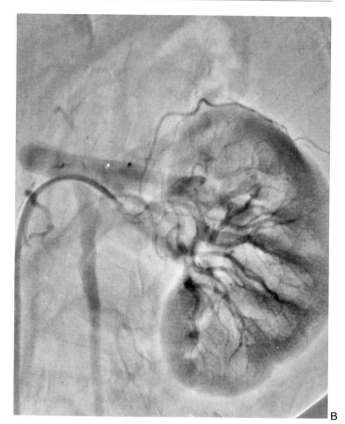

B

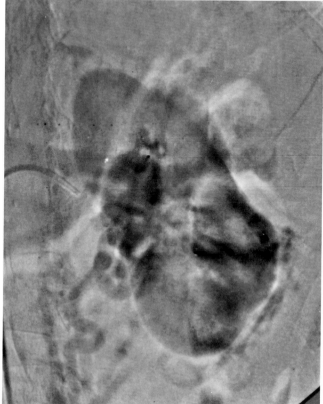

C

Figure 12–44. Sequence of images from a renal arteriogram. **(A)** During an early arterial phase, there is early filling of the left renal vein. **(B)** A second later the contrast is also seen in the left gonadal vein. **(C)** In the later phase a large venous network is opacified, adapting to the overfilling of the venous system. Similar findings would be expected in renal vein occlusion, except there would not be early venous filling.

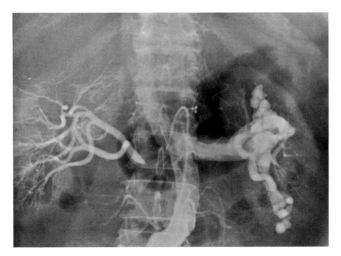

Figure 12–45. Large AVM fills the entire left renal sinus during early arterial phase. The degree of shunting must be severe since the inferior vena cava has opacified even though there is still contrast in the descending aorta and right renal arteries. There is marked underfilling of the left renal arteries for the lack of adequate perfusion pressure, a situation known as a "steal phenomenon." Renal underperfusion may be a cause of hyperreninemia and high blood pressure.

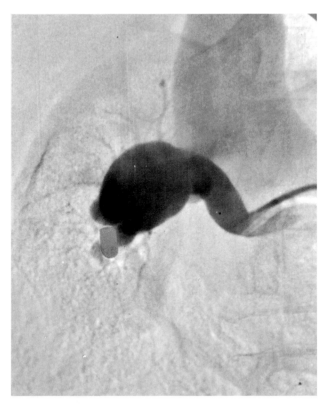

Figure 12–46. Selective renal arteriogram (subtraction angiography) on a patient with a history of a bullet wound sustained 15 years earlier. Patient is completely asymptomatic in regard to the renal fistula. Notice the bullet at the apex of the fistula, early filling of the vena cava, and arterial underperfusion of the kidney. Treatment was surgical.

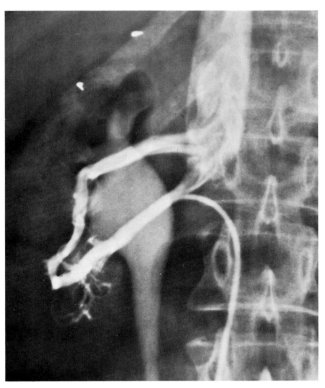

Figure 12–47. Two right renal veins almost equal in caliber are seen on this retrograde renal vein venogram. Unlike the arteries, intrarenal veins freely communicate at the arcuates.

In addition, the left renal vein in particular has communicating channels with the periureteral venous plexus.

Imaging Modalities

Ultrasound in particular is capable of demonstrating the main trunks of right and left renal vein, including the inferior vena cava. Duplex and color Doppler ultrasound may demonstrate blood velocity within the vessel.

Computerized axial tomography is of value if contrast is used. In addition to the vein itself, the adjacent areas to the vessel are scrutinized in the best possible way (Fig. 12–51).

Because of the blood flow within the renal veins, magnetic resonance images excellently demonstrate the vessel lumen, collateral circulation, intraluminal filling defects, and displacements.

Congenital Anomalies

1. *Circumaortic venous ring.* Congenital abnormalities of the left renal vein in particular are rela-

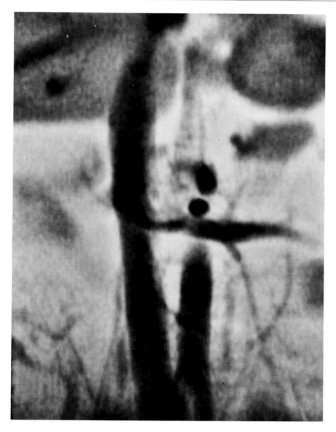

Figure 12–48. MR image of the inferior vena cava and left renal vein in the coronal plane. The renal vein crosses anterior to the aorta. Celiac and superior mesenteric arteries are seen in a cross-section just as they emerge from the aorta. Note the left inferior adrenal vein as well as left gonadal vein. Right gonadal vein is seen entering the inferior vena cava.

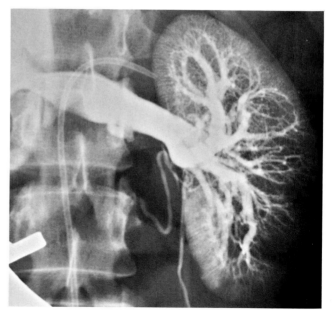

Figure 12–49. Detailed vascular anatomy of the left renal vein. The examination is epinephrine-assisted left retrograde renal vein venogram. The arterial catheter is used to deliver epinephrine just before retrograde injection of the contrast into the renal vein. Decreased renal blood flow permits retrograde reflux of the contrast into the arcuates, interlobular, and even into subcapsular stelate veins. This procedure has lost its popularity since there is seldom a need to visualize deep venous structures in such detail.

tively common (4.4%).[34] Most common is circumaortic venous ring where a slightly inferior retroaortic channel develops which may or may not be a dominant channel (Fig. 12–52). Frequently, a left gonadal vein drains into this slightly inferiorly positioned vessel.

2. *Retroaortic left renal vein.* Less commonly one will find a simple left retroaortic renal vein (1.8%) (Figs. 12–53, 12–54).

3. *Vena cava anomalies.* Rare anomalies also include the inferior vena cava, such as transposition or duplication (Fig. 12–55).[35–38]

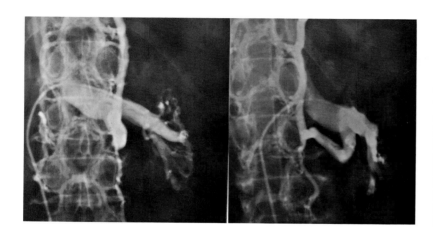

Figure 12–50. Communicating lumbar vein connecting left renal vein with the ascending lumbar vein (later to become hemiazygos). Renal carcinoma frequently extends into the renal vein and may also extend into the gonadal, inferior adrenal, and even into the lumbar vein. Rich collateral pathways of the left renal vein make it less susceptible to deleterious effects of renal vein occlusion compared with its counterpart on the right.

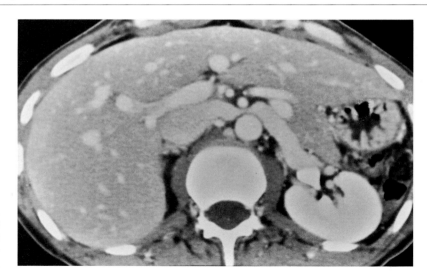

Figure 12–51. Variant of normal. Although the left renal vein appears narrowed as it transits between the aorta and superior mesenteric artery, this is a frequent normal finding.

4. *Renal vein valves.* Although the renal vein is commonly considered valveless, valves or remnants of the valvular structures within the left renal vein have been described but are considered extremely rare.

5. *Renal vein varix.* Usually involves left renal vein and is very rare (Fig. 12–53).[39] May thrombose.[40]

Renal Vein Thrombosis

Etiology. Children: dehydration, volume depletion, febrile illness.

Adults: nephrotic syndrome, hypercoagulable states, postpartum.

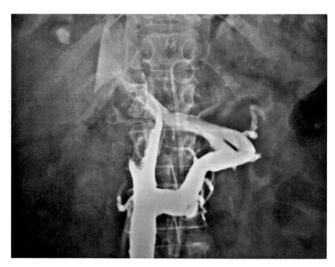

Figure 12–52. Circumaortic left renal vein. Catheter is in the aorta while an inferior vena cavogram is performed. Two vessels are seen arising from the left kidney. The upper crosses the aorta anteriorly, the way a normal vein does. The lower limb, which is dominant in this case, transverses slightly inferiorly and extends posterior to the aorta. Both limbs and the inferior vena cava form a circumaortic ring. There is also a large intracaval tumor originating from a large right renal carcinoma.

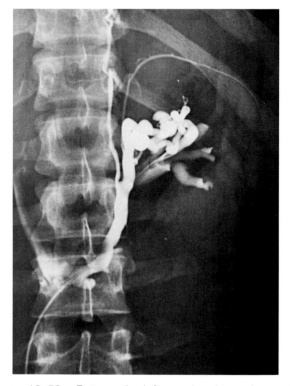

Figure 12–53. Retroaortic left renal vein and peculiar venous varicosities in the region of the left renal hilum.

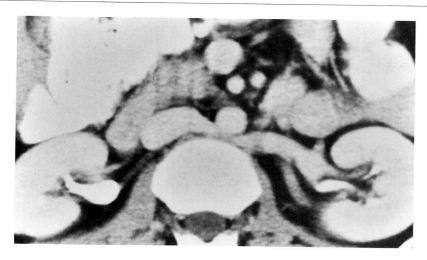

Figure 12–54. Retroaortic left renal vein seen on contrast-enhanced CT.

Clinical Presentation.

1. *Subclinical.* The lumen of the renal vein is still patent despite the presence of a silent thrombus. These patients present with proteinuria and nephrotic syndrome. The nephrotic syndrome is likely the result of a primary glomerular disease. With proteinuria there is loss of coagulation-inhibiting factors from circulating plasma.

2. *Acute.* Venous outflow from the affected kidney is severely compromised, leading to acute venous stasis. Flank pain, tenderness, proteinuria, and hematuria are present.

Clinical manifestations vary, depending on whether the process is unilateral or bilateral, and whether the occlusion is partial or complete.

Radiological Findings. Ultrasound examination has for some time been the primary mode for detection of this disease in children[41] and is probably the primary method for initial investigation in adults. Color Doppler or duplex ultrasound may become the method of choice.[42] In the acute stage the kidney enlarges and the renal vein is dilated proximal to the point of obstruction. The thrombus may be demonstrated in the lumen of the renal vein and even extending into the inferior vena cava.[43]

On contrast examinations, such as EXU, CT, and arteriogram, renal enlargement is again demonstrated. Decreased nephrographic density and loss of corticomedullary differentiation are common in the acute stage.[44] Appearance of contrast in the collecting system may be delayed and concentration is poor. Because of renal enlargement and swelling, the infundibula are stretched and spidery in appearance. When and if collateral venous circulation develops, pelvic and ureteral notchings and "cobwebs" in perinephric space[45] may be seen.

Cortical subcapsular rim sign, representing a dense outer nephrogram only a few millimeters thick, has been described in renal vein thrombosis,[46] although this sign is almost pathognomonic for renal artery occlusion.

Low-density nonenhancing thrombus may be identified on CT in somewhat dilated renal vein.[47] MR imaging is still of unknown value.[48]

Cavography and retrograde venography demonstrate intraluminal filling defects (Figs. 12–56, 12–57). Although retrograde venography is the gold standard,[49] the diagnosis is usually established by ultrasound or CT.

Systemic or transcatheter fibrinolytic therapy (either transarterial or retrograde venous) has been successfully tried on a limited number of patients with acute renal vein thrombosis.[50–52]

Long-term sequela of unrecognized renal vein thrombosis, particularly in infancy, may be a small, smooth kidney without calyceal clubbing, discovered later in life.

Renal Vein Tumor Thrombus

Upon detection, some 5% of renal carcinomas will have extended into the renal vein and may propagate along the venous channel into the inferior vena cava, right atrium, right ventricle, pulmonary outflow tract, opposite renal vein, and, in retrograde fashion, into the lower IVC, lumbar vein, and gonadal vein.[53,54] Less well known is the fact that tumors other than a renal cell carcinoma may also extend along the pathway of the renal vein. Metastatic leiomyosarcoma to the kidney, adrenal carcinoma, transitional cell carcinoma, osteosarcoma, and spindle cell sarcoma (Fig. 12–58) are examples.

Most commonly there is no invasion of the venous

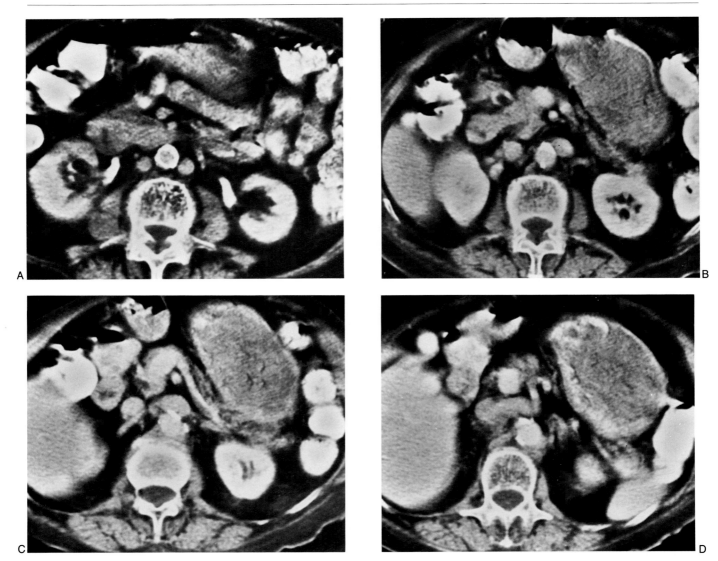

Figure 12–55. Selected slices from a CT scan in a patient with double inferior vena cava. **(A)** The most inferior cut shows a calcified aorta flanked by a vessel on both sides. **(B)** A cut more cephalad, the left inferior vena cava starts to move medially and anteriorly to the aorta. **(C)** Even more cephalad, the left limb is now anterior to the aorta and at this point has joined with the left renal vein. **(D)** Finally, on the next cephalad cut the left inferior vena cava joins the right.

wall by the propagating intraluminal tumor. On the contrary, the majority of tumor thrombi are shelled out with relative ease at surgery.

In choosing the appropriate surgical approach, including placing the patient on a cardiovascular pump, the surgeon must be aware of the true extensions of the tumor, particularly the limits of its cephalad extension. Relation to the hepatic veins and right atrium is of particular importance.

MR imaging appears to be somewhat better than CT and ultrasound in demonstrating venous tumor extension. In addition, MR imaging particularly well demonstrates the extent of collateral venous circula-

tion and unusual propagation of the tumor into the communicating lumbar or gonadal veins.[55–57]

Ultrasound in a controlled prospective study was also capable of demonstrating renal vein or inferior vena cava involvement. The major drawback of ultrasound is its difficulty in demonstrating lymph node or other organ involvement.

Periureteral Venous Varices

Periureteral venous plexus is a network of veins that occasionally may enlarge and cause impressions and

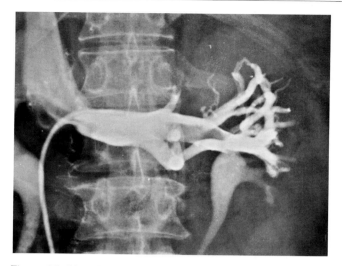

Figure 12–56. A thrombus of moderate size is present in the mid left renal vein.

notching upon the ureter (see Fig. 15–40).[58] The exact etiology of formation of these varices is unknown and the majority of patients will have no predisposing disease, such as occlusion of the left renal vein by pancreatic carcinoma. These vessels usually can be confirmed by selective venography of the renal vein.[58,59] It is usually a segmental branch

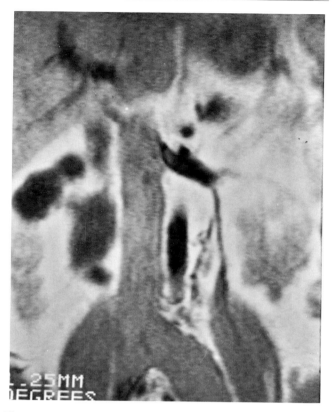

Figure 12–58. Spindle cell sarcoma filling and expanding the entire inferior vena cava and both iliac veins. Left renal vein is partially obstructed, although free of tumor. Collaterals have developed.

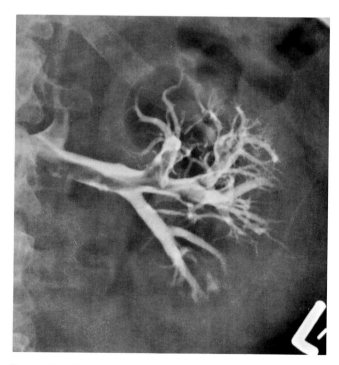

Figure 12–57. A more extensive left renal vein thrombus bifurcating into the segmental branches and even into the inferior adrenal vein.

that will fill in a retrograde fashion. Clinically, these patients may present with hematuria and most likely will require no treatment.

Nutcracker Syndrome (Mesoaortic Compression of the Left Renal Vein)

This is an interesting and well-documented phenomenon where the left renal vein upon crossing the aorta is compressed by the superior mesenteric vein. This compression is sufficient to cause elevation of blood pressure within the renal vein. Periureteral and gonadal vein collaterals frequently develop (Fig. 12–59 A,B). The patients are usually middle-aged slender females. Clinical findings are chronic incapacitating left flank pain and occasional intermittent hematuria.

Diagnosis can only be made by retrograde venography and pressure measurements in the proximal and distal portion of the renal vein. A pressure gradient of only 6 cm H_2O is considered significant. Surgery consists of separating the left renal vein from

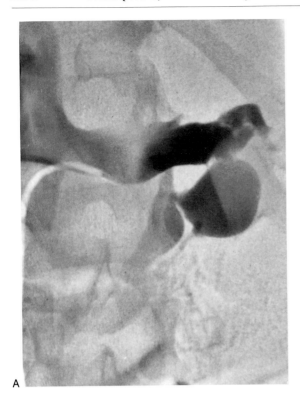

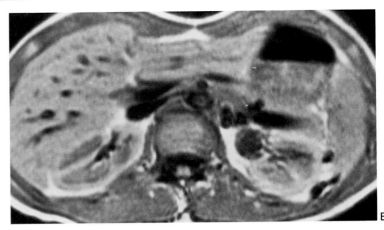

Figure 12–59A,B. This patient presents with incapacitating chronic left flank pain and hematuria. Both retrograde renal vein venogram and MR imaging demonstrate some varicose collateral circulation from the left renal vein. It was difficult to negotiate the selective catheter to the left of the aorta, but once this was achieved the pressure gradient was high. Surgery was curative.

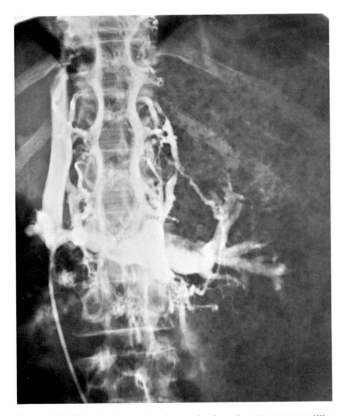

Figure 12–60. Left renal vein occlusion due to pancreatitis.

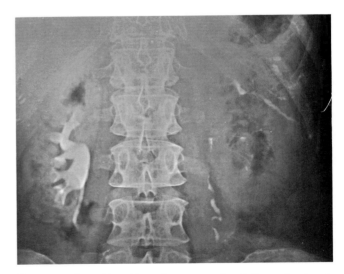

Figure 12–61. Renal lymphoma causing left renal vein occlusion. The left kidney is enlarged with poor nephrogram and spidery calyces. These findings, however, may be due to lymphoma or renal vein occlusion. Ureteral notching is present and suggests venous periureteral enlargement, since the ureter is notched both from the lateral and medial aspect.

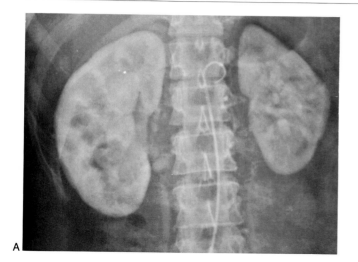

A

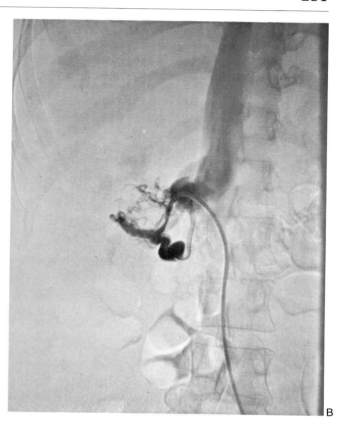

B

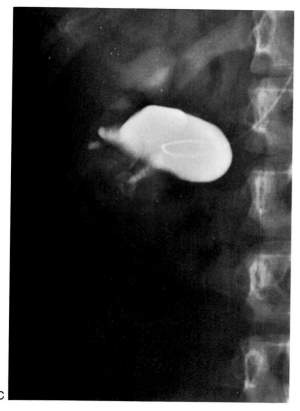

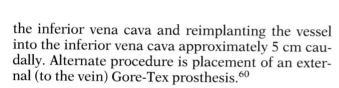

C

Figure 12–62. This young female presented with chronic right flank pain. **(A)** Renal angiography was performed because a mass lesion was discovered in the kidney. The kidney is enlarged and there is a radiolucent mass in the lower pole. Also, collateral venous circulation is detected between renal hilus and spine. **(B)** Retrograde renal vein venogram was done to clarify status of the renal vein and was found to be obstructed. **(C)** Since the mass was cystic on sonography a cyst puncture was performed during the same session. The cyst was causing partial obstruction to the venous outflow.

the inferior vena cava and reimplanting the vessel into the inferior vena cava approximately 5 cm caudally. Alternate procedure is placement of an external (to the vein) Gore-Tex prosthesis.[60]

Other Causes of Renal Vein Occlusion

Pancreatitis (Fig. 12–60), neoplastic processes (Fig. 12–61), and even renal cyst (Fig. 12–62) may cause renal vein obstruction.

Collaterals to Renal Veins

Collaterals to the renal vein may develop in patients with portal hypertension. This is usually seen on the left and must be very rare on the right (Fig. 12–63).

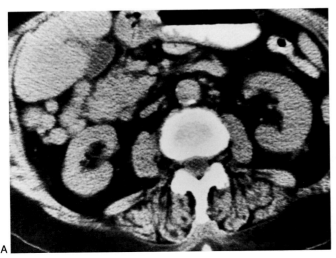
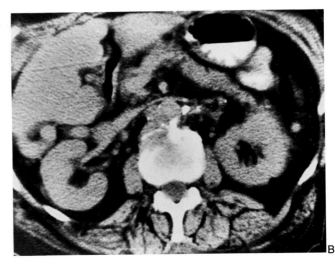

Figure 12–63. Large venous collaterals are present between the right kidney and the liver **(A)**, which can be traced to the right renal vein **(B)**. This was also confirmed on sonography. (Photograph courtesy of Dr. M. Bein.)

REFERENCES

1. Frank PH, Nuttall J, Brander WL, Prosser D. The cortical rim sign of renal infarction. Br J Radiol 1974; 47:875–878.
2. Glazer GM, Francis IR, Brady TM, Teng SS. Computed tomography of renal infarction: clinical and experimental observations. AJR 1983; 140:721–727.
3. Eliska O. The perforating arteries and their role in the collateral circulation of the kidneys. Acta Anat (Basel) 1968; 70:184–201.
4. Ranninger K, Abrams E, Bordent A. Pseudotumor resulting from a fresh renal infarct. Radiology 1969; 92:343–344.
5. Sussman SK, Baker ME, Saeed M, Stickel DL. Polar infarct in a transplanted kidney: cause of a pseudomass. Urol Radiol 1987; 9:42–44.
6. Belville JS, Morgantaler A, Loughlin KR, Tumeh SS. Spontaneous perinephric and subcapsular renal hemorrhage: evaluation with CT, US and angiography. Radiology 1989; 172:733–738.
7. Kendall AR, Senay BA, Cill ME. Spontaneous subcapsular renal hematoma: diagnosis and management. J Urol 1988; 139:246–250.
8. Schaner EG, Balow JE, Doppman JL. Computed tomography on the diagnosis of subcapsular and perirenal hematoma. AJR 1977; 129:83–88.
9. Hilton S, Bosniak MA, Megibow AJ, Ambos MA. Computed tomographic demonstration of a spontaneous subcapsular hematoma due to small renal cell carcinoma. Radiology 1981; 141:743–744.
10. Staab GE, Tegtmeyer CJ, Constable WC. Radiation-induced renovascular hypertension. AJR 1976; 126:634–637.
11. Thornbury JR, Stanley JC, Fryback DG. Hypertensive urogram: a nondiscriminatory test for renovascular hypertension. AJR 1982; 138:43–49.
12. Wenting GJ, Tan-Tijong HL, Derkx FH, et al. Split renal function after captopril in unilateral renal artery stenosis. Br Med J 1984; 288:886–890.
13. Dunnick NR, Svetkey LP, Cohan R, et al. Intravenous digital subtraction renal angiography: use in screening for renovascular hypertension. Radiology 1989; 171:219–222.
14. Bookstein JJ, Abrams HL, Buenger RE, et al. Radiologic aspects of renovascular hypertension. III. Appraisal of arteriography. JAMA 1972; 221:368–374.
15. Harrison EG Jr, McCormack LJ. Pathologic classification of renal arterial disease in renal vascular hypertension. Mayo Clin Proc 1971; 46:161–167.
16. Lewis IIIVD, Meranze SG, McLean GK, et al. The midaortic syndrome: diagnosis and treatment. Radiology 1988; 167:111–113.
17. Perry MO. Hypertension and dissecting aneurysm of the renal artery. Arch Surg 1971; 102:216–217.
18. Sos TA, Tegtmeyer KG. Techniques of renal angioplasty. Radiology 1986; 161:577–586.
19. Sos TA, Pickering TG, Sinderman KW, et al. Percutaneous transluminal renal angioplasty in renovascular hypertension due to atheroma or fibromuscular dysplasia. N Engl J Med 1983; 309:274–279.
20. Archibald GR, Beckmann CF, Libertino JA. Focal renal artery stenosis caused by fibromuscular dysplasia: treatment by percutaneous transluminal angioplasty. AJR 1988; 151:593–596.
21. Klinge J, Mali WPTM, Puijlaert CBAJ, et al. Percutaneous transluminal renal artery angioplasty: initial and long-term results. Radiology 1989; 171:501–506.
22. Reuter SR. Embolic control of hypertension caused by segmental renal artery stenosis. AJR 1976; 127:389–392.
23. Adler J, Einhorn R, McCarthy J, et al. Gelfoam embolization of the kidneys for treatment of malignant hypertension. Radiology 1978; 128:45–48.
24. Eliscu EH, Haire HM. Control of malignant renovascular hypertension by percutaneous transluminal angioplasty and therapeutic renal embolization. AJR 1980; 134:815–817.
25. Nanni GS, Hawkins IF Jr, Orak JK. Control of hypertension by ethanol renal ablation. Radiology 1983; 148:51–54.

26. Hoard TD, O'Brien DP III. Simple renal cyst and high renin hypertension cured by cyst decompression. J Urol 1976; 115:326–327.
27. Mena E, Bookstein JJ, Holt JF, Fry WJ. Neurofibromatosis and renovascular hypertension in children. Am J Roentgenol 1973; 118:39–45.
28. Silverthorn K, George D. Renal cirsoid arteriovenous malformation masquerading as neoplasia. J Can Assoc Radiol 1988; 39:277–279.
29. Saito S, Iigaya T, Koyama Y. Transcatheter embolization for the rupture of congenital arteriovenous malformation of the kidney in pregnancy. J Urol 1987; 137:964–965.
30. Morton MJ, Charboneau JW. Arteriovenous fistula after biopsy of renal transplant: detection and monitoring with color flow and duplex ultrasonography. Mayo Clin Proc 1989; 64:531–534.
31. Middleton WD, Erickson S, Melson GL. Perivascular color artifact: pathologic significance and appearance on color Doppler US images. Radiology 1989; 171:647–652.
32. Middleton WD, Kellman GM, Melson GL, Madrazo BL. Postbiopsy renal transplant arteriovenous fistulas: color Doppler US characteristics. Radiology 1989; 171:253–257.
33. Barzilai IM, Braden GL, Ford LD, et al. Renal angiomyolipoma with arteriovenous shunting. J Urol 1987; 137:483–484.
34. Reed MD, Friedman AC, Nealey P. Anomalies of the left renal vein: analysis of 433 CT scans. J Comput Assist Tomogr 1982; 6:1124.
35. Fisher MR, Hricak H, Higgins CB. Magnetic resonance imaging of developmental venous anomalies. AJR 1985; 145:705.
36. Kellman GM, Alpern MB, Sandler MA, Craig BM. Computed tomography of vena caval anomalies with embryologic correlation. Radiographics 1988; 8:533–566.
37. Mayo J, Gray R, St Louis E, et al. Anomalies of the inferior vena cava. AJR 1983; 140:339–345.
38. Chuang VP, Mena EC, Hoskins PA. Congenital anomalies of the inferior vena cava. Review of embryogenesis and presentation of simplified classification. Br J Radiol 1974; 47:206–213.
39. Beckmann CF, Abrams HL. Idiopathic renal vein varices: incidence and significance. Radiology 1982; 143:649–652.
40. Curry NS, Frangos DN, Stanley JH. Thrombosed right renal vein varix simulating a renal pelvic mass. Urol Radiol 1987; 9:36–38.
41. Lam AH, Warren PS. Ultrasonographic diagnosis of neonatal renal vein thrombosis. Ann Radiol 1981; 24:7–12.
42. Reuther G, Wanjura D, Bauer H. Acute renal vein thrombosis in renal allografts: detection with duplex Doppler US. Radiology 1989; 170:557–558.
43. Braun B, Weileman LS, Weigand W. Ultrasonographic demonstration of renal vein thrombosis. AJR 1980; 138:157–160.
44. Coel MN, Talner LB. Obstructive nephrogram due to renal vein thrombosis. Radiology 1971; 101:573–574.
45. Winfield A, Gerlock AJ, Schaff MI. Perirenal cobwebs: a CT sign of renal vein thrombosis. J Comput Assist Tomogr 1981; 5:705–707.
46. Hann L, Pfister RC. Renal subcapsular rim sign: new etiologies and pathogenesis. AJR 1982; 138:51–54.
47. Gatewood OMB, Fishman EK, Burrow CR, et al. Renal vein thrombosis in patients with nephrotic syndrome: CT diagnosis. Radiology 1986; 159:117–120.
48. Honda H, Yuh WT, Lu CC. Magnetic resonance imaging of renal vein and inferior vena cava thrombosis in a patient with glomerulonephritis: a case report. J Comput Assist Tomogr 1988; 12:147–149.
49. March TL, Halpern M. Renal vein thrombosis demonstrated by selective renal phlebography. Radiology 1965; 81:958–961.
50. Crowley JP, Matarese RA, Quevedo SF, Garella S. Fibrinolytic therapy for bilateral renal vein thrombosis. Arch Intern Med 1984; 144:159–160.
51. DiMarco PL, Sheinfeld J, Gutierrez OH, Cockett ATK. Direct fibrinolytic therapy for renal vein thrombosis: radiographic followup. J Urol 1984; 132:966–968.
52. Vogelzang RL, Moel DI, Cohn RA, et al. Acute renal vein thrombosis: successful treatment with intra-arterial urokinase. Radiology 1988; 169:681–682.
53. Handel DB, Heaston DU, Uorobrinm, et al. Circumaortic left renal vein with tumor thrombus. CT diagnosis with angiographic and pathologic correlation. AJR 1983; 141:97.
54. Schweru WD, Schweru WN, Rdeck G. Venous renal tumor extension. Prospective US evaluation. Radiology 1985; 156:449.
55. Hricak H, Theoni RF, Carroll PR, et al. Detection and staging of renal neoplasms: a reassessment of MR imaging. Radiology 1988; 166:643–649.
56. Fein AB, Lee JKT, Balfe DM, et al. Diagnosis and staging of renal cell carcinoma: A comparison of MR imaging and CT. AJR 1987; 148:749–753.
57. Patel SK, Stack CM, Taner DA. Magnetic resonance imaging in staging of renal cell carcinoma. Radiographics 1987; 7:703–716.
58. Beinart C, Sniderman UW, Saddekni S, Weiner MA, Vaughan ED, Sos TA. Left renal vein hypertension: A cause of occult hematuria. Radiology 1982; 145:647.
59. Beckmann CF, Abrams HC. Idiopathic renal vein varices: Incidence and significance. Radiology 1982; 143:649.
60. Barnes RW, Fleisher HL 3d, Redman JF, et al. Mesoaortic compression of the left renal vein (the so-called nutcracker syndrome): repair by a new stenting procedure. J Vasc Surg 1988; 8:415–421.

13

Renal Failure

ACUTE RENAL FAILURE

Etiology. *Prerenal:* Renal hypoperfusion due to heart failure, hypotension, dehydration, shock (blood loss, sepsis).

Primary renal: Nephrotoxins (aminoglycosides, cyclosporine, amphotericin B, cisplatin, radiologic contrasts); endogenous nephrotoxins (myoglobin, myeloma proteins); glomerulonephritis; interstitial nephritis; bacterial nephritis; renal artery occlusion; renal neoplasm; cystic renal disease.

Postrenal: Ureteral obstruction, outflow bladder obstruction, outflow conduit obstruction, nephrostomy tube obstruction.

Clinical Presentation. Oliguria, anuria, manifestation of primary disease, uremia, fatigue, malaise.

Laboratory Findings. Elevated serum creatinine and BUN, electrolyte imbalance, hypoglycemia.

Radiological Findings

Prerenal failure. Causes of prerenal failure such as cardiac failure, hypotension, septic shock, or severe dehydration are usually clinically obvious.

Primary Renal Versus Postrenal Failure. Sonography is considered the method of choice for differentiating these two entities after prerenal failure has been excluded with reasonable certainty on clinical grounds.

The absence of any urinary tract dilatation is presumptive evidence against urinary obstruction. This, however, is not always the case. Instances of complete reversal of renal failure after empirical nephrostomy placement in a nondilated system have been described.[1,2] Other instances of obstruction without dilatation have been reported.[3-5] Therefore, ultrasound should not be completely trusted in this regard. If clinical suspicion of nondilated obstruction exists, diuretic Tc-99M DTPA scintigraphy should be considered.[6]

Along the same lines, dilatation of the collecting system and ureters may be present on ultrasound examination and be unrelated to obstruction.

Ultrasound is very useful in demonstrating the number of kidneys present and their size. Generally, large kidneys are associated with an acute renal process leading to temporary or permanent functional loss (Fig. 13–1). The notable exceptions to this rule are polycystic renal disease and the early stages of renal amyloidosis.

The finding of bilateral small kidneys with an echo texture greater than that of the liver is indicative of irreversible chronic renal disease. In general, most diffuse parenchymal renal diseases are associated with higher echo textures than the normal kidney's. A few will behave quite the opposite and present with decreased echo texture. This is probably related to edema, as in renal vein thrombosis or acute pyelonephritis.

In the absence of ultrasound equipment, similar information may be obtained using CT without contrast. Renal size and number, as well as the presence (or absence) of pelvocalyceal dilatation may be seen very well. In addition, presence of nephrocalcinosis, renal masses, retroperitoneal pathology, etc., may be detected (Fig. 13–2). Despite markedly reduced function, even small kidneys may concentrate urine (Fig. 13–3).

In rare instances bilateral renal embolus may be suspected if there are predisposing factors, such as atrial fibrillation or left atrial myxoma (Fig. 13–4). Bilateral renal artery stenosis may reach a critical point of narrowing, precipitating occlusion. In the unlikely event of bilateral acute thrombosis, urgent angiography is required, followed by an attempt to either aspirate visible thrombi, to begin infusion of

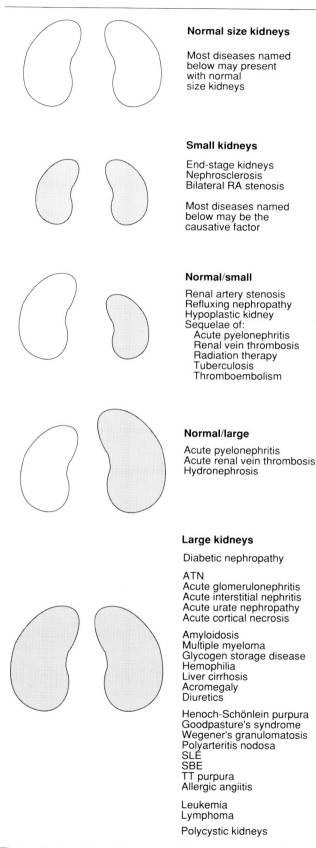

Normal size kidneys

Most diseases named below may present with normal size kidneys

Small kidneys

End-stage kidneys
Nephrosclerosis
Bilateral RA stenosis

Most diseases named below may be the causative factor

Normal/small

Renal artery stenosis
Refluxing nephropathy
Hypoplastic kidney
Sequelae of:
    Acute pyelonephritis
    Renal vein thrombosis
    Radiation therapy
    Tuberculosis
    Thromboembolism

Normal/large

Acute pyelonephritis
Acute renal vein thrombosis
Hydronephrosis

Large kidneys

Diabetic nephropathy

ATN
Acute glomerulonephritis
Acute interstitial nephritis
Acute urate nephropathy
Acute cortical necrosis

Amyloidosis
Multiple myeloma
Glycogen storage disease
Hemophilia
Liver cirrhosis
Acromegaly
Diuretics

Henoch-Schönlein purpura
Goodpasture's syndrome
Wegener's granulomatosis
Polyarteritis nodosa
SLE
SBE
TT purpura
Allergic angiitis

Leukemia
Lymphoma

Polycystic kidneys

Figure 13–1. Diagnostic possibilities associated with kidneys of different sizes.

streptokinaze or urokinaze, or to perform embolectomy.

ACUTE TUBULAR NECROSIS (ATN)

Etiology. Tubular damage due to nephrotoxic agents, including radiographic contrasts.

Preglomerular ischemia caused by hypotension, shock, dehydration, shock injuries, etc., causing tubular damage. ATN is commonly associated with ischemia during transplantation and some types of renal and vascular surgery.

Pathology. Interstitial edema and cellular infiltration. Microscopically tubular cells may appear normal or show varying degrees of necrosis. Cellular debris is present in the tubular lumen causing dilatation.

Clinical Presentation. Oliguric renal failure, usually reversible in 1 to 3 weeks. History of exposure to a nephrotoxic agent or other precipitating event.

Radiological Findings. On sonography, the kidney may be somewhat enlarged, but otherwise its appearance is usually normal. The main purpose of this examination is to exclude obstruction as the main cause of acute renal failure.

Radionuclide scan demonstrates unimpaired renal blood flow.

Prolonged and relatively dense nephrogram is a common finding on radiological examinations using intravascular contrast. Contrast may persist for more than 24 hours and is particularly well seen on CT. Varying degrees of intrarenal tubular obstruction by cellular debris responsible for abnormal nephrogram (Fig. 13–5). The collecting system may become faintly opacified, depending on the severity of tubular obstruction. Contrast examinations are not indicated for evaluation of the kidney in this condition, but may be a necessary part of other examinations, such as angiography or CT.

GLOMERULAR SCLEROSIS

"Loss of renal function begets further loss of renal function."[7]

Age-Related Glomerular Sclerosis. Glomerular sclerosis refers to morphological changes, which may begin as vacuolization of epithelial cells, foot process fusion, and expansion of mesangial matrix. Eventually, hyalinization, sclerosis, and disappear-

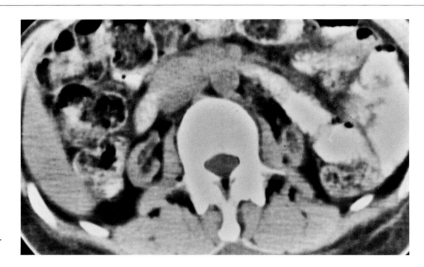

Figure 13–2. Small kidneys in a patient with renal failure.

ance of glomerulus and the entire nephron ensues. In this process there is a gradual and continual decrease in the number of nephrons over a lifetime. Of course, this by itself is of little clinical significance, since total nephron reserve is so large.[8]

Glomerular Capillary Hypertension. In the presence of sustained increase in capillary hydraulic pressure, however, the process of glomerular sclerosis markedly accelerates.

Loss of substantial amount of kidney parenchyma, such as following nephrectomy, results in significant rise in renal blood flow and glomerular filtration rate in the remaining kidney. If more than three-fourths of the total renal mass is removed, morphological changes heralding glomerulosclerosis appear.[9]

High protein diet also induces increased glomerular capillary pressures. The changes heralding

glomerulosclerosis are significantly amplified in experimental animals with 25% or less renal mass remaining, if subjected to a high protein diet.[10–12]

Renal mass loss need not be from nephrectomy. Loss of functioning renal parenchyma in refluxing nephropathy, different types of glomerulonephritis, etc., subject the unaffected glomeruli to hyperperfusion and capillary hypertension. The greater the loss, the more pronounced the capillary pressure. Once the threshold is reached, the progression to glomerulosclerosis is irreversible.[13]

Another example of glomerulosclerosis is seen in diabetic nephropathy. The early stages of this disease are characterized by hyperfiltration, increase in re-

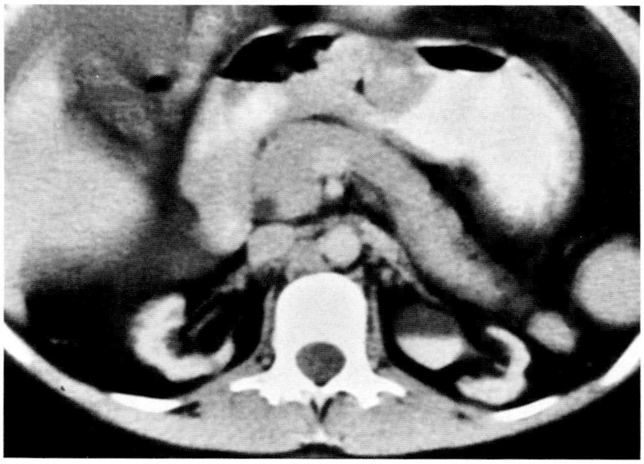

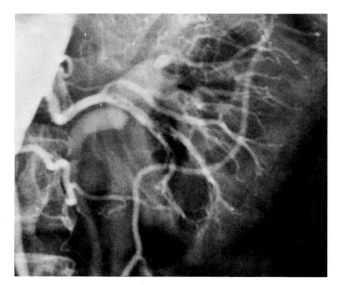

Figure 13–4. Typical appearance of renal artery emboli. Intra-arterial "filling defects" are seen. There has been at least one report of successful catheter aspiration of the bilateral renal emboli.

Figure 13–3. Nephrogram and a fluid-fluid level between urine and excreted contrast are seen in tiny kidneys in a patient on hemodialysis.

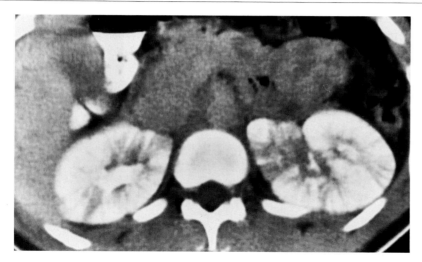

Figure 13–5. Contrast-enhanced CT performed on a young woman to elucidate the symptoms of acute abdominal pain she developed in the middle of a 10 K race. There is a very dense nephrogram with patchy areas of nephrogram absence. The collecting system is opacified. In retrospect creatinine was 3 mg/dl about the time the study was obtained. Two days later, creatinine level was down to 1.6 mg/dl and the patient had an uneventful recovery. This was probably ATN due to dehydration.

nal plasma flow, and renal enlargement. Associated elevation in capillary pressure is thought to be responsible for eventual glomerular sclerosis.[13]

In patients with renal injury, in addition to specific therapy for the primary disease, such as diabetes or hypertension, therapy should also be directed toward decreasing glomerular capillary pressure.

GLOMERULONEPHRITIS

Mechanism of Glomerular Injury

1. Usually the process begins as an antigen-antibody reaction and the formation of immune complexes.

2. Immune complexes are deposited either in glomerular mesangium or subepithelium. There they activate chemical mediators, which induce proliferation (hypercellularity) of resident cells.

3. Leukocytes are attracted to the deposits, possibly damaging capillary endothelium in the process. Endothelial damage and platelet aggregation occur. Glomerular permeability is adversely affected by local release of cationic proteins.

4. In some instances *crescent formations* develop within Bowman's space. These are accumulations of macrophages, fibroblasts, and fibrin.

5. In the later stages there is a buildup of glomerular basement material, which obliterates ultrafiltration surface area.

Clinical Manifestations

Most patients with glomerular disease present with similar clinical findings, which may differ only in acuteness or insidiousness of onset. Renal biopsy is the most reliable diagnostic method for establishing the diagnosis. The most important consequence of glomerulonephritis is progressive renal failure. Since loss of 30% or more of glomerular filtration rate (GFR) is required before there is a rise in serum creatinine, early loss of renal function is easily overlooked.

Cellular casts, red and white blood cells, and proteinuria are present in all patients.

Proteinuria and Nephrotic Syndrome

Proteinuria is always associated with glomerulonephritis. Increased permeability of the glomerular wall permits loss of larger protein molecules in addition to normal loss of light chain molecules.

When urinary loss of protein exceeds proximal tubular reabsorption and liver production capacity, hypoalbuminemia and hyperlipidemia ensue. Reduction in oncotic pressure and decrease in vascular volume activate renin-angiotensin-aldosterone axis and antidiuretic hormone. Vast amounts of salt and water are thus retained, but because of low oncotic pressure the vascular volume is not expanded. Retained fluid results in interstitial edema. This set of events is referred to as nephrotic syndrome, and all glomerulopathies are capable of producing it.

Urinary loss of immunoglobulins and coagulation inhibitors places these patients at increased risk of infections and thromboembolic events. Examples are pneumonia, peritonitis, or acute and silent renal vein thrombosis, and pulmonary emboli.

Acute Postinfectious Glomerulonephritis (APGN)

Although initially described with group A beta-hemolytic streptococcal infections, the most common association today is with nonstreptococcal infections, including bacterial endocarditis, pneumonia, abdominal abscesses, and infected prosthesis.

Antigen against infectious organism provides for formation of immune complexes, which deposit into glomeruli. Clinically, APGN is manifested one to several weeks following infection. Acute renal failure is usually reversible. APGN is probably more common than generally recognized, since most cases are probably mild and never come to clinical attention.

Rapidly Progressive (Crescentic) Glomerulonephritis (RPGN)

RPGN has an insidious onset and if left untreated results in end-stage renal disease in 1 to 2 years. Most of glomeruli contain cellular crescents. Causes of RPGN can be systemic lupus erythematosus, vasculitis, and production of autoantibody to glomerular basement membrane (anti-GMB antibody disease).

Mesangial Proliferative Glomerulonephritis (IgA Nephropathy)

This is a common glomerulonephritis. There is an increase in number of mesangial cells and amount of mesangial matrix. The most common form is IgA nephropathy, which also has mesangial deposits of IgA and C3 immune complex aggregates.

Membranoproliferative Glomerulonephritis (MPGN)

Hypercellularity and immune deposits are present at the basement membrane, which appears dense and shows "double contour." There is marked reduction in serum C3 complement, which is due to the presence of an autoantibody (nephritic factor). MPGN often results in renal failure.

Membranous Nephropathy

This is one of the most common causes of nephrotic syndrome in nondiabetic adults. There is thickening of the glomerular basement membrane but (unlike MPGN) there is no hypercellularity. Subepithelial deposits of IgA and C3 are present. Many patients eventually develop end-stage renal disease.

Lipoid Nephrosis (Minimal Change Glomerular Disease)

More common in children. Etiology unknown, possibly due to an aberration in T-cells. It may be seen in

patients with Hodgkin's disease. There are lipid-containing vacuoles in tubular cells on light microscopy and widespread effacement of foot processes on electron microscopy.

Focal Segmental Glomerular Sclerosis

Etiology unclear. Most glomeruli are normal on light microscopy. Others are segmentally solidified by basementlike material and show foci of hyalinosis, or exhibit mesangial cellular hyperplasia. Prognosis is poor in the presence of repeated episodes of renal failure. A very severe form of this disease has been described in heroin addicts and patients with AIDS.[14,15]

Lupus Glomerulonephritis

Antigen-antibody complexes are formed with DNA. Kidney is frequently affected.[16] Diagnosis by renal biopsy is difficult, since the findings resemble other glomerular diseases. These range from mild mesangial changes to proliferative lesions with crescents. Biopsy may be needed to differentiate proliferative from mesangial form, since treatment for these two forms differs. Clinical presentation is variable, ranging from isolated hematuria to RPGN and nephrotic syndrome.

Goodpasture's Syndrome

This is a rare disease mostly affecting young men. It is caused by production of antiglomerular basement membrane antibody, resulting in severe glomerulonephritis.[17] There are simultaneous severe pulmonary changes consisting of alveolar hemorrhage, hemoptysis, and diffuse air-space consolidation. The lung changes are most likely caused by the same antibody, since there is close antigenic similarity between basement membrane and alveoli. Outcome is usually poor.

VASCULITIDES

Polyarteritis Nodosa

Incidence. Most common in third and fourth decades. More common in males.

Pathology. Segmental or diffuse thrombotic and necrotizing glomerulonephritis. Glomerular capillary inflammation is the major manifestation. Tubular damage and interstitial infiltrate of mixed cells is frequent.[18]

Segmental inflammation of medium sized arteries and arterioles is found in less than 30% of renal biopsies. Inflammatory infiltrate may destroy arterial wall, resulting in thrombosis, occlusion, small aneurysms, and occasionally acute hemorrhage.

Clinical Presentation. Multisystem illness. Fever, weight loss, arthralgia, cutaneous rash. In patients with predominantly glomerular capillary disease, renal failure may become the dominant feature with a high mortality rate in the first year (sepsis, hemorrhage, etc.).[18] In patients with predominant involvement of the smaller vessels, neurologic, cardiac, and gastrointestinal symptoms are seen more often.

Radiological Findings. Contrast radiographic examinations such as CT and angiography may demonstrate areas of hypoperfusion and infarctions. These appear as patchy defects in nephrographic phase of the examination (Fig. 13–6).

On angiography, and sometimes on CT,[19] aneurysms measuring several millimeters in diameter are seen arising from small arterial branches in the kidney (Fig. 13–7), liver (Fig. 13–8),[20] and mesenteric arteries. The intralobar and arcuate arteries may be irregular, with areas of narrowing and obstruction. These findings may also be seen in necrotizing angiitis, systemic lupus erythematosus, intravenous drug abuse, and bacterial endocarditis. Therefore the findings of small aneurysms and vessel irregularity are not pathognomonic for polyarteritis nodosa.

Severe retroperitoneal hemorrhage from the kidney or even renal rupture have been described.[21–23] As might be expected, the severity of the acute disease correlates with positive angiographic findings and the presence of aneurysms.[24]

Occasionally, the ureter may become involved and narrow sufficiently to produce obstruction.[25] Notching of the ureter, presumably produced by periureteral aneurysms, has been shown to disappear after adequate systemic therapy.[26]

Henoch-Schönlein Purpura

Henoch-Schönlein purpura is associated with acute vasculitis and is characterized by nonthrombocytopenic rash, arthritis, and gastrointestinal disease,

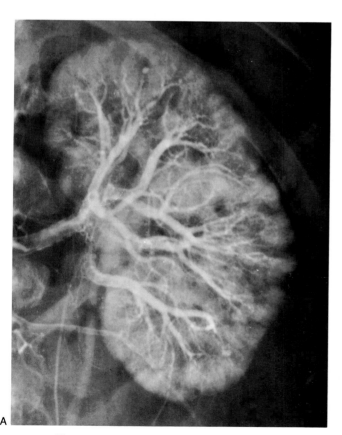
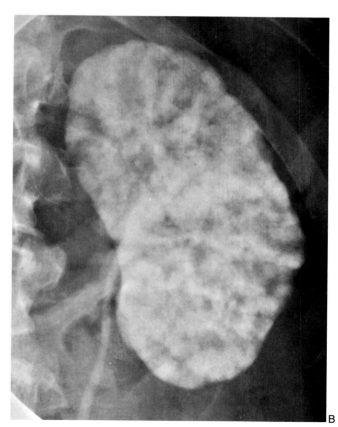

A

B

Figure 13–6. **(A)** On the arterial phase, the renal vessels are narrowed and irregular and some are completely occluded. Only one or two small aneurysms can be seen. **(B)** The nephrogram is patchy with areas of hypoperfusion due to narrowing and obstruction of the small vessels.

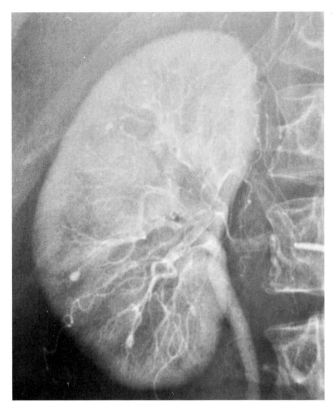

Figure 13–7. Classic small renal artery aneurysms in polyarteritis nodosa.

including intussusception. It is usually a childhood disease, but may occur in adults.

Focal glomerulonephritis may be present in 20% of cases.[27] Mesangial IgA deposits are present in the renal biopsy. Prognosis as far as nephropathy is concerned is good.[27,28]

Testicular torsion, epididymal involvement,[29] and ureteral obstruction[30] may also be associated with the syndrome.

Hemolytic Uremic Syndrome (HUS)

Microangiopathy, hemolytic anemia, thrombocythopenia, and acute renal failure are the principal findings. Peak incidence is at 3 years of age and is more common in females. Hemolysis apparently occurs as the red blood cells transit the glomerular capillary bed, resulting in glomerular damage and tubular obstruction. Small cysts, less than 2 mm, may be identified in the kidneys on occasion. Other organs may be affected. Diarrhea, often bloody, vomiting, and symptoms related to the central nervous system may be the presenting symptoms.

DIABETIC NEPHROPATHY

Incidence. Fifty percent of all insulin-dependent and juvenile-onset diabetics (Type I) develop clinically significant renal disease 20–30 years after onset.

Etiology. It appears that both metabolic and genetic factors may be contributory.

Normal kidneys transplanted into a diabetic patient develop changes suggestive of diabetic nephropathy within several years.

Kidney harvested from a diabetic with diabetic nephropathy (by biopsy) showed reversal of the changes (on repeated biopsy) after being transplanted into a nondiabetic patient.

Pathology. All glomeruli are involved in a process referred to as *diffuse intercapillary glomerulosclerosis*. The characteristic feature is an increase in PAS positive, eosinophilic material in the mesangial region, which encroaches on adjacent capillaries. Acellular *nodules* may form at the periphery of the glomerulus, a pathognomonic sign of diabetic nephropathy. There is *glomerular basement membrane thickening*. Eventually, glomeruli become *hyalinized* and the nephron is lost. Varying degrees of *arteriolosclerosis* may be present.

In the early stage there is an increase in kidney size and weight due to an increase in glomerular volume and capillary luminal area.[31,32] Increase in size is speculated to be due to intermittent or persistent elevation in growth hormone.[33] In the late stage kidneys are small.

Intrarenal vascular changes, particularly in the vasa recta, may cause ischemic changes leading to papillary necrosis.

Clinical Presentation. For many years after onset of diabetes, renal function is normal despite positive findings on renal biopsy. In the very early stage there are increases in renal plasma flow (RPF) and glomerular filtration rate (GFR), which coincide with an increase in renal size and weight.

In a later stage the onset of proteinuria heralds progressive impairment of renal function. Within several years, 50% of patients with proteinuria progress to end-stage kidney disease.

Laboratory Findings. Exercise-provoked proteinuria (early finding), proteinuria, rise in creatinine.

Radiological Findings. Diffuse renal enlargement is commonly present in the early stage of the disease. In fact, early diabetic nephropathy is the most common cause of bilateral nephromegaly, comprising some 50% of all newly discovered enlarged kidneys

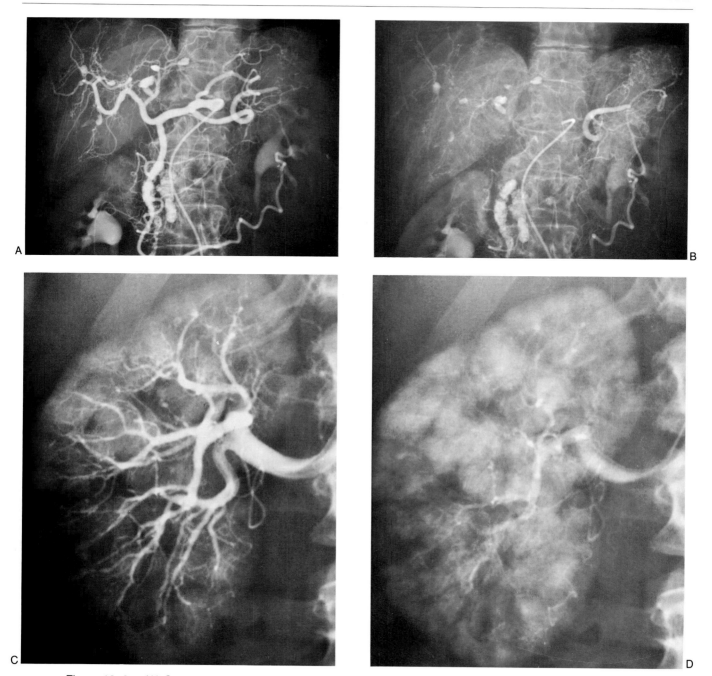

Figure 13–8. (A) Celiac angiogram demonstrates several aneurysms in the liver. (B) The contrast lingers in the aneurysms while it clears the arteries. (C) Irregular narrowing and occlusion of many smaller vessels, and only a few very small aneurysms are present in the kidneys. (D) Patchy nephrogram is due to hypoperfusion and infarction of the smaller arterioles.

by any imaging modality (Fig. 13–9).[34] Later the kidneys are small.

There is an increased incidence of urinary tract infection associated with diabetes mellitus. Gas-forming organisms may be responsible for *emphysematous cystitis and emphysematous pyelonephritis.*

Papillary necrosis may also be present, sometimes presenting with ureteral obstruction.

Neurogenic bladder dysfunction may contribute to urinary tract infection. Bladder has enlarged capacity, appears smooth on cystography, and there is a large postvoid residual.

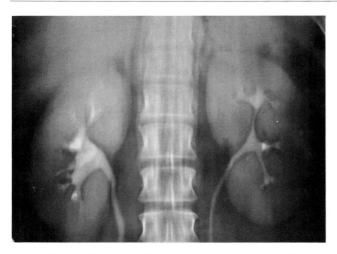

Figure 13–9. Bilateral diffuse renal enlargement. Although this finding is seen in many other diseases, statistically, when discovered as a serendipitous finding, the diagnosis is most likely diabetes.

INTERSTITIAL NEPHRITIS

Acute Interstitial Nephritis

Etiology. Allergic reactions due to hypersensitivity to a number of drugs. The more common ones include ampicillin, penicillin, methicillin, diphenylhydantoin, etc.

Direct toxicity to tubular cells may be associated with drugs such as cephalosporins, neomycin, amphotericin B, and gentamycin.

Pathology. Varying degrees of tubular cell necrosis. Tubular damage evokes interstitial changes. These consist of interstitial edema and infiltration with inflammatory mononuclear or polymorphonuclear cells.

Clinical Presentation. Renal failure, usually reversible. Fever and rash may be part of the clinical picture.

Radiological Findings. Imaging is geared to exclude postrenal causes of renal failure, namely, obstruction. Ultrasound is the examination of choice. Kidneys may be normal in size or may be enlarged. Increased echogenicity may be detected on ultrasound, but the finding is nonspecific.[35]

Alport's Syndrome

Alport's syndrome consists of hereditary chronic nephritis associated with high-tone nerve deafness and ocular anomalies.[36] Hematuria is the prominent fea-ture. There is a higher incidence of severe renal disease in affected males. There is extensive thickening and splitting of the glomerularbasement membrane (GBM). Eventually, glomerulosclerosis ensues, further compromising renal function. Clinical expression ranges from mild (usually in females) to severe (in most males) and may result in end-stage kidney disease.[37–39] Families with hematuria without ocular or hearing anomalies have also been described.

ANALGESIC NEPHROPATHY (ANALGESIC ABUSE)

Incidence. Seen in some parts of the world more often, perhaps because of local habits ("addiction to powders"). In Australia, end-stage renal failure due to analgesic nephropathy in 1979 was 25%, in 1987, 13%.[40] In the United States the incidence is probably much smaller. Definite female predominance.

Etiology. Excessive ingestion of analgesics, particularly mixed powders. Phenacetin (now banned), acetaminophen,[41,42] and mixed analgesics are the main causative factors. Aspirin works synergistically. Dehydration potentiates renal damage. Many other pharmacological and industrial compounds have papillotoxic effects on experimental animals.[43,44]

Pathogenesis. Not entirely understood. Relatively chronic process associated with human analgesic abuse need not be identical to the acute experimental animal models. Theories range from occlusion of vasa recta to increase in concentration of intermediate (biologically reactive) metabolites of phenacetin and acetaminophen.[43] Concentration of the intermediaries produces an increase of free radicals that cause oxidative damage. Medullary interstitial cells appear to be affected first, followed by loops of Henle.

Pathology. Interstitial nephritis and papillary necrosis ensue. Sloughed papilla may cause ureteral obstruction. Transitional cell dysplasia, which predisposes to neoplasia, is widespread.[45] Transitional cell carcinoma has been described.[46]

Clinical Presentation. Early on, there may be symptoms related to gastrointestinal tract and anemia. Intermediate symptoms include urinary tract infection, hematuria, nocturia, lower back pains, and symptoms due to transit of the sloughed papilla through the ureter, including obstruction. End-stage renal disease is inevitable if abuse continues.

Laboratory Findings. Defective acidification and concentration of urine, proteinuria, hematuria.

Radiological Findings. Diagnosis of analgesic nephropathy is probably best made by paying attention to detailed patient histories. When morphological changes of papillary necrosis become evident on radiological studies, the disease is already severe (Fig. 13–10). Impaired renal function does not allow for adequate concentration of contrast material on excretory urography, so that very early and even late macroscopic changes are difficult to see. If creatinine is above 1.2 mg/dl, there may be some risk of contrast material nephrotoxicity.

Nevertheless, discovering evidence for papillary necrosis on excretory urography or retrograde pyelography (Fig. 13–11) is an important contribution to the establishment of the diagnosis (see also papillary necrosis).

Papillary necrosis "in situ" may be suspected on sonography when renal papillary calcifications surrounding the central sinus complex in a complete or incomplete garland pattern are seen.[47] However, when these changes are seen on sonography, the damage to the kidney is already severe.

Obstruction caused by a sloughed papilla needs to be corrected as soon as possible to prevent further

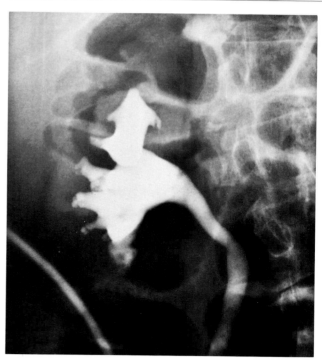

Figure 13–11. Another case of papillary necrosis seen on retrograde pyelogram. Carefully search the papillary areas for small contrast-filled cavities.

loss of functioning renal parenchyma. Filling defects representing papillary tissues may be seen in the ureter or renal pelvis on contrast examinations (Fig. 13–12).[48]

In the later stages kidney size decreases and clubbed calyces are present.

Finally, one must remember the possible increased incidence of transitional cell carcinoma in this patient population. When a contrast examination of the urinary tract is obtained, all uroepithelial-bearing surfaces should be scrutinized for irregularities or filling defects (Fig. 13–13).

SICKLE CELL DISEASE

Sickle Cell Nephropathy

Etiology. S-hemoglobinopathy.

Pathogenesis. Medullary ischemia caused by sickling. Hypoxic conditions as well as hypertonicity in the medulla promote sickling. Ischemic changes result in vascular congestion and edema.

Pathology. Papillary necrosis, glomerular enlargement, tubular atrophy, and interstitial fibrosis. Spi-

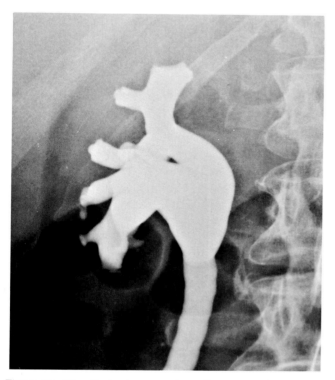

Figure 13–10. Early changes of papillary necrosis are seen on a retrograde pyelogram. Small cavities filled with contrast are seen in the papillary regions, particularly at the lower pole.

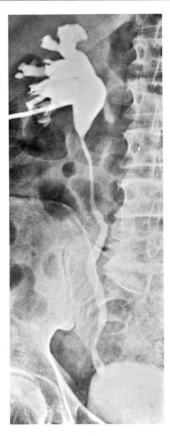

Figure 13–12. Sloughed papilla can be seen in the distal right ureter as a radiolucent "filling defect." Previously, complete distal ureteral obstruction necessitated placement of a percutaneous nephrostomy tube for drainage and preservation of renal function. At the present time, no obstruction is present. Note subtle changes of papillary necrosis in the kidney.

raling and obliteration of smaller renal vessels is possible. Vasa recta are irregular or obliterated.

Clinical Findings.   Hematuria, proteinuria, eventually renal failure, retarded growth, hypertension.

Radiological Findings.   Caution should be exercised when radiographic contrasts are used. Ionic contrasts cause sickling, nonionic contrasts less so.[49]

1. *Renal size.* Global renal enlargement is present in the early stages. This is probably related to glomerular engorgement and hypertrophy of the unaffected parenchyma. Later, in the chronic stages the kidneys are small and scarred.

2. *Papillary necrosis.* This expression of the disease may present as several different morphological types (see papillary necrosis). It is probably the most destructive aspect of the disease, since the cortical tissues served by the affected papilla are eventually

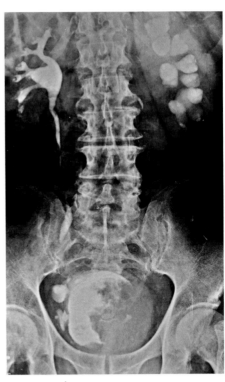

Figure 13–13. Concomitant transitional cell carcinoma (TCC) of the bladder and renal papillary necrosis in the right kidney. The left ureter is obstructed by TCC, causing left hydronephrosis.

replaced by a scar.[50] Early detection of papillary necrosis is therefore of considerable importance.

3. *Clubbed calyces.* Clubbing of the calyces may be the end result of papillary necrosis or of retractile fibrosis of the media. Scarring may or may not be present.

4. *Calcifications.* Three types may be present: a) retained sloughed papilla may calcify along periphery ("ring sign"); b) morphologically unchanged necrotic papilla may calcify (papillary necrosis "in situ"); and c) cortical calcifications may be due to cortical necrosis and seen as early as 8 weeks after an ischemic event.[51]

5. *Perinephric hemorrhage.* This is a rare event.[52]

6. *Striated nephrogram.* This finding has been described on CT and may represent either tubular obstruction or a reflection of interstitial changes.[53]

Patients with sickle cell disease are probably most commonly (and most effectively) evaluated by CT during painful abdominal episodes. A variety of findings, including splenic and liver infarction, splenic rupture, retained intrahepatic gallstones, and abdominal abscesses, may be detected (Fig. 13–14).[53] CT is too insensitive to detect papillary necrosis, however.

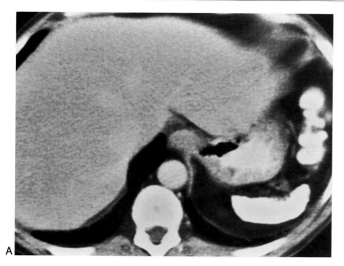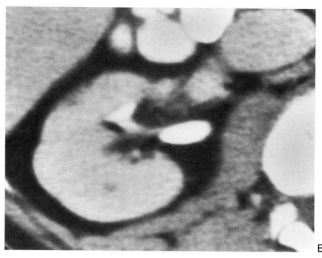

Figure 13–14. (A) Small calcified spleen in a patient with sickle cell disease. (B) Small radiolucent areas in the kidney may represent small areas of hypoperfusion due to small infarcts.

Sickle cell nephropathy may recur in a transplanted kidney.[54]

Sickle Cell Glomerulopathy

Nephrotic syndrome occurs in 4% of patients with sickle cell anemia. Of these, a majority develop renal failure, and half die within 2 years.[55] Glomerulopathy is characterized microscopically by mesangial expansion and GBM duplication. This setting differs from common sickle cell nephropathy, which is a tubulointerstitial disease.

RENAL PAPILLARY NECROSIS

Etiology. The following are causes of renal papillary necrosis:

1. Diabetes mellitus.
2. Analgesic abuse. Phenacetin, acetaminophen (paracetamol),[41,42] naproxen. Aspirin and dehydration are contributing factors.
3. High-dose nonsteroidal anti-inflammatory drug therapy.[56]
4. Sickle cell anemia.
5. Infection: pyelonephritis, tuberculosis, candidiasis.
6. Others: renal vein thrombosis, obstructive uropathy, chronic alcoholism, severe jaundice.

Pathogenesis. Papillary necrosis is probably the end expression of different pathophysiological processes. In diabetes mellitus and sickle hemoglobinopathy, occlusion of vasa recta and resultant ischemia are the likely causes. Biologically reactive intermediate metabolites of phenacetin and acetaminophen are implicated in analgesic nephropathy. Proteolytic destruction and endotoxins may be responsible for papillary necrosis in some infectious diseases. The cause for papillary necrosis found occasionally in other above-mentioned entities is still unclear.

Treatment. Placing the primary disease under control, discontinuing abuse. If there is ureteral obstruction caused by a sloughed papilla, it must be promptly treated (ureteroscopic removal, nephrostomy, etc.).[57]

Radiological Findings. When early changes become visible to the naked eye, moderate destruction of the papillary tissue is already present. The only practical way to detect these changes is by excretory urography or retrograde pyelography (Fig. 13–15).

This, of course, is problematic, since many patients affected may already have reduced renal function and intravenous injection of radiographic contrast may not be advisable. Also, diabetics have higher incidence of contrast-induced nephrotoxicity. Sickling may be induced in the presence of radiographic contrasts.

For these reasons, papillary necrosis is more often discovered incidentally, usually in a patient being worked-up for hematuria or flank pain.

There are three early morphological appearances of papillary necrosis (Fig. 13–16):

1. *Medullary type.* The early destructive changes occur on the tip of the papilla and a small cavity

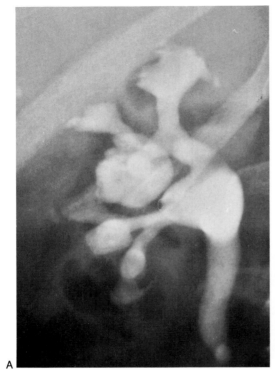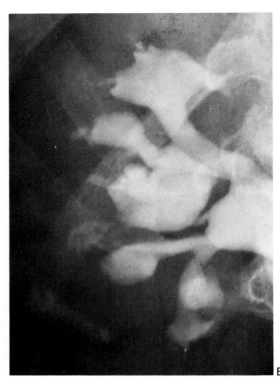

Figure 13–15. **(A)** Papillary necrosis is clearly seen in the upper and middle calyceal groups as small contrast-filled cavities. An infundibular diverticulum is also present, diverting attention from the really important finding. **(B)** If in doubt, a different projection is usually helpful. Papillary necrosis is seen better on this LPO projection of the right kidney.

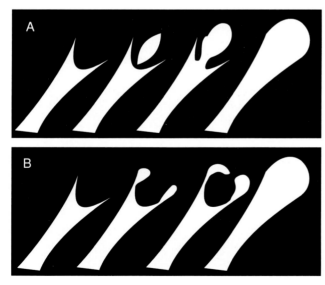

Figure 13–16. Schematic drawing of **(A)** medullary and **(B)** papillary types of papillary necrosis, the latter resulting in a sloughed papilla.

forms in the center of the papilla. Contrast from the collecting system fills the cavity, rendering it visible on radiographs.

2. *Papillary type.* Necrosis and cavitation occur at the periphery, in the forniceal area, circumferential around the papilla. As the necrotic process continues, the papilla is sloughed. If retained on the calyx or in the collecting system, the sloughed papilla may present as a filling defect and may calcify at the periphery. A calcified sloughed papilla usually has a triangular appearance. The calyx where the sloughing occurred is clubbed, reflecting the loss of papillary tissues. In the acute stage the cortex above it may still be of normal thickness. Eventually, atrophy and scarring take place and the clubbed calyx is indistinguishable from scarring seen in refluxing nephropathy. Acute ureteral obstruction may take place during the transit of a sloughed papilla (Fig. 13–17). Radiographic findings of ureteral obstruction are present, as well as changes in the other papillae in

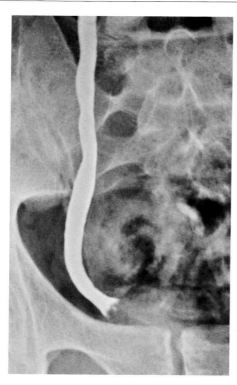

Figure 13–17. Sloughed papilla causing complete ureteral obstruction for which a percutaneous nephrostomy was placed.

different stages of development. A radiolucent "filling" defect may be identified in the ureter.

3. *In situ.* Necrotic papilla is morphologically unchanged on excretory urography. Diffuse faint calcifications may be present. The diagnosis may be impossible by radiography.

The Role of Ultrasound. Very early changes are impossible to detect by ultrasound. Later on, nonspecific changes such as clubbed calyx, obstruction, and calcified papilla may be identified.

Diffuse faint calcification in the papilla may be detected in some cases as an increase in echogenicity in the area in a garland pattern around the central sinus.[58]

REFLUXING NEPHROPATHY

Incidence. Familial predisposition, less common in black children.[59] If mild, the reflux may decrease or disappear entirely with age.

Pathophysiology. *Vesicoureteral reflux* is an abnormality, in which urine from the bladder reenters the ureter and the collecting system. Reflux is usually seen during active voiding when bladder pressure is highest. Some strains of *E. coli* produce endotoxins, which may paralyze ureteral smooth muscle and promote or make reflux appear more severe.

Pathology. *Primary vesicoureteral reflux* is most likely the result of maldevelopment of the ureterovesical junction. Gaping ureteral orifices with short intramural segment are present. *Secondary ureterovesical reflux* may be induced by a diverticulum at the ureterovesical junction (Hutch diverticulum) or by increased intravesical pressure, such as in neurogenic bladder or other types of outflow bladder obstruction.

Orifices of the collecting tubules differ morphologically in the upper calyceal group, compared to the rest of the kidney. In the upper papillae the openings are round and gaping in contrast to the oval, slit-type openings found elsewhere. Compound papillae are also more likely to have gaping orifices. Reflux from the pelvocalyceal system into the collecting tubules is thus more likely to occur in the upper pole papillae. Reflux into the collecting tubules is referred to as *intrarenal reflux.*

Focal areas of renal scarring develop where *intrarenal reflux* occurs. Scarring may be the end result of:

1. Hammerhead ("big bang") effect as sterile refluxing urine, suddenly, repeatedly, and under pressure, enters the collecting tubules. This once-popular theory is now largely discredited.
2. Reflux of infected urine into the renal pelvis and collecting tubules produces focal or diffuse acute pyelonephritis, the end-result of which is a scar. The scars most commonly involve the upper pole. For many years, this clinical entity was inaccurately referred to as *chronic pyelonephritis.* Proper term is *refluxing nephropathy.*

Clinical Presentation. Frequent urinary tract infections, flank pain, fever. Mild to moderate reflux usually disappears spontaneously after treatment for urinary tract infection and over a period of years. Only more severe reflux is likely to produce progressive renal damage, almost always before 5 years of age.[60]

Following significant renal mass reduction progressive renal insufficiency may develop even if the reflux and infection have been corrected. This is very likely due to increased glomerular capillary pressure in the remaining but overworked glomeruli. Glomerular hypertension leads to glomerulosclerosis and further reduction in the number of functioning nephrons. Eventually, this may progress to irreversible renal failure and associated hypertension.

This clinical setting of focal scarring and hypertension was once thought to be a separate disease entity labeled *segmental renal hypoplasia* or *Ask-Upmark kidney.*[61-64]

Laboratory Findings.   Pyuria, bacteriuria, diminishing renal function.

Radiological Findings.

1. *Renal scar.* Normal parenchymal thickness is drastically reduced in the affected areas as the functioning tissues are replaced by scar tissue. The distance between interpapillary line and renal outline is drastically reduced in the focal areas (Fig. 13–18).

2. *Calyceal clubbing.* Scar involves both cortex and medulla so that papillary impression eventually disappears, leaving a "blunted" calyx. There may be only a paper-thin fibrous tissue separating the calyx from the perinephric space (Fig. 13–19, 13–20).

3. *Pseudotumor.* Nephrons in unaffected areas may hypertrophy. Hypertrophied parenchyma surrounded by scarred tissues occasionally resemble a mass.

4. *Ureteral dilatation.* Repeated reflux may result in ureteral dilatation despite absence of obstruction.

Detecting and Grading Vesicoureteral Reflux

Voiding Cystourethrogram (VCUG).   The purpose of this examination is to visualize the bladder and urethral anatomy and to affirm or exclude the presence of vesicoureteral reflux.[65-67] Bladder is catheterized under sterile conditions and residual urine volume is determined. Bladder is filled to capacity with contrast material. Patient is instructed to void, preferably in an upright position. Males use a urinal while female patients catch urine in a cystogram kit tray, which they hold between the thighs. In infants and small children the examination is performed in the supine oblique position.

Spot or 100 mm films are obtained in the RPO and LPO projection to visualize reflux in the distal ureteral segment (which may be obscured behind the bladder on the frontal projection). If reflux into the upper system is detected, a spot film of the kidney is obtained to confirm presence of contrast in the kidney and to obtain "free" anatomical information as to the calyceal clubbing, presence of renal scarring, and caliber of the ureter.

Needless to say, urethra and bladder are carefully scrutinized for presence of ureterocele, ectopic ureter, urethral and ureteral and bladder diverticula, thickness and trabeculation of the bladder wall, or any other anomalies. Some of these findings may be seen only on a postvoid radiograph.

As in all contrast examinations, a scout film is

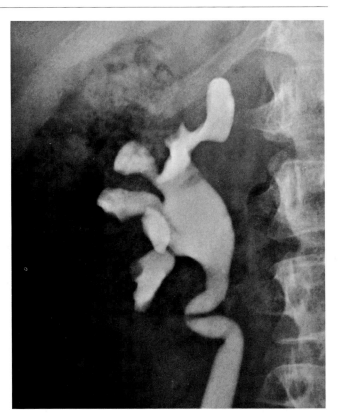

Figure 13–19.   Clubbed calyces, particularly the upper pole calyx, in refluxing nephropathy.

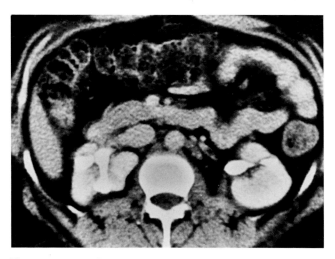

Figure 13–18.   Severe renal parenchymal scarring. Visualized calyces in both kidneys have no parenchyma above them, only a thin scar tissue. Remaining nephrons are unaffected and have normal function.

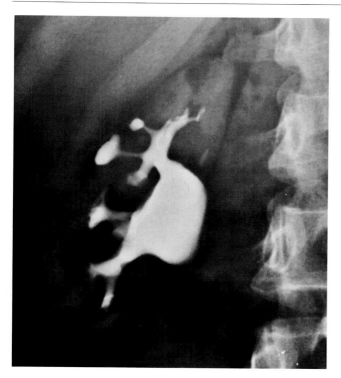

Figure 13–20. Another, less severe example of calyceal clubbing of the upper pole calyces.

obtained prior to contrast installation. Urinary tract calculi should not be missed.

Radionuclide Cystogram. This study is usually performed as the follow-up study. The radiation exposure is less than that of VCUG. Anatomical detail, however, is not as revealing but the test is quite sensitive for detection of reflux. Bladder is catheterized and filled with Tc-99m pertechnetate. Presence or absence of reflux is determined on sequential scintigrams obtained on a gamma camera.[68]

Grading. As seen on VCUG, vesicoureteral reflux is classified into four groups:

- Group I: Minimal reflux into distal ureter.
- Group II: Reflux into proximal ureter and nondilated renal pelvis.
- Group III: Reflux into dilated pelvocalyceal system.
- Group IV: Documented intrarenal (intratubular) reflux.

Reimplantation (Ureteroneocystotomy). Ureteroneocystotomy is rarely performed after the age of 5 years. After surgical reimplantation, there should be no vesicoureteral reflux or obstruction at the reimplantation site. Certain types of operations may

make it more difficult or impossible to catheterize the ureter in a retrograde fashion.[69]

REFERENCES

1. Curry NS, Bogien RP, Schabel SI. Minimal dilatation obstructive nephropathy. Radiology 1982; 143:531–534.
2. Naidich JB, Rackson ME, Mossey RT, Stein HL. Nondilated obstructive uropathy: percutaneous nephrostomy performed to reverse renal failure. Radiology 1986; 160:653–657.
3. Maillet PJ, et al. Nondilated obstructive acute renal failure. Radiology 1986; 160:659–662.
4. Rascoff JH, et al. Nondilated obstructive nephropathy. Arch Intern Med 1983; 143:696–698.
5. Spital A, Valvo JR, Segal AJ. Nondilated obstructive uropathy. Urology 1988; 31:478.
6. Goldfarb R, Ongseng F, Finestone H, Garcia H. Nondilated obstructive uropathy. (Letter.) Urology 1989; 33:257.
7. Brenner BM, Anderson S. Why kidneys fail: an unifying hypothesis. Trans Am Clin Climatol Assoc 1986; 98:59–70.
8. Anderson S, Brenner BM. Effects of aging on the renal glomerulus. Am J Med 1986; 80:435.
9. Hostetter TH, Olson JL, Rennke HG, et al. Hyperfiltration in remnant nephrons: a potentially adverse response to renal ablation. Am J Physiol 1981; 241:85.
10. Brenner BM, Meyer TW, Hostetter TH. Dietary protein intake and the progressive nature of kidney disease. N Engl J Med 1982; 307:652–655.
11. Mizuiri S, Hayashi I, Ozawa T, et al. Effects of an oral protein load on glomerular filtration rate in healthy controls and nephrotic patients. Nephron 1988; 48:101–106.
12. Hostetter TH, Meyer TW, Rennke HG, et al. Chronic effects of dietary protein on renal structure and function in the rat with intact and reduced renal mass. Kidney Int 1986; 30:509.
13. Hostetter TH, Rennke HG, Brenner BM. The case for intrarenal hypertension in the initiation and progression of diabetic and other glomerulopathies. Am J Med 1982; 72:375.
14. Rao TKS, Fillipone EJ, Nicastri AD, et al. Associated focal and segmental glomerulosclerosis in acquired immunodeficiency syndrome. N Engl J Med 1984; 310:669–673.
15. Schaffer RM, Schwartz GE, Becker JA, et al. Renal ultrasound in acquired immunodeficiency syndrome. Radiology 1984; 153:511–513.
16. Stanley JH, Cornella R, Loevinger E, et al. Sonography of systemic lupus nephritis. Am J Roentgenol 1984; 142:1165–1168.
17. Weber M, Kohler H, Manns M, et al. Identification of Goodpasture target antigens in basement membranes of human glomeruli, lung, and placenta. Clin Exp Immunol 1987; 67:262–269.
18. Adu D, Howie AJ, Scott DG, Bacon PA, et al. Polyarteritis and the kidney. Q J Med 1987; 62:221–237.
19. Wilms G, Oyen R, Wear M, et al. CT demonstration of aneurysms in polyarteritis nodosa. J Comput Assist Tomogr 1986; 10:513.

20. Peterson C Jr, Willerson JT, Doppman JL, Decker J. Polyarteritis nodosa with bilateral renal artery aneurysms and perirenal hematomas: angiographic and nephrotomographic features. Br J Radiol 1970; 43:62.

21. Kirkali Z, Finci R, Eryigit M, Ozdemir C. Spontaneous kidney rupture in polyarteritis nodosa. Report of four cases. Eur Urol 1988; 15:153–155.

22. Cornfield JZ, Johnson ML, Dolehide J, Fowler JE Jr. Massive renal hemorrhage owing to polyarteritis nodosa. J Urol 1988; 140:808–809.

23. Miller CM, Reiber K, Waxman J, et al. Massive intraabdominal bleeding in polyarteritis nodosa. Mt Sinai J Med 1987; 54:512–515.

24. Ewald EA, Griffin D, McCune WJ. Correlation of angiographic abnormalities with disease manifestations and disease severity in polyarteritis nodosa. J Rheumatol 1987; 14:952–956.

25. Hefty TR, Bonafede P, Stenzel P. Bilateral ureteral stricture from polyarteritis nodosa. J Urol 1989; 141:600–601.

26. Cochran ST, Kanter SA. Ureteric changes in polyarteritis nodosa. Br J Radiol 1978; 52:504–506.

27. Stewart M, Savage JM, Bell B, McCord B. Long term renal prognosis of Henoch-Schönlein purpura in an unselected childhood population. Eur J Pediatr 1988; 147:113–115.

28. Koskimies O, Sevi M, Rapola J, Vilska J. Henoch-Schönlein nephritis: long term prognosis of unselected patients. Arch Dis Child 1981; 56:482–484.

29. Ross WB, Davis-Reynolds LM. Epididymal involvement in Henoch-Schönlein purpura mimicking testicular torsion. J R Col Surg Edinb 1987; 32:247.

30. Powell JM, Ware H, Williams G. Recurrent ureteric obstruction in association with Henoch-Schönlein purpura. Postgrad Med J 1987; 63:699–701.

31. Zatz R, Brenner BM. Pathogenesis of diabetic microangiopathy: the hemodynamic view. Am J Med 1986; 80:443.

32. Mogensen CE, Anderson MJF. Increased kidney size and glomerular filtration rate in early juvenile diabetes. Diabetes 1973; 22:706.

33. Kahn CB, Raman PG, Zic Z. Kidney size in diabetes mellitus. Diabetes 1974; 23:788–792.

34. Segel MC, Lecky JW, Slasky BS. Diabetes mellitus: the predominant cause of bilateral renal enlargement. Radiology 1984; 153:341–362.

35. Rosenfield AT, Siegel NJ. Renal parenchymal disease: histopathologic-sonographic correlation. AJR 1981; 137:793–798.

36. Alport AC. Hereditary familial congenital hemorrhagic nephritis. Br Med J 1927; 1:504–506.

37. Gubler M, Habib R. Alport's syndrome—a report of 58 cases and a review of the literature. Am J Med 1981; 70:493–505.

38. Flinter FA, Cameron JS, Chantler C, et al. Genetics of classic Alport's syndrome. Lancet 1988; 2:1005–1007.

39. Grunfeld JP, Charbonneau R, Grateau G, Noel LH. Alport's syndrome and related hereditary nephropathies. Contrib Nephrol 1988; 61:82–90.

40. Kincaid-Smith P. Analgesic nephropathy. Aust N Z J Med 1988; 18:251–254.

41. Segasothy M, Suleiman AB, Puvaneswary M, Rohana A. Paracetamol: a cause for analgesic nephropathy and end-stage renal disease. Nephron 1988; 50:50–54.

42. Björck S, Svalander CT, Aurell M. Acute renal failure after analgesic drugs including paracetamol (acetaminophen). Nephron 1988; 49:45.

43. Bach P, Gregg NJ. Experimentally induced renal papillary necrosis and upper urothelial carcinoma. Int Rev Exp Pathol 1988; 30:1–53.

44. Levy M. Adverse reactions to over-the-counter analgesics: an epidemiological evaluation. Agents Actions (Suppl) 1988; 25:21–31.

45. Blohme I, Johansson S. Renal pelvic neoplasms and atypical urothelium in patients with end-stage analgesic nephropathy. Kidney Int 1981; 20:671–675.

46. Chapple CR, Newman J, O'Brien JM, Considine J. Analgesic nephropathy complicated by transitional cell carcinoma of the renal pelvis. Br J Urol 1987; 59:89.

47. Weber M, Braun B, Kihler H. Ultrasonic findings in analgesic nephropathy. Nephron 1985; 39:216–222.

48. Andriole GL, Bahnson RR. Computed tomographic diagnosis of ureteral obstruction caused by a sloughed papilla. Urol Radiol 1987; 9:45–46.

49. Rao VM, Rao AK, Steiner RM, et al. The effect of ionic and nonionic contrast media on the sickling phenomena. Radiology 1982; 144; 219–293.

50. Vaamonde CA. Renal papillary necrosis in sickle cell heminoglobinopathy. Semin Nephrol 1984; 4:48–62.

51. Mapp E, Karasick S, Pollack H, et al. Uroradiological manifestations of S-hemoglobinopathy. Semin Roentgenol 1987; 22:186–194.

52. Sickles EA, Korobkin M. Perirenal hematoma as a complication of renal infarction in sickle cell trait. AJR 1974; 122:800–803.

53. Magid D, Fishman EK, Charache S, Siegelman SS. Abdominal pain in sickle cell disease: the role of CT. Radiology 1987; 163:325–328.

54. Miner DJ, Jorkasky DK, Perloff LJ, et al. Am J Kidney Dis 1987; 10:306–313.

55. Bakir AA, Hathiwala SC, Ainis H, et al. Prognosis of the nephrotic syndrome in sickle glomerulopathy. A retrospective study. Am J Nephrol 1987; 7:110–115.

56. Bach PH, Bridges JW. Chemically induced renal papillary necrosis and upper urothelial carcinoma. CRC Crit Rev Toxicol 1985; 15:331–441.

57. Salo JO, Talja T, Lehtonen T. Ureteroscopy in the treatment of ureteral obstruction caused by papillary necrosis. Eur Urol 1987; 13:140–141.

58. Weber M, Braun B, Kihler H. Ultrasonic findings in analgesic nephropathy. Nephron 1985; 39:216–222.

59. Sirota L, Hertz M, Laufer J, et al. Familial vesicoureteral reflux: study of 16 families. Urol Radiol 1986; 8:22–25.

60. Brown JH, McGeown MG. Reflux nephropathy as a cause of end-stage renal failure. Clin Nephrol 1988; 29:103–105.

61. Ask-Upmark E. Uber juvenile malignan nephrosklerose ung ihr vehaltnis zu storungen in der nierenentwicklung. Acta Pathol Microbiol Scand 1929; 6:383–442.

62. Fikri E, Hanrahan JB, Stept LA. Renovascular hypertension in a child. Ask-Upmark kidney. J Urol 1973; 110:728–731.

63. Benz G, Willick E, Svharer. Segmental renal hypoplasia in childhood. Pediatr Radiol 1976; 5:86–92.

64. Pfister RC. Case records of the Massachusetts General Hospital: hypertension and a small kidney in a 17-year-old. N Engl J Med 1973; 289:736–743.

65. Lebowitz RL. Detection of vesicoureteral reflux in the child. Invest Radiol 1986; 21:519–524.

66. Lebowitz RL, Mandell J. Urinary tract infection in children: putting radiology in its place. Radiology 1987; 165:1–4.

67. Blickman JG, Taylor GA, Lebowitz RL. Voiding cystourethrography: initial radiologic study in children with urinary tract infections. Radiology 1985; 156:659–662.

68. Zhang G, Day DL, Loken M, et al. Grading of reflux by radionuclide cystography. Clin Nucl Med 1987; 12:106–109.

69. Mezzacappa PM, Price AP, Kassner EG, et al. Cohen ureteral reimplantation: sonographic appearance. Radiology 1987; 165:851–852.

14

Renal Transplants

RENAL TRANSPLANTATION

Frequency. About 10 000 transplants/year in the United States.

Allograft Survival. Cadaveric allograft survival rates are about 80% at 1 year. Sibling-related 1 year allograft survival rate is close to 100%.

Donor Workup

Radiologic workup of living-related donor ensures that the donor will be left with a normal kidney and that the harvested kidney is anatomically and functionally normal. This is most efficiently accomplished by an excretory urogram.

Arteriography determines the number of renal arteries, length of the main renal artery segment before bifurcation, and presence of arterial disease (e.g., fibromuscular dysplasia). Catheter position during the aortogram must be high enough so that an upper pole aberrant renal artery, if present, is not missed. The filming sequence should be extended long enough to visualize the renal vein, usually 12 to 16 seconds after the injection. Arteriography will dictate the choice of the kidney to be harvested in approximately 24% of prospective renal donors.[1] This simple examination can be performed on an outpatient basis.[2]

A cadaver kidney requires no radiological workup.

Acute Tubular Necrosis (ATN)

Etiology. Ischemia related to transplantation surgery.

Pathology. Tubular cell necrosis ranging from very mild to severe. Tubular debris.

Clinical Presentation. Transient renal failure usually apparent within the first 48 hours after transplant surgery.

Radiological Findings. Morphologically, renal allograft appears normal on ultrasound. In mild cases renal blood flow is usually altered only slightly by any imaging modality. In more severe cases blood flow decreases. It is very difficult or impossible to differentiate mild cases of rejection from ATN on imaging findings alone.

Acute Rejection

Pathology. *Cellular (interstitial) rejection* is the result of cellular immune reaction. Edema is present in the interstitium. Intertubular capillaries, venules, and lymphatics in the cortex are infiltrated with mononuclear cells. Tubular cells are swollen. Glomeruli, arterioles, and arteries are usually spared. Cortex thickens.

Acute vascular rejection is the result of both humoral and cellular immune reaction. Arterioles and small and medium-sized arteries are involved. Endothelial swelling, subendothelial space infiltration, fibrinoid necrosis, fibrin, and platelet adhesion to damaged endothelium are present. Thrombosis and obliteration of blood flow are possible.

Depending on the severity of rejection, the kidney may be normal in size, or mildly or markedly enlarged in both types of rejection. As the outward expansion becomes restricted by the capsule, inward enlargement compresses on renal sinus, making it small. Mononuclear cell infiltration may also involve renal sinus fat, renal pelvis, and ureter. Rapid and massive enlargement may result in parenchymal rupture and bleeding. Lymph production is accelerated.

Clinical Presentation. Commonly apparent in the first 7 days after transplantation. May be evident within hours following surgery (hyperacute rejection). *Acute cellular rejection* may occur at any time, even years after transplantation. Late *vascular rejection* is rare. Varying degrees of renal insufficiency are found, depending on the severity of the process. Local tenderness may be present, probably because of pressure exerted on adjacent tissues by the enlarging allograft (allograft nerves are severed at harvest and the pain is not renal).

Radiological Findings. The principal finding by any imaging modality is renal enlargement. This finding is not specific, however, and is also present in acute pyelonephritis, renal vein thrombosis, acute glomerulonephritis, and may be present even in ATN. Furthermore, allografts tend to hypertrophy over a period of time and are 20% larger in 2 to 3 weeks than at harvest.[3,4]

Sonography (Fig. 14–1).

- *Size.* In moderate to severe rejection there may be an increase in renal volume 30% over baseline value. In mild rejection this change may be imperceptible.
- *Cortex.* There is an increase in cortical thickness. Cortex may be either hypoechoic or hyperechoic, so that, except for the thickness, the echo texture provides no significant contribution to diagnosis.[4]
- *Medulla.* In moderate to severe rejection the medullary pyramids are enlarged and hypoechoic.[5] The enlarged, broadened pyramids may appear rectangular.
- *Corticomedullary junction (CMJ).* CMJ frequently becomes indistinct or, in other words, the echo

textures of both cortex and medulla blend so that these structures are no longer easily discriminated from each other.
- *Central echo complex (CEC).* CEC represents all there is in the renal sinus. In the absence of hydronephrosis CEC is echogenic. As edema and infiltration by polymorphonuclear cells ensue, there may be a decrease in, or even absence of, CEC echogenicity.[6]
- *Renal pelvis.* The collecting system may also respond to rejection. Edema, as well as cellular infiltration, may be observed. Thickened collecting system wall may be seen on ultrasound, although the finding is nonspecific.

Duplex Doppler Sonography. Duplex Doppler sonography visually displays blood velocity within the arteries (or veins) during a cardiac cycle. In general, there is a decrease in renal blood flow during an episode of acute rejection. However, this is true of most other pathological conditions affecting the allograft. Also there is a question of the severity of the process.

In general, one might expect early decrease in height of the diastolic component, followed by further loss of diastolic and systolic components. Pulsatility index (height of the peak systolic component minus height of the end-diastolic component divided by height of the peak systolic component) or other indices may become abnormal.

Preferably, measurements are obtained from arcuates or lobar arteries.

Nuclear Medicine. Tc-99m DTPA injected as a bolus provides information regarding perfusion of the transplanted organ. The sequential images may be

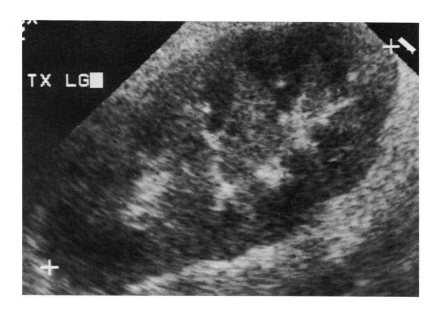

Figure 14–1. Acute rejection on sonography. There is an increase in size and cortical thickness and pyramids are hypoechoic. There is decreased echogenicity of the renal cortex. (Photograph courtesy of Dr. Rita Perella.)

viewed in analog form or may be analyzed and presented as a time-activity curve. Somewhat delayed images provide information regarding glomerular filtration and concentrating function. In rejection there is diminished renal blood flow and this is well reflected on scintigraphy, sometimes several days prior to the clinical findings of rejection. However, the findings are nonspecific and may be observed in ATN. The true value in Tc-99m DTPA scintigraphy is in the serial follow-up studies.[7]

Tc-99m MAG$_3$ will probably become the agent of choice for estimating blood flow and functional insufficiency. This compound compares favorably to I-131-orthoiodohippurate in both glomerular filtration and tubular secretion with all the advantages of imaging with gamma energy level of technetium.

MR Imaging. Enlargement and loss of CMJ are the principal findings.[8] Renal sinus may be obliterated, and even the thickened collecting system wall may be identified. In general, these findings parallel those seen on ultrasound. However, identical changes may be seen in infection, renal vein thrombosis, obstruction, and even acute tubular necrosis. Mild cases of rejection frequently appear normal.[9] Because it is an expensive examination, ultrasound and nuclear medicine studies are the preferred procedures.

Renal Angiography. Renal angiography is obviously not the primary, or even secondary, method of diagnosing allograft rejection. However, during a workup of renal artery stenosis or arteriovenous fistula, angiographic features of acute rejection may be observed. Pruning and focal areas of narrowing of the vessels are seen associated with blotchy nephrogram.

Cyclosporin A (Cs) Nephrotoxicty

Pathogenesis. Renal vasoconstriction and vasculopathy caused by direct endothelial cell damage and platelet aggregation. In chronic stage there may be interstitial fibrosis and mononuclear cell infiltration.

Pathology. Diagnosis of exclusion, i.e., histopathologic features of acute rejection are absent on biopsy.

Clinical Presentation. There is slow rise in serum creatinine, usually 4 to 5 weeks after surgery. Hypertension.

Laboratory Findings. High serum Cs (100–250 ng/ml, or more).

Treatment. Cs therapy is discontinued or the dose is adjusted.

Renal Allograft Dysfunction: Workup

The imaging workup of a patient with renal allograft dysfunction should begin with sonography. Presence or absence of ureteral obstruction, major arterial occlusion, or perinephric fluid collection can be easily established. If obstruction is excluded and patency of major vessels established, further management is dependent on clinical and laboratory findings.

For instance, if the clinical course is compatible with ATN, or if the serum Cs is high, or if there is evidence of infection, it may be prudent to institute supportive therapy, discontinue Cs, or treat urinary tract infection. If allograft dysfunction is still unexplained, renal transplant biopsy is obtained. This usually determines specific pathologic diagnosis and permits prompt institution of therapy.

Duplex Doppler sonography has generated considerable interest, but it appears to be an inaccurate method for establishing the nature or degree of renal allograft dysfunction.[10–12] While decreased diastolic blood flow velocity is a sensitive sign of increased vascular resistance in the kidney, it cannot be used to diagnose underlying pathological causes (Table 14–1).[13,14] Since change in the resistive index (RI) value does not reflect the pathologic process in the kidney, nor its severity, this test should not determine initial patient management. After biopsy and appropriate therapy have been instituted, RI may be useful in following the progression of the disease.

Scintigraphy reportedly can differentiate acute rejection from cyclosporine nephrotoxicity.[15] MR imaging demonstrates renal enlargement and loss of corticomedullary differentiation but is at the present time nonspecific (Table 14–2).[8]

Table 14–1. Reported Value in Duplex Doppler Sonography in Acute Rejection

MODALITY	INDICATION	RESULT	REFERENCE
US	Acute rejection/other causes	Poor	Hoddick et al.,[10] 1986
Doppler US	Acute rejection/Cs NT*	Not possible	Linkowski et al.,[11] 1987
Doppler US	Acute rejection/normal	Excellent	Steinberg et al.,[12] 1987
Doppler US	Acute rejection/other causes	Poor	Genkins et al.,[13] 1989
Doppler US	Acute rejection/other causes	Poor	Don et al.,[14] 1989

*Cs: cyclosporine; NT: nephrotoxicity.

Table 14-2. Reported Value of Scintigraphy and MR Imaging in Acute Rejection

MODALITY	INDICATION	RESULT	REFERENCE
Scintigraphy	Acute rejection/Cs NT*	Good	Kim et al.,[15] 1986
MR imaging	Acute rejection (mild)/normal	Difficult	Mitchell et al.,[9] 1986
MR imaging	Acute rejection/other causes	Poor	Hricak et al.,[8] 1987

*Cs: cylosporine; NT: nephrotoxicity.

Chronic Rejection

Pathology. Mononuclear cellular infiltrates and intimal fibrosis. Kidney is usually decreased in size.

Clinical Presentation. Gradual decline in renal function, usually months or years after transplantation surgery.

Radiological Findings. The kidney is usually decreased in size. Cortex may become hypoechoic and corticomedullary junction indistinct (Fig. 14–2). Decreases in blood flow velocities[14] parallel the angiographic findings of arterial narrowing, irregularities, and reduction in number.[16] Effective renal blood flow (ERBF) decreases steadily over time. Sonography is of no particular value in differentiating normal kidney from chronic rejection in children.[17]

Recurrence of the Primary Disease in Allograft

Renal failure following transplantation may be due to recurrent glomerulopathy, which led to end-stage native kidneys in the first place. In general, the more severe and rapid deterioration of the native kidneys, the greater the chances of recurrence in allograft.[18]

Among patients with primary glomerulonephritis, those with focal segmental glomerulosclerosis and membranous nephropathy have the greatest chance of losing their allograft due to recurrence.

Diabetic nephropathy reoccurs in all allografts, but it takes many years, perhaps 20, before allograft function is irreversibly lost.

In any event, 1 to 2% of allograft failures are due to recurrent primary disease that caused loss of the native kidneys and should be considered in differential diagnosis.

Arterial Complications

ACUTE POSTOPERATIVE RENAL ARTERY OCCLUSION

Acute renal artery thrombosis (Fig. 14–3), intimal dissection (Fig. 14–4), or severe kink (Fig. 14–5) may all cause complete renal artery occlusion in the postoperative period. Several hours of ischemia will result in irreversible loss of renal function and it is urgent to establish correct diagnosis. Anuria is the main clinical presentation. Differential diagnosis includes ATN, ureteral obstruction, and, occasionally, hyperacute rejection. There is no perfusion on Tc-

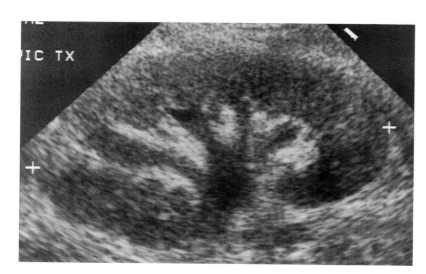

Figure 14–2. Chronic rejection (biopsy) and mild hydronephrosis. CMJ is indistinct. Findings are nonspecific.

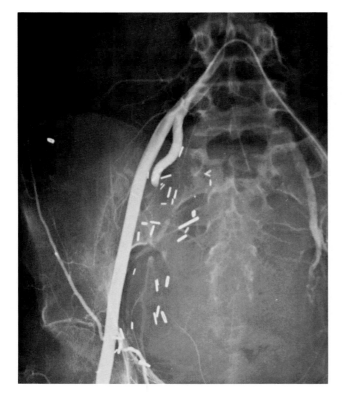

Figure 14–3. Acute occlusion at the arterial anastomotic site. Patient presents with acute anuria.

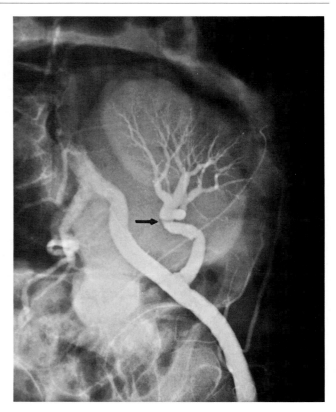

Figure 14–5. Severe kink in the distal renal artery (arrow) in a patient with severe hypertension. End-to-side anastomosis (renal to external iliac artery) is patent.

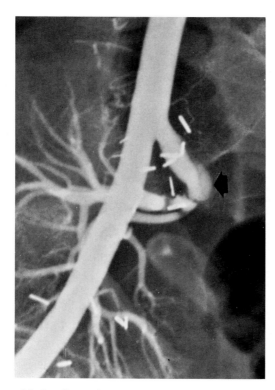

Figure 14–4. Stenosis and spontaneous dissection at the end-to-end (renal to hypogastric artery) anastomotic site. Contrast is seen outside the arterial lumen (arrow).

99m DTPA flow scan. Duplex Doppler ultrasound demonstrates lack of flow and is the examination of choice. Angiography is diagnostic. Treatment is surgical.

RENAL ARTERY STENOSIS

Incidence. Five to 16%.

Etiology. Postoperative stricture, vessel wall rejection, extrinsic compression, kink in the vessel, dissection, atherosclerosis.

Clinical Presentation. Diminishing renal function, hypertension.

Radiological Findings. If functionally significant obstruction is present, there is delay in perfusion on Tc-99m DTPA flow scan. A marked reduction in pulse amplitude is present on duplex Doppler ultrasound scan.[19,20] In severe cases a reverse in the flow pattern may occasionally be identified. Angiography is the definitive diagnostic method and angioplasty may be performed during the same session (Fig. 14–6).

Prior to beginning an angiographic examination on a renal allograft, it is important to know what type

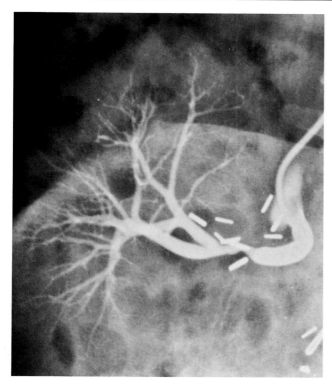

Figure 14–6. Stenosis at the anastomotic site seen on selective arteriogram.

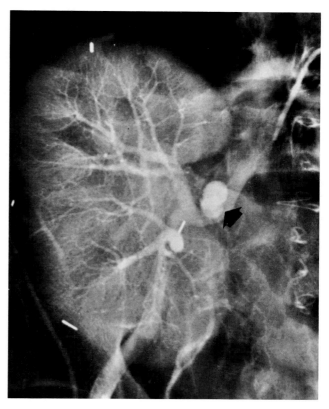

Figure 14–7. Pseudoaneurysm at end-to-end anastomosis. Small pocket of pus was found in the area.

of arterial anastomosis is present. Basically, there is end-to-end renal artery-hypogastric artery anastomosis as well as end-to-side renal artery-iliac (common or external) artery anastomosis. In the first instance the patient should be positioned in steep ipsilateral oblique projection in order to place both the renal artery and hypogastric artery parallel to the film and "open" the anastomotic site for viewing. In the second, the patient has to be placed in an almost lateral projection, since the renal artery is usually anastomosed to the anterior wall of the common or external iliac artery. If angioplasty is anticipated in the same session, in the first instance the contralateral femoral approach is usually technically easier. The ipsilateral femoral approach may be easier in end-to-side anastomosis.

Angioplasty success rate is as high as 87%.[21–23] Surgical correction is usually very difficult because of dense fibrous tissues surrounding the area of anastomosis.

RENAL ARTERY PSEUDOANEURYSM

Aneurysm of the allograft renal artery is rare. The pseudoaneurysm at the anastomotic site may be a complication of surgery or may result from an infection in the area (Fig. 14–7). These aneurysms are dangerous and may rupture unexpectedly. Ultrasound is the diagnostic method of choice. CT may also demonstrate the lesion.[24] Angiography is the gold standard. Treatment is surgical.

AV FISTULAS

Arteriovenous fistulas in the renal allograft are usually a complication of renal biopsy. Asymptomatic fistulas are very common in the immediate postbiopsy period and spontaneously close within weeks or months. Acute or chronic hemorrhage may be present in others. Some patients may develop renin-mediated hypertension because of the "steal" phenomenon. Duplex Doppler ultrasound may demonstrate the fistula.[25–27] Angiography is the examination of choice if ultrasound is negative and the patient is symptomatic (hematuria or hypertension) (Fig. 14–8). Symptomatic AV fistulas may be treated successfully by transcatheter embolization.

Renal Vein Occlusion

Allograft renal vein anastomosis is usually end-to-side to common or external iliac vein. The most

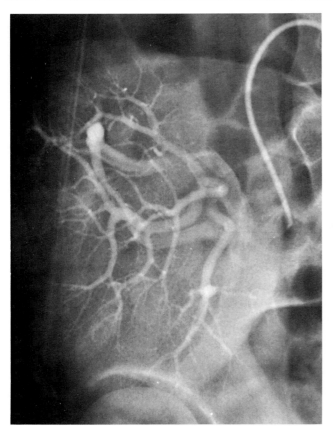

Figure 14–8. Postbiopsy arteriovenous fistula in the upper pole of the renal allograft. Renal and iliac veins are opacified by contrast during the arterial phase.

common causes of renal vein occlusion are various peritransplant fluid collections producing extrinsic compression upon the vessel. External and common iliac vein may also be affected. Patients are likely to present with significant proteinuria.

Primary acute allograft renal vein thrombosis is probably rare and difficult to diagnose. Most occur in the first 3 days following surgery. Retrograde diastolic flow was observed at the level of the arcuate arteries following peak systolic frequency shift.[28] The kidney may be enlarged. Ultrasound may or may not be successful in demonstrating the intravascular thrombus.[29] Retrograde venography is difficult, since the anastomotic site may be difficult to cross even in normal patients. MR and CT are untested in this area.

Complications Involving Ureter and Bladder

URETERAL OBSTRUCTION

Obstruction at the ureterovesical anastomosis is the most common site and is either related to postsurgi-

cal edema, stricture, vascular ischemia, rejection, relative position of the kidney (Fig. 14–9), or extrinsic compression (Fig. 14–10). Long ureteral segments may be involved (Fig. 14–11). Obstruction at the ureteropelvic junction (UPJ) may sometimes be seen when an allograft for technical reasons had to be inverted upside-down. There may be disproportionate dilatation of the calyces compared with that of the renal pelvis.

Diagnosis of the obstruction may be difficult. On contrast or isotope imaging, there is no opposite kidney to compare function and this method is generally unreliable. Sequential ultrasonography is reasonably accurate if progressive dilatation of the collecting system is detected. In some instances, even in the presence of severe obstruction, there may be no dilatation of the collecting system or the ureter.

If the dilemma of physiologic versus anatomic dilatation cannot be resolved, antegrade pyelography, a mininephrostomy, or a Whitaker pressure-flow study may be necessary (see Chapter 7, "Urinary Tract Obstruction").

About 50% of patients with obstruction may be treated by percutaneous methods, ranging from percutaneous drainage, balloon dilatation, and antegrade stent placement.[30–36]

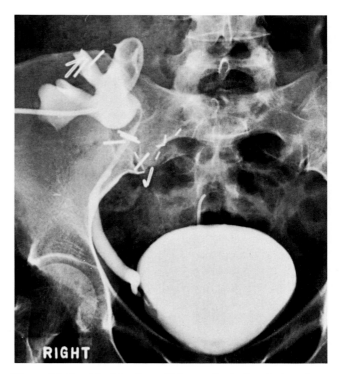

Figure 14–9. Upside-down kidney oriented so that ureteropelvic junction is pointing cephalad. Mild obstruction was present at the UPJ and distal ureteral anastomotic site.

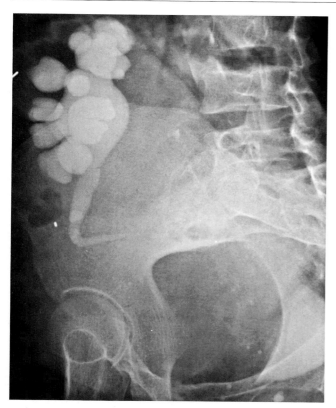

Figure 14–10. Large lymphocele presents as a pelvic mass and displaces bladder posteriorly and ureter superiorly. Partial ureteral obstruction is caused by extrinsic compression.

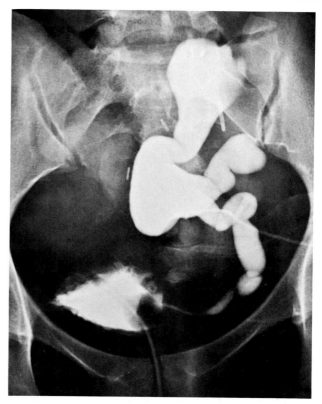

Figure 14–11. Long distal ureteral stricture. Site of anastomosis of the ureter to the bladder may be seen in most patients as a filling defect and is a normal finding.

URINE LEAKS

Ureteroneocystostomy is the common site for urine extravasation. If extravasation is minimal, an antegrade or retrograde ureteral stent may promote healing and eliminate the need for surgical intervention.

Other sites of extravasation are from a ruptured kidney, after a biopsy, necrosed ureter (Fig. 14–12), or from an incompletely closed bladder incision. In searching for urinary extravasation, a cystogram should be the first examination (Fig. 14–13).

Antegrade pyelography is more accurate than sonography or nuclear scintigraphy in detecting urine leaks.[34]

Peritransplant Fluid Collections

URINOMA

Presence of urine in the perinephric areas or in the peritoneal cavity implies disruption of the ureterovesical anastomosis, incomplete bladder closure, or rupture of the pelvocalyceal system. If the leak is active at the time of nuclear medicine or radio-graphic intravenous contrast examination, the urine collection may become visible over a period of time. Precise location usually cannot be identified. A cystogram may confirm or exclude leak from the bladder. If leak is absent, the "cold" mass may be identified on nuclear medicine study. Ultrasound may identify the fluid collection but is nonspecific as to its character. Signal characteristics on MR are those of urine in the adjacent bladder.

LYMPHOCELE

Lymphatics along the iliac vessels disrupted at surgery and renal lymphatics disrupted at harvesting may continue to pour lymph into the area for days and even months. Increased lymph production is present during episodes of rejection and may accelerate lymphocele formation, and association between these two entities is high. Small lymphoceles are commonly found in the peritransplant area and are usually inconsequential. Lymphoceles may attain a large size and may have an adverse effect on the allograft, its vascular supply, ureter, and bladder (Fig. 14–10).

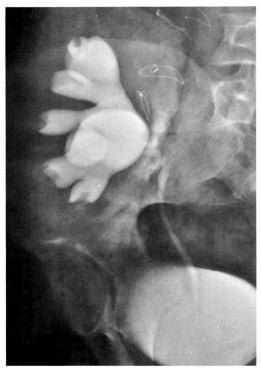

Figure 14–12. Urine extravasation in the region of the proximal ureter.

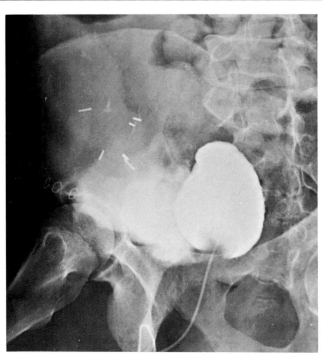

Figure 14–13. Extraperitoneal leak from vesical incision site.

Peritransplant fluid collection is most readily detected by ultrasound. Multiple septations are commonly seen.[37] On MR imaging, the protein-rich lymph is usually of low signal intensity (dark) on T1-weighted and of high signal intensity (bright) on T2-weighted sequences. The common problem in differentiating a urinoma from a lymphocele may be solved by a simple percutaneous aspiration and fluid analysis (Fig. 14–14).

Percutaneous drainage is the treatment of choice (Fig. 14–15). The draining catheter is left in place until several days after cessation of lymph flow. Instillation of sclerosing agents, such as solution of tetracycline or 50 cc of 10% povidone-iodine (Betadine), will facilitate the healing process.[37–39] Secondary infection may promote the healing process but may also be associated with significant morbidity. Differential diagnosis includes ovarian cysts.

HEMATOMA

Hematomas may be postsurgical or secondary to allograft rupture during an episode of severe acute rejection. On MR imaging hematoma is usually seen as a bright (hyperintense) mass on both T1- and T2-weighted sequences. Layering may also be identified. Other imaging modalities are nonspecific. On sonography acute hematoma is anechoic, in subacute stage, hyperechoic, and in a lysed stage (seroma), anechoic.

ABSCESS

Abscess in the renal transplant region may be devastating in the immediate post-transplant period. Pseudoaneurysm at the arterial anastomosis site and exsanguination are possible. Nephrectomy may be the only solution. Otherwise, the abscess may be

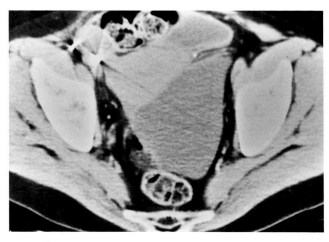

Figure 14–14. Large lymphocele seen on CT.

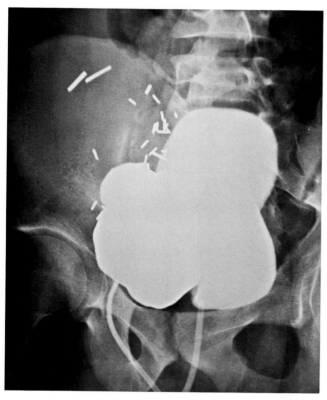

Figure 14–15. Percutaneous drainage of a lymphocele (anterior and to the right). Contrast is also present in the bladder.

drained percutaneously, but only if there is a fluid component present (Fig. 14–16). A complex mass is found on ultrasound. Gas within the abscess may be identified on CT or ultrasound (bright echoes).

Differential features are presented in Table 14–3.

Less Common Complications of Renal Transplantation

Papillary necrosis may be seen on occasion and even cause ureteral obstruction.

Infection may be seen in the presence of indwelling catheters.

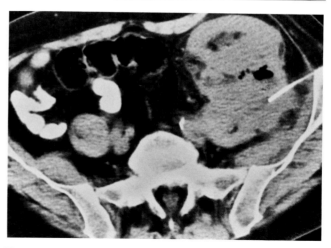

Figure 14–16. Percutaneous drainage of a retrorenal abscess.

Gas in the transplant may be associated with infection (emphysematous pyelonephritis) or may be seen in complete renal artery occlusion (similar to that sometimes found in a dead fetus).[40]

Urolithiasis is rare but should be considered in differential diagnosis of ureteral obstruction (Fig. 14–17).[41]

Autonephrectomy refers to dead, small, calcified renal allograft.

Pseudoaneurysm of the iliac artery may develop after removal of a dead transplant (Fig. 14–18).

Hypertension in Renal Transplant Patients

In the presence of normally functioning renal allograft and normal renal artery surgical anastomotic site, the native diseased kidneys are suspected of producing high renin levels. Transcatheter embolization may be considered. The procedure is usually simple and the postinfarction syndrome is mild, since the native diseased kidneys are usually small.[42,43]

Table 14–3. Differential Features of Peritransplant Fluid Collections

	US	CT	MR	TC-99M DTPA
Urinoma	Anechoic	Enhancing if leaking	T1 dark T2 brighter	"Hot" if leaking
Lymphocele	Anechoic Fine septa	Not enhancing	T1 dark T2 very bright	"Cold"
Hematoma	Hypoechoic Hyperechoic	40–60 HU	T1 bright T2 bright	"Cold"
Abscess	Complex	Complex	T1 dark T2 bright	"Cold"

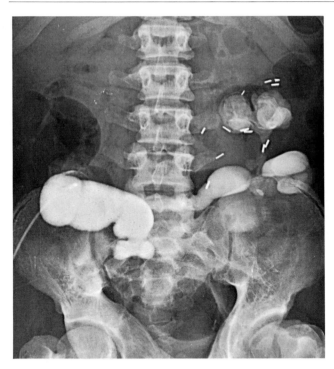

Figure 14–17. Renal allograft more than 15 years old and ileal loop diversion. Renal pelvis is scarred and contracted (purse-string sign). Laminated calculi are present in the upper pole calyces, renal pelvis, and in the ileal loop (scout not shown). Stones were removed using percutaneous approach.

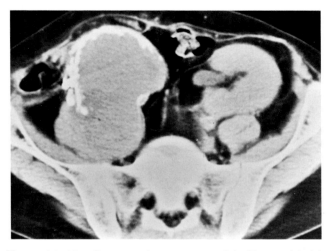

Figure 14–18. Same patient presented in Figure 14–14. Large calcified pseudoaneurysm has developed at the site of a failed allograft which was removed. The new transplant on the left is normal except for asymptomatic lymphocele.

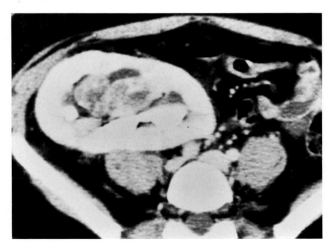

Figure 14–19. Renal carcinoma in a renal allograft.

Cyclosporine-Induced Lymphoproliferative Disorders

The incidence of malignancy in transplant patients is 100 times that for age-matched general population (Fig. 14–19).[44]

Cyclosporine is a suppressor of T-cells. Depression of immune system may result in a variety of infectious diseases and increased incidence of some cancers, such as Kaposi's sarcoma and lymphoma-like lesions. The risk of lymphoma increases in the presence of some viral infections (Epstein-Barr virus).

Lymphoproliferative disorders may resolve spontaneously if the patient is taken off cyclosporine. Enlarged lymph nodes or involvement of liver or other organs may be detected.[45,46]

Pulmonary Infections

Patients on cyclosporine immunosuppression may develop opportunistic infections. Cytomegalovirus (CMV), *Pneumocystis carinii*, *Legionella*, and *Pseudomonas* are the most common. Single- or multiple-organism infections are possible. In general, on chest radiographs, focal consolidation and pleural effusion favor bacterial or fungal origin. Diffuse interstitial or reticulonodular pattern favors CMV or *Pneumocystis* infection.[47]

REFERENCES

1. Walker TG, Geller SC, Delmonico FL, et al. Donor renal angiography: its influence on the decision to use the right or left kidney. AJR 1988; 151:1149–1151.

2. Spencer W, Streem SB, Geisinger MA, et al. Outpatient angiographic evaluation of living renal donors. J Urol 1988; 140:1364–1366.
3. Burgener FA, Schabel SI. The radiographic size of renal transplants. Radiology 1975; 117:547–550.
4. Hricak H, Cruz C, Eyler WR, et al. Acute post-transplantation renal failure: differential diagnosis by ultrasound. Radiology 1981; 139:441–449.
5. Heckman R, Rehwald U, Jakubowski HD, et al. Sonographic criteria for renal allograft rejection. Urol Radiol 1982; 4:15–18.
6. Hricak H, Romanski RN, Eyler WR. The renal sinus during allograft rejection. Sonographic and histopathologic findings. Radiology 1982; 142:693–699.
7. McConnell JD, Sagalowsky AI, Lewis SE, et al. Prospective evaluation of renal allograft dysfunction with Tc 99m-DTPA renal scans. J Urol 1984; 131:875–878.
8. Hricak H, Terrier F, Marotti M, et al. Posttransplant renal injection: comparison of quantitative scintigraphy, US, and MR imaging. Radiology 1987; 162:685–688.
9. Mitchell DG, Roza AM, Spritzer CE, et al. Acute renal allograft rejection: difficulty in diagnosis of histologically mild cases by MR imaging. J Comput Assist Tomogr 1986; 11:655–663.
10. Hoddick W, Filly RA, Backman U, et al. Renal allograft rejection: US evaluation. Radiology 1986; 161:469–473.
11. Linkowski GD, Warvariv V, Filly RA, Vincenti F. Sonography in the diagnosis of acute renal allograft rejection and cyclosporine nephrotoxicity. AJR 1987; 148:291–295.
12. Steinberg HV, Nelson RC, Murphy FB, et al. Renal allograft rejection: evaluation by Doppler US and MR imaging. Radiology 1987; 162:337–342.
13. Genkins SM, Sanfilippo FP, Carroll B. Duplex Doppler sonography of renal transplants: lack of sensitivity and specificity in establishing pathologic diagnosis. AJR 1989; 152:535–539.
14. Don S, Kopecky KK, Filo RS, et al. Duplex Doppler US in renal allografts: causes of elevated resistive index. Radiology 1989; 171:709–712.
15. Kim EE, Pjeura G, Lowry P, et al. Cyclosporin-A nephrotoxicity and acute cellular rejection in renal transplant recipients: correlation between radionuclide and histologic findings. Radiology 1986; 159:443.
16. Kaude JV, Hawkins IF Jr. Angiography of renal transplant. Radiol Clin North Am 1976; 14:295–308.
17. Babcock DS, Slovis TL, Han BK, McEnery P, McWilliams DR. Renal transplants in children: long term follow-up using sonography. Radiology 1985; 156:165–167.
18. Mathew TH. Recurrence of disease following renal transplantation. Am J Kidney Dis 1988; 12:85–96.
19. Taylor KJW, Morse SS, Rigsby CM, Bia M, Schiff M. Vascular complications in renal allografts: detection with duplex Doppler US. Radiology 1987; 162:31–38.
20. Stringer DA, O'Halpin D, Daneman A, et al. Duplex Doppler sonography for renal artery stenosis in the post-transplant pediatric patient. Pediatr Radiol 1989; 19:187–192.
21. Sinderman KW, Sprayregen S, Sos TA, et al. Percutaneous transluminal angioplasty in renal transplant arterial stenosis for relief of hypertension. Transplantation 1980; 30:440–444.
22. Raynaud A, Bedronsian J, Perry P, et al. Percutaneous transluminal angioplasty of renal transplant artery stenosis. AJR 1986; 146:853–857.
23. Gerlock AJ, MacDonell RC, Smith CW, et al. Renal transplant arterial stenosis: percutaneous transluminal angioplasty. AJR 1983; 140:325–331.
24. Raval B, Balsara V, Kim EE. Computed tomography detection of transplant renal artery pseudoaneurysm. J Comput Assist Tomogr 1985; 9:149–150.
25. Morton MJ, Charboneau JW. Arteriovenous fistula after biopsy of renal transplant: detection and monitoring with color flow and duplex ultrasonography. Mayo Clin Proc 1989; 64:531–534.
26. Middleton WD, Erickson S, Melson GL. Perivascular color artifact: pathologic significance and appearance on color Doppler US images. Radiology 1989; 171:647–652.
27. Middleton WD, Kellman GM, Melson GL, Madrazo BL. Postbiopsy renal transplant arteriovenous fistulas: color Doppler US characteristics. Radiology 1989; 171:253–257.
28. Reuther G, Wanjura D, Bauer H. Acute renal vein thrombosis in renal allografts: detection with duplex Doppler US. Radiology 1989; 170:557–558.
29. Taylor KJW, Morse SS, Rigsby CM, et al. Vascular complications in renal allografts: detection with duplex Doppler US. Radiology 1987; 162:31–38.
30. Barbaric ZL, Thompson KR. Percutaneous nephropyelostomy in the management of obstructed renal transplants. Radiology 1978; 126:639–642.
31. Curry N, Cochran ST, Barbaric ZL, et al. Interventional radiological procedures in renal transplants. Radiology 1984; 152:647–653.
32. Glanc S, Rotter MR, Gordon DH, et al. Interventional radiologic procedures in the management of renal transplant patient. Urol Radiol 1985; 7:97–101.
33. Steem SB, Novic AC, Steinmuller DR, et al. Percutaneous techniques for the management of urological renal transplant complications. J Urol 1986; 135:456–501.
34. Smith TP, Hunter DW, Letourneau JG, et al. Urinary obstruction in renal transplants: diagnosis by antegrade pyelography and results of percutaneous treatment. AJR 1988; 151:507–510.
35. Lang EK, Glorioso LW III. Antegrade transluminal dilatation of benign ureteral strictures: long term results. AJR 1988; 155:131–134.
36. Voegli DR, Crummy AB, McDermott JC, Jensen SR. Percutaneous dilatation of ureteral strictures in renal transplant patients. Radiology 1988; 169:185–188.
37. von Sonnenberg E, Wittich GR, Casola G, et al. Lymphoceles: imaging characteristics and percutaneous management. Radiology 1986; 161:593–596.
38. Cohan RH, Saeed M, Sussman SK, et al. Percutaneous drainage of pelvic lymphatic fluid collections in the renal transplant patients. Invest Radiol 1987; 22:864–867.
39. White M, Mueller PR, Ferrucci JT Jr, et al. Percutaneous drainage of postoperative abdominal and pelvic lymphoceles. AJR 1985; 145:1065–1069.
40. Potter JL, Sullivan BM, Flournoy JG, Gerza C. Emphysema in the renal allograft. Radiology 1985; 155:51–55.
41. Cho DK, Zackson DA, Cheig J, et al. Urinary calculi in renal transplant recipients. Transplantation 1988; 45:899.
42. Fletcher EWL, Thompson JF, Chalmers DHK, et al. Embolization of host kidneys for the control of hyper-

tension after renal transplantation: radiological aspects. Br J Radiol 1984; 57:279–284.

43. Thompson JF, Wood RFM, Taylor HM, et al. Control of hypertension after renal transplantation by embolization of host kidneys. Lancet 1984; 2:424–427.

44. Penn I. Tumor incidence in human allograft recipients. Transplant Proc 1979; 11:1047–1051.

45. Harris KM, Schwartz ML, Slasky BS, et al. Posttransplantation cyclosporine-induced lymphoproliferative disorders: clinical and radiologic manifestations. Radiology 1987; 162:697–700.

46. Honda H, Franken EA Jr, Barloon TJ, Smith JL. Hepatic lymphoma in cyclosporine-treated transplant recipients: sonographic and CT findings. AJR 1989; 152:501–503.

47. Moore EH, Webb WR, Amend WJC. Pulmonary infections in renal transplantation patients treated with cyclosporine. Radiology 1988; 167:97–103.

15

Ureter

URETERAL DISPLACEMENT

Normal ureters are 24–30 cm long and are bound to be affected by numerous adjacent pathological processes that occur along the way. A word of caution: absence of ureteral displacement does not exclude any disease enumerated below and normal variants

in regard to ureteral position may invoke false-positive diagnosis of retroperitoneal disease. Regarding displacement, the ureter is a treacherous waterway (Fig. 15–1):

1. Enlarged para-aortic lymph nodes typically displace upper ureters laterally (Fig. 15–2), while

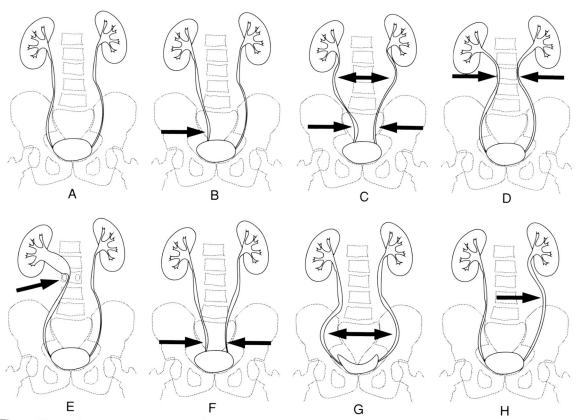

Figure 15–1. Schematic drawings of various types of ureteral displacement. **(A)** Normal; **(B)** normal variant in females, iliac lymph node enlargement, or iliac artery aneurysm; **(C)** massive lymph node enlargement; **(D)** retroperitoneal fibrosis; **(E)** retrocaval ureter; **(F)** hypertrophied psoas muscles, normal after AP resection, iliac lymph node enlargement; **(G)** pelvic mass; and **(H)** aortic aneurysm, any primary retroperitoneal tumor or fluid collection.

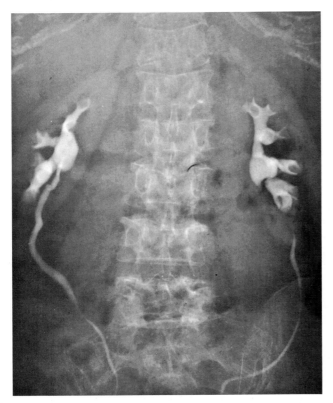

Figure 15–2. Lateral ureteral displacement due to massive para-aortic lymph node enlargement.

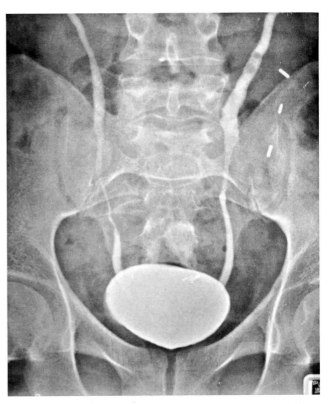

Figure 15–3. Medial ureteral displacement by enlarged iliac nodes in a patient with lymphoma.

enlarged iliac chain lymph nodes displace ureters medially (Fig. 15–3).

2. Retroperitoneal fibrosis typically retracts mid-ureters medially.
3. Any retroperitoneal mass, such as lymphoma, abdominal aorta or iliac artery aneurysm, hematoma, abscess, lymphocele, urinoma, or primary retroperitoneal tumor, may displace the ureter in a particular direction, depending on the origin of the mass. If the displacement is in anteroposterior direction, it may not be detected without oblique views.
4. Pelvic masses originating from female reproductive organs typically displace ureters laterally and posteriorly.
5. After abdominoperineal resection, distal ureters migrate medially (Fig. 15–4).
6. Bladder diverticulum may originate and enlarge so that the distal ureteral segment is displaced medially.
7. Normal variants: a) Distal right ureteral segment in females may be normally positioned medially to the extent that it mimics displacement by a tumor mass (Fig. 15–5).[1] This variant of normal is also rarely seen on the left side; b) proximal ureter

may normally cross the psoas anteriorly and abruptly, so that it resembles displacement by a mass; c) in younger muscular athletes both ureters may be displaced medially by hypertrophied psoas muscle (Figs. 15–6, 15–7); d) it just happens (Fig. 15–8).

8. Instrumentation and various ureteral catheters may displace or "tent" the ureter (Fig. 15–9).

WIDE URETER

Abnormal dilatation of the ureter need not be the result of a mechanical ureteral obstruction.[2] Other causes may be responsible and are enumerated below.

Polyuria. Classic example is upper system dilatation in association with diabetes insipidus where enormous quantities of urine may overwhelm the capacity of the system over a period of time. Complicating factor is the almost inevitable development of increased bladder pressures which may lead to reflux, infection, and "non-neurogenic neurogenic bladder."

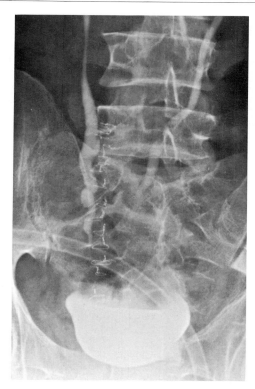

Figure 15–4. Normal medial position of the ureters after abdominoperineal resection.

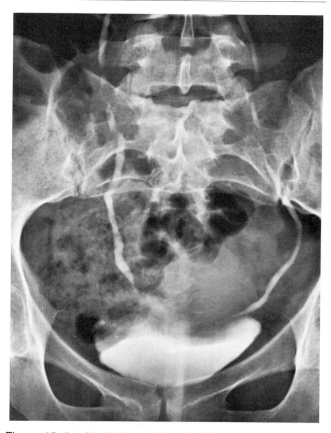

Figure 15–5. Medially positioned right ureter in a female patient was a normal variant. However, one should be concerned about possible iliac lymph node enlargement or other pathology.

Infection. Bacterial toxins may have paralytic effect on ureteral peristalsis and wide ureter is often seen associated with infection.[3]

Obstruction. Obstruction is the most common cause of ureteral dilatation.

Primary Megaureter. This disease entity is described below.

Outflow Bladder Obstruction. Increased bladder pressure transmits across ureterovesical junction, which in turn causes ureteral dilatation.

Dysplasia. Poor or incomplete development of ureteral smooth muscles also results in ureteral dilatation.

Reflux. Vesicoureteral reflux is a common cause of ureteral dilatation. High vesical pressures during voiding contribute to ureteral dilatation.

Ectopic Ureter and Ureterocele. Both malformations may be associated with varying degrees of obstruction and dilatation.

Pregnancy. Ureters are affected during pregnancy in several ways. They become lax and dilated, proba-

bly as a result of increased progesterone levels and the compression of the enlarged uterus against pelvic brim. Gonadal veins enlarge severalfold in diameter and may impress on the ureter.

LOCALIZED URETERAL NARROWING

Stricture. Ureteral narrowing due to fibrosis is a common form of narrowing (Fig. 15–10). Stricture may be the result of an inflammatory disease, impacted ureteral calculus (Fig. 15–11), localized periureteral fibrosis, tuberculosis, schistosomiasis, iatrogenic injury, adjacent surgery, radiation injury, and polyarteritis nodosa.[4] The cause may not be readily known (Fig. 15–12). Rare congenital strictures have been described in infants.

Treatment of ureteral strictures may involve retrograde or antegrade balloon dilatation (Fig. 15–13). Depending on the size of the patient, 4 to 10 mm

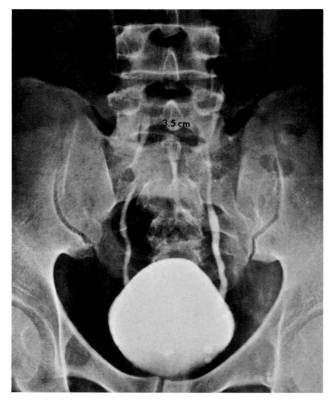

Figure 15–6.   A young athlete with medial ureters due to psoas hypertrophy.

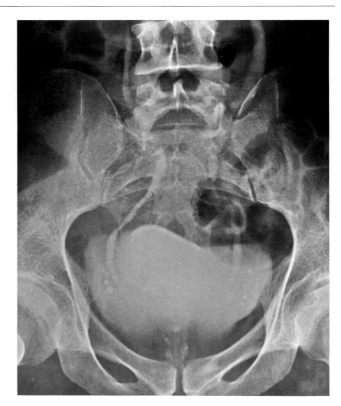

Figure 15–7.   An Olympic weightlifter with medial ureters due to psoas hypertrophy.

balloon diameters may be used, followed by 4 to 6 weeks of stenting, preferably by a 10 F stent. Long-term success rates for different anatomical sites and types of strictures are presented in Table 1.[5–8]

Metastases.   Metastases to the ureter from a distant source (not extension from an adjacent tumor) are indistinguishable from other causes of localized ureteral narrowing (Fig. 15–14). The most common are metastases from the breast, colon, thyroid, prostate (Fig. 15–15), cervix (Fig. 15–16), rectum, and melanomas (Fig. 15–17). Lymphoma is rare.[9] Metastases do not necessarily involve the mucosa and hematuria is infrequent. Therefore ureteral brushing and urine cytology need not produce malignant cells.

CT may demonstrate smooth, localized thickening of the ureter with disappearing lumen, without evidence of a periureteral mass.[10,11]

Amyloidosis.   A rare cause of ureteral narrowing is localized amyloid deposit beneath the mucosa. Hematuria and obstruction are possible.[12,13]

Primary Megaureter.   This entity is described elsewhere in this chapter.

Vessel Crossings.   Normal vessels which may make an imprint on the ureter, thereby making it narrow, are: a) aberrant lower pole renal artery; b) right gonadal vein (Fig. 15–18); c) left gonadal vein; and d) iliac arteries. Gonadal vessels are anterior to the ureter. Iliac vessels are posterior to the ureter.

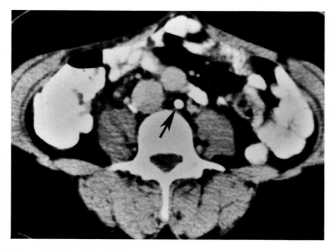

Figure 15–8.   The left ureter deviates medially and for several centimeters is seen posterior to the abdominal aorta (arrow). This is not circumaortic ureter and is an incidental finding.

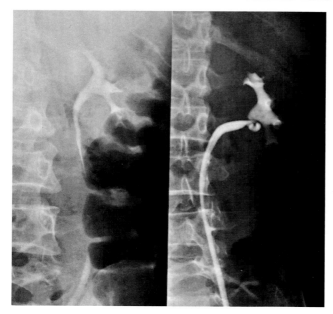

Figure 15–9. Normal EXU (left) and "tenting" of the ureter (right) produced by a stiff retrograde catheter.

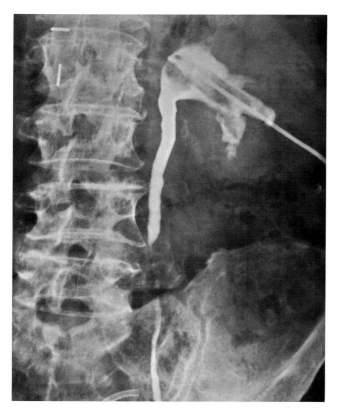

Figure 15–10. Short mid-ureteral stricture causing partial obstruction. Percutaneous nephrostomy is in place surrounded by a blood clot, which appears as a radiolucent filling defect.

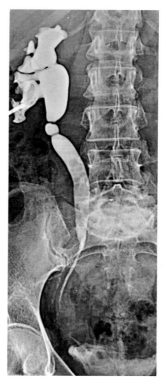

Figure 15–11. Long distal ureteral stricture in a patient with prior calculous disease. The bands of apparent narrowing in the proximal ureter may be regarded as ureteral valves and are of no clinical significance.

Extrinsic Compression. In addition to vessels, apparent ureteral narrowing may be due to extrinsic compression by enlarged lymph nodes (Fig. 15–19), primary retroperitoneal tumors, lower pole renal masses, retroperitoneal fluid collections, etc. (Fig. 15–20).

Endometriosis. Possibly a lesion that may be diagnosed by MR imaging. Endometriosis usually appears hyperintense on both T1- and T2-weighted images. Otherwise, a mass indistinguishable from other neoplasms is seen.[14]

Congenital Bands. Congenital bands are rare and may occasionally cause ureteral obstruction.

Malakoplakia. Malakoplakia most commonly involves the bladder but may be present in the ureter and produce narrowing sufficient to cause obstruction.[15]

PRIMARY MEGAURETER

Incidence. Four times more common in males. Bilateral in 20% and almost always in males.

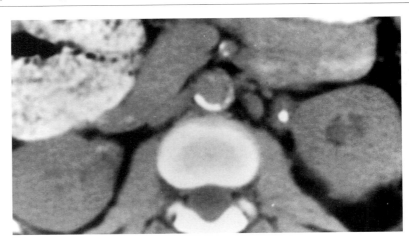

Figure 15–12. Nonenhanced CT. Retrograde stent is in place, transverses an area where a ureteral stricture is present. The fibrotic process probably involves more than the wall of the ureter and may be termed periureteral fibrosis. Differentiation from primary tumor or metastases is not possible. MR imaging may provide additional insight. Old fibrotic tissue is hypointense on T2-weighted sequences as opposed to malignant tissues, which are hyperintense.

Pathology.   Abnormal dilatation of the ureter with the exception of the very distal juxtavesical aperistaltic segment. Histologically, aperistaltic distal ureteral segment may exhibit: a) muscular hypoplasia; b) mural fibrosis; c) collagenous infiltration; d) abnormal smooth muscle orientation; or e) it may be normal.

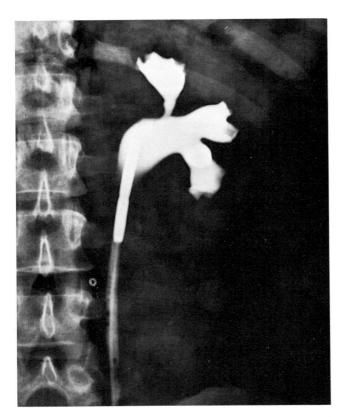

Figure 15–13.   Retrograde dilatation of a UPJ. (Photograph courtesy of Dr. G. Fuchs.)

Pathophysiology.   Neuromuscular dysfunction of the aperistaltic distal ureteral segment eventually causes distention and inefficient peristaltic activity in the rest of the ureter.

Clinical Presentation.   Asymptomatic, infection, pain, hematuria, urolithiasis.

Treatment.   Ureteroneocystotomy if clinically indicated.

Radiological Findings.   Primary megaureter is the diagnosis of exclusion. Other numerous causes for distal ureteral obstruction must be dismissed. These include ureteral calculi, strictures, neoplasms, ureteroceles, ectopic insertion, iatrogenic injury, etc. Vesicoureteral reflux and long-standing prior obstruction, now resolved, may also be associated with a dilated ureter. Outflow bladder obstruction from whatever cause must also be excluded.

On radiographic examination, the ureter is dilated, ending with a bulbous appearance at or just above the bladder (Fig. 15–21).[16–18] The upper segment may be less distended than the lower. The collecting system may also be dilated (Fig. 15–22). The aperistaltic segment is rarely seen. The relatively diagnostic feature is the funneling of the ureter from the dilated segment into the aperistaltic segment, which may be seen only in an oblique projection and only intermittently (Fig. 15–23).

Retrograde ureterography will demonstrate absence of mechanical obstruction and the catheter will pass with ease through the aperistaltic ureteral segment.

Vesicoureteral reflux has been described in patients with primary megaureter (Fig. 15–24).[19]

Primary megaureter may be also seen in association with megacalyces[20,21] and ureteropelvic (UPJ) obstruction (Fig. 15–25).[22,23]

Table 15-1.   Long-Term Success in Percutaneous Treatment of Ureteral Strictures

	%	REFERENCES
Ureteroenteric strictures	16	Shapiro et al.[5]
UPJ percutaneous pyeloplasty	85	Lang and Glorioso;[6] Beckmann et al.[7]
Acquired strictures less than 3 months old	90	Beckmann et al.;[7] Chang et al.[8]
Acquired strictures older than 3 months	54	Beckmann et al.[7]

SIMPLE URETEROCELE

Pathology. Dilatation of the intramural ureteral segment caused by congenital or acquired stenosis at the distal ureteral orifice. Dilated segment protrudes into the bladder. Calculi within the ureterocele are common.

Clinical Presentation.   Most ureteroceles are small and asymptomatic. Calculi may form within the ureterocele. Obstruction and infection involving the upper system may be the presenting symptoms. On occasion, ureterocele may cause outflow bladder obstruction, particularly if it is large.

Radiological Findings.   "Cobra head" appearance is the pathognomonic radiographic finding on excretory urography (Fig. 15–26). Radiographic contrast in the bladder is separated from the contrast within the dilated ureterocele by a thin radiolucent line representing bladder and ureteral mucosa.

An intraluminal bladder filling defect is seen if bladder but not ureterocele is filled with contrast. Ureteral calculus is identified on the preliminary radiograph (Fig. 15–27).

Ultrasound is well suited to diagnose not only ureteroceles but also the presence of calculi and the degree of the obstruction of the upper system, if any.

In infants the ureterocele may become very large and fill the entire bladder or cause outflow bladder obstruction. Under these circumstances, the diagnosis may be difficult, since the ureterocele may be mistaken for a normal bladder.

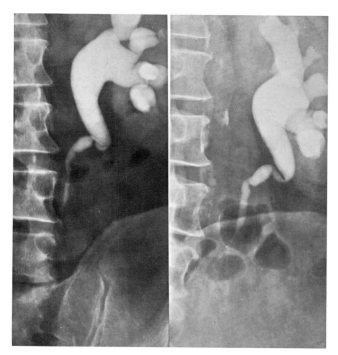

Figure 15–14. Carcinoma of the prostate with a distant localized metastasis in the ureter.

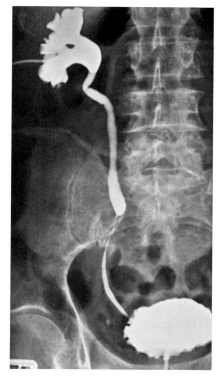

Figure 15–15. Metastasis from carcinoma of the prostate causing ureteral narrowing.

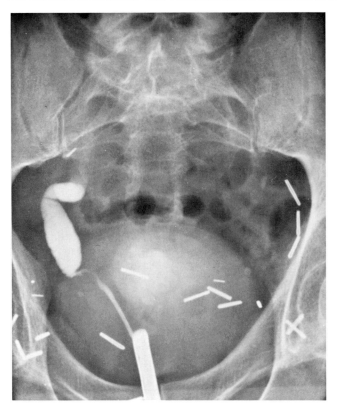

Figure 15–16. Cervical carcinoma involving the distal ureter and causing obstruction.

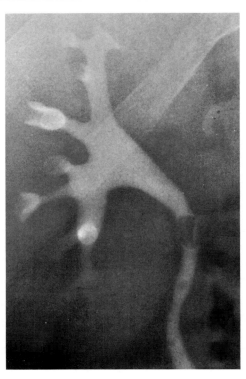

Figure 15–17. Ureteral metastasis from malignant melanoma. This particular metastasis presented as a filling defect rather than ureteral narrowing. Differential diagnosis includes TCC, blood clot, radiolucent calculus, sloughed papilla, and other entities.

ECTOPIC URETER AND URETEROCELE

Incidence. Relatively rare. More frequent in children and young adults. Definite female preponderance.

Pathology. Anomalous distal ureteral insertion is most commonly associated with complete duplication.[24] The ureter of the lower moiety inserts into the bladder more superiorly and laterally in relation to its counterpart. The upper moiety ureter usually crosses the lower ureter twice while coursing toward the bladder. Bladder insertion of the upper moiety ureter is more distal and medial.

The two ureteral orifices are usually in close proximity and in no way interfere with function.

However, intramural portion of the lower moiety ureter is usually short, an anatomical mishap, which results in increased incidence of vesicoureteral reflux in that system.

Ureteral insertion of the upper moiety may be ectopic and empty low in the bladder, posterior urethra and vagina, uterus, seminal vesicle, ejaculatory duct, and vas deferens. Such an ectopic orifice is

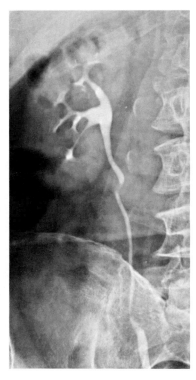

Figure 15–18. Vascular impression upon the right ureter by gonadal vein and common iliac vessels.

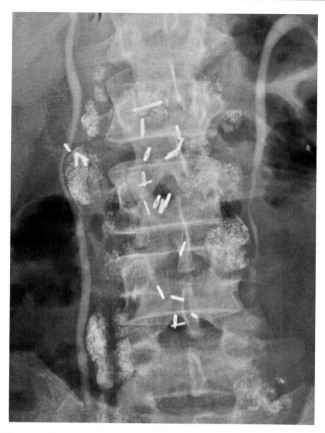

Figure 15–19. Localized ureteral narrowing caused by lymph node enlargement. Lymphangiogram has been done to render lymph nodes visible.

more likely to become obstructed or associated with constant urine leak and dribbling.

Ectopic ureterocele is commonly associated with upper moiety ureteral insertion.

Clinical Presentation. Urinary tract infection, loss of urine (dribbling), dysuria, and flank pain.

Radiological Findings

Ectopia Without Obstruction. In this situation the ureteral orifice is either in the low position in the bladder or in the proximal urethra (Fig. 15–28). Other ectopic sites are usually associated with obstruction. On an excretory urogram, it may be possible to identify the ectopic insertion site. While catheterizing the bladder, the catheter may be inadvertently inserted into the ectopic ureter, which empties into urethra.

Ectopia With Obstruction. The upper moiety ureter is more commonly obstructed than the lower. Nonfunctioning hydronephrotic and dysplastic segment may change the orientation of the functioning lower moiety. The mass effect of such a hydronephrotic segment may displace the pelvocalyceal system of the lower moiety, resulting in pathognomonic *drooping lily* sign on urography or pyelography (Fig. 15–29). Dilated upper moiety ureter is likely to cause impressions on the lower ureter.

Ultrasound is an excellent diagnostic method for detecting dilated obstructed system and may also estimate the thickness of the renal parenchyma and frequently the site of the ectopic insertion.[25] The functional reserve of the obstructed and probably dysplastic system deserves consideration, since a functionally recoverable segment may be preserved by ureteroneocystotomy of the ectopic ureter. Tc-99m-DTPA or Tc-99m-MAG₃ functional evaluation may be considered. If the segment is small and hydronephrotic with thin parenchyma, this is unnecessary, and partial nephrectomy and ureterectomy are indicated.

An important part of the radiologic evaluation is determination of the exact insertion site. Frequently, this cannot be accomplished by any other means but antegrade pyelography.

Ectopic Ureterocele. Most ectopic ureteroceles are associated with obstruction (Fig. 15–30). Mass effect in the bladder may be observed on contrast examination or the cystic dilatation is seen on ultrasound. Bulging ureterocele may partially protrude into the vagina and become palpable on physical examination. Needle aspiration and retrograde contrast injection into the ureterocele (retrograde ureterocelegram) may help pinpoint the exact site of distal insertion (Fig. 15-31).

If the upper moiety is severely dysplastic and afunctional, there need not be any dilatation of the upper part of the system, an entity referred to as *ureterocele disproportion* (Fig. 15–32).[26]

In rare instances an ectopic ureterocele may prolapse through the urethra and be visible on physical examination. Outflow bladder obstruction may be the presenting symptom.[27]

PSEUDOURETEROCELE

Inflammation, neoplasm, or calculus may produce distal ureteral dilatation that resembles a ureterocele (Fig. 15–33). Differentiating feature is a relatively thick wall in pseudoureterocele compared with a very thin wall seen in true ureterocele. This is an important point, since neoplasm enters in the differential diagnosis of pseudoureterocele.[28,29]

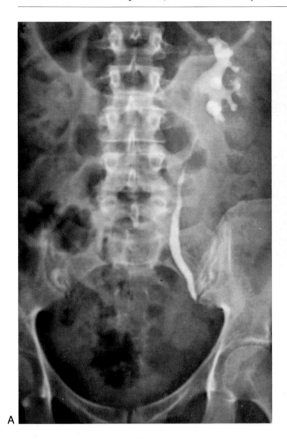

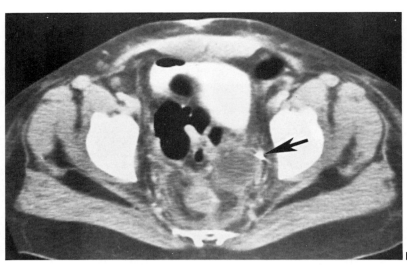

Figure 15–20. (A) Left ureteral narrowing causing mild obstruction in the solitary kidney seen on EXU. (B) Extrinsic compression on the ureter (arrow) is caused by a localized periureteric hematoma which resulted from recent pelvic surgery.

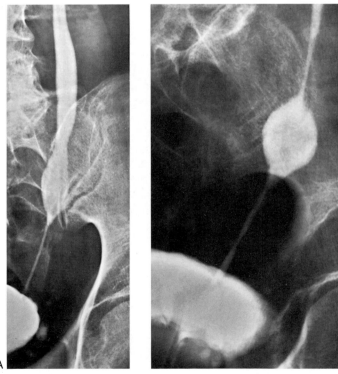

Figure 15–21. Primary megaureter. (A) Retrograde ureterogram demonstrates dilated upper ureter ending in a bulbous segment, which tapers into a narrow segment. (B) Under fluoroscopy peristalsis was seen in the entire ureter with the exception of the very distal segment. Here the peristaltic wave has reached the distal ureter but no contrast is being expelled. There was no difficulty in introducing the retrograde catheter, another feature of this disease.

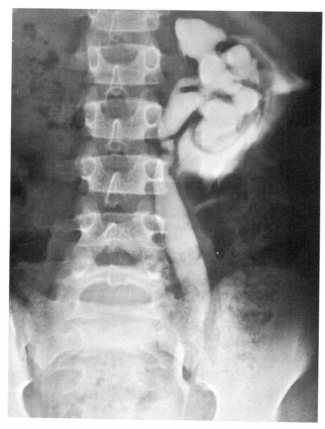

Figure 15–22. Primary megaureter resulting in moderate hydronephrosis and loss of renal function. When the ureter becomes so dilated, peristalsis is ineffectual in propelling urine through the afunctional segment. This is an antegrade pyelogram and some contrast extravasation is seen around the kidney, allowing us to judge the extent of renal parenchyma atrophy.

RETROCAVAL URETER

Retrocaval ureter is a rare congenital anomaly in which the ureter passes posterior to and around the inferior vena cava (Fig. 15–34). The anomaly occurs when the infrarenal vena cava segment is formed from the subcardinal vein.[30] Such entrapment may cause significant ureteral obstruction. Diagnosis is made on retrograde pyelogram. Ureter is seen looping medial to the vertebral pedicle at L-2 and L-3 level (Figs. 15–1E, 15–35). CT may also demonstrate retrocaval ureter if the ureteral lumen is opacified.[31] With sonography, the diagnosis is somewhat more difficult.[32] Ureteral division and reanastomosis is the accepted method of treatment if obstruction is present. Some have proposed division and reanastomosis of the inferior vena cava.

Left retrocaval ureter has been described associated with anomalous presence of the left inferior vena cava.

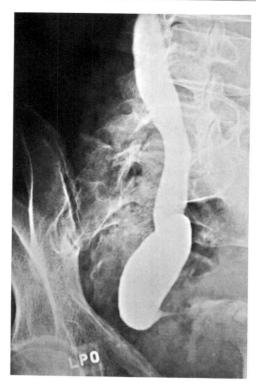

Figure 15–23. Primary megaureter in an adult patient with benign prostatic hypertrophy.

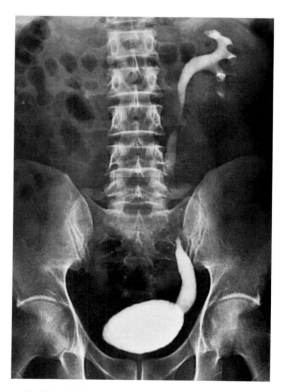

Figure 15–24. Primary megaureter and coexisting vesicoureteral reflux. The diagnosis may be confirmed by performing an EXU while keeping the bladder empty with a draining catheter.

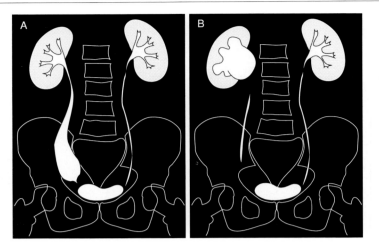

Figure 15–25. Schematic drawing of primary megaureter (**A**) and coexisting megaureter and ureteropelvic junction obstruction (UPJO) (**B**). In this case the UPJO is more dominant and the ureter is not dilated as seen on EXU.

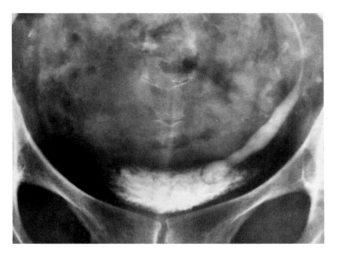

Figure 15–26. Small simple ureterocele.

A rare transcaval ureter has also been described. The ureter splits the inferior vena cava and medial deviation is less than in retrocaval ureter.[33]

RETROILIAC URETER

Retroiliac ureter is very rare and it is usually only detected when it is complicated by obstruction.[34] This entity is somewhat more difficult to diagnose, since there is no significant ureteral deviation from the expected pathway. The normal vascular impression frequently seen on excretory urography or retrograde studies may appear somewhat more exaggerated. The diagnosis may be arrived at unequivocally if there is a radiopaque retrograde ureteral

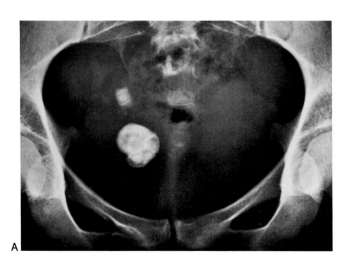

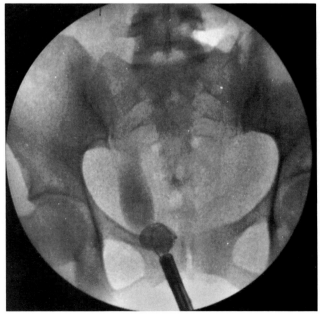

Figure 15–27. Simple ureterocele containing a calculus. (**A**) Preliminary radiograph. The larger stone is in the ureterocele, the smaller in the ureter above. (**B**) Endoscopic manipulation of the calculus. (Photograph courtesy of Dr. G. Fuchs.)

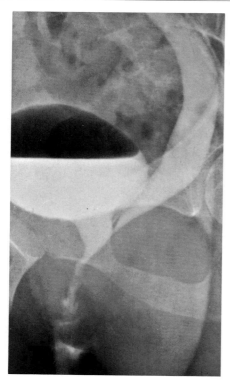

Figure 15–28. VCUG in upright position. Ectopic insertion of the left ureter into the urethra. Reflux into the ureter (urethroureteral reflux) is present only during voiding.

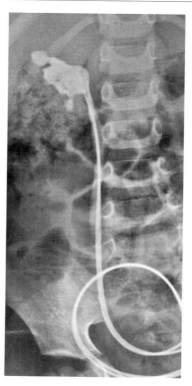

Figure 15–29. Drooping lily sign. Hydronephrotic upper moiety is responsible for peculiar displacement of the contrast-filled lower moiety.

catheter in place and a limited CT is done over the crossing area.

CONGENITAL URETERAL DIVERTICULA

Solitary ureteral diverticulum probably represents a blind-ending ureter, formed during an attempted but failed duplication (abortive ureter) (Fig. 15–36). Patients are usually asymptomatic. On retrograde ureterography or excretory urography, the appearance is that of a blind-ending ureter of various lengths (Fig. 15–37). Transitional cell carcinoma or urolithiasis may be found.[35,36]

ABNORMAL VASCULAR IMPRESSIONS

Arterial supply to the ureter is from segmental renal arteries (Fig. 15–38), lumbar arteries, and internal iliac branches. Ureteric arteries freely anastomose along the entire length of the ureter and serve as an important collateral pathway in renal artery stenosis.

Venous drainage parallels that of arterial supply. In addition to the common finding of ureteral impressions caused by normal vascular structures, such as gonadal veins and iliac vessels, several pathological processes may be diagnosed or suggested because of this finding.

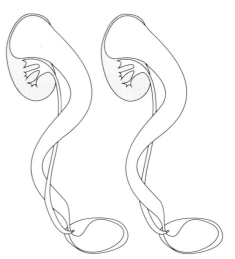

Figure 15–30. Schematic drawings of ectopic ureteroceles with upper moiety obstruction.

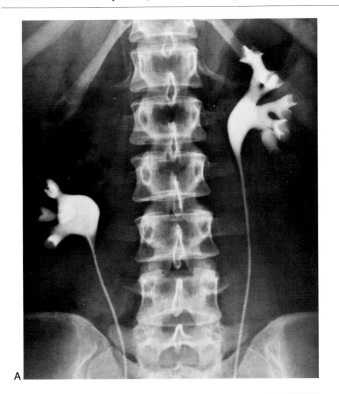

A

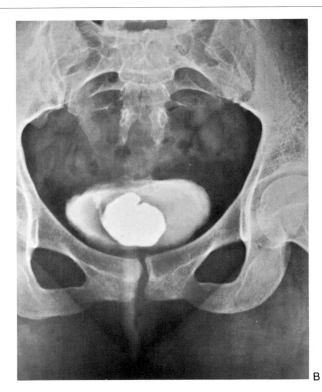

B

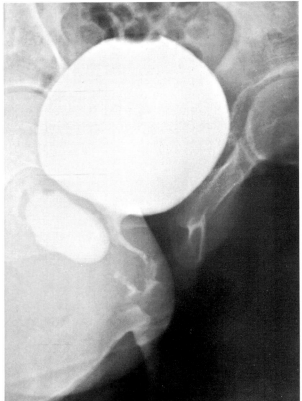

C

Figure 15–31. (A) Retrograde pyelogram demonstrates only the lower moiety on the right side. Only one ureteral orifice was identified on cystoscopy. (B) A cystic mass was palpated posterior to urethra, punctured with a small needle, and injected with contrast. (C) Only an oblique projection demonstrates a ureterocele and its relation to the urethra where the ectopic orifice was meant to be.

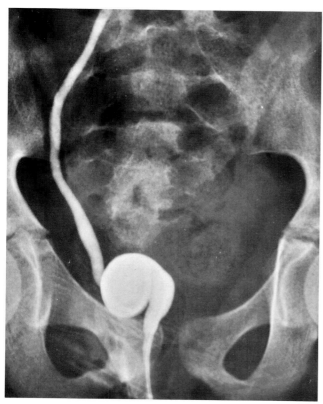

Figure 15–32. Retrograde ureterogram in a boy with an ectopic ureter draining into prostatic urethra. A part of the distal ureter is dilated and probably can be classified as a ureterocele. Above it, the ureter leading to a small dysplastic segment appears to be nonobstructed.

Periureteral Venous Varices

The ureter is surrounded by a plexus of veins incorporated in the areolar periureteral tissues known as Waldeyer's sheet. This venous plexus may enlarge spontaneously (Fig. 15–39) or it may enlarge because of increased left renal venous pressures, such as can be present in the nutcracker syndrome or presence of an intravenous tumor (Fig. 15–40). Enlarged venous channels impress upon the ureter, causing 1–2 cm indentations. Unlike impressions by enlarged lymph nodes, impressions by enlarged veins are seen on both sides of the ureter and may disappear if external ureteral compression is applied. The enlarged periureteral venous plexus should not be confused with gonadal veins.

The right ovarian vein varices usually seen postpartum may partially obstruct the right ureter, a condition referred to as *ovarian vein syndrome.*

Periureteral Arterial Collaterals

Arterial collaterals develop in association with renal artery stenosis and may impress upon ureters causing ureteral "notching" (see Fig. 12–21). This is one of the findings seen in renal vascular hypertension.

Polyarteritis Nodosa

In rare instances polyarteritis nodosa may involve periureteral vessels and produce ureteral "notching."[37]

URETERITIS CYSTICA

Etiology. Unknown, seen in patients with recurrent urinary tract infection.

Pathology. Multiple small cystic structures involving the bladder (cystitis cystica), and occasionally ureter and renal pelvis (pyelitis cystica). Histologically, they represent downward proliferating urothelium and metaplasia of Von Brunn's nests.

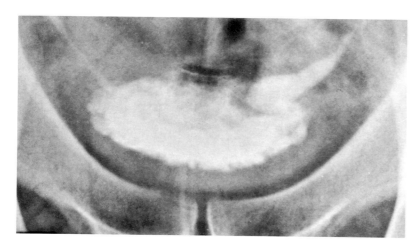

Figure 15–33. Pseudoureterocele caused by a small transitional cell carcinoma at the ureteral orifice. Carcinoma is seen as a negative "filling" defect at the tip of the ureterocele.

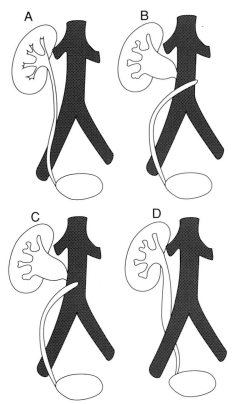

Figure 15–34. Schematic drawing of ureteral relations to major veins. **(A)** Normal; **(B)** retrocaval ureter; **(C)** transcaval ureter; and **(D)** retroiliac ureter.

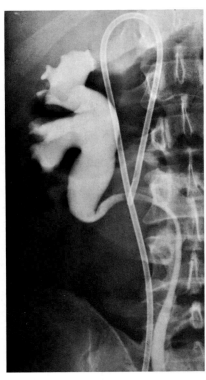

Figure 15–35. EXU in a patient with a retrocaval ureter. An enormous catheter has been placed in the inferior vena cava by a urologist (in the old days urologists were contemplating doing angiography).

Clinical Presentation. Recurrent urinary tract infections. More common in women. Small cystic changes persist for a long time after eradication of infection.

Radiological Findings. Small multiple intraluminal filling defects may be seen in the pelvis (Fig. 15–41), ureters (Figs. 15–42, 15–43) and bladder.[38–40] These should not be confused with ureteral notching seen in renal vascular hypertension or periureteral venous varices or with other types of intraluminal filling defects, including transitional cell carcinoma (Fig. 15–44).

URETERAL PSEUDODIVERTICULOSIS

Pathology. Reactive hyperplasia of transitional epithelium secondary to inflammation.[41,42] The diverticula represent downward proliferation of epithelium into the loose connective tissue of the lamina propria, producing outpouchings. These do not con-

tain all layers of the ureter, nor are they mucosal protrusions through the muscular wall.

Clinical Presentation. Incidental finding. Patients may have a risk factor for transitional cell carcinoma and interval follow-up is suggested.

Laboratory Findings. Urinalysis may show nonspecific atypical cells seen in 30%.

Radiological Findings. Multiple diverticular outpouches are seen on urography or pyelography (Fig. 15–45).[41] These measure only 1–2 mm in diameter and may be difficult to identify (Fig. 15–46). Bilateral disease is seen in 70%. Solitary pseudodiverticula are seen in 9%.[43] Retrograde ureterography and pyelography may be necessary to exclude transitional cell carcinoma.

SPONTANEOUS URETERAL PERFORATION

The most common site of pelvocalyceal extravasation is the fornix. Spontaneous perforation of the

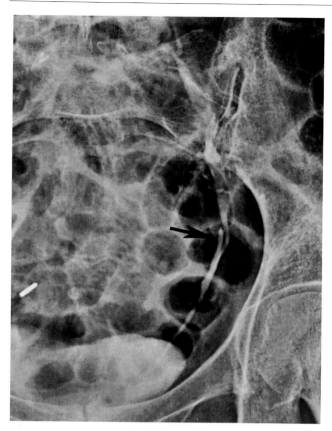

Figure 15–36. Ureteral diverticulum or abortive ureter.

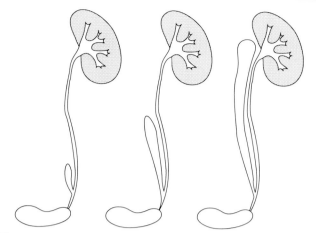

Figure 15–37. Schematic drawing of ureteral diverticuli of different sizes.

common site for local recurrence of the rectal carcinoma for which the abdominoperineal resection was performed (Fig. 15–49). Differential diagnosis may be difficult and thin needle aspiration biopsy of the lesion may be necessary.[51]

ureter without obstruction is rare and incompletely understood (Fig. 15–47). The common denominator is increased diuresis.

URETERAL HERNIATION

Sciatic hernia is the most common (Fig. 15–48).[44–46] Rarely, the ureter may herniate into the scrotum,[47,48] inguinal or femoral canal. Ureteral herniation may or may not be associated with obstruction. "Curlicue" sign may be seen on urography.[49]

ABDOMINOPERINEAL RESECTION

Following abdominoperineal resection, the ureters normally migrate medially because of the lack of supportive tissues (Fig. 15–4).[50] Occasionally, one of the ureters may cross the midline. Ureteral injury is most likely to occur during dissection of the site where the sigmoid mesocolon crosses the left ureter and may result in ureteral stricture. This is also a

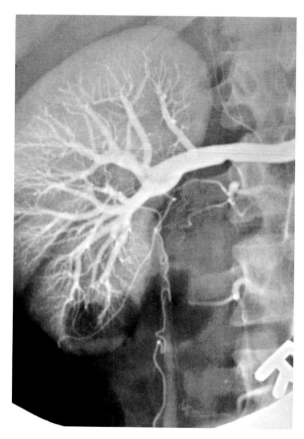

Figure 15–38. Ureteric artery supplying upper third of the ureter is seen arising from segmental arterial branches. Tortuous course is normal.

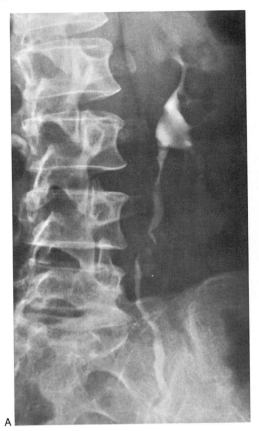
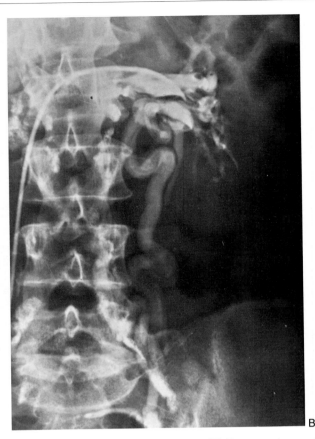

A   B

Figure 15–39. (A) Ureteral notching due to varicose enlargement of periureteral veins. (B) Retrograde renal vein venogram demonstrates large, tortuous periureteric veins that originate from segmental venous branches and should not be confused with gonadal vessels. Otherwise the renal vein was normal.

PRIMARY URETERAL TUMORS

Incidence. Transitional cell carcinoma is the most common urothelial neoplasm in the ureter and represents 2.5% of all uroepithelial tumors of the urinary tract. Occurs in the fourth through seventh decades of life. Male predominance. High frequency of transitional cell carcinoma has been reported in endemic areas, associated with interstitial nephritis (Balkan nephropathy).[52]

Pathology

Epithelial. Benign: inverted papilloma,[53,54] polyp, adenoma.

Malignant: transitional cell carcinoma (TCC), squamous cell carcinoma, adenocarcinoma.

Mesodermal. Benign: fibroma, hemangioma, myoma, lymphangioma.

Malignant: sarcoma, angiosarcoma, carcinosarcoma (mixed).[55]

Metastases are in the regional lymph nodes, liver, axial skeleton, lungs, kidney, and adrenal glands. Early lymphatic invasion. TCC is more common in the distal ureter.

Clinical Presentation. Hematuria, ureteral obstruction.[56] Transitional cell carcinoma may be simultaneously present in the renal pelvis, opposite ureter,[57] and the bladder.

Laboratory Findings. Hematuria. Positive cytology in voided specimens (16%), and ureteral washings (50%).[58]

Radiological Findings. Excretory urography is the examination of choice. This is the only quick and practical way to opacify a pair of long narrow tubular structures such as ureters (Fig. 15–50). In any patient where urothelial malignancy is suspected ureters must be filled with contrast and preferably viewed in several different projections. This is particularly true in patients presenting with hematuria or a known transitional cell carcinoma of the bladder or renal

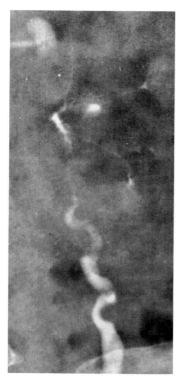

Figure 15–40. Venous impressions upon the ureter in a patient with a tumor thrombus in left renal vein. Enlarged periureteral veins allow for renal venous outflow.

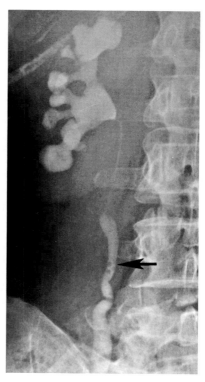

Figure 15–42. Ureteritis cystica in a patient with a staghorn calculus and recurrent infections. Only few small lesions are evident in the somewhat dilated mid-ureter (arrow).

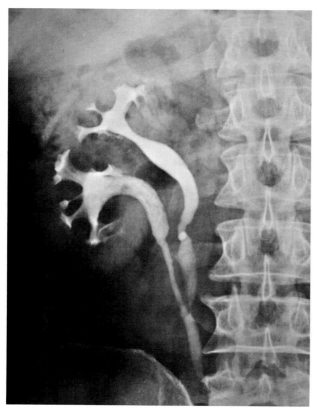

Figure 15–41. Very subtle changes of pyelitis and ureteritis cystica in the lower moiety. Small rounded mucosal protrusions are detected.

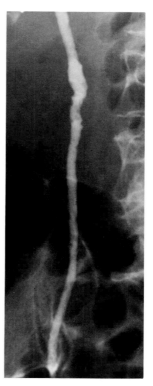

Figure 15–43. Ureteritis cystica involving the entire ureter (close-up).

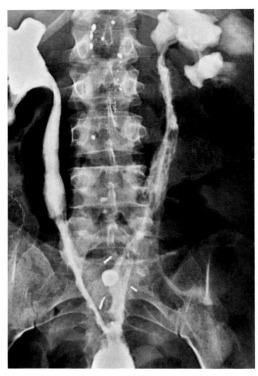

Figure 15–44. Severe ureteritis cystica involving the left ureter in a patient with ureteral stent and diversion.

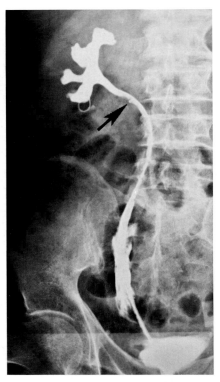

Figure 15–46. Subtle changes of pseudodiverticulosis (arrow) in a patient with urine cytology positive for atypical cells. Diagnosis of pseudodiverticulosis was not made prior to retrograde endoscopy performed to find the source of atypical cells. During this procedure, there was ureteral perforation. Contrast is seen in the periureteral tissues around the distal ureter.

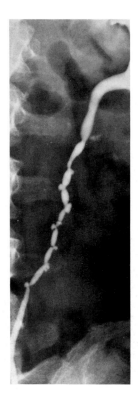

Figure 15–45. Ureteral pseudodiverticulosis. (From Cochran et al.[41] Reprinted with permission.)

pelvis. These neoplasms are multicentric and the entire transitional-bearing epithelial surfaces must be thoroughly examined (Fig. 15–51).

Urothelial malignancy commonly presents as an intraluminal filling defect with marginal cupping immediately above and below the lesion (Fig. 15–52). Proximal ureter need not be dilated and is frequently normal in appearance. Differential diagnosis for intraluminal filling defects includes ureteral calculus, blood clot, sloughed papilla, and fungus ball.

Second type of presentation is associated with ureteral obstruction where renal function may be inadequate to visualize the ureter at the point of the obstruction.

Retrograde ureterography allows for more controlled administration of the contrast material and in general a more thorough examination. Frequently, the retrograde catheter may coil within the somewhat expanded ureter just distal to the tumor (Bergman sign) (Fig. 15–53).[59] This is opposite to the ureteral calculus where the ureter immediately distal

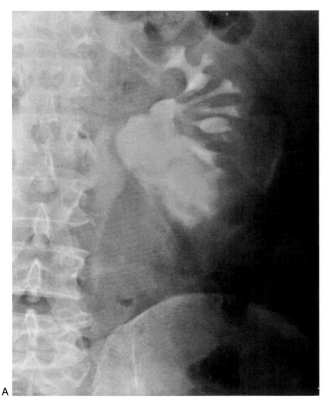
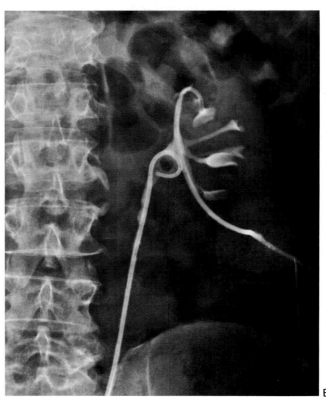

A

B

Figure 15–47. (A) EXU in a patient with sudden onset of left flank pain. Contrast is present in what is essentially nondilated collecting system. A large amount of contrast is outside the renal pelvis, in the renal sinus and retroperitoneum. (B) A nephrostomy tube and a retrograde stent were eventually placed without difficulty. No stone was ever found and the kidney had normal appearance after all the tubes were discontinued.

to the calculus is narrow, probably because of edema and spasm. Retrograde ureteroscopy, brush biopsy, ureteral washings, and thorough visual inspection of the bladder are all accomplished during this somewhat invasive study.

Air bubbles are inadvertently injected into the ureter or pelvis during retrograde examination and may present diagnostic problems. Change in patient position and additional injection of the contrast may help to resolve the dilemma of whether the filling defect is an air bubble or a genuine filling defect.

Ureteral tumors may be pedunculated and protrude through the ureteral orifice into the bladder or change in position on retrograde ureterography.

CT is helpful in instances where the ureter is incompletely visualized by either of the methods

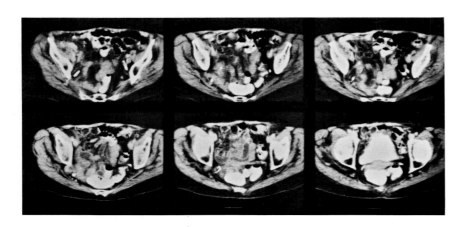

Figure 15–48. Composite of CT images showing sciatic ureteral hernia on the right. Right ureter is opacified and can be traced from image to image into the hernia and into the bladder.

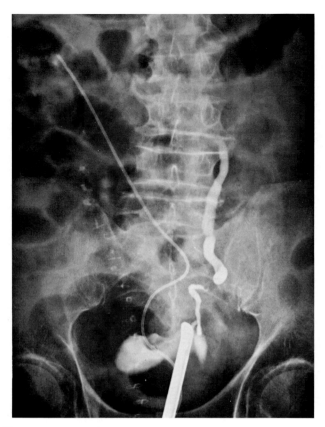

Figure 15–49. Medially drawn ureters after AP resection. Narrowing is present at the distal left ureter, which may be either tumor recurrence or a stricture. (From Barbaric et al.[50] Reprinted with permission.)

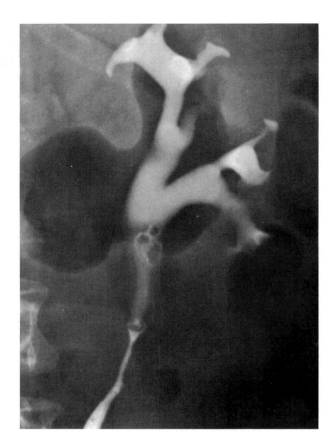

Figure 15–51. Multicentric transitional cell carcinoma presenting as multiple small, irregular filling defects. Note cupping (vine glass) just distal to the most inferior tumor.

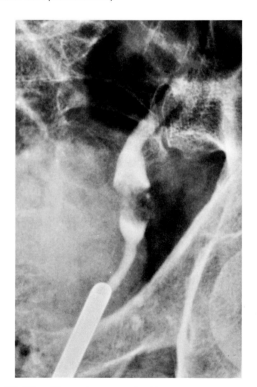

Figure 15–50. Ureter is expanded by noncalcified intraluminal mass.

306

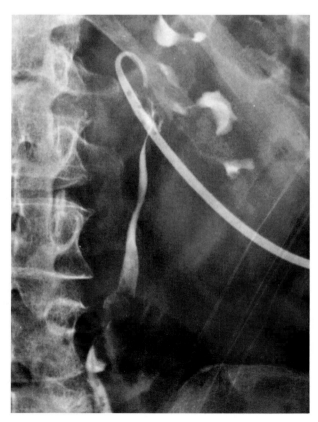

Figure 15–52. Intraluminal TCC with distal cupping. Nephrostomy was placed because of obstruction.

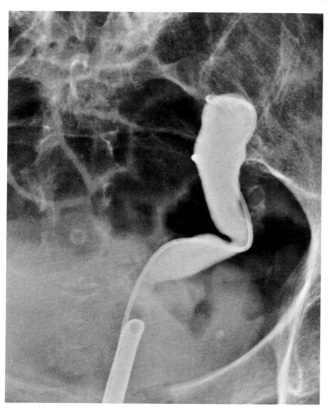

Figure 15–53. Bergman sign. The retrograde catheter coils in dilated ureteral segment just below the tumor.

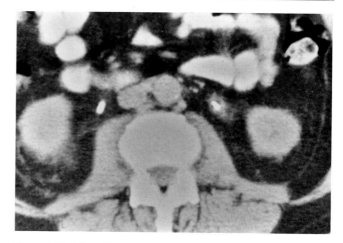

Figure 15–54. CT through the ureters and lower poles of both kidneys. Contrast is seen in the right ureter. Ureteral wall is not normally perceivable on CT. On the left there is a double "J" stent in place that passes through an area of abnormal ureteral thickness. The difference from the opposite side is striking. Differential diagnosis, however, includes periureteral fibrosis, metastasis, and other diseases.

described above.[60,61] Several thin cuts over the area of interest frequently disclose an intraluminal filling defect, density of which is higher than that of urine (Fig. 15–54). On the postcontrast scans, smaller lesions may be easily missed because of volume averaging.

CT is very helpful in distinguishing radiolucent stones from soft tissue filling defects.[62]

Ureteral Stump

Treatment for upper tract transitional cell carcinoma is nephroureterectomy, including removal of a bladder cuff. In some instances the very distal ureter is left behind for technical reasons. Recurrence of ureteral tumor within the stump is common and these patients require periodical cystoureteroscopy for follow-up. Retrograde ureterography is the method of choice for demonstrating the presence of a recurrent tumor.[63] If retrograde ureterography proves impossible for technical reasons, CT, MR imaging,[64] and perhaps even ultrasound may demonstrate intraluminal tumor within the stump.

REFERENCES

1. Kabakin HA, Armenian HK, Deeb ZL, et al. Asymmetry of the pelvic ureters in normal females. Am J Roentgenol 1976; 127:723–727.
2. Whitaker RH, Johnston JH. A simple classification of wide ureters. Br J Radiol 1976; 47:781–787.
3. Hellstrom M, Jodal U, Marild S, et al. Ureteral dilatation in children with febrile urinary tract infection or bacteriuria. AJR 1987; 148:483–484.
4. Hefty TR, Bonafede P, Stenzel P. Bilateral ureteral stricture from polyarteritis nodosa. J Urol 1989; 141:600–601.
5. Shapiro MJ, Banner MP, Amendola MA, et al. Balloon catheter dilatation of ureteroenteric strictures: Long-term results. Radiology 1988; 168:385–387.
6. Lang EK, Glorioso LW III. Antegrade transluminal dilatation of benign ureteral strictures: long-term results. AJR 1988; 150:131–134.
7. Beckmann CF, Roth RA, Bihrle W III. Dilatation of benign ureteral strictures. Radiology 1989; 172: 437–441.
8. Chang R, Marshal FF, Mitchell S. Percutaneous management of benign ureteral strictures and fistulas. J Urol 1987; 137:1126–1131.
9. Bruneton JN, Drouillard J, Normand F, et al. Nonrenal urological lymphomas. Fortschr Rontgenstr 1987; 146:42–46.
10. Puech JL, Song MY, Joffre F, et al. Ureteral metastases—computed tomographic findings. Eur J Radiol 1987; 7:103–106.
11. Mitty HA, Droller MJ, Dikman SH. Ureteral and renal pelvic metastases from renal cell carcinoma. Urol Radiol 1987; 9:16–18.
12. Lee KT, Deeths TM. Localized amyloidosis of the ureter. Radiology 1976; 120:60.

13. Yalowitz PA, Kelalis PP. Primary amyloidosis of the ureter. J Urol 1966; 96:668–670.

14. Lucero SP, Wise HA, Kirsh G, et al. Ureteric obstruction secondary to endometriosis: report of three cases with review of the literature. Br J Urol 1988; 61:201.

15. Latimer J, Feggetter JGW. Malakoplakia as a cause of ureteric obstruction. Br J Urol 1988; 61:365.

16. Pfister RC, Hendren WH. Primary megaureter in children and adults; clinical and pathophysiological features of 150 ureters. Urology 1978; 12:160–176.

17. Mellins HZ. Cystic dilatation of the upper urinary tract: a radiologist's developmental model. Radiology 1984; 153:291–301.

18. Hamilton S, Fitzpatrick JM. Primary non-obstructive megaureter in adults. Clin Radiol 1987; 38:181–189.

19. Blickman JG, Lebowitz RL. The coexistence of primary megaureter and reflux. AJR 1984; 143:1053–1057.

20. Vargas B, Lebowitz RL. The coexistence of congenital megacalyces and primary megaureter. AJR 1986; 147:313–316.

21. Mandell GA, Snyder HM III, Heyman S, et al. Association of congenital megacalycosis and ipsilateral segmental megaureter. Pediatr Radiol 1987; 17:28–31.

22. Wood BP, Ben-Ami T, Teele RL, Rabinowitz R. Ureterovesical obstruction and megaloureter: diagnosis by real-time US. Radiology 1985; 156:79–80.

23. McGrath MA, Estroff J, Lebowitz RL. The coexistence of obstruction at the ureteropelvic and ureterovesical junctions. AJR 1987; 149:403–406.

24. Mandell J, Colodny AH, Lebowitz R, et al. Ureteroceles in infants and children. J Urol 1980; 123:921–926.

25. Nussbaum AR, Dorst JP, Jeffs RD, et al. Ectopic ureter and ureterocele: their varied sonographic manifestations. Radiology 1986; 159:227–235.

26. Share JC, Lebowitz RL. Ectopic ureterocele without ureteral and calyceal dilatation (ureterocele disproportion): findings on urography and sonography. AJR 1989; 152:567–571.

27. Hochhauser L, Alton DJ. Prolapse of an ectopic ureterocele into both urethra and ipsilateral ectopic ureter. Pediatr Radiol 1986; 16:167.

28. Mitty HA, Schapira HE. Ureterocele and pseudoureterocele: cobra versus cancer. J Urol 1977; 117:557–561.

29. Thornbury JR, Silver TM, Vinson RK. Ureteroceles vs. pseudoureteroceles in adults. Urographic diagnosis. Radiology 1977; 122:81–84.

30. Kenawi MM, Williams DI. Circumcaval ureter. A report of four cases in children with a review of the literature and a new classification. Br J Urol 1976; 48:183–192.

31. Murphy BJ, Casillas J, Becerra JL. Retrocaval ureter: computed tomography and ultrasound appearance. CT 1986; 11:89–91.

32. Schaffer RM, Sunschine AG, Becker JA, et al. Retrocaval ureter: sonographic appearance. J Ultrasound Med 1985; 4:199–200.

33. Rosen MP, Walker TG, Brennan JF, et al. Transcaval ureter with hydronephrosis: radiologic demonstration. AJR 1989; 152:793–794.

34. Hanna MK. Bilateral retro-iliac artery ureters. Br J Urol 1972; 44:339–344.

35. Harrison GSM. Transitional cell carcinoma in congenital ureteral diverticulum. J Urol 1983; 129:1231–1232.

36. Roodhooft AM, Boven K, Gentens P, et al. Abdominal colic due to ureteric diverticulum with stone formation. Pediatr Radiol 1987; 17:252–253.

37. Cochran ST, Kanter SA. Ureteric changes in polyarteritis nodosa. Br J Radiol 1978; 52:504–506.

38. Mahboubi S, Duckett JN, Spackman TJ. Ureteritis cystica after treatment of cyclophosphamide-induced hemorrhagic cystitis. Urology 1976; 7:521–523.

39. Kamens L. Ureteritis cystica: Diagnosis by antegrade pyelography. Urology 1975; 6:209–211.

40. Cory DA, Tarver RD, Baker MK, et al. Subepithelial pyeloureteric lesions in patients with nephrostomy tubes. Br J Radiol 1987; 60:449–453.

41. Cochran ST, Waisman J, Barbaric ZL. Radiographic and microscopic findings in multiple ureteral diverticula. Radiology 1980; 137:631–636.

42. Wasserman NF, Posalaky IP, Dykoski R. The pathology of ureteral pseudodiverticulosis. Invest Radiol 1988; 23:592–598.

43. Wasserman NF, La Pointe S, Posalaky IP. Ureteral pseudodiverticulosis. Radiology 1985; 155:561–566.

44. Lebowitz R. Ureteral sciatic hernia. Pediatr Radiol 1973; 1:178–182.

45. Gaffney CM. Case profile: bilateral inguinal herniation of ureter. Urology 1987; 29:665.

46. Oyen R, Gielen J, Baert L, et al. CT demonstration of a ureterosciatic hernia. Urol Radiol 1987; 9:174–176.

47. Mallough C, Pellman CM. Scrotal herniation of ureter. J Urol 1971; 106:38–41.

48. Rocklin MS, Apelgren KN, Slomski CA, Kandzari SJ. Scrotal incarceration of the ureter with crossed renal ectopia: case report and literature review. J Urol 1989; 142:366–368.

49. Ney C, Miller HL, Gardimer H. Preinguinal canal herniation of the ureter: Value of curlicue sign direction. Arch Surg 1972; 105:633–634.

50. Barbaric ZL, Wolfe DE, Segal AJ. Urinary tract after abdominoperineal resection. Radiology 1978; 128:345–348.

51. Lee JKT, Stanley RJ, Sagel SS, Levitt RG, McClennan BL. CT appearance of the pelvis after abdomino-perineal resection for rectal carcinoma. Radiology 1981; 141:737–741.

52. Petkovic SB. Epidemiology and treatment of renal, pelvic and ureteral tumors. J Urol 1975; 114:858–865.

53. Nadel S, St. Amour TE, Kyriakos M. Asymptomatic woman with unilateral urethelial lesions. Urol Radiol 1987; 9:57–61.

54. Kimura G, Tsuboi N, Nakajima H, et al. Inverted papilloma of the ureter with malignant transformation: a case report and review of the literature. The importance of the recognition of the inverted papillary tumor of the ureter. Urol Int 1987; 42:30–36.

55. Fleming S. Carcinosarcoma (mixed mesodermal tumor) of the ureter. J Urol 1987; 138:1234–1235.

56. Mills CM, Vaughan ED. Carcinoma of the ureter: natural history, management and 5-year survival. J Urol 1983; 129:275–277.

57. Talavera JM, Carney JA, Kelalis PP. Bilateral, synchronous, primary transitional cell carcinoma of the ureter: report of 2 cases and review of literature. J Urol 1970; 104:679–683.

58. Nakada T, Umeda K, Koike H, et al. Clinical analysis of ureteral tumours with or without renal pelvic neoplasms. Int Urol Nephrol 1987; 19:377–384.

59. Bergman H, Friedenberg RM, Sayegh V. New roentgenologic signs of carcinoma of the ureter. Am J Roentgenol 1961; 86:707–717.
60. Kenney PJ, Stanley RJ. Computed tomography of ureteral tumors. J Comput Assist Tomogr 1987; 11:102–107.
61. Baron RL, McClennan BL, Lee JK, Lawson TL. Computed tomography of the transitional cell carcinoma of the renal pelvis and ureter. Radiology 1982; 144:125–130.
62. Parienty RA, Ducellier R, Pradel J, et al. Diagnostic value of CT numbers in pelvocalyceal filling defects. Radiology 1982; 145:743–747.
63. Pollack HM, Banner MP, Popky GL. Radiologic evaluation of ureteral stump. Radiology 1982; 144:225–230.
64. Jaffe J, Friedman AC, Seidmon EJ, et al. Diagnosis of ureteral stump transitional cell carcinoma by CT and MR imaging. AJR 1987; 149:741–742.

16

Retroperitoneum

INTRODUCTION

Of all areas in the body the retroperitoneum was one of the most difficult to image until the introduction of CT. Presence of a retroperitoneal tumor, for example, could only be inferred on classic radiographic imaging by indirect evidence, such as displacement of kidney, ureters, and bowel. The "psoas sign" (loss of psoas outline due to adjacent fat replacement by either tumor or fluid) is still considered by many to be an important indicator in retroperitoneal pathology, although the value of this sign is limited.[1,2]

It is not surprising that techniques such as retroperitoneal air insufflation were developed in an attempt to render retroperitoneal pathology visible.

RETROPERITONEAL FIBROSIS

Etiology. Methysergide (Sansert),[3] idiopathic,[4] familial (rare).[5]

Pathology. Local or massive proliferation of fibrous tissues, engulfing great vessels and ureters. Spectrum ranges from a marked chronic inflammatory infiltrate mixed with fibroblast to collagenous fibrous tissue with a few inflammatory cells. Rectractile fibrosis may cause ureteral and vena cava obstruction.

Clinical Presentation. Renal failure, hypertension, anemia, proteinuria.

Radiological Findings. The fibrosis may encapsulate the inferior vena cava, aorta, and ureters, which may become obstructed. Characteristically, ureters are drawn medially by the cicatrizing mass and the site of obstruction has a rat tail appearance. Obstruction is a late sequel of retroperitoneal fibrosis and

may not be present at the time the diagnosis is made (Fig. 16–1).

CT[6,7] and MR imaging[8] are the methods of choice for making the diagnosis, for determining the extent of the disease process and the level of ureteral obstruction. Bolus contrast injection is necessary to demonstrate great vessels within the mass on CT study. Fibrotic mass may appear hypointense, (dark) on T2-weighted images and thus can be differentiated from retroperitoneal metastases, which are of high signal intensities (bright) on the same imaging sequences (Fig. 16–2).

Retroperitoneal fibrosis need not displace (retract) ureters medially and may be localized around a single ureter causing unilateral obstruction. Fibrotic process may in rare instances surround the kidneys.[8]

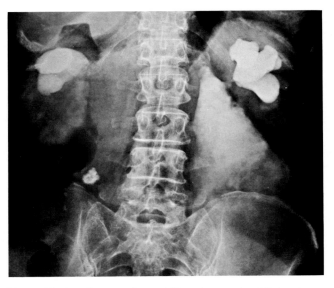

Figure 16–1. Retroperitoneal fibrosis causing bilateral ureteral obstruction and rupture of the left collecting system. (Photograph courtesy of Dr. R.B. Smith.)

T1-weighted   T2-weighted

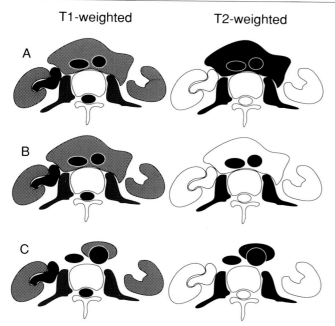

Figure 16–2. Schematic drawing of **(A)** retroperitoneal fibrosis; **(B)** malignant retroperitoneal fibrosis; and **(C)** periaortic fibrosis as they would appear on T1- and T2-weighted spin echo sequences.

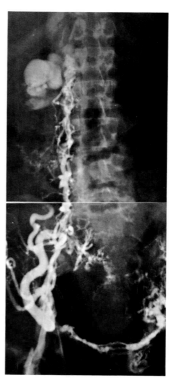

Figure 16–3. Composite image of an attempted inferior cavogram. Contrast was injected into the right external iliac vein. Common iliac vein and inferior vena cava are completely obstructed and collateral pathways via ascending lumbar vein have developed. The left kidney is not functioning, having been obstructed for a long time. The right kidney is obstructed (hydronephrosis, delayed function) and also retracted medially.

Obstruction of the inferior vena cava is unusual (Fig. 16–3). Slow cicatrizing process allows development of collateral circulation. Inferior vena cavogram or iliac vein venogram is the diagnostic method of choice. Obstruction of the inferior vena cava may cause pelvic edema, resulting in a peculiar bladder appearance known as *"inverted pear-shape or tear-shape bladder."*

Differential diagnosis includes *perianeurysmal fibrosis* or *periaortic fibrosis* which looks similar on CT, except that there is no medial retraction of the ureters. Retroperitoneal malignant lymphoma, melanoma, etc., must also be considered. In the presence of malignancy, aorta is often displaced anteriorly, a finding not seen in idiopathic retroperitoneal fibrosis.[7]

Recently, a case of amyloidosis diffusely involving the retroperitoneum was described.[9] Its appearance mimicked retroperitoneal fibrosis.

PERIAORTIC FIBROSIS (INFLAMMATORY AORTIC ANEURYSM)

Etiology. Unknown.

Incidence. May be as high as 5–23% of all abdominal aortic aneurysms.

Pathology. Thickened aortic wall surrounded by dense fibrotic mass infiltrated with lymphocytes, plasma cells, and histiocytes.[10] Ureters, duodenum, inferior vena cava, and renal veins may be incorporated into, or adhered to, the inflammatory mass. Aneurysm may or may not be present. May represent a different clinical manifestation of retroperitoneal fibrosis.

Clinical Presentation. Back pain.

Treatment. Surgical morbidity and mortality are higher than with simple aortic aneurysms.[11] Preoperative steroids may be tried and response observed using cross-sectional imaging.

Radiological Findings. CT may reveal calcified or thickened aortic wall. Aneurysm may or may not be present. Inflammatory/fibrotic mass surrounds the aorta and commonly spares the posterior aortic wall.[12] The mass is seen as a soft tissue density that may enhance slightly on dynamic CT scan. The lesion should not be confused with a false lumen of a dissecting aortic aneurysm.

On ultrasound, the mass is hypoechoic. The thickened aortic wall appears hyperechoic.

The appearance of the mass on MR imaging probably depends on the relative amounts of fibrous versus inflammatory tissues. The old fibrous tissues appear dark on T2-weighted sequences, while the inflammatory tissues are more likely to appear gray or bright (Fig. 16–2).

MALIGNANT RETROPERITONEAL FIBROSIS

Etiology. Infiltration of the retroperitoneum by malignant cells.

Pathology. Most common metastases are from breast, stomach, colon, and lung. Desmoplastic reaction and sclerosis are induced in the retroperitoneum by metastatic deposits.

Clinical Presentation. Differentiation from idiopathic retroperitoneal fibrosis is difficult. History of malignancy favors malignant retroperitoneal fibrosis. Biopsy or surgery may be necessary.

Radiological Findings. Diagnosis of malignant retroperitoneal fibrosis is impossible on the basis of morphological changes alone. On CT, a soft tissue mass may be identified causing ureteral obstruction at times. Contrast enhancement is similar to benign retroperitoneal fibrosis.

It appears MR imaging may be the examination of choice. If the retroperitoneal soft tissue mass is homogeneous, exhibits low signal intensity (dark), and is well marginated, it is probably a benign retroperitoneal fibrosis. If the mass is inhomogeneous, with areas of increased signal intensity (bright) on T2-weighted images, and has ill-defined margins, it is most likely malignant retroperitoneal fibrosis (Fig. 16–2).[13] Biopsy may still be necessary, since benign retroperitoneal fibrosis may also exhibit high signal intensity and inhomogeneity on T2-weighted sequences, depending on the age of the fibrosis.

LYMPHADENOPATHY

Pathological enlargement of the lymph node is the only diagnostic imaging criterion on CT. If the lymph node is larger than 1 cm in the longest axis, it is considered abnormal, and if it is larger than 1.5 cm, it is definitely pathological. As always, comparison

with old, previous examinations is of help in detecting interim changes in size.

Within the abdomen and pelvis, CT and MR imaging are about equal in their ability to detect lymph node enlargement (Figs. 16–4, 16–5, 16–6). Neither is able to differentiate inflammatory from malignant lymph nodes. CT has somewhat better resolution, while MR clearly differentiates vascular structures from the lymph nodes. Dynamic CT scanning may be employed if differentiation from vascular structures is difficult.

Substantive lymph node enlargement may affect adjacent organs, including ureters (Figs. 16–7, 16–8). Displacement or encasement may result in obstruction. In general, enlarged para-aortic lymph nodes displace proximal ureters laterally, while enlarged iliac lymph nodes displace distal ureters (and occasionally the bladder) medially.

In addition to displacement, the lymph nodes can also make impressions upon the ureters, referred to as *"ureteral notching."* Ureteral notching may also be caused by periureteral venous varices and venous collaterals.

Searching for a 1–2 cm mass among multiple normal lymph nodes on hundreds of thoracic, abdominal, and pelvic CT cuts and comparing these to prior examinations is very time-consuming and difficult. It demands concentration, patience, and a thorough knowledge of cross-sectional anatomy.

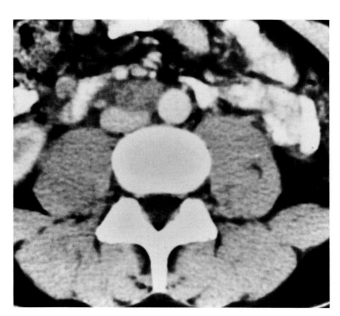

Figure 16–4. Enlarged lymph node nestled between aorta, inferior vena cava, and superior mesenteric vessels. All vessels are enhanced and contrast is seen in third portion of duodenum on adjacent slices.

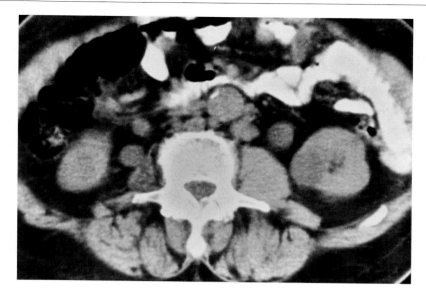

Figure 16–5. Enlarged left para-aortic lymph node is adjacent to and just posterior to the aorta. A few other small lymph nodes are seen posterior to the aorta and vena cava. Both ureters are dilated due to outflow bladder obstruction by carcinoma of the prostate. Note mass in the left kidney medially and unusual atrophy of the psoas on the right.

LYMPHANGIOGRAPHY

This radiographic examination takes 2 days to complete. On the first day, a small amount of methylene blue is injected into the intradigital web of the third, fourth, and fifth toes. A 1 cm incision is made under local anesthesia in the dorsum of the foot where dye-containing lymphatics are identified, carefully isolated and cannulated using a 28 gauge needle. Ligatures are placed around the needle and the lymphatic is infused with oily contrast (Lipoidol) with the help of an infusion pump. It may take 1 to 2 hours for the contrast to reach para-aortic lymph channels, at which time the infusion is terminated. Radiographs taken at the time the infusion is terminated

show the *flow phase* during which only lymphatic channels are seen.

On the second day, a set of radiographs is obtained to demonstrate contrast within the lymph nodes, referred to as the *storage phase* (Fig. 16–9). Two distinct types of morphological abnormalities are found:

1. Diffuse enlargement with "lacy pattern" is seen in lymphomas.
2. Focal defect within the lymph node implies replacement of normal tissues with either metastases or a fibrofatty tissue. At times, the node may be totally replaced and invisible on this examination. Differentiating between metastases and fibrofatty tissues within the lymph node may also

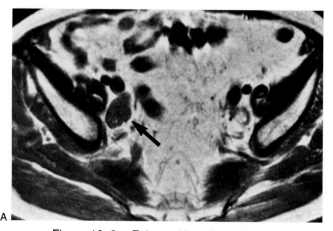
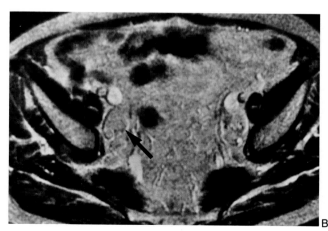

Figure 16–6. Enlarged lymph node (arrows) along the right internal iliac chain in a patient with prostatic carcinoma is of low signal intensity on T1-weighted sequence (**A**) and of intermediate intensity on T2-weighted sequence (**B**).

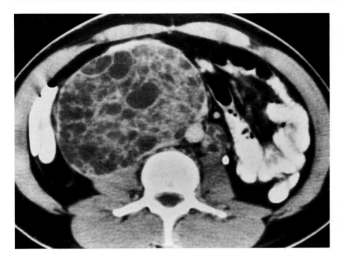

Figure 16–7. Mature testicular teratoma with a large metastasis to the right and a small metastasis to the left of the aorta. A cystic component as is seen here is also seen in primary mature teratomas of the retroperitoneum.

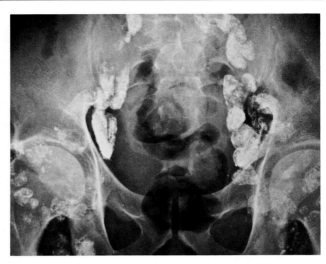

Figure 16–9. Storage phase of a lymphangiogram showing diffuse nodal enlargement and lacy pattern typical of lymphoma.

be difficult and sometimes a skinny needle biopsy is necessary.

Absence of a focal filling defect within the lymph node does not preclude metastases, since microscopic deposits may be present.

LYMPHOCELE

Retroperitoneal collection of lymphatic fluid is usually a result of retroperitoneal surgery (Fig. 16–10), such as radical lymph node dissection or renal trans-

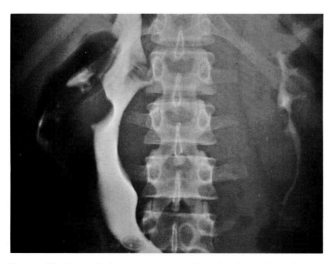

Figure 16–8. Inferior cavogram. Massive lymph node enlargement in a young patient with metastatic seminoma. Kidneys, ureters, and vena cava are displaced.

plants. Extravasation of the lymphatic fluid is due to transection of the lymphatic channel, and if it is a small residual, it is usually clinically inconsequential. Massive accumulations of fluid are observed on ultrasound, CT, or MR imaging. A large lymphocele may cause displacement of various organs, including kidneys, and may also cause ureteral obstruction, particularly in renal transplants. MR imaging will demonstrate cystic masses, exhibiting low signal intensity on T1-weighted and high signal intensity on T2-weighted images.

Repeated aspirations may be required to drain lymphoceles, but they usually reaccumulate. Percutaneous instillation of sclerosing agents, such as a solution of tetracycline, and prolonged drainage may be highly effective.[14–16] Rarely, surgical exploration will be needed.

RETROPERITONEAL CYSTIC LYMPHANGIOMA

Etiology. Probably developmental hamartoma.

Pathology. Dilated lymphatics containing serous or chylus fluid, lined with endothelium and usually communicating with the lymphatic system.[17] The neck, where the lesion is known as cystic hygroma, is the most common site (75%), followed by the axilla (20%) and elsewhere in the body (5%).

Clinical Presentation. Mass lesion may be palpable or may interfere with function of other organs because of its bulk.

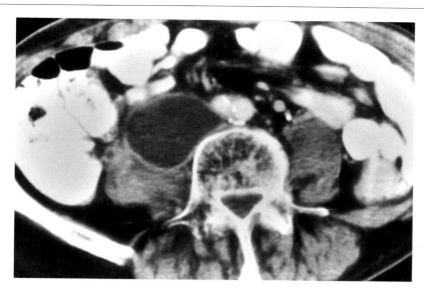

Figure 16–10. Right lymphocele anterior to psoas appeared after right radical nephrectomy. The fluid is surrounded by a pseudocapsule.

Radiological Findings. A fluid-filled mass is demonstrated by ultrasound, CT, or MR imaging (Fig. 16–11). Percutaneous aspiration confirms the presence of protein-rich fluid. Lymphangiography may demonstrate puddling of contrast within the cyst,[18] but this examination is probably unnecessary.

Percutaneous drainage is usually ineffective because of constant replenishment of the lymph via connecting channels and frequent infections.

RETROPERITONEAL HEMATOMA

Etiology. Trauma, instrumentation, biopsy, postoperative, anticoagulant therapy, ruptured aneurysm, polyarteritis nodosa, spontaneous.

Radiological Findings. On CT, fresh blood is hyperdense compared to the kidney and muscle, often reaching values as high as 60 HU (Fig. 16–12). Within a week or two, the organizing hematoma becomes gradually radiolucent, sometimes forming a pseudocapsule. More often, the extravasated blood dissects between the fascial and septal layers and is often contained in the perinephric space by the renal fascia. Kidney and ureters are frequently displaced (Fig. 16–13).

On MR imaging, signal intensities change significantly as the hematoma ages and as oxyhemoglobin degrades to deoxyhemoglobin, methemoglobin, ferritin, and hemosiderin (Fig. 16–14).[19] These changes need not be uniform within the mass formed by extravasated blood (Fig. 16–15).

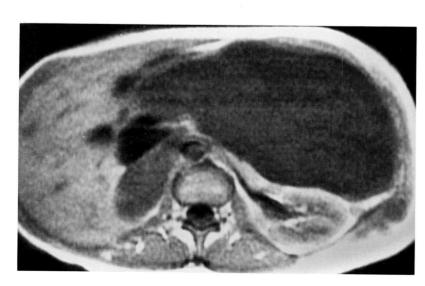

Figure 16–11. Retroperitoneal cystic lymphangioma in a young woman.

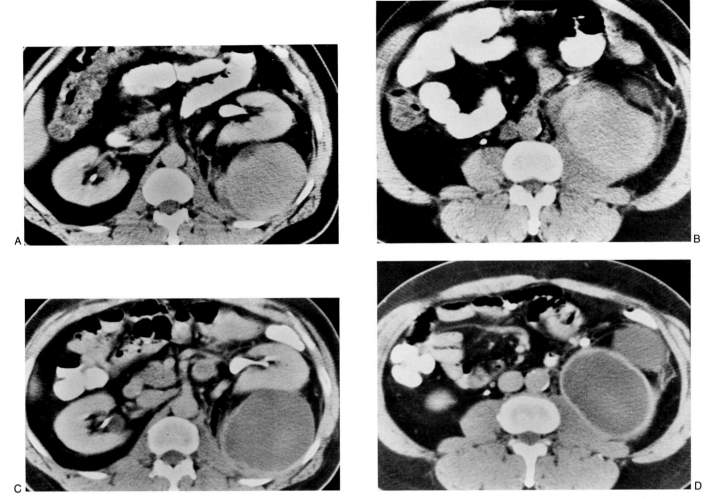

Figure 16–12.   Acute retroperitoneal hemorrhage extending posterior **(A)** and inferior **(B)** to the left kidney. It is hyperdense. Two months later **(C,D)** the hematoma is radiolucent with a thick pseudocapsule.

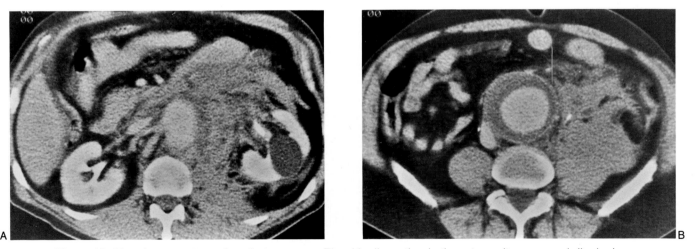

Figure 16–13.   Acute rupture of aortic aneurysm. Blood is dissecting in the retroperitoneum and displacing the kidney **(A)**. Radiolucent thrombus is seen between the intraluminal contrast and outer wall of the aneurysm **(B)**. Note displacement of the vena cava and a cyst in the left kidney.

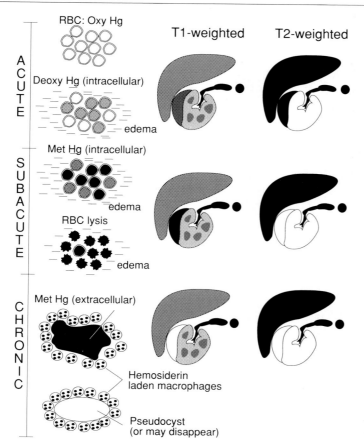

Figure 16–14. Schematic drawing of MR signal characteristic of a subcapsular hematoma over a period of time on spin echo T1- and T2-weighted sequences.

CHYLURIA

Etiology. Infestation with filarial worm (filariasis),[20] lymphadenectomy, metastases to the lymph nodes, pregnancy, trauma, congenital.[21]

Pathology. Occlusion of lymphatic cephalad to the kidneys or bladder, retrograde flow of lymph to the kidney or bladder with lymph extravasation in urine.

Clinical Presentation. Milky urine. May be mistaken for pyuria.

Laboratory Findings. Larvae of *Wuchereria bancrofti* in blood (blood must be drawn at night when microfilariae are active). Proteinuria, nonglobular fat in urine with high triglyceride component. Treatment is specific for filariasis or other primary cause.

Radiological Findings. On lymphangiography contrast is seen flowing in retrograde fashion to the kidney from the retroperitoneal lymphatic channels.[22] Eventually, contrast is seen extravasating into the collecting system and can be seen in the ureter and bladder (Fig. 16–16).

PRIMARY RETROPERITONEAL TUMORS

Incidence

Malignant. Common: Malignant fibrous histiocytoma, liposarcoma, leiomyosarcoma. Less common: Neurofibrosarcoma, neuroblastoma, hemangiopericytoma, fibrosarcoma, malignant germ cell, rhabdomyosarcoma, etc.[23]

Benign. Common: Paraganglioma, neurofibroma, neurilemoma. Less common: Hemangioma, lipoma, teratoma, desmoid, ganglioneurinoma, etc.[24]

Radiological Findings. Excretory urography and other projectional radiological examinations may discover a retroperitoneal tumor by virtue of organ displacement, such as kidney or ureter (Fig. 16–17). CT and MR imaging are by far superior, not only in detecting, but also being able to suggest specific diagnosis at times, and also defining local extension (Fig. 16–18). Suggestive but nonspecific radiological findings are presented in Table 16–1.

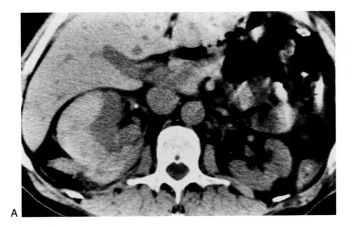

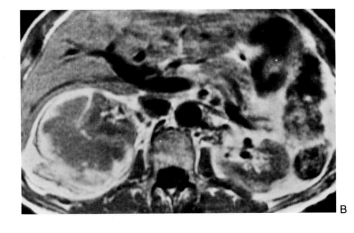

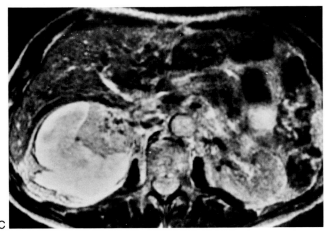

Figure 16–15. Spontaneous subcapsular hematoma in a healthy young man with no history of trauma, proteinuria, hematuria, or clotting abnormalities. **(A)** In the acute phase a hyperdense right subcapsular and perinephric hematoma are evident. **(B)** In the subacute phase on T1-weighted sequence the outer part of hematoma is of strong signal intensity, while the inner portion is still of low intensity (dark). **(C)** On T2-weighted sequence the outer part still exhibits a strong signal (bright), and the inner part is of medium signal intensity (gray). Looking at Figure 16–14, one can surmise that the outer part of hematoma is already in chronic stage, and the inner portion is in transition from acute to chronic.

Malignant Fibrous Histiocytoma

Incidence. Most common primary retroperitoneal malignancy.

Pathology. Mixed population of histiocyte-like cells in a fibrous stroma. May contain dystrophic calcifications.

Clinical Presentation. Abdominal mass, abdominal pain, anemia.

Radiological Findings. May attain large size. Inhomogeneous appearance on CT is common. Calcifications may be present.[23,24]

Hemangiopericytoma

Incidence. All ages, equal sex distribution.

Pathology. Neoplastic proliferation of pericytes and abundant presence of thin wall sinusoidal vascular channels with numerous branchings. May be benign or malignant. Local recurrence and hematogenous and lymphatic metastases in lung, bone, and liver. May be encapsulated.

Clinical Presentation. Pelvic or retroperitoneal mass. May be associated with hypoglycemia.[24]

Treatment. Surgical removal. May be unresectable. Embolization prior to surgery may be considered. Five-year survival is 50%.

Radiological Findings. Bulky tumors arising in the retroperitoneum commonly displace adjacent organs.[23,24] Margins are usually well differentiated (Fig. 16–19). The distinguishing feature is marked hypervascularity. On angiography, the tumors are hypervascular with prominent feeding arteries, usually lumbar or hypogastric.[26–28]

The tumor is obviously hypervascular with areas of enhancement following contrast injection.[24] Inhomogeneous areas of tumor necrosis or intratumoral hemorrhage may be seen.[29] Other retroperitoneal tumors are seldom, if ever, hypervascular and preoperative diagnosis is therefore possible.

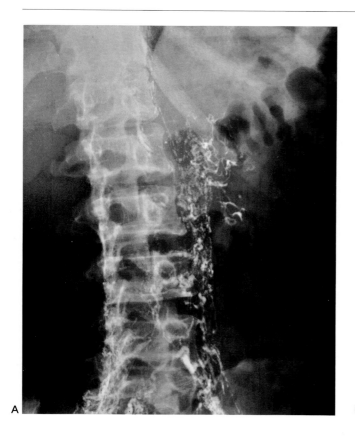

A

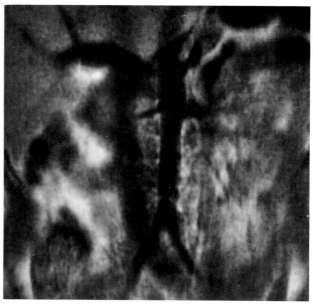

B

Figure 16–16.   Filariasis. **(A)** In the flow phase of lymphangiogram contrast is seen in dilated para-aortic lymphatics. Because of the more cephalad obstruction, the flow is diverted toward the kidney where contrast is seen entering lower pole calyx. **(B)** On T1-weighted coronal sequence in the same patient, dilated para-aortic lymphatics (in retrospect) are recognized.

Liposarcoma

Incidence.   Eleven percent of all primary retroperitoneal tumors. Male preponderance.

Pathology.   Subtypes are: a) Well-differentiated liposarcoma; b) myxoid liposarcoma; and c) pleomorphic liposarcoma.

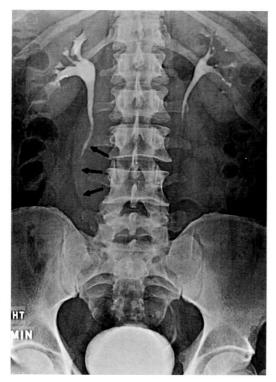

Figure 16–17.   A small retroperitoneal tumor is suspected because of minimal lateral displacement of the left ureter (arrows).

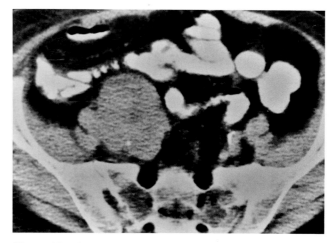

Figure 16–18.   Recurrent retroperitoneal leiomyosarcoma.

Table 16–1.   Suggestive but Nonspecific Radiological Findings in Primary Retroperitoneal Tumors

Heterogeneous mass with areas of fat	Liposarcoma
Homogeneous fat mass	Lipoma
Mixed fat, calcifications, soft tissue	Teratoma
Calcifications (adult)	Malignant fibrous histiocytoma
Calcifications (child)	Neuroblastoma
Hypervascular	Hemangiopericytoma, hemangioma
Para-aortic location (catecholamine excess)	Paraganglioma
Homogeneous, low density	Neurofibroma
Dark (hypointense) on T2-weighted sequence	Fibrosarcoma, rhabdomyosarcoma

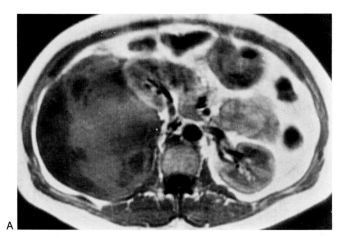
A

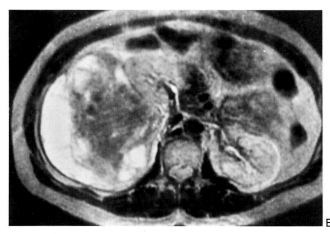
B

Figure 16–19A,B.   Large hemangiopericytoma appears well demarcated and inhomogeneous. Areas of hemorrhage are present and appear dark on T1- and bright on T2-weighted sequences.

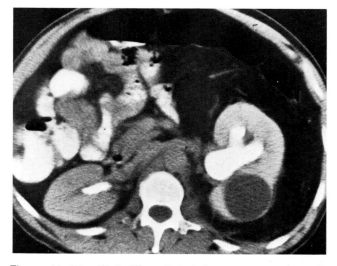

Figure 16–20.   Well-differentiated liposarcoma surrounds and displaces the left kidney and intestines. The tumor is predominantly of fat density. Renal cyst is an incidental finding.

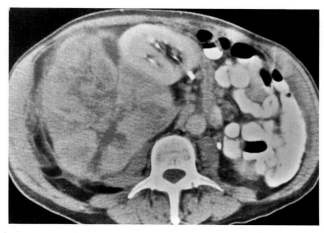

Figure 16–21.   Large retroperitoneal pleomorphic liposarcoma is predominantly of soft tissue density. The right kidney is displaced anteriorly and medially.

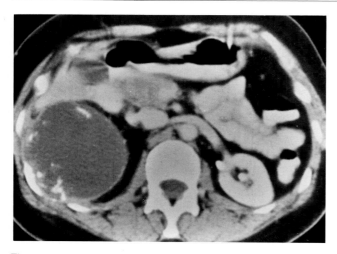

Figure 16–22. Chondrosarcoma originating from the rib extends into right retroperitoneum.

Clinical Presentation. Palpable abdominal mass, abdominal pain.

Radiological Findings. On CT and MR imaging, the tumor is predominantly of fat density (high signal intensity on T1- and T2-weighted sequences) (Fig. 16–20). Pleomorphic liposarcoma is of soft tissue density and may have areas of necrosis (Fig. 16–21).[23]

Mature Teratoma

Incidence. Rare. Female to male ratio is 3 to 1. Peak occurrence in first 6 months of life and early adulthood.

Radiological Findings. Well-circumscribed tumors with solid and cystic components. Fat may be identified in 60% of mature teratomas. Calcification is present in the majority of tumors.[24,30]

Secondary Tumors

Besides nodal metastases and malignant retroperitoneal fibrosis, various neoplastic processes may invade retroperitoneum by direct extension from the adjacent structures (Fig. 16–22).

REFERENCES

1. Elkin M, Cohen G. Diagnostic value of the psoas shadow. Clin Radiol 1962; 13:210–217.
2. Williams SM, Hultman SA, Harned RK, Quaife MA. The psoas sign: a reevaluation. Radiographics 1985; 5:525–536.
3. Damstrup L, Jensen TT. Retroperitoneal fibrosis after long-term daily use of ergotamine. Int Urol Nephrol 1986; 18:299–301.
4. Baker LR, Mallinson WJ, Gregory MC, et al. Idiopathic retroperitoneal fibrosis. A retrospective analysis of 60 cases. Br J Urol 1987; 60:497–503.
5. Doolin EJ, Goldstein H, Kessler B, et al. Familial retroperitoneal fibrosis. J Pediatr Surg 1987; 22:1092–1094.
6. Smith SJ, Bosniak MA, Megibow AJ, et al. CT demonstration of rapid improvement of retroperitoneal fibrosis in response to steroid therapy. Urol Radiol 1986; 8:104–107.
7. Degesys GE, Dunnick NR, Silverman PM, et al. Retroperitoneal fibrosis: use of CT in distinguishing among possible causes. AJR 1986; 146:57–60.
8. Yancey JM, Kaude JV. Diagnosis of perirenal fibrosis by MR imaging. J Comput Assist Tomogr 1988; 12:335–337.
9. Glynn TP Jr, Kreipke DL, Irons JM. Amyloidosis: diffuse involvement of the retroperitoneum. Radiology 1989; 170:726.
10. Walker DI, Bloor K, Williams G, Gillie I. Inflammatory aneurysms of the abdominal aorta. Br J Surg 1972; 59:609–614.
11. Baskerville PA, Blakeney CG, Young AE, Browse NL. The diagnosis and treatment of periaortic fibrosis ("inflammatory" aneurysms). Br J Surg 1980; 70:381–385.
12. Cullenward MJ, Scanlan KA, Pozniak MA, Acher CA. Inflammatory aortic aneurysms (periaortic fibrosis): radiologic imaging. Radiology 1986; 159:75–82.
13. Arrivé L, Hricak H, Tavares NJ, Miller TR. Malignant versus nonmalignant retroperitoneal fibrosis: differentiation with MR imaging. Radiology 1989; 172:139–143.
14. Cohan RH, Saeed M, Sussman SK, et al. Percutaneous drainage of pelvic lymphatic fluid collections in the renal transplant patients. Invest Radiol 1987; 22:864–867.
15. von Sonnenberg E, Wittich GR, Casola G, et al. Lymphoceles: imaging characteristics and percutaneous management. Radiology 1986; 161:593–596.
16. White M, Mueller PR, Ferrucci JT Jr, et al. Percutaneous drainage of postoperative abdominal and pelvic lymphoceles. AJR 1985; 145:1065–1069.
17. Leonidas JC, Brill PW, Bhan I, Smith TH. Cystic lymphangioma in infants and children. Radiology 1978; 127:203–208.
18. Castellino RA, Finkelstein S. Lymphangiographic demonstration of a retroperitoneal lymphangioma. Radiology 1975; 115:355–356.
19. Gomori JM, Grossman RI. Mechanisms responsible for the MR appearance and evolution of intracranial hemorrhage. Radiographics 1988; 8:427–440.
20. Udonsi JK. Bancroftian filariasis in the Igwun basin, Nigeria: an epidemiological, parasitological, and clinical study in relation to the transmission dynamics. Folia Parasitol 1988; 35:147–155.
21. Greig JD, MacKenzie JR, Azmy AA. Congenital pyelolymphatic fistula in a child with chyluria. Br J Urol 1989; 63:550–551.
22. Chen KC. Lymphatic abnormalities in patients with chyluria. Urology 1971; 106:111–114.

23. Lane R, Stephens DH, Reiman HM. Primary retroperitoneal neoplasms: CT findings in 90 cases with clinical and pathologic correlation. AJR 1989; 152:83–89.

24. Goldman SM, Hartman DS, Weiss SW. Varied radiographic manifestations of retroperitoneal malignant fibrous histiocytoma revealed through 27 cases. Radiology 1986; 135:33–38.

25. Yasuda Y, Kasahara K, Tenmoku S, et al. Retroperitoneal hemangiopericytoma associated with hypoglycemia: report of a case. Jpn J Surg 1979; 9:350–358.

26. Smith RB, Machleder HI, Rand RW, Bentson J, Toubas P. Preoperative vascular embolization as an adjunct to successful resection of large retroperitoneal hemangiopericytoma. J Urol 1976; 115:206–208.

27. Levin DC, Watson RC, Baltaxe HA. Arteriography of retroperitoneal masses. Radiology 1973; 108:543–551.

28. Smullens SN, Scotti DJ, Osterholm JL, Weiss AJ. Preoperative embolization of retroperitoneal hemangiopericytomas as an aid to their removal. Cancer 1982; 50:1870–1875.

29. Alpern MB, Thorsen MK, Kellman GM, et al. CT appearance of hemangiopericytoma. J Comput Assist Tomogr 1986; 10:264–267.

30. Schey WL, Vesely JJ, Radkowski MA. Shard-like calcifications in retroperitoneal teratomas. Pediatr Radiol 1986; 16:82–83.

17

Urinary Tract Trauma

RENAL TRAUMA

Mechanism of Injury. Renal injury resulting from blunt trauma is primarily due to motor vehicle accidents and less frequently to sports injuries, falls, or assaults. Blunt trauma accounts for 70 to 80% of all renal injuries.[1] The right kidney is slightly less susceptible to injury compared to its counterpart, since it has added protection provided by the liver mass.

Penetrating renal injury caused by gunshot or knife wounds accounts for 20 to 30% of all renal trauma, more in some urban areas.

Predisposing Factors. Preexisting conditions such as renal tumor, hydronephrosis, ureteropelvic junction obstruction, solitary kidney, horseshoe kidney, ectopic kidney, and polycystic kidney make the kidney more susceptible to injury even in less severe trauma.[2] Kidneys in children are injured more frequently and more severely than in adults, probably because they are larger and less well protected.[3,4] Also, preexisting conditions are more frequently encountered in children.

Associated Injuries. Associated soft tissue injuries, such as splenic rupture, liver laceration, subcapsular hematoma of the liver, and injuries to the small and the large bowel, stomach, and pancreas, are seen in 20–30% of blunt renal trauma victims. Bone fractures are present in almost half of these patients. Injuries to other organs are substantially higher in penetrating injuries.[5]

Classification. Classification presented (Fig. 17–1) is but one of several different proposals.[6,7]

Clinical Presentation. Microscopic and gross hematuria, flank pain, tenderness, hypotension, shock. Severity of clinical findings may range from very mild to severe. Preexisting conditions, such as renal tumors, and hydronephrosis, may be mistakenly attributed to trauma.

Radiological Workup

Who Needs It? This question is difficult to answer, in part because management issues regarding category II injuries are still unresolved.[7] Some urologists advocate a conservative approach, supportive therapy, and observation.[8,9] For these, imaging is secondary to the clinical presentation. Others advocate immediate surgical intervention and for those surgeons radiologic imaging contributes significant information regarding the extent of injury, condition of the opposite kidney, and injury to the other organs.[10]

Unstable patients may have no radiographic studies whatsoever, if their condition requires an immediate exploration.

In stable patients with blunt trauma and microscopic hematuria, without suspected associated injuries or fractures, the yield of radiological contrast examination in detecting significant renal injury is low.[11,12]

In stable patients with blunt trauma and gross hematuria, or microscopic hematuria with more than 25–50 red blood cells per high field, the yield of radiological contrast examinations is sufficiently high to influence further therapy.

Patients with suspected injuries to other organs, such as the spleen, are likely to have a CT examination anyway.

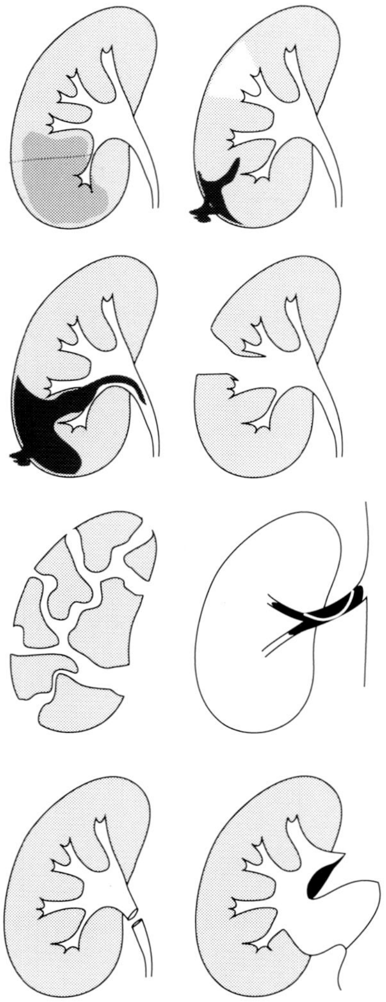

	Category & frequency	Description	Treatment
	I	•Contusions	Expectant
		•Parenchymal lacerations which are usually small and do not communicate with the collecting system	Expectant
	80%	•Small or medium size infarcts	Expectant
	II	•Parenchymal lacerations which extend and communicate with the collecting system	Controversial. Some advocate immediate surgery, others conservative management
	15%		
	III	Catastrophic injuries	
		•Shattered kidney	Surgery
	5%	•Injuries to vascular pedicle	Surgery within 2-12 h
	IV	•UPJ avulsion	Surgery
		•Laceration of the renal pelvis	Surgery or stenting
	rare		

Figure 17–1. Renal trauma classification.

Suspected renal injury should be investigated as soon as possible. In cases of complete arterial occlusion, renal function is irreversibly lost after 2 hours of ischemia in over 90% of cases. This is a very short period of time when considering the time lost in transportation to the emergency room, initial physical examination, and laboratory workup.

In a stable patient with suspected renal injury the first and foremost question is: is injury to other abdominal organs suspected? followed by: are both kidneys present? and if so, are they functioning?

CT. If the answer to the first question is yes, the radiological examination of choice is contrast-enhanced CT. CT is the method of choice for examining parenchymal organs, such as liver, spleen, and pancreas (Figs. 17–2, 17–3, 17–4). Intraperitoneal and retroperitoneal hemorrhage, as well as free intraperi-

toneal air, are easily demonstrated. Duodenal hematoma, thickened bowel wall, and dilated loops of bowel may be seen. Fractures are also well demonstrated. In patients with suspected head injuries, head CT may be performed in the same session (probably prior to the abdomen).

Whether the other abdominal organs are injured or not, CT will determine if both kidneys are present and if function is absent in one or both kidneys or in a part of one kidney.

Intravenous Pyelography. Even if no injury to the other organs is suspected, CT is still an excellent method for evaluating the extent of renal trauma. Unsuspected injuries to other organs are common and are likely to be revealed on this examination much more readily than by any other modality.

Excretory urogram has a place when injuries to

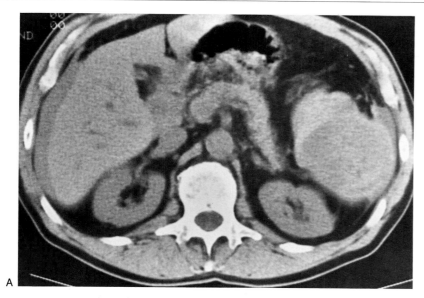

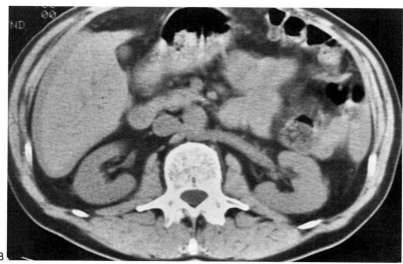

Figure 17–2. (A) Splenic rupture and splenic hematoma are detected several days after trauma on nonenhanced scan. (B) Intraperitoneal fluid is seen around the liver and in the left paracolic gutter. Also note left retroaortic renal vein.

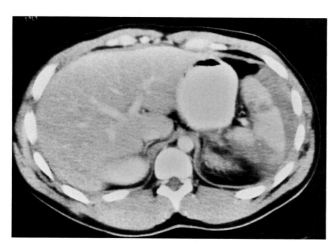

Figure 17–3. Splenic laceration. Parts of the spleen are still well perfused with contrast. Hematoma appears to be contained. Stomach is displaced medially.

other organs are not suspected and injury to the kidney is not too severe. Since this is a simple, quick, and readily available study, the question of whether both kidneys are functioning and present may be promptly answered. If a nonfunctioning kidney is discovered, either CT or angiography may be necessary to decide on the cause and to guide further management.

Frequently, linear tomography or larger than usual dose of radiographic contrast is necessary for better delineation of the kidneys.

Limited excretory urography may be very useful in the operating room when retroperitoneal hematoma or other signs of renal injury are encountered during exploration of the abdomen.

Angiography. Angiographic evaluation of traumatized kidney may be indicated as a prelude to surgery

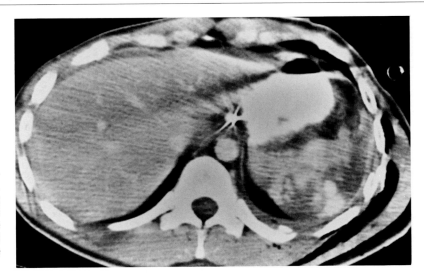

Figure 17–4. Major splenic laceration. Splenic contour is disrupted. Active bleeding is present judging by the appearance of extravasated contrast in the posterior part of the spleen. There are several fractured ribs as well as soft tissue air outside of the rib cage.

in cases of a nonfunctioning kidney, presumably due to vascular occlusion. Surgeon may need to have a clear definition of the level and completeness of vascular occlusion, in which case angiography should be urgently done. Of course, one must keep in mind the inevitable loss of time involved in bringing the angio team to the hospital and time necessary to complete the procedure.

The second indication for angiography is in situations where there is continuous bleeding from the kidney, either from a severed smaller artery or from a traumatic arteriovenous fistula. Transcatheter supraselective embolization of the bleeding vessel is a very effective means of arresting hemorrhage, thus allowing the patient to stabilize without surgery.

Sonography and Nuclear Medicine. These imaging methods may be considered in patients who are sensitive to radiographic contrast. Sonography may answer questions related to morphology such as subcapsular or perinephric fluid, and displacement. Scintigraphy may answer questions relating to renal perfusion and function and is useful for follow-up.

Radiological Findings

RENAL CONTUSION

This is the most common type of renal trauma. Renal contusion may be very mild and need not be recognized on radiographic examination. More severe cases demonstrate mild renal enlargement and somewhat decreased function on urography and angiography (Fig. 17–5). Inhomogeneous perfusion of an area with preserved perfusion of immediate surrounding parenchyma is suggestive (Fig. 17–6).[13]

Striated nephrogram may be present and detected on all contrast examinations.[14] Blood flow may be slower than normal. The entire kidney or part of the kidney may be affected. The collecting system may become spidery due to parenchymal edema and renal enlargement.

RENAL LACERATION

"Fracture" through renal parenchyma frequently occurs between major vascular branching so that two fragments may be widely separated with surprisingly little associated hemorrhage (Fig. 17–7).[15] Normal nephrogram may be seen, either on CT, EXU, or angiography, in both fragments thus separated with

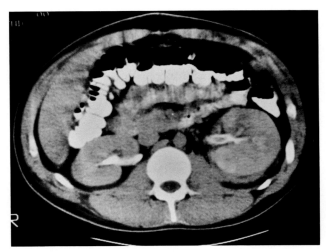

Figure 17–5. Left renal contusion. Kidney is enlarged due to edema. Small perinephric hematoma is present posterior to the kidney. A blood clot in the renal pelvis is seen as a "filling defect."

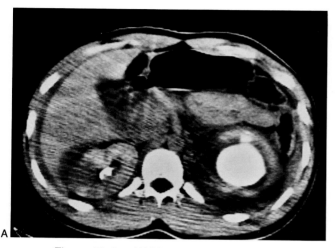 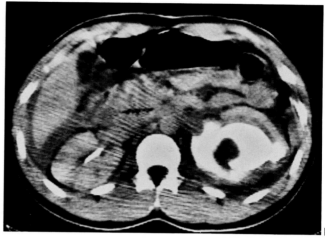

Figure 17–6. **(A)** Mild contusion of the right kidney is manifested as inhomogeneous nephrogram. **(B)** At first glance the left kidney looks alarming since it appears there is a major laceration. However, the contrast is well contained in what is obviously a hydronephrotic functioning kidney. Congenital ureteropelvic junction obstruction was confirmed at surgery. Note free intraperitoneal fluid around the liver.

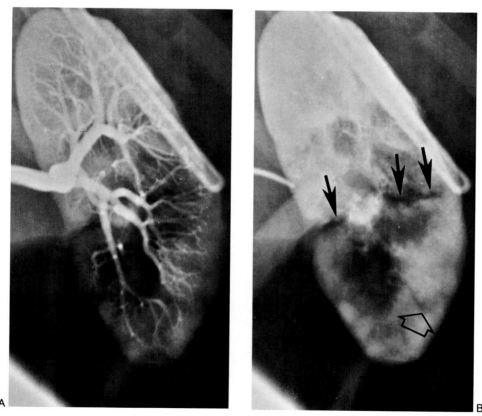

Figure 17–7. **(A)** Major renal laceration has propagated between major vessels, leaving them intact. **(B)** The fissure (arrows) separating the upper and lower parts of the kidney is not wide and is in a plane so that it may easily remain undetected on CT scan. A smaller laceration is seen in the lower pole (open arrow). Underperfused area in the lower fractured segment medially probably represents segmental infarct. This patient was successfully treated conservatively.

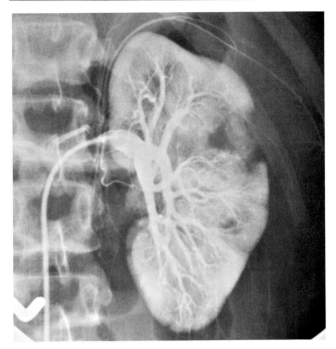

Figure 17–8. Renal laceration is wide and filled with a clot. Large perinephric hematoma is detected because of displacement of capsular arteries.

blood clot between (Figs. 17–8, 17–9). Contrast extravasation from ruptured pelvocalyceal system usually signifies major disruption of renal parenchyma and places the injury in category II (Fig. 17–10).

A very large collection of radiographic contrast, especially if located medial to the kidney, is suggestive of pelvocalyceal or ureteral tear. This is particularly true if the renal parenchyma does not appear

disrupted and the distal ureter does not opacify with contrast.[16]

RENAL ARTERY OR SEGMENTAL BRANCH OCCLUSION

Injury to the renal artery or branch artery can be due to sudden elongation or intimal flap elevation. Blood flow through the injured artery is significantly diminished or arrested. Thrombosis of the vessel follows, resulting in segmental or total renal infarction.

Nonfunctioning kidney is discovered on either CT, intravenous urography, or radionuclide scan. Triangular or wedge-shaped nonperfused area is seen in segmental infarction.[15] *Cortical subcapsular rim sign* represents 2 to 3 mm thick dense outer nephrogram overlying the infarcted segment (Fig. 17–11).[17,18] This sign is pathognomonic for infarction if only part of the kidney is involved. If there is global involvement of the entire kidney, main renal artery occlusion is the most likely diagnosis, although this sign has been described in renal vein thrombosis, acute cortical necrosis, and acute tubular necrosis.

Retrograde flow of contrast into the renal vein may be detected in renal artery occlusion or avulsion (Fig. 17–12).[19,20]

Stretched and irregular renal artery may be demonstrated on an angiogram leading to the obstructed branch. There is lingering of radiographic contrast in the proximal part of the obstructed artery (Fig. 17–13).

HEMATOMA

Subcapsular hematoma is usually self-limiting. The diagnosis is generally obvious on CT scan (Fig. 17–

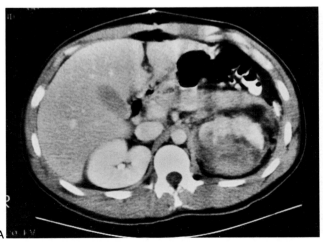

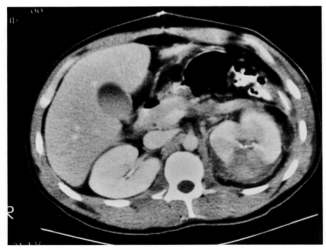

Figure 17–9. Major renal laceration extending from the upper pole **(A)** to the midpart of the kidney **(B)**. There is surprisingly little perinephric hematoma.

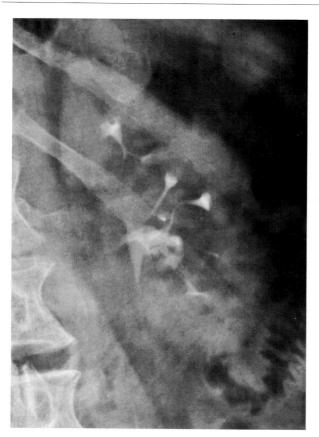

Figure 17–10. Since the collecting system is so well protected by surrounding parenchyma, any extravasation of the radiographic contrast not only confirms pelvocalyceal tear, but also suggests parenchymal laceration.

14). Renal parenchyma is usually flattened immediately under the collected blood.

Intrarenal hematoma is seen as poorly perfused areas demonstrating patchy or absent nephrogram on contrast studies (Fig. 17–15). Acute hematoma is hyperdense to the kidney on nonenhanced scan (Fig. 17–16).

Perirenal hematoma is commonly seen in major renal trauma. Renal fascia prevents diffusion of blood into the retroperitoneum and is thought to have a tampon effect, thus restricting and to a certain degree arresting the hemorrhage. Indeed if the renal fascia is opened during surgery without having the renal artery and vein secured, major hemorrhage is likely to ensue. Perirenal and retroperitoneal hemorrhage is readily discovered on CT (Fig. 17–17). Blood may track to the opposite perirenal spaces along a communicating plane anterior to the lower aorta and inferior vena cava.[21]

On angiography, perinephric hematoma is suspected because of displacement and stretching of capsular arteries (Fig. 17–8). If displaced anteriorly by a large hematoma, the kidney may appear enlarged on projectional contrast examinations due to geometric magnification.

All types of hematomas described above may be discovered as solitary findings or may be associated with contusion, laceration, or infarction of the smaller vessels.

RENAL TORSION

This a rare occurrence and usually associated with a severe multisystem trauma. If the condition permits a radiological examination, a nonfunctioning kidney is discovered.

AVULSION

Renal pedicle avulsion and associated major vessel tear usually result in death before the patient reaches the hospital.

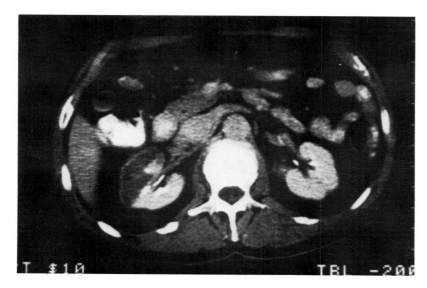

Figure 17–11. Segmental renal infarct following a trauma whereby the patient fell onto a ski pole. Triangular nonperfused area and cortical subcapsular rim sign are pathognomonic findings. (Photograph courtesy of Dr. Kevin Kelly.)

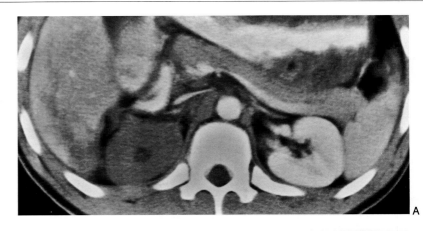

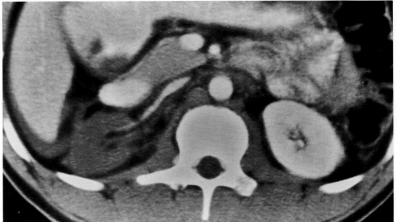

Figure 17–12. (A) Nonfunctioning right kidney following blunt abdominal trauma. There is liver laceration. (B) Retrograde flow of contrast from inferior vena cava into the right renal vein suggests marked decrease in blood outflow from the kidney.

HYPOTENSION AND SHOCK

In severe hypotension, such as in shock, the kidneys are small and although a nephrogram may be present, due to lack of filtration pressure there is no excretion of the contrast into the collecting system. Administration of contrast material to severely hypotensive patients is contraindicated, but at times this may not be recognized or the patient may become hypotensive immediately after contrast delivery (Fig. 17–18). Once blood pressure is normalized, the kidney resumes its normal size and contrast excretion.[22]

AFTERMATH OF RENAL TRAUMA

Chronic changes caused by renal trauma may be manifested years later as renal deformity, Page kidney, pseudocysts, etc. (Fig. 17–19). Hypertension is rare and apparently may appear years after the trauma.

URETERAL TRAUMA

Mechanism of Injury. Ureteral trauma is comparatively rare. Despite their length, ureters are well protected from the effects of blunt trauma. More common is penetrating injury due to knife or bullet wound. The most common type of injury to the ureter is the result of surgical trauma, such as inadvertent ligation, clipping, contusion, laceration, and periureteral hematoma. Some reports claim 0.5% or more incidence of ureteric injury during abdominal hysterectomy, higher in extensive abdominal gynecologic operations.[23] Injury due to retrograde or antegrade endourological procedures is also on the rise.

Clinical Presentation. Acute symptoms are related to ureteral obstruction or urine extravasation. Extravasation may be retroperitoneal or intraperitoneal. Both types may cause signs of peritoneal

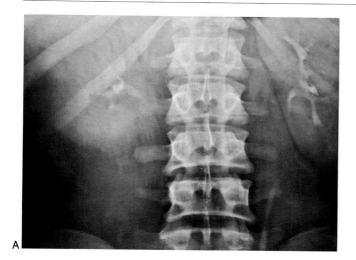

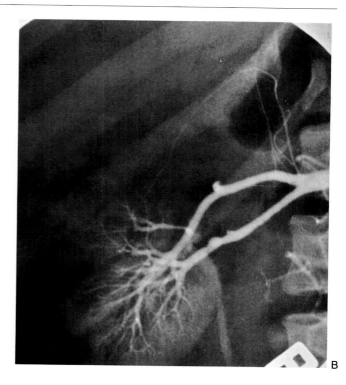

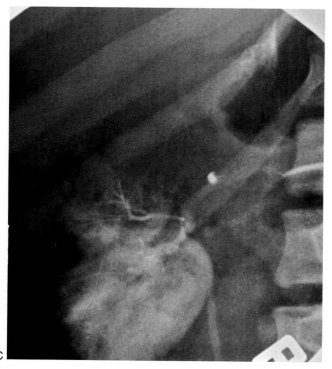

Figure 17–13. **(A)** The extent of renal injury is difficult to ascertain from the EXU alone. What can be determined is that the left kidney is normal, and that some function does remain in the right kidney. There is probably a large retroperitoneal hematoma obliterating right psoas outline. **(B)** Selective right renal arteriogram demonstrates complete occlusion of the segmental branches supplying the upper pole. Slight wavering in the caliber of the most lower segmental branch suggests injury due to overstretching. Inferior adrenal branches are intact and normal adrenal blush is evident. **(C)** Lingering of the radiographic contrast for several seconds in an acutely occluded branch is a very common finding. This type of injury is beyond surgical repair as far as restitution of blood flow to the kidney is concerned. This patient was treated conservatively.

irritation. Hematuria may or may not be present. Ureterocutaneous fistula may be present following surgery.

Ureteral injury may result in ureteral stricture, hydronephrosis, and loss of renal function.

Radiological Findings

Penetrating Trauma. Many patients with penetrating abdominal wounds end up in the operating room before there is time to adequately assess the urinary tract system. Ureteral transection may be overlooked if the retroperitoneum is left unexplored. Retroperitoneal urinoma may be diagnosed later in the postoperative period.

Both CT and excretory urography are excellent diagnostic modalities for discovering and assessing the level and severity of ureteral injury. Retrograde pyelography may also be needed for determining the precise location and possible retrograde stent placement. CT excels in discovering perirenal and periureteral fluid collections. Concentrated radiographic contrast is found in the retroperitoneum, implying ureteral laceration, avulsion, or transection (Fig. 17–20). Although primary repair is usually necessary, percutaneous drainage combined with stent

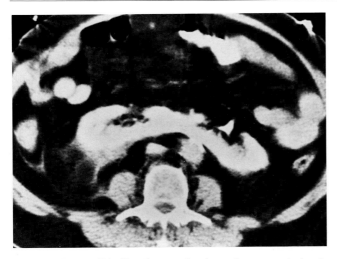

Figure 17–14. Small subcapsular hematoma posterior to the right horseshoe kidney following blunt trauma.

placement has been successful in some instances (Fig. 17–21).

Iatrogenic Surgical or Endourological Trauma. Excretory urography is the examination of choice. Retroperitoneal extravasation, if present, is readily detected and so is the location of the injury. An abnormal fluid collection detected by any imaging modality may be related to unsuspected ureteral urine leak. Obstruction may be complete or partial.

Iatrogenic trauma to the ureter is a common indication for percutaneous nephrostomy. Usually it is placed to buy time before corrective surgery or as a means for placing antegrade ureteral stents.

BLADDER TRAUMA

Incidence. Present in 10% of patients with pelvic fracture. Lower and upper urinary tract injury are seldom seen together, usually only in very severe trauma.

Mechanism of Injury. Pelvic fracture is the most common cause. Also common are blunt trauma, such as seat belt injury and blow to the lower abdomen.[24] Chances of rupture increase if the bladder is distended. Point of weakness is usually at the dome.

Less common are penetrating injuries, such as bullet and knife wounds, puncture by a bone fragment associated with a pelvic fracture, instrumentation, biopsy, and abdominal surgery.

Obstetrical injuries are extremely rare and are

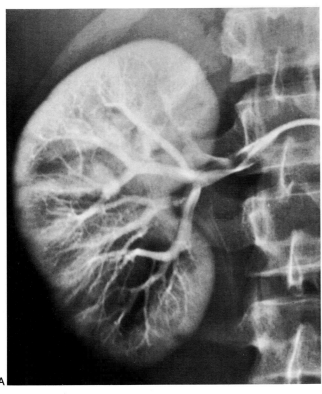
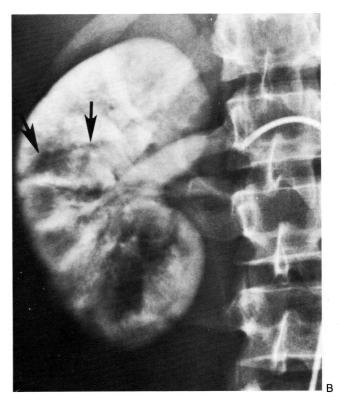

Figure 17–15. Intrarenal hematoma is present in the lower pole of the right kidney displacing lobar branches (A) and appearing as a nonperfused area on later phase (B). Note parenchymal laceration (arrows).

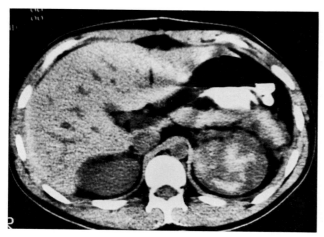

Figure 17–16. Acute left upper pole intrarenal hematoma on nonenhanced CT scan is hyperdense compared to the renal parenchyma.

caused by compression of the bladder against the pubis by the fetal head, or combination of uterine and bladder rupture during a prolonged and difficult delivery.

Associated Injuries. Pelvic fractures, urethral injury (male), and injuries to other abdominal organs are common.[25]

Clinical Presentation. Hypotension, gross hematuria, blood clots in urine, abdominal distention, lower abdominal, or suprapubic pain.[26,27] Patient may be unable to urinate.

Radiological Workup and Findings

Cystogram remains the method of choice for determining the extent of bladder injury.[28] This should be

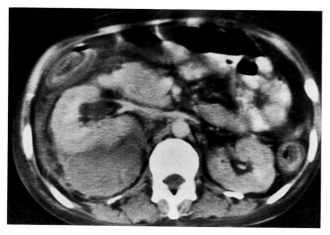

Figure 17–17. Acute perinephric hematoma following renal biopsy. (Photograph courtesy of Dr. Mark Mehringer.)

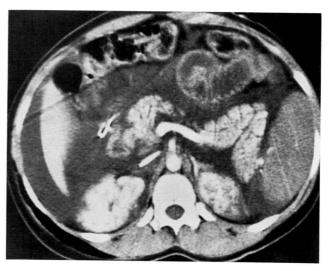

Figure 17–18. Contrast-enhanced CT in a patient with a major trauma with intraperitoneal bladder rupture and large amounts of intraperitoneal fluid. Sometime during the examination, the patient became hypotensive. There is lingering of contrast in the major vessels. The spleen is underperfused, probably due to vasoconstriction in shock. Kidneys are small and show inhomogeneous areas of cortical hypoperfusion. Left adrenal is densely stained. "Buckled" tail of pancreas is a normal variant.

done in increments of 50 to 100 cc between exposures, since there is no need to fill the entire peritoneal cavity should there be intraperitoneal rupture. Bladder should never be catheterized if a urethral injury is suspected. Under these circumstances, the examination of choice is retrograde urethrogram followed by a cystogram only if the urethra is found to be normal. If time is of the essence, it is permissible to perform urography and cystography simultaneously. Otherwise urography should precede cystography.

Small extraperitoneal ruptures may not be clearly visible without oblique views. This usually is a difficult task, since turning a patient with major pelvic trauma may be painful. On occasion, the extravasated contrast may be observed only on the postevacuation radiograph. It is possible to completely miss a bladder rupture despite technically well-executed cystogram.[29]

Many patients will undergo CT scanning of the abdomen and pelvis for evaluation and diagnosis of injury to other organs following a major abdominal trauma. One should be aware that bladder rupture may be missed on CT if the bladder is decompressed by a catheter or if it is incompletely filled.[30]

PERIVESICAL HEMATOMA

Perivesical hematoma is commonly seen with major pelvic fractures (Fig. 17–22). Accumulated blood

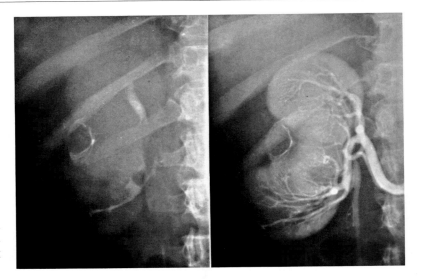

Figure 17–19. Renal angiogram many years after trauma demonstrates calcified remnants of a hematoma in the region of what must have been a major renal laceration.

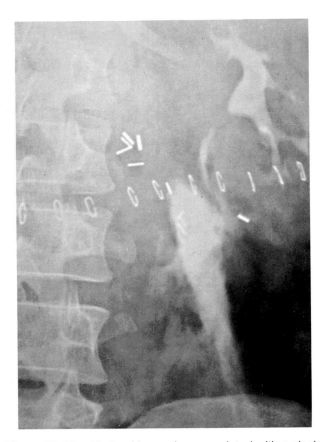

Figure 17–20. Ureteral laceration associated with a slashing anterior abdominal wound caused by a broken industrial knife. Despite exploration and repair of bowel injuries, the ureteral laceration was only recognized several days after surgery.

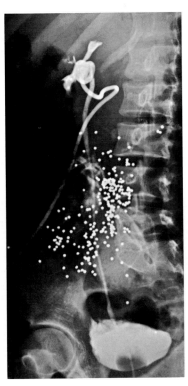

Figure 17–21. Shotgun wound through anterior abdominal wall resulted in ureteral laceration which remained undiscovered until after abdominal surgery for bowel injury. Percutaneous nephrostomy and ureteral stent were used as the treatment of choice. Ureter was patent on a 1-year follow-up.

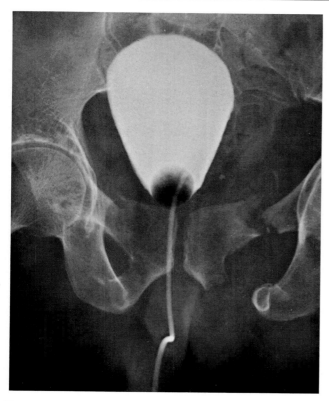

Figure 17–22.   Perivesical hematoma associated with major fractures of the bony pelvis.

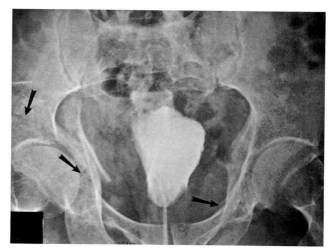

Figure 17–23.   Inverted pear sign and elevated bladder base in the presence of skeletal fractures is indicative of perivesical hematoma. Although the major fracture fragment within the right pelvis is obvious, other fractures are more subtle (arrows).

compresses upon the extraperitoneal part of the bladder, narrowing it at the base. An *inverted teardrop* sign or *inverted pear* sign is present on cystogram, indicating the presence of extraperitoneal fluid. Bladder is usually elevated (Fig. 17–23). Asymmetrical bladder displacement is more common in penetrating wounds (Fig. 17–24). Hematoma is well visualized on CT.

EXTRAPERITONEAL BLADDER RUPTURE

This is an anterior bladder floor injury usually due to separation of symphysis pubis. During cystographic examination of the bladder, contrast is seen in streaky pattern outside the bladder. More importantly, the extraluminal contrast is stationary and persists in the same area unchanged over a period of time (Fig. 17–25). If small, this type of bladder injury may under certain circumstances be treated only by an indwelling catheter.

INTRAPERITONEAL BLADDER RUPTURE

This is usually a more serious injury, which is likely to require open bladder surgery. The contrast is seen

to freely enter the peritoneal cavity and form small triangles between the bowel loops (Fig. 17–26). Contrast is likely to be seen in the dependent parts of the abdominal cavity first. These are pouch of Douglas, right paracolic gutter, and Morison's pouch. Liver and spleen may also be outlined (Fig. 17–27). Since intraperitoneal contrast is reabsorbed into systemic circulation, the kidneys and ureters are likely to become visible just as they are during excretory urography. On CT, rupture may be missed unless the bladder is well distended. If a bladder catheter is present, it should be temporarily clamped following

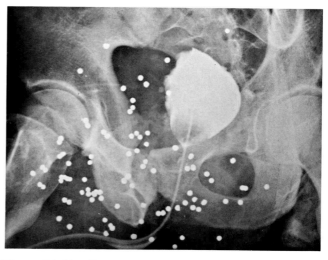

Figure 17–24.   Perivesical hematoma following a gunshot wound.

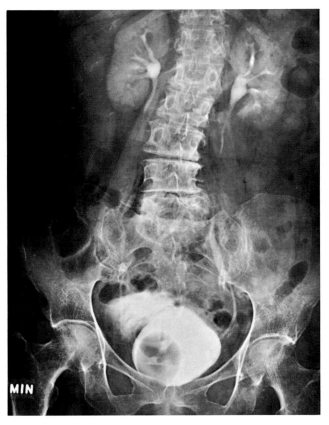

Figure 17–25. Extraperitoneal bladder perforation seen on simultaneously performed urogram and cystogram. Extravasated contrast remains stationary for prolonged period. Oblique projection will show contrast to be anterior in location.

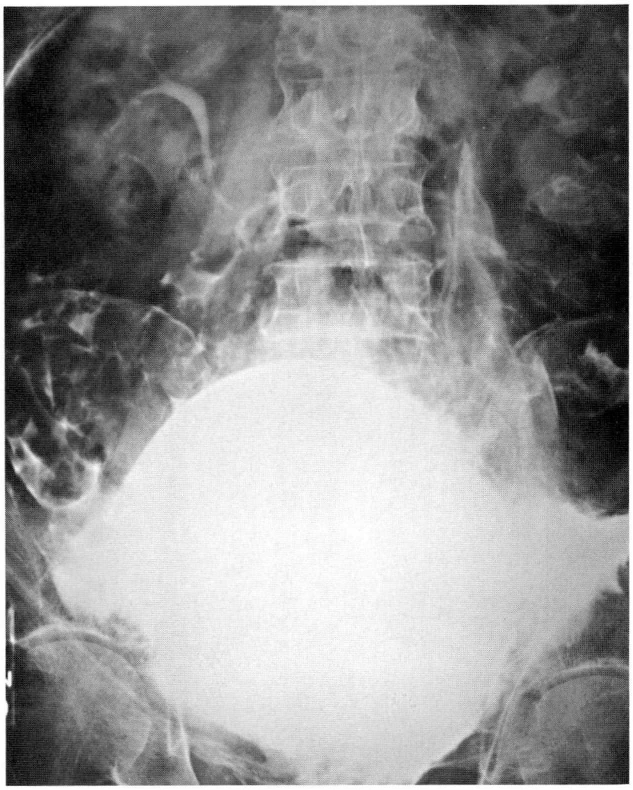

Figure 17–26. This cystogram (and the one in Figure 17–27) is presented as an example of how not to perform this study on a patient with suspected intraperitoneal bladder rupture. Instead of being filled in small increments, the bladder was filled to capacity all at once. Moderate amount of contrast is seen within the peritoneal cavity where it assumes triangular shapes between loops of bowel.

intravenous injection of contrast (Fig. 17–28) or one could consider filling the bladder with contrast (expensive CT cystogram).

Iatrogenic perforation is most commonly associated with bladder biopsy (Fig. 17–29).

INTRALUMINAL CLOTS

Intraluminal blood clots may be associated with primary bladder injury but may also form in any patient with gross hematuria (Fig. 17–30).

BLADDER AND PELVIC HEMORRHAGE

In some instances intractable hemorrhage from the bladder and traumatized pelvis may be life threatening and surgery ineffectual or not feasible. Angiographic demonstration of the bleeding vessel may be necessary, followed by therapeutic embolization. Selective hypogastric (internal iliac) arteriograms are performed one at a time. Bleeding site is diagnosed when a localized puddle of contrast appears during arterial phase of the angiogram (Fig. 17–31).

If hemorrhage is detected, the tip of the catheter should be placed beyond the takeoff of the gluteal arteries and preferably selectively into the bleeding artery followed by embolization with particular matter for hemorrhage control.[31,32] Embolization of the gluteal arteries may result in skin necrosis in elderly and diabetic individuals with compromised systemic circulation.

URETHRAL TRAUMA

Incidence. Present in 5 to 10% of males with pelvic fractures.[33] Rare in females.[34] Associated bladder injury may be seen in 10 to 20% of the patients with posterior urethral injuries.[35]

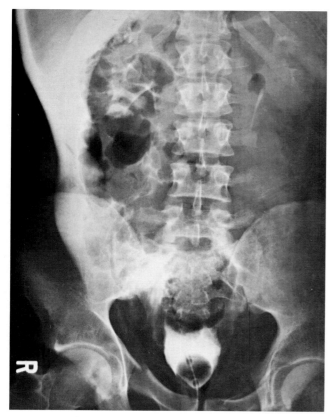

Figure 17–27. Cystogram demonstrating intraperitoneal bladder rupture. Large amount of contrast is in the peritoneal cavity filling right paracolic gutter (right colon is displaced from properitoneal stripe) and surrounding the liver. Contrast is reabsorbed from the peritoneal surface and excreted by the kidneys.

Mechanism of Injury. Anterior urethra: Straddle injury (crush upon pubic arch), gunshot wound, iatrogenic, human bite, intercourse.[36]

Posterior urethra: Pelvic fractures, gunshot and knife wounds.

Classification

Anterior urethra: Incomplete or complete.
Posterior urethra (Fig. 17–32):[37,38]

- Type I: Urethra stretched
- Type II: Tear above urogenital diaphragm
- Type III: Tear at urogenital diaphragm, which is disrupted

Clinical Presentation. Inability to urinate. Blood may be seen at the meatus. "Floating" or "high-riding" prostate on physical examination.

Treatment. Placement of a suprapubic tube. Incidence of impotence after immediate primary repair is high. Incidence of impotence and other complications decreases dramatically if the primary repair is delayed 3 to 4 months.[39,40]

Radiological Findings. Retrograde urethrogram is the examination of choice.[41,42] It is important to obtain radiographs in oblique projections. This may be difficult in the presence of pelvic fractures, but is nonetheless required in order to determine the type and extent of the injury. Radiographic contrast should be about 25–30% and judicious amounts should be used. Too much extravasated contrast may delay the healing process, too little contrast may be insufficient for diagnosis.

In type I posterior urethral injury one may identify urethral elongation. In type II either partial or complete urethral tear above the urogenital diaphragm will show as contrast outside the urethral lumen above the urogenital diaphragm only (Figs. 17–33, 17–34). In type III rupture contrast must be seen below the urogenital diaphragm, although it may be seen at both sides and in the bladder, depending on completeness of the tear (Fig. 17–35).

Both types II and III posterior urethral rupture may be partial or complete. Partial tear may be

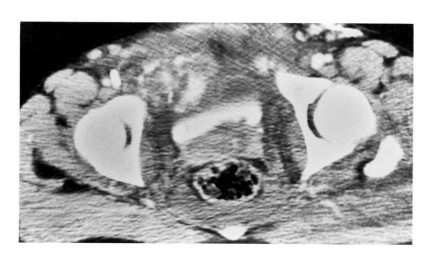

Figure 17–28. Intraperitoneal bladder rupture due to blunt trauma. Contrast is seen leaking into the peritoneal cavity at the anterior bladder wall.

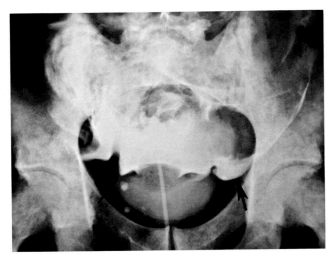

Figure 17–29. Intraperitoneal bladder perforation after a bladder biopsy. The Foley catheter was inadvertently passed through the perforation into the peritoneal cavity and secured by inflating the balloon. Contrast was thereafter infused into the peritoneal cavity instead of the bladder (transvesical peritoneogram?). Lateral pelvic recesses are well seen filled with contrast (arrows). The classic "dog ears" sign involves accumulation of peritoneal fluid in these. Also note diffuse osteoblastic metastases.

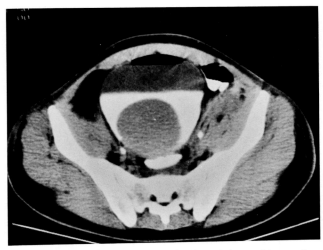

Figure 17–30. Large bladder clot from left renal laceration.

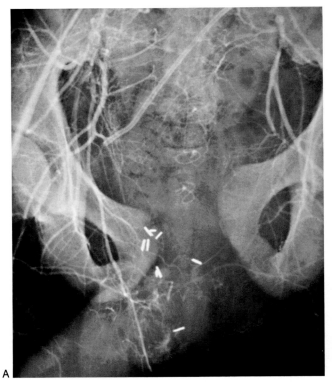

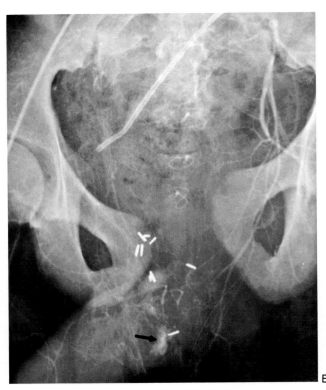

Figure 17–31. Acute hemorrhage from the right internal pudendal artery associated with pelvic fractures and bladder rupture. **(A)** Early arterial phase; **(B)** Late arterial phase shows puddling of the contrast (arrow). Transcatheter embolization is frequently the treatment of choice.

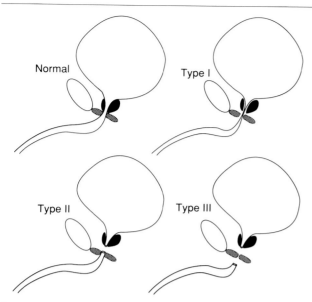

Figure 17–32. Classification of posterior urethral injury based on the urethrographic appearance. Types II and III may be partial or complete.[37]

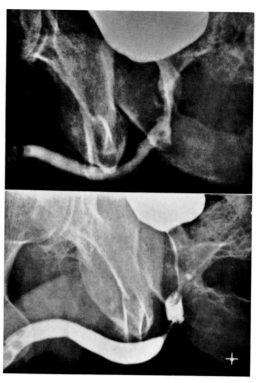

Figure 17–33. Partial tear above urogenital diaphragm (top) resulting in stricture after several months of suprapubic drainage (bottom).

inadvertently made complete by attempting retrograde bladder catheterization (Fig. 17–36). Although both result in strictures, those associated with partial tears may be treated without major surgery, i.e., urethrotomy or dilatation.[43] Therefore retrograde urethrogram should precede bladder catheterization whenever urethral injury is suspected.

In straddle injury causing anterior urethral tear, contrast may be seen in the scrotum and penis. Contrast extravasation depends on whether Buck's fascia is intact or ruptured.

SCROTAL TRAUMA

Traumatized scrotum is probably best examined by ultrasound.[44] Copious amounts of ultrasound jelly coupling allows examination without actually touching the patient.

Hydroceles of varying size are common following scrotal trauma, as is hematocele. Pyocele is less common and requires exploration if its presence is suspected. Hematocele and pyocele are indistinguishable on ultrasound examination. Enlarged and hyperechoic epididymis may be observed as an extratesticular mass.

Testicular hematoma is recognized as localized or extensive areas of increased echogenicity within the testicle.

Testicular rupture or laceration is suspected when the testicle cannot be visualized or when there is

poorly marginated testis with inhomogeneous internal echoes (Fig. 17–37). This is an indication for immediate exploratory surgery.

Summary

Ultrasound examination of the traumatized scrotum may influence the method of therapy. Surgical intervention is indicated if intratesticular hemorrhage, rupture, laceration, torsion, or pyocele are present. If intact testes are unequivocally demonstrated, an enlarged epididymis, hydrocele, or testicular contusion could be treated conservatively.

PENILE TRAUMA

Trauma to the penis may result in rupture of corpus cavernosum, laceration of tunica albuginea, and arteriovenous fistula (Fig. 17–38). Cavernosogram may exclude laceration of the tunica albuginea. Priapism may result from arteriocorporeal fistula and may require angiography and possible embolization.

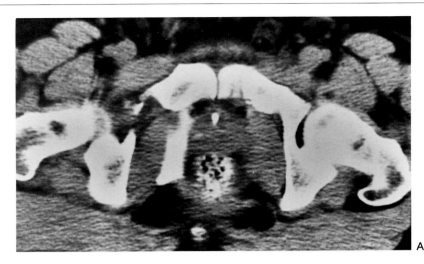

A

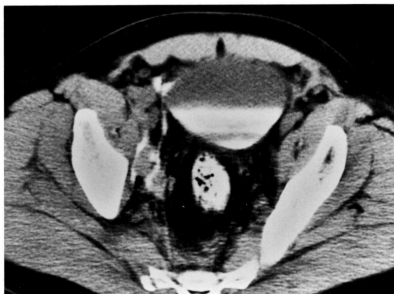

Figure 17–34. CT in a patient with type II urethral rupture 15 minutes after a urethrogram and suprapubic catheter placement. Extravasated contrast (from RUG) is propagating along the right internal obturator (**A**) and along the vascular and higher up in the extraperitoneal space (**B**). Blood is seen layering in the bladder after suprapubic catheter placement.

B

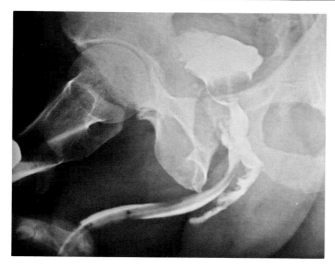

Figure 17–35. Type III urethral rupture, contrast is seen below the urogenital diaphragm. Tear is partial and (luckily) the bladder catheter was successfully negotiated into the bladder. This, of course, should not be attempted if urethral injury is suspected as it could be converted into a complete rupture and complicate management.

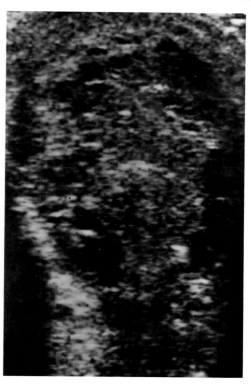

Figure 17–37. Testicular rupture and hematoma. The normal echotexture is replaced with inhomogeneous internal echoes. Hyperechoic spots probably represent areas of hemorrhage. (Photograph courtesy of Dr. David Cho.)

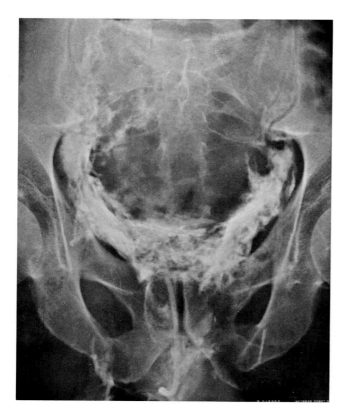

Figure 17–36. Unsuspected urethral tear was made worse when the Foley catheter was inflated at the posterior urethral rupture site. The examiner thought the catheter was in the bladder. Fifty cubic centimeters of radiographic contrast intended for cystography were injected and demonstrate extraperitoneal extravasation.

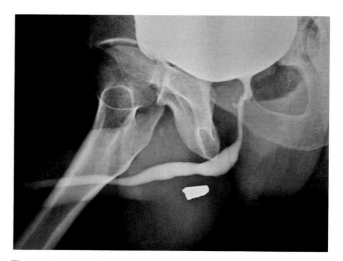

Figure 17–38. Bullet fragment lodged in corpus spongiosum just ventral to the bulbous urethra.

REFERENCES

1. Hai MA, Pontes JE, Pierce JM Jr. Surgical management of major renal trauma: a review of 102 cases treated by conservative surgery. J Urol 1977; 118:7–9.
2. Brower P, Paul J, Brosman SA. Urinary tract abnormalities presenting as a result of blunt abdominal trauma. J Trauma 1978; 18:719–722.
3. Waxman J, Belman B, Kass EJ. Traumatic amputation of the left lower renal pole in children. J Urol 1985; 134:114–117.
4. Taylor GA, Eichelberger MR, Potter BM. Hematuria: a marker of abdominal injury in children after blunt trauma. Ann Surg 1988; 208:688–693.
5. Sagalowski AI, McConnell JD, Peters PD. Renal trauma requiring surgery: an analysis of 185 cases. J Trauma 1983; 23:128–131.
6. Federle M. Evaluation of renal trauma. In Clinical Urography (Pollack HM, ed). Philadelphia: Saunders 1989:1472–1494.
7. Pollack HM, Wein AJ. Imaging of renal trauma. Radiology 1989; 172:297–308.
8. Evins SC, Thomason WB, Rosenblaum R. Non-operative management of severe renal lacerations. J Urol 1980; 123:247–249.
9. Yale-Loehr AJ, Kramer SS, Quinlan DM, et al. CT of severe renal trauma in children: evaluation and course of healing with conservative therapy. AJR 1989; 152:109–113.
10. Cass AS. Immediate radiological evaluation and early surgical management of genitourinary injuries from external trauma. J Urol 1979; 122:772–774.
11. Lieu TA, Fleisher GR, Mahboubi S, Schwartz JS. Hematuria and clinical findings as indications for intravenous pyelography in pediatric blunt renal trauma. Pediatrics 1988; 82:216–222.
12. Hardeman SW, Husman DA, Chinn HKW, Peters PC. Blunt urinary trauma: identifying those patients who require radiological diagnostic studies. J Urol 1987; 138:99–101.
13. Lang EK. Assessment of renal trauma by dynamic computed tomography. Radiographics 1983; 3:566–584.
14. Rubin BE, Schliftman R. The striated nephrogram in renal contusion. Urol Radiol 1979; 1:119–121.
15. Scaflani SJA, Becker JA. Radiological diagnosis of renal trauma. Urol Radiol 1985; 7:192–200.
16. Kenney PJ, Panicek DM, Witanowski LS. Computed tomography of ureteral disruption. JCAT 1987; 11:480–484.
17. Frank PH, Nuttall J, Brander WL, Prosser D. The cortical rim sign of renal infarction. Br J Radiol 1974; 47:875–878.
18. Glazer GM, Francis IR, Brady TM, Teng SS. Computed tomography of renal infarction: clinical and experimental observations. AJR 1983; 140:721–727.
19. Steinberg DL, Jeffrey RB, Federle MP, McAninch JW. The computerized tomography appearance of renal pedicle injury. J Urol 1984; 132:1163–1164.
20. Cates JD, Foley WD, Lawson TL. Retrograde opacification of renal vein: a CT sign of renal artery avulsion. Urol Radiol 1986; 8:92–94.
21. Kneeland JB, Auh YH, Rubenstein WA, et al. Perirenal spaces: CT evidence for communication across the mid-line. Radiology 1987; 164:657–664.
22. Katzberg RW, Schabel SI. Bilaterally small kidneys in shock. JAMA 1976; 235:2213–2214.
23. Daly JW, Higgins KA. Injury to the ureter during gynecological surgical procedures. Surg Gynecol Obst 1988; 167:19–22.
24. Sandler CM, Hall TJ, Rodriquez MB, Coriere JN Jr. Bladder injury in blunt pelvic trauma. Radiology 1986; 158:633–638.
25. Flancbaum L, Morgan AS, Fleisher M, Cox EF. Blunt bladder trauma: manifestation of severe injury. Urology 1988; 31:220–222.
26. Cass AS, Luxenberg M. Features of 164 bladder ruptures. J Urol 1988; 138:743–745.
27. Hardeman SW, Husmann DA, Chinn HK, Peters PC. Blunt urinary tract trauma: identifying those patients who require radiological diagnostic studies. J Urol 1987; 138:99–101.
28. Peterson NE, Schulze KA. Selective diagnostic uroradiography for trauma. J Urol 1987; 137:449–451.
29. Lieberman AH, Walden TB, Bogash M, Pollack HM, Kendall AR. Negative cystography with bladder rupture; presentation of 2 cases and review of the literature. J Urol 1980; 124:428–430.
30. Mee SL, McAninch JW, Federle MP. Computerized tomography in bladder rupture: diagnostic limitations. J Urol 1987; 137:207–209.
31. Lang EK, Deutch JS, Goodman JR, et al. Transcatheter embolization of hypogastric branch arteries in the management of intractable bladder hemorrhage. J Urol 1979; 121:30–36.
32. Ring EJ, Athanasoulis C, Waltman AC, et al. Arteriographic management of hemorrhage following pelvic fracture. Radiology 1973; 109:65–70.
33. Palmer JK, Benson GS, Corriere JN Jr. Diagnosis and initial management of urological injuries associated with 200 consecutive pelvic fractures. J Urol 1983; 130:712–714.
34. Spirnak JP. Pelvic fracture and injury to the lower urinary tract. Surg Clin North Am 1988; 68:1057–1069.
35. Cass AS, Gleich P, Smith C. Simultaneous bladder and prostatomembranous urethral rupture from external trauma. J Urol 1984; 132:907–908.
36. Pierce JM Jr. Disruptions of the anterior urethra. Urol Clin North Am 1989; 16:329–334.
37. Colapinto V, McCallum RW. Injury to the male posterior urethra in fractured pelvis. A new classification. J Urol 1977; 118:575–580.
38. Sandler CM, Harris JH Jr, Corriere JN Jr, Toombs BD. Posterior urethral injuries after pelvic fracture. AJR 1981; 137:1233–1237.
39. Ellison M, Timberlake GA, Kerstein MD. Impotence following pelvic fracture. J Trauma 1988; 28:695–696.
40. Morehouse DD, MacKinnon KJ. Management of prostatomembranous urethral disruption: 13 year experience. J Urol 1980; 123:173–174.
41. Sandler CM, Corriere JN Jr. Urethrography in the diagnosis of acute urethral injuries. Urol Clin North Am 1989; 16:283–289.
42. Barbagli G, Selli C, Stomaci N, et al. Urethral trauma: radiological aspects and treatment options. J Trauma 1987; 27:256–261.
43. Cass AS. Urethral injury in the multiple-injured patient. J Trauma 1984; 24:901–906.
44. Lupetin AR, King W III, Rich PJ, Lederman RB. The traumatized scrotum. Ultrasound evaluation. Radiology 1983; 148:203–207.

18

Urinary Diversions and Bladder Augmentation

ILEAL LOOP DIVERSION (BRICKER LOOP)

This is a common, simple, and effective type of urinary tract diversion that has the disadvantage of an external collecting bag placed over a stoma.[1] Imaging is used to check the result of surgery, as a follow-up, and to evaluate complications. Both ureters are implanted into an isolated loop of small bowel. The loop is brought to the skin where a stoma is created.

Loopogram

Loopogram is a simple retrograde procedure. A 10 F Foley catheter is introduced into the ileal loop and the balloon is gently inflated. This should be done under fluoroscopic control, ensuring that the balloon is within the loop's lumen and does not distend the stoma. Contrast (30%) is infused under no more than 30 cm hydrostatic pressure and spot or overhead films are obtained in frontal and oblique projections. Some authors object to insertion of the Foley catheter and to the balloon inflation within the loop for fear of inadvertent injury. Instead, they promote a technique whereby the inflated balloon is held by the patient outside the stoma while only the leading tip of the catheter is within the stoma (Fig. 18–1). External compression prevents leaks. Either technique is acceptable if done gently and carefully. The loop is somewhat foreshortened in frontal projection, since it is usually oriented in the anteroposterior direction.

To optimally visualize this structure, the radiograph should be taken from the right overhead lateral position. In this position the loop is both parallel and closer to the film.

Normal Radiographic Findings. The loop will distend and peristalsis can be seen under fluoroscopy. In 95% of patients, the contrast material will freely reflux into both ureters and collecting systems. Varying degrees of dilatation may be present, perhaps related to an obstructive process that may have been present before the diversion (Fig. 18–2).

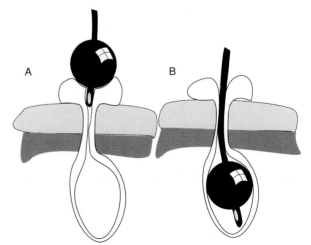

Figure 18–1. Two methods for performing retrograde loopogram. If the balloon is inflated in the loop, it must be beyond the abdominal wall musculature and the balloon inflated gently, while the catheter is slowly moved to make sure the viscus itself is not injured.

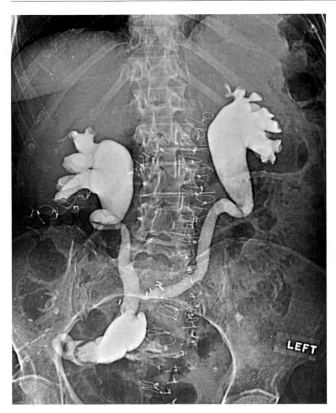

Figure 18–2. Loopogram. Free reflux into both ureters and upper collecting system is present, ensuring that there is no obstruction in the system. Hydrostatic pressure should never exceed 30 cm H$_2$O and the examination should be terminated if the patient feels discomfort.

Abnormal Radiographic Findings

1. *Absence of reflux* into one or both ureters and collecting systems implies ureteral obstruction.

2. *Ureteral narrowing and hydronephrosis.* Obstruction is most commonly due to postoperative edema or stricture at the anastomotic site. Strictures are also common at the point where the left ureter is brought into the peritoneal cavity.

3. *Contrast extravasation* into the abdominal cavity, retroperitoneum, or adjacent bowel. Loop necrosis, perforation, disruption of ureteral anastomotic site, or bowel fistula are possible diagnoses (Fig. 18–3).

4. *Narrow, rigid, and tubular loop* without folds is diagnostic of loop vascular ischemia (Fig. 18–4).

5. *Abnormal distention* of the loop and upper urinary tract system is seen in stomal stenosis.

6. *Filling defects* at the base of the loop are suggestive of local recurring carcinoma (transitional cell carcinoma of the bladder, for example).

7. *Loop displacement* by a mass suggests an adjacent abscess, hematoma, or malignancy. CT is the examination of choice.

8. *Calculi,* encrusted stents, and other foreign objects may be encountered (Fig. 18–5).

Excretory Urogram. Cystectomy for treatment of transitional cell carcinoma of the bladder is the most common reason for ileal loop diversion. Since this tumor tends to be multicentric, the remaining transitional cell epithelium should be examined as thor-

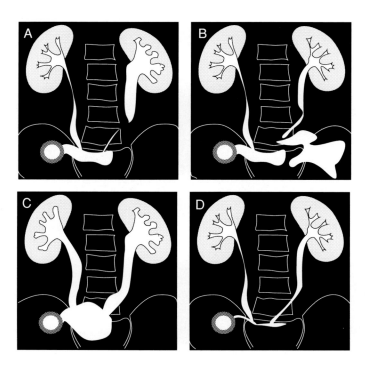

Figure 18–3. Schematic drawing of several possible complications involving the ileal loop diversion. Clockwise from upper left: normal; leak from ureteroileal anastomotic site; ischemic loop; and outflow loop obstruction.

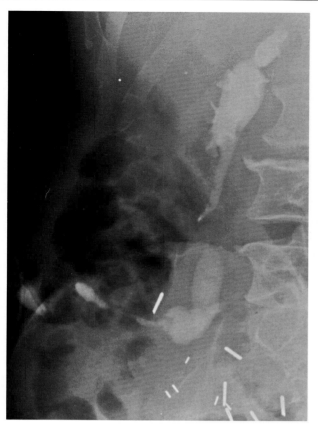

Figure 18–4. Loopogram. The loop is best visualized in an oblique or overhead lateral projection when it is parallel to the film. In this patient there is narrowing of the loop, a finding pathognomonic for chronic vascular ischemia which has resulted in fibrosis.

oughly as possible. This is why projectional contrast examinations (loopogram or IVP) are preferable to ultrasound or even CT. Any mucosal irregularities or intraluminal filling defects within the upper urinary tract should be regarded as new tumors.

It is common to find some degree of obstruction at anastomotic sites, even 6 months after surgery. This is probably caused by postoperative edema and, if mild, is usually of no concern. There are two common obstruction sites resulting from strictures: at the anastomoses and at the point where the ureters are brought into the peritoneal cavity (particularly the left ureter) (Fig. 18–6). Ureteral calculi are commonly missed in the distal ureteral segments, since these are obscured by the spine. The distal left ureteral segment is best seen in right lateral overhead projection (like the loop). In this position the contrast from the left kidney falls under the influence of gravity into the now dependent distal left ureter (Fig. 18–7).

Most patients may be followed with serial sonography to detect increasing hydronephrosis.[2]

Interventional Procedures— Special Considerations

Antegrade stent placement may be somewhat difficult because of the surgical technique for creating an anastomosis. It involves bringing the ureter under and in front of the loop, creating two additional compound curves. Once the guidewire is passed in antegrade fashion through the loop and stoma, stent placement is very easy because one controls both ends of the wire. The stent can be threaded in a retrograde manner and later replaced via the same route.

Treatment of ureteral strictures at the anastomotic site may involve retrograde or antegrade balloon dilatation.[3] Depending on the size of the patient, 4 to 10 mm balloon diameters may be used, followed by 4 to 6 weeks of ureteral stenting preferably by a 10 F stent. Long-term (1.5 years or more) success rates, however, are only 16 to 20%.[4]

The most disastrous complication is loop necrosis or disruption of the ureteral anastomosis, resulting in abdominal or perineal fistula (Fig. 18–8). If the patient isn't a candidate for an immediate revision, percutaneous nephrostomies are placed to divert the urine and allow healing. These may not be enough to prevent antegrade flow of urine and detachable balloons may have to be placed into the ureter, or the ureter may be permanently obstructed by some other percutaneous method.

ILEAL LOOP UNDIVERSION

Some 15 years ago many paralyzed patients underwent ileal loop diversion in the hope of eliminating the myriad problems associated with neurogenic bladder. The results for this group of patients were dismal. Many patients developed renal calculi, obstruction, urinary tract infection, and sepsis. In the interim, knowledge and management of neuropathic bladder disorders have vastly improved.

Undiversion is a surgical procedure where the ileal loop is anastomosed with the bladder, reasserting the bladder's role as the reservoir (Figs. 18–9, 18–10).[5]

COLONIC LOOP

Occasionally, for technical reasons, it is impossible to use the small bowel as a conduit and a segment of the large bowel is used as a substitute. All diagnostic imaging and procedures are the same as those for the ileal loop. The colonic loop is usually high in the abdomen.

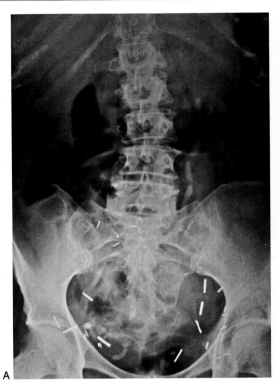

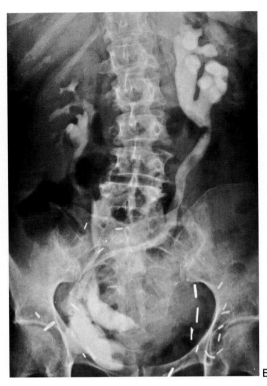

A

B

Figure 18–5. **(A)** On the preliminary radiograph, the radiolucent stent which is in the left ureter and in the loop is seen only because it is partially calcified. **(B)** On EXU surrounding contrast makes the stent, even the calcified portion, relatively radiolucent. There is partial ureteral obstruction.

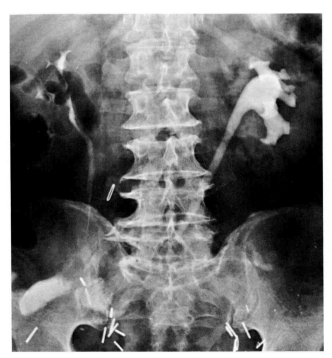

Figure 18–6. EXU. The left ureter is dilated and partially obstructed at the point where it was brought into the peritoneal cavity.

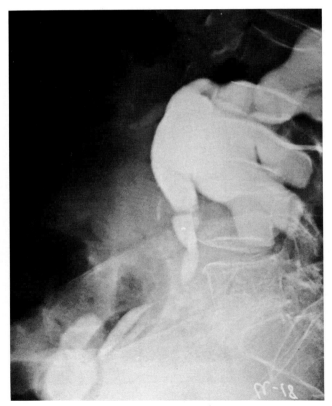

Figure 18–7. Nephrostogram. Overhead lateral projection may be needed to demonstrate the ureter distal to mid-ureteral obstruction. The stricture in this patient is also at the site where the ureter is brought into the peritoneal cavity.

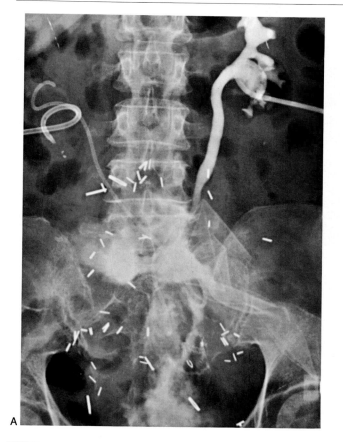

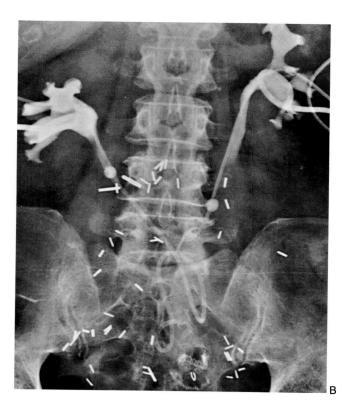

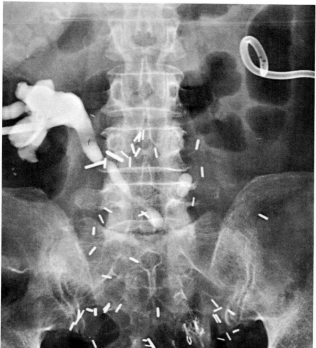

Figure 18–8. (A) Ileal loop disruption and perineal fistula have formed in radiated field. Bilateral percutaneous nephrostomies were placed but are still insufficient to completely divert urine flow away from the loop. Patient is too ill to withstand general anesthesia or surgery. (B) Antegrade occlusive balloon catheters are placed in an attempt to seal the ureters and, although ureteral occlusion is achieved, the maintenance of these fragile catheters proves difficult. (C) Finally the ureters are occluded with detachable balloons filled with solidifying radiopaque material. This is a permanent occlusion which will be dealt with in the future when the loop is revised, when and if the patient's general condition improves.

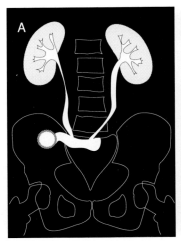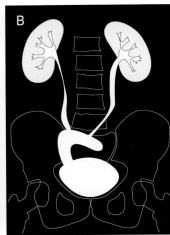

Figure 18–9. Schematic drawing of an ileal loop before (**A**) and after (**B**) undiversion.

ILEAL URETER

A segment of the ileum is isolated and anastomosed to the renal pelvis and the bladder (Fig. 18–11A). Antegrade peristaltic activity prevents reflux from the bladder to the kidney (Fig. 18–12). The procedure is usually done to help chronic stone formers get rid of renal calculi without associated ureteral colic. Usually, the ureter is left in place and is frequently seen during contrast examination. Radiological examinations are usually carried out to exclude anastomosis leakage after surgery. Occasionally, the ileal ureter may herniate (Fig. 18–13).

URETEROSIGMOIDOSTOMY

Implantation of the ureters into the sigmoid colon is a method of urinary tract diversion that completely eliminates a stoma bag or self-catheterization (Fig. 18–11B). Complications are hyperchloremic acidosis, obstruction at the anastomotic site (Fig. 18–14), reflux of bowel contents into the kidney, and urinary tract infection. After a prolonged period of time, there is a significant increase in incidence of colon carcinoma at the site of ureteral implantation.[6] Barium enemas and antegrade stent placements are contraindicated.

CONTINENT POUCHES

Camey Pouch

This conduit is constructed of a single isolated segment of ileum, and both ureters are implanted at one

end. The opposite end of the ileal segment is closed. A side-to-end anastomosis is made between the midpart of the segment and the trigone or the very proximal urethra (Fig. 18–15).[7] Continence and spontaneous voiding are common.

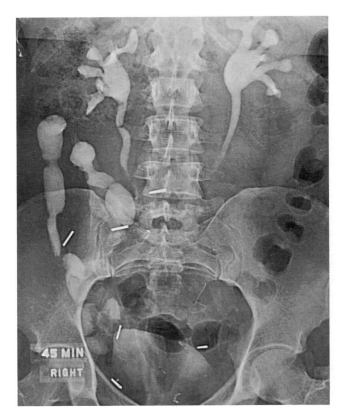

Figure 18–10. Ileal loop undiversion. Cutaneous stoma was removed and an additional ileal segment was interposed between the original loop and the bladder. This made for a somewhat redundant segment that needs more time to fill with contrast material.

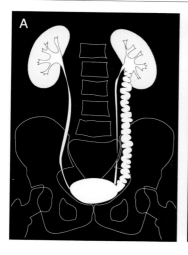
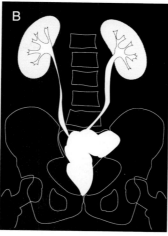

Figure 18–11.   (A) Schematic drawing of an ileal ureter interposed between renal pelvis and the bladder. Native ureter is usually left intact. (B) Schematic drawing of ureterosigmoidostomy.

Kock Pouch (Continent Ileal Urinary Reservoir)

This is an ingenious although somewhat complicated conduit and reservoir. Ureters are led to an intussuscepted segment of the small bowel. This segment protrudes (nipple) and empties into a larger reservoir (pouch) made of a 40 cm segment of ileum (Fig.

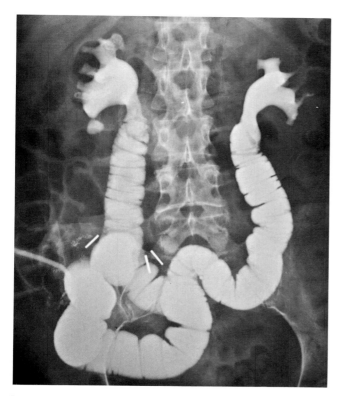

Figure 18–12.   Bilateral ileal ureters ending in an ileal loop. Although antegrade peristaltic activity prevents reflux into the kidney, this can be overcome if necessary by filling the loop or bladder to capacity.

18–16). Another nipple is interposed between the pouch and the skin or between the pouch and the prostatic urethra.[8] Nipples are oriented to prevent reflux from the pouch into the ureters and to maintain continence (Fig. 18–17). The patient empties the pouch through self-catheterization several times a day. Since the pouch is continent, there is no need for an external bag.

Complications include extravasation at the anastomotic site, fistulas, urinary obstruction, and calculi within the pouch.[9,10]

In attempting antegrade stent placement from the kidney into the pouch, one must be sure that the distal end of the catheter has passed and cleared the nipple. Otherwise, it may be difficult to retrieve the stent at a later date.

Continent Ileo-Cecal Cutaneous Diversion (Indiana Pouch, King Pouch, Mainz Pouch, Penn Pouch, UCLA Pouch)

The continent ileo-cecal pouch with cutaneous diversion is made from the right colon and part of the ileum. There are a number of variations as to how the pouch is constructed (Fig. 18–18).[11] In one version the ureters are implanted directly into what was the colon wall. Ileum is intussuscepted so that only one nipple is created. Since most complications involving the pouch are related to the nipples, eliminating one decreases the chances of complications (Fig. 18–19).

Complications include incontinence (Figs. 18–20, 18–21), intraluminal mucosal aggregates, ureteral strictures, and leaks at the anastomotic site.

Pouch calculi are also a common nuisance. They are initially formed as encrustation on a bare surface of an exposed staple (Fig. 18–22).

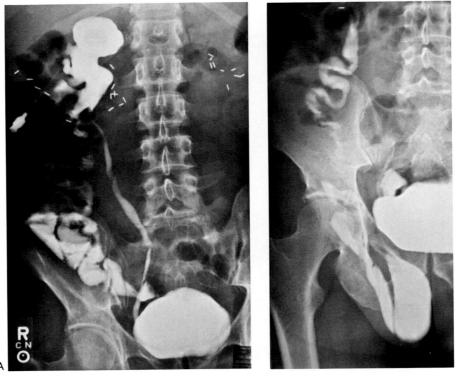

Figure 18–13. (A) Redundant ileal ureter looped in the right lower quadrant is seen on this antegrade pyelogram. Hydronephrosis and clubbed calyces from previous obstructions, urolithiasis, and infection are seen. The native ureter is left in place and is not obstructed at the moment. (B) In the upright position the redundant ileal ureter herniates through the inguinal canal.

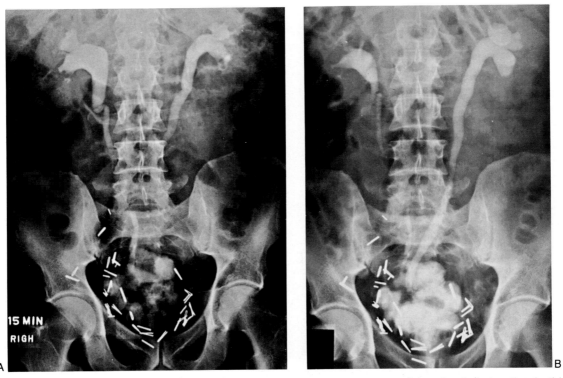

Figure 18–14. (A) Slight dilatation of the left collecting system suggests mild ureteral obstruction in this patient with ureterosigmoidostomy. (B) Delayed radiographs are needed primarily to opacify the colorectal segment with contrast material. Increased incidence of colon carcinoma at the implantation site and inability to perform a barium enema make this the only practical contrast examination. "Standing column" is present, diagnostic of partial obstruction at the anastomosis site.

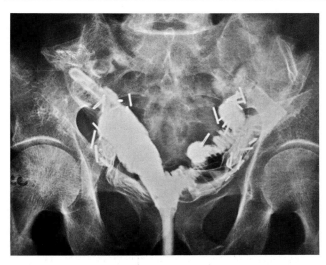

Figure 18–15. Pouchogram in a Camey pouch in the post-operative period.

URETEROCUTANEOUS STOMA

This is a quick method of urinary tract diversion and is usually used in very small children to buy time for a more definitive diversion procedure, or in patients with short life expectancy. The bag is carried over the stoma. Stricture and premature closure are far too common and limit the value of the procedure. Obstruction and sepsis are common complications.

TRANSURETEROURETEROSTOMY (TUU)

In some situations it is permissible to create an anastomosis with a short proximal ureter to the normal contralateral ureter. The anastomosis is end-to-side (Fig. 18–25). Several complications are possible, including obstruction and disruption of the anastomotic site. In case of obstruction of the common ureter both kidneys become hydronephrotic (Fig. 18–26).

PSOAS HITCH

When a distal ureteral segment becomes unusable, the bladder can be brought to the middle ureteral segment for anastomosis (Fig. 18–23). To prevent tension on the anastomotic site, the bladder is fixed with a suture to the psoas muscle and assumes a tented appearance to one side. Occasionally, when a simple approximation is not enough, a flap is carved out of the bladder and made into a tube. This tubular structure, or *Boari flap,* is brought to the free end of the high ureter (Fig. 18–24).

SUPRAPUBIC CATHETER

This is a common postoperative or emergency vesical diversion method used for bypassing outflow bladder obstruction or fresh surgical anastomosis. The problems associated with this catheter are rare and include hemorrhage and catheter dislodgement. If uncertain of the catheter position, a suprapubic catheter cystogram in a lateral projection will best show its relation to the bladder.

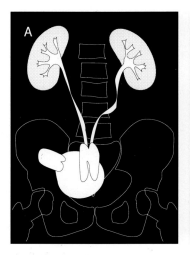
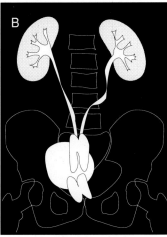

Figure 18–16. Schematic drawing of a Kock pouch. Continent nipple may be at the anterior abdominal wall (**A**) or urethra (**B**).

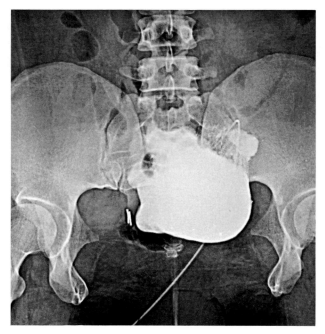

Figure 18–17.   Pouchogram in a Kock pouch. Pouchogram is easier to perform than loopogram, since the patient is usually able to accomplish self-catheterization. Note marked epispadia.

It may become necessary to exchange the suprapubic tube for a large one. This may be accomplished by progressive dilatation under fluoroscopic control using either balloon or rigid dilaters (Fig. 18–27).

BLADDER AUGMENTATION
Enterocystoplasty

Augmentation enterocystoplasty is an operation which increases bladder capacity by an addition of a

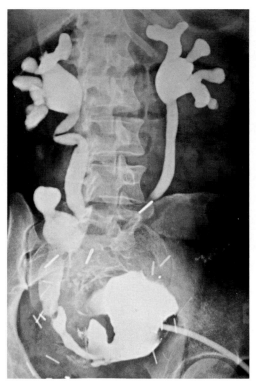

Figure 18–18.   One of many versions of a continent pouch. In this patient, failure of the antirefluxing nipple (at the bottom right of the pouch) is demonstrated on the retrograde pouchogram. Long segment leading to the nipple is an undiverted ileal loop.

bowel segment to the bladder (Fig. 18–28).[12,13] Cystogram or other radiological examinations are performed to evaluate the anastomosis between the bladder and the augmented segment and to evaluate the upper system.[12,14,15] A narrow anastomosis may result in underfilling or in incomplete emptying of the augmented segment, providing excellent sur-

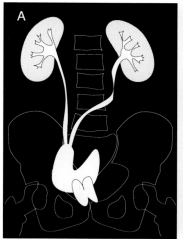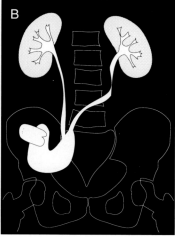

Figure 18–19.   Schematic drawing of a continent pouch with continent nipple only, to the skin (A) and urethra (B).

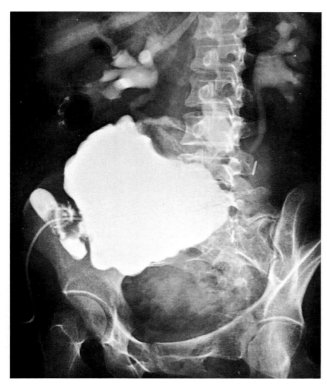

Figure 18–20. Failure of the continent nipple is demonstrated during a retrograde pouchogram with the catheter in place.

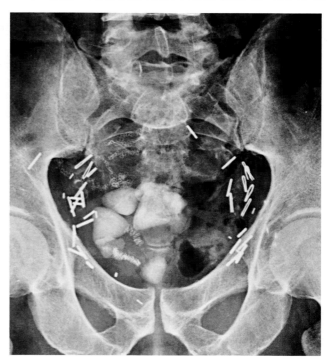

Figure 18–22. Plain radiograph in a patient with multiple radiopaque calculi in the continent pouch. Bare staples form a nidus. Patients frequently find free staples in the urine. Most patients can be treated by retrograde endourological methods.

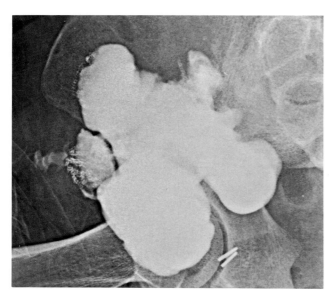

Figure 18–21. Failure of the continent nipple without the retrograde catheter in place. This image demonstrates the mucosal folds of intussuscepted small bowel, a necessary step in creating a nipple. Many surgical bowel staples are in the area.

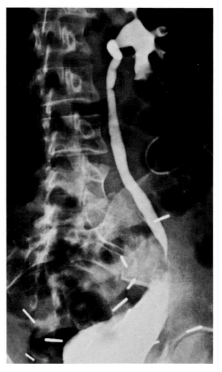

Figure 18–23. Left nephrostogram. Typical appearance of the bladder after a psoas hitch procedure. Some residual edema is present at the ureteral implantation site which still creates mild obstruction to the flow of urine.

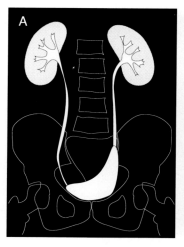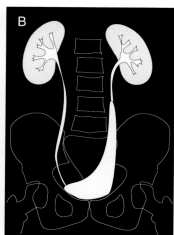

Figure 18–24. Schematic drawing of psoas hitch **(A)** and Boari flap **(B)**. The latter is usually reserved for connecting the bladder to the high proximal ureter. Radiographically, it is usually difficult to differentiate between the two.

roundings for an infection (Fig. 18–29). Ureters may be reimplanted or left intact, depending on circumstances. Vesicoureteral reflux may complicate the outcome (Fig. 18–30). Other complications are rare (Fig. 18–31).

Ileocystoplasty

An isolated loop of small bowel is incised along the antemesenteric border, cupped, and anastomosed with its free margin to the bladder cuff.

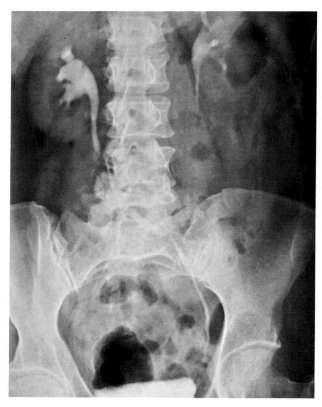

Figure 18–25. Excretory urogram in a patient with transureteroureterostomy. The right ureter is anastomosed end-to-side with the left.

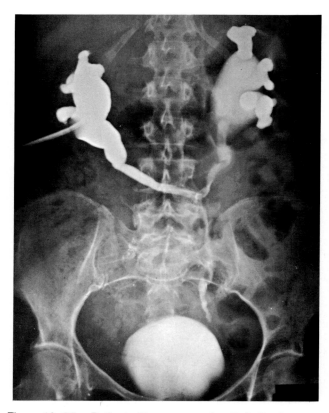

Figure 18–26. Patient with a now resolved left distal ureteral obstruction and transureteroureterostomy. Single percutaneous nephrostomy drained both kidneys successfully during the period of the obstruction. Some bilateral residual hydronephrosis still remains.

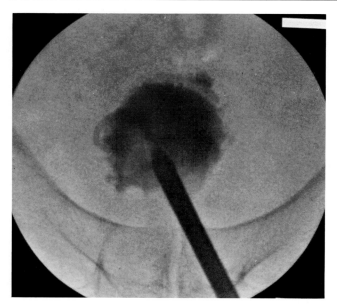

Figure 18–27. Progressive enlargement of a suprapubic tube tract using dilators for placement of a large suprapubic tube. Suprapubic tube is much better tolerated than a comparable indwelling urethral catheter.

Cecocystoplasty

Cecum is isolated from the fecal stream either above or below the ileocecal valve. Anastomosis with the bladder cuff is performed after appendectomy (Fig. 18–32).

Ileocecocystoplasty

This operation is similar to cecocystoplasty except that a segment of ileum is included. Ureters are usually anastomosed to the ileal segment. Ileocecal valve prevents ureteral reflux.

Sigmoidocystoplasty

A segment of sigmoid colon is isolated from the fecal stream, divided along the antemesenteric border, and anastomosed to the bladder cuff.

Enterourethroplasty

Rarely, after cystectomy, any enteric segment may be anastomosed to the proximal urethra. In males the procedure is known as enteroprostatoplasty.

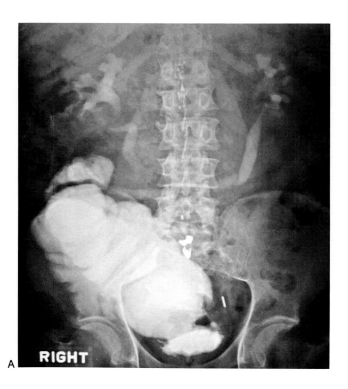

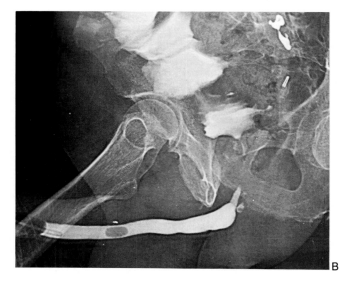

Figure 18–28. EXU (**A**) and retrograde urethrogram (**B**) in a patient with an augmentation cystoplasty. There is a relatively narrow segment between the bladder remnant and the augmented segment which could result in moderate postvoid residual.

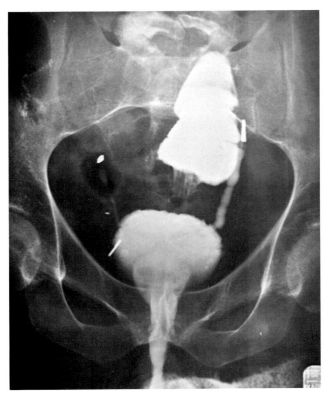

Figure 18–29. Narrow segment, moderate postvoid residual, and reflux into the left ureter are present in this patient with augmentation cystoplasty. As seen by the appearance of the bladder neck during voiding, gross incontinence is apparent and no simple solution readily avails itself.

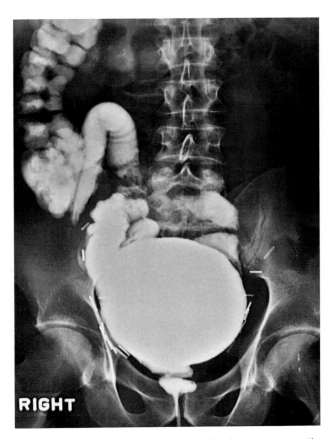

Figure 18–31. Vesicoileal fistula following augmentation cystoplasty. The augmented segment is underfilled but the terminal ileum and cecum fill with radiographic contrast during cystography.

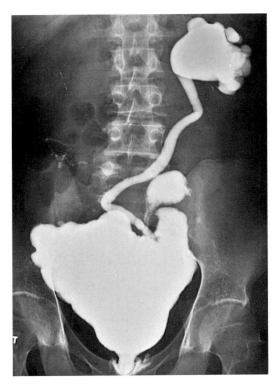

Figure 18–30. Severe vesicoureteral reflux in a patient with augmentation cystoplasty during cystography.

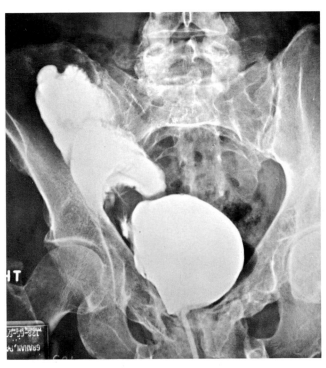

Figure 18–32. Cecocystoplasty, one of several augmentation procedures. This patient has sustained a major injury to the pelvis with several healed bone fractures visible. Augmentation relieved symptoms related to small bladder capacity. There is an apparent narrowing at the anastomosis site.

REFERENCES

1. Bricker EM. Bladder substitution after pelvic evisceration. Surg Clin North Am 1950; 30:1511–1521.
2. Cronan JJ, Amis ES Jr, Scola FH, Schepps B. Renal obstruction in patients with ileal loops: ultrasound evaluation. Radiology 1986; 158:647–650.
3. Kramolowsky EV, Clayman RV, Weyman PJ. Endourological management of ureteroileal anastomotic strictures: is it effective? J Urol 1987; 137:390–394.
4. Shapiro MJ, Banner MP, Amendola MA, et al. Balloon catheter dilatation of ureteroenteric strictures: long-term results. Radiology 1988; 168:385–387.
5. Amis ES Jr, Pfister RC, Hendren WH. Radiology of urinary undiversion. Urol Radiol 1981; 3:161–169.
6. Spence HM, Hoffman WW, Fosmire GP. Tumor of the colon as a late complication of ureterosigmoidostomy for extrophy of the bladder. Br J Urol 1979; 51:466–470.
7. Camey M. Bladder replacement by ileocystoplasty following radical cystectomy. Semin Urol 1987; 5:8–14.
8. Kock NG. Intra-abdominal "reservoir" in patients with permanent ileostomy. Arch Surg 1969; 99:223–231.
9. Ralls PW, Barakos JA, Skinner DG, et al. Imaging of the Kock continent ileal reservoir. Radiology 1986; 161:477–483.
10. Skinner DG, Lieskovsky G, Boyd SD. Continuing experience with the continent ileal reservoir (Kock pouch) as an alternative to cutaneous urinary diversion: an update after 250 cases. J Urol 1987; 137:1140–1145.
11. Amis ES Jr, Newhouse JH, Olsson CA. Continent urinary diversions: review of current surgical procedures and radiologic imaging. Radiology 1988; 168:395–401.
12. Pagani JJ, Barbaric ZL, Cochran ST. Augmentation enterocystoplasty. Radiology 1979; 131:321–326.
13. Gil-Vernet JM Jr. The ileocolic segment in urologic surgery. J Urol 1965; 94:418–426.
14. Hertzberg BS, Bowie JD, King LR, Webster GD. Augmentation and replacement cystoplasty: sonographic findings. Radiology 1987; 165:853–856.
15. Goldwasser B, Webster GD. Augmentation and substitution enterocystoplasty. J Urol 1986; 135:215–224.

19

Bladder

Urologic practice deals mainly with diseases involving the lower urinary tract. Radiological diagnosis of these disorders is perhaps more mundane than detection and accurate diagnosis of upper urinary tract disease but is arguably more important, more difficult, and probably serves a much larger patient population. What follows are the common radiological findings concerning the bladder.

Perivesical Fat Stripe. This is a useful anatomical landmark that helps to outline the bladder on the plain radiograph. Differentiation of an enlarged bladder from a supravesical mass can be made because the fat stripe can be identified between the mass and top of the bladder. The stripe disappears or is displaced superiorly when the bladder is full (Fig. 19–1).

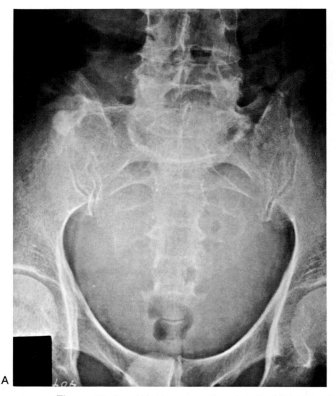

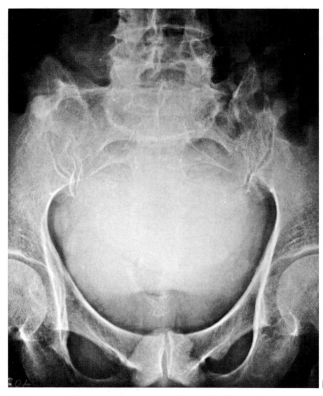

Figure 19–1. (A) Absence of perivesical fat stripe implies that the pelvic mass is an overdistended bladder that fills with contrast (B) on EXU.

Impressions and Displacement. Impressions upon the bladder can be made by the uterus (Fig. 19–2), small bowel, sigmoid colon, and low-lying cecum (Fig. 19–3). Enlarged prostate displaces trigone superiorly together with distal ureteral segments ("J" hook or fish hook). Urethral diverticulum in a female patient may be of such size as to impress upon the base of the bladder, resembling median prostatic lobe enlargement in males.

Pelvic masses originating from the female reproductive system, such as ovarian neoplasms and cysts, uterine fibroids, uterine neoplasms, etc., may displace the bladder (Fig. 19–4) and in some instances invade it as well. Other neoplasms may do the same (Fig. 19–5).

A perivesical hematoma, urinoma, or a lymphocele may impress upon the bladder, depending on its location (Fig. 19–6).[1]

The Pear-Shaped or Inverted Teardrop Bladder. In many instances these perivesical fluid collections elevate the bladder by compressing its base, forming a striking resemblance to an inverted pear. Other pathological processes that may produce this sign

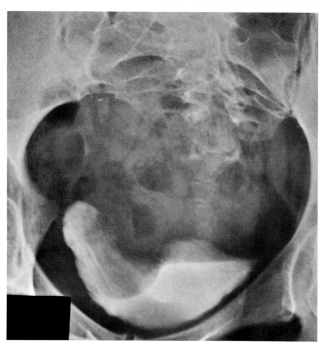

Figure 19–3. Impression upon the bladder by a low-lying cecum.

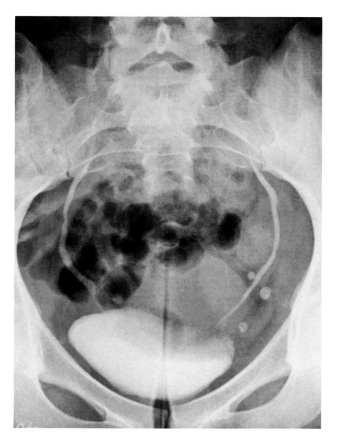

Figure 19–2. Uterine impression upon the bladder dome.

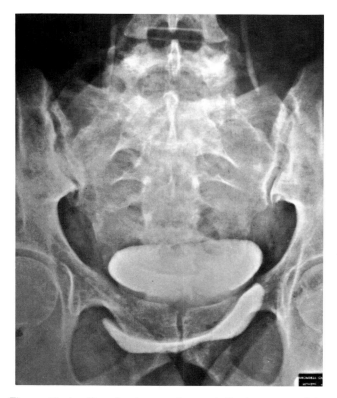

Figure 19–4. Peculiar impression and displacement of the bladder by a pelvic mass. The mass is compressing the bladder in the middle, forming two contrast-filled compartments.

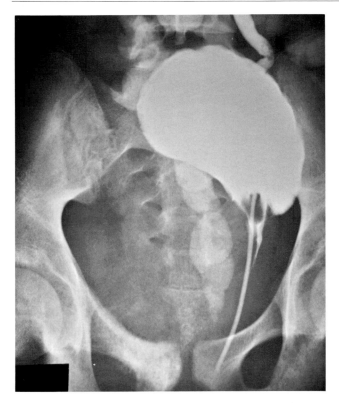

Figure 19–5. Massive bladder displacement by a soft tissue component of an Ewing's sarcoma.

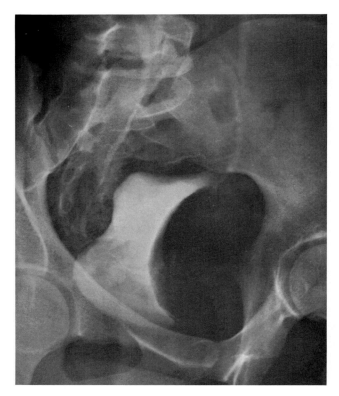

Figure 19–6. Perivesical hematoma displacing the bladder after pelvic surgery.

are pelvic lipomatosis (Fig. 19–7), massive lymph node enlargement (Figs. 19–8, 19–9), and infiltrating pelvic neoplasm. Pelvic edema due to inferior vena cava obstruction (tumor invasion or encroachment by retroperitoneal fibrosis) may also produce this sign.[2] Large ileopsoas muscles in younger athletes may displace distal ureters medially and the bladder may also assume the inverted pear appearance.[3]

Filling Defects. Tumors, blood clots (Figs. 19–9, 19–10), bladder calculi (Figs. 19–11, 19–12, 19–13), sloughed papilla, foreign bodies, ureterocele are some intraluminal "filling" defects that may be encountered.

Thick Bladder Wall. Thick bladder wall may be identified on any contrast examination, ultrasound, or MR imaging. Thickening may be due to:

1. *Edema,* such as in acute bacterial cystitis, bullous edema, chemical cystitis
2. *Infiltration,* such as in eosinophilic cystitis, neoplasm, schistosomiasis
3. *Outflow bladder obstruction,* such as BPH, urethral strictures, urethral valves, neuropathic bladder

Trabeculation. More severe and long-standing outflow obstruction produces hypertrophy of the detru-

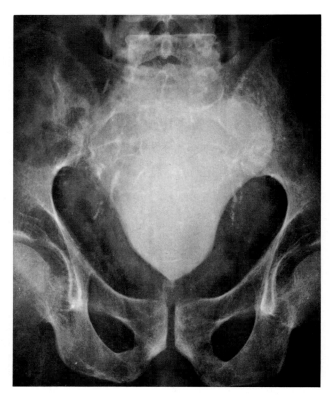

Figure 19–7. "Inverted pear" bladder in a patient with pelvic lipomatosis.

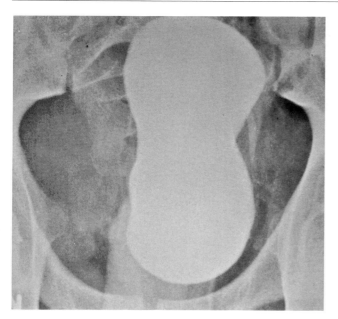

Figure 19–8. Change in bladder appearance due to massive pelvic lymph node enlargement.

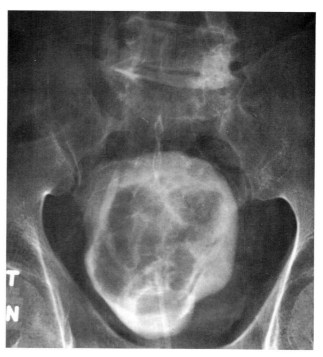

Figure 19–10. Many bladder clots are present. Foley catheter is also in place.

sor muscle bundles. These are seen as irregularities of the contrast-filled bladder and may be termed mild, moderate, or severe. Cystoscopic examination is more sensitive than radiography in detecting mild forms of trabeculation.

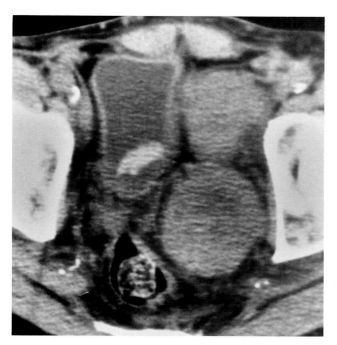

Figure 19–9. Bladder displacement by enlarged left pelvic lymph nodes. Hyperdense intravesical "filling" defect is a fresh blood clot.

Diverticula. As the outflow bladder obstruction continues, the mucosal layer invaginates in between the hypertrophied muscle bundles and protrudes outward. It is covered by serosal bladder layer and its wall contains no smooth muscles. A diverticulum is usually very smooth and frequently fails to empty on the postvoid radiograph. Transitional cell carcinoma and bladder calculi may originate in the diverticulum and any irregularity should raise suspicion. Because of a narrow mouth or unusual and inaccessible location, the inside of the diverticulum is often impossible to evaluate cystoscopically. In these instances, radiography or ultrasound may be the only diagnostic method available.

Calcifications. Calcifications involving the wall of the bladder are rare. Commonly known are schistosomiasis (Fig. 19–14),[4] tuberculosis, radiation cystitis, and amyloidosis.[5] Adenocarcinoma of the bladder may also calcify, but unlike previously described entities, the calcifications are usually psammomatous and within well-delineated tumor mass.[6] Psammomatous calcifications in the mass at the dome of the bladder strongly favor urachal carcinoma. Rare cause is alkaline encrusting cystitis.[7]

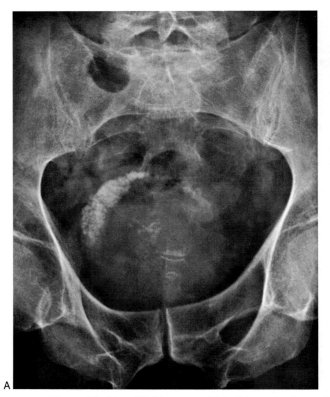

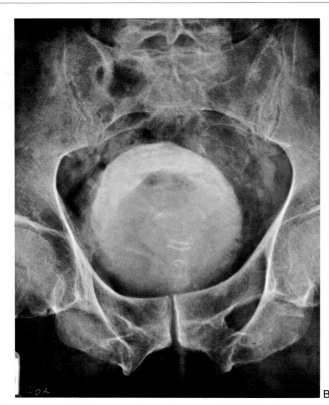

A   B

Figure 19–11. **(A)** Many small bladder calculi are displaced superiorly by an enlarged prostate. **(B)** Calculi blend with contrast and become invisible.

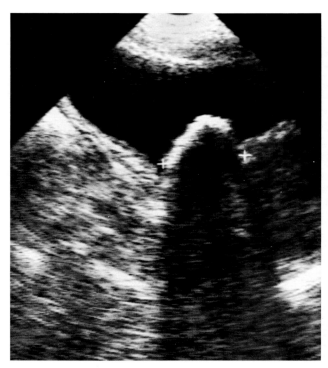

Figure 19–12. Sonographic appearance of a bladder calculus. The echodense outline of the calculus is seen together with marked acoustical shadowing. Most of the calculus is hidden from view within the acoustical shadow.

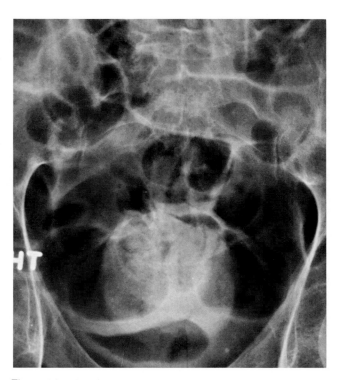

Figure 19–13. A bladder calculus may be easily overlooked on plain radiography if only mildly radiopaque.

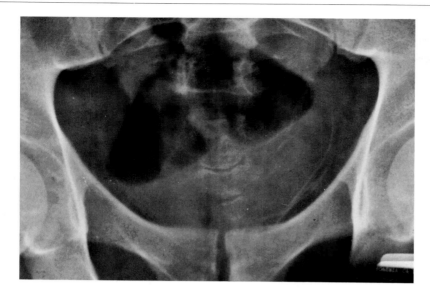

Figure 19–14. Faint thin calcification of the bladder wall in schistosomiasis.

BLADDER DUPLICATION

Sagittal Septal Divisions

Complete. Sagittal septum may be muscular and/or mucosal. Only one urethra is present and only one chamber is usually drained. The chamber without the urethra is obstructed and its kidney hydronephrotic and dysplastic (Fig. 19–15).

Incomplete. Septum does not completely isolate two bladder chambers.

Sagittal Duplication

Complete. Complete bladder duplication is the most common type of multichambered bladder. Two completely separated bladders have their separate urethras and ureters (Fig. 19–16).

Incomplete. Incomplete duplication is less common. Two chambers are partially separated by a peritoneal fold, each having its own ureter. There is a common urethra.

Transverse Septal Divisions

Complete. Unlike sagittal division where there is a left and right bladder, when a transverse septum exists, an anterior and a posterior chamber are present. Each chamber usually has its own ureter. More commonly, a single urethra is present draining the anterior chamber. The undrained chamber may enlarge and its kidney becomes hydronephrotic and dysplastic (Fig. 19–17).

Incomplete (hourglass). Incomplete septum allows communication between the chambers. A variant of the incomplete transverse septal division is the hourglass bladder where an upper and a lower chamber are identified.

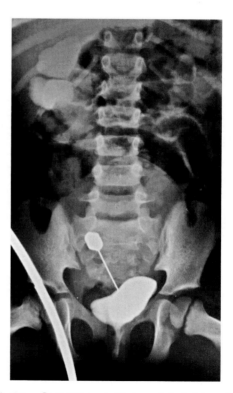

Figure 19–15. Complete sagittal septal division. Blind left bladder compartment was percutaneously punctured and filled with contrast. Some contrast is present in the right compartment (EXU) and can be seen in the urethra. Dilated right collecting system is present. The left kidney draining into the blind compartment is not functioning.

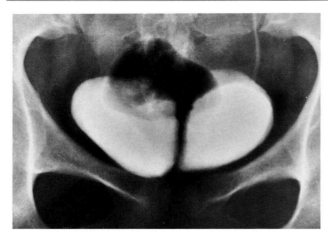

Figure 19–16. Complete sagittal duplication.

It is obvious from the description of the duplication anomalies that the complete divisions are associated with more severe urinary tract dysfunction. Ipsilateral obstruction and dysplastic kidney are associated with blind, nondraining chambers. The blind chamber may enlarge and cause outflow bladder obstruction or obstruction of the opposite ureter. As in other congenital anomalies of the urinary tract, there are numerous associated congenital anomalies of the reproductive system and of other organs.[8–11]

Exstrophy—Epispadic Complex

Congenital separation of the pubic bones by more than 1 cm may be associated with bladder exstrophy, epispadias without exstrophy, and duplication and anorectal anomalies. Undescended testicle is common, as is bilateral inguinal hernia. Absence of the anterior bladder wall is seen in classic exstrophy.

Radiological Findings. Pubic separation is the principal finding on plain radiographs (Fig. 19–18). There is outward rotation of the inominate bone, "squaring" of the iliac notch, and mild separation of the inferior aspect of sacroiliac joint on plain radiog-

raphy. Prenatal diagnosis by sonography is possible.[12]

URACHAL ANOMALIES

Patent Urachus

There is persistent opening of the bladder in the umbilicus. The bladder may be in a normal or abnormal position. Patency may be demonstrated either by cystography or retrograde injection of contrast into the umbilical opening. Lateral projection is required. Outflow bladder obstruction should be excluded or corrected if present.

Partially Patent Urachus

Partially patent urachus may have its opening at the bladder dome or at the umbilical end and may be of varying length. The opposite end is atretic. Cystogram or retrograde sinogram are the methods of examination, just as in patent urachus.

Urachal Cyst

Closure at both ends and incomplete obliteration of the urachal lumen allows formation of a urachal cyst. These usually develop in the distal third of the urachus and close to the bladder dome. The urachal cyst may be small but may also attain enormous size and produce symptoms of an intra-abdominal mass.[13] These may appear in adulthood and for no apparent reason. Since there is no communication with the bladder, only indirect signs of the presence of a mass can be detected because of posterolateral bladder displacement (Fig. 19–19). Cross-sectional imaging provides direct evidence for a fluid-filled mass in the characteristic anterior location.

If one is confident of the diagnosis, aspiration and perhaps instillation of sclerosing agents may be considered.

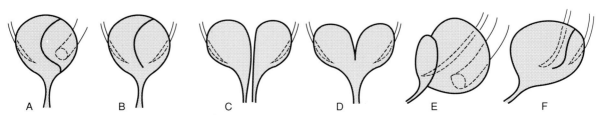

Figure 19–17. **(A)** Complete sagittal septal division. **(B)** Incomplete sagittal septal division. **(C)** Complete sagittal duplication. **(D)** Incomplete sagittal duplication. **(E)** Complete transverse septal division. **(F)** Incomplete sagittal septal division.

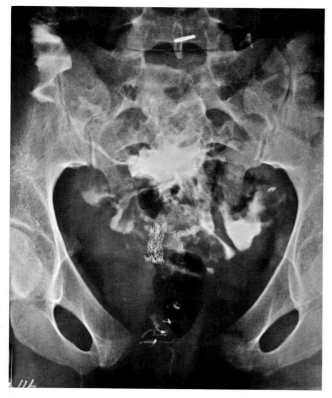

Figure 19–18. A patient with bladder exstrophy after diversion and creation of a continent pouch.

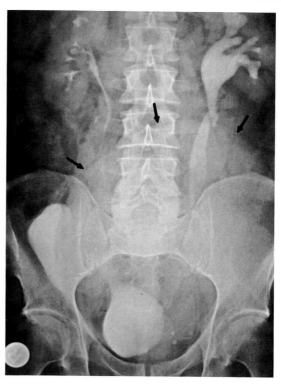

Figure 19–19. A large urachal cyst is displacing bladder to the right. (From Spataro et al.[13] Reprinted with permission.)

Urachal cysts may become infected. Severe lower abdominal pain, fever, and dysuria may be presenting symptoms.[14]

Urachal Neoplasms

Mucinous adenocarcinoma is the most common tumor, followed by nonmucinous-producing adenocarcinoma, sarcomas, squamous cell carcinoma, and transitional cell carcinoma. Hematuria is a common presenting sign. Adenocarcinoma is usually observed in the midline, at the dome of the bladder, and is several centimeters large when first detected. Either cystic or solid tumors may be observed on CT.[15,16] Calcifications within the tumor are common (Fig. 19–20).[17] Local invasion into the bladder, abdominal wall, regional lymph nodes and peritoneum is common at the time of diagnosis.[18] Local recurrence after excision is also common. Prognosis is worse than that of bladder carcinoma. CT is the examination of choice. Bladder involvement may perhaps be better judged on MR study, using T2-weighted sequences and sagittal plane.

BLADDER NECK CONTRACTURE (IDIOPATHIC BLADDER NECK OBSTRUCTION)

Etiology. Congenital or acquired. Postoperative.

Incidence. Rare. Probably more common in males.

Pathology. Submucosal fibrosis of the bladder neck, hypertrophied smooth muscles, or inflammatory changes.[19–21]

Clinical Presentation. Outflow bladder obstruction. Hydronephrosis. Renal failure.

Radiological Findings. The hypertrophied bladder wall is present because of outflow obstruction (Fig. 19–21). Often it will be impossible or difficult to pass the catheter into the bladder. "Jet effect" may be seen on retrograde urethrogram. Dilatation of the upper system may also be present (Fig. 19–22). Diagnosis is made on cystoscopy. Treatment is transurethral resection (TUR).

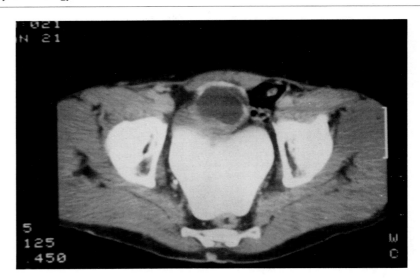

Figure 19–20. Relatively radiolucent urachal carcinoma with peripheral calcification.

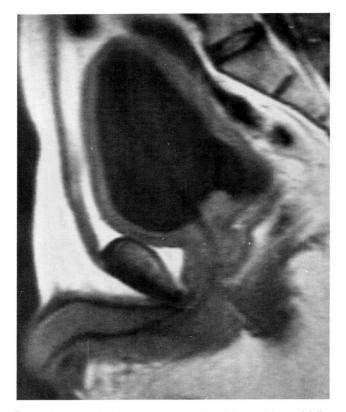

Figure 19–21. Markedly thickened bladder wall in a middle-aged patient with outflow bladder obstruction. Prostate is not enlarged. Edematous posterior trigonal line is seen just posterior to the internal orifice. Prostatic urethra is visualized on this T1-weighted sequence because of presence of the Foley catheter. A "mini" TURP procedure resulted in a complete cure.

ACUTE BACTERIAL CYSTITIS

Etiology. *E. coli, Klebsiella, Enterobacter, Proteus, Pseudomonas aeruginosa, Serratia,* enterococcus, *Candida albicans, Cryptococcus neoformans.*

Incidence. Generally 10–20% of women will experience urinary tract infection. Common following bladder catheterization. In girls, bacteriuria is found in 1.2%, and in boys, 0.003%.

Clinical Presentation. Dysuria, frequency, urgency, gross hematuria, pyuria, malodorous urine. Frequently asymptomatic.

Laboratory Findings. Bacteriuria (100,000 colonies/ml) from midstream urine specimen, preferably on several occasions. Pyuria, hematuria.

Radiological Workup. There is no indication for radiographic workup in female patients with lower urinary tract infection. In the vast majority, cystography and excretory urography are normal.

Excretory urography, cystography, or sonography is recommended to reveal or exclude obstructive uropathy, congenital anomalies, foreign bodies, vesicoureteric reflux, or neurogenic bladder dysfunction in the following situations:

1. Repeated lower urinary tract infections in a female
2. Lower urinary tract infections in a male
3. Bacteriuria unresponsive to antimicrobial therapy

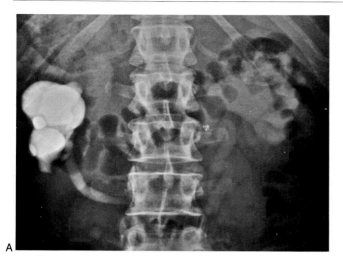

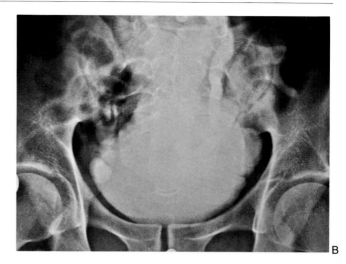

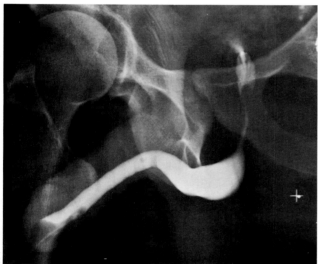

Figure 19–22. A young athletic man presents with markedly decreased stream. **(A)** On EXU there is delay in function and bilateral dilatation of the upper system compatible with obstruction. **(B)** Markedly trabeculated bladder, almost Christmas tree in appearance, eventually fills with contrast, suggesting outflow bladder obstruction and neurogenic bladder. However, no neurological disorder was found. **(C)** Retrograde urethrogram demonstrates normal urethra with the exception of a very tight bladder neck where a retrograde "jet" phenomenon may be identified. Indeed, even a small catheter could not be passed into the bladder. A "mini" TURP was curative.

4. Urinary tract infection in the presence of urolithiasis
5. Infection in the presence of voiding dysfunction

EMPHYSEMATOUS CYSTITIS

Etiology. *E. coli, Proteus, Pseudomonas, Candida albicans.*

Pathology. Inflammatory changes in the bladder wall associated with gas vesicles in mucosa, detrusor muscle, or in the bladder lumen.

Clinical Presentation. Frequency, urgency, dysuria, suprapubic pain. Most patients are diabetic and elderly. Unlike emphysematous pyelonephritis, patients are not very ill and symptoms are surprisingly mild.

Radiological Findings. Gas is seen in the bladder wall and occasionally in the bladder lumen. Diagnosis is made by cystoscopy, cystography,[22] and positive urinalysis, including bacterial culture. As expected, its gaseous appearance looks spectacular on CT,[23,24] although this is not the examination of choice. Sonography shows acoustical shadowing.[25] Cobblestone effect is seen along the interface between mucosa and contrast-filled bladder in the early stage on cystogram (Fig. 19–23). In a more pronounced case the gas is seen in the bladder wall and in the bladder lumen. Gas may also be seen in subserosa and occasionally around the bladder.

Differential diagnosis, if intraluminal gas is present, includes vesicoenteric or vesicocolic fistula.

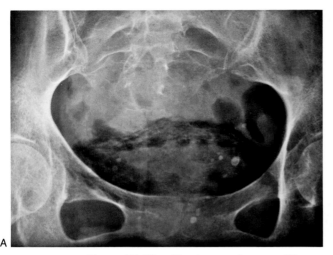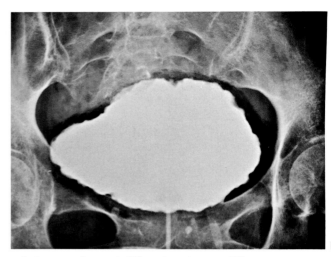

Figure 19–23.   Emphysematous cystitis seen on preliminary radiograph (**A**) and cystogram (**B**).

CYSTITIS CYSTICA

Etiology.   Unknown; seen in patients with recurrent urinary tract infection.

Pathology.   Multiple small cystic structures involving the bladder and occasionally ureter (ureteritis cystica) and renal pelvis (pyelitis cystica). Histologically they represent downward proliferating urothelium and metaplasia of Von Brunn's nests.[26–28]

Clinical Presentation.   Recurrent urinary tract infections. More common in women. Small cystic changes persist for a long time after eradication of infection.

Radiological Findings.   Multiple small intraluminal filling defects may be seen in the bladder, ureters, and pelvis (Fig. 19–24). Diagnosis is made by cystoscopy.

CYSTITIS GLANDULARIS

Etiology.   Chronic and repeated urinary tract infections and foreign body irritation.

Pathology.   Mucosal metaplasia resulting from glandular formation of Von Brunn's nests. The lesion may be premalignant and is associated with adenocarcinoma of the bladder.[29]

Clinical Presentation.   Chronic urinary tract infection, bladder calculi. May be associated with pelvic lymphedema and pelvic lipomatosis.[30] May produce distal ureteral obstruction.[31]

Radiological Findings.   Radiolucent filling defects and thickening of the bladder wall are the only findings and are quite nonspecific.[32]

EOSINOPHILIC CYSTITIS

Eosinophilic cystitis is an inflammatory bladder disease characterized by eosinophilic infiltration of the bladder wall with polypoid lesions extending into the bladder. The disease may be of allergic origin. Diagnosis is made by biopsy. Thick bladder wall is seen on radiographic examinations.[33,34]

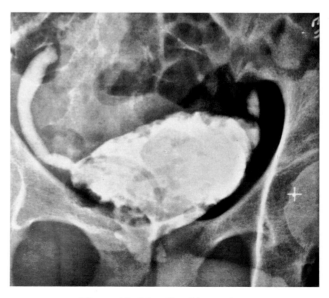

Figure 19–24.   Cystitis cystica.

GRANULOMATOUS CYSTITIS

This is a rare bladder disease that may be seen in children with chronic granulomatous disease. This is a chronic hereditary disease characterized by chronic infections involving multiple organ systems. Urinary tract involvement is rare. Bladder becomes thickened, a nonspecific finding that may be identified on sonography or other imaging modalities.[35]

INTERSTITIAL CYSTITIS

Interstitial cystitis is an incapacitating bladder disease of unknown etiology, characterized by severe bladder pain, frequency, and progression to bladder contracture and limited bladder capacity (Fig. 19–25).[36,37] The disease is more common in females and is progressive. Increases in number of mast cells (detrusor mastocytosis) are found on bladder biopsy.[38] Hunner's ulcers may be seen on cystoscopy.[39] These are small stellate lesions with central ulceration and tendency to hemorrhage on bladder distention and are seen in later stage of disease. Treatment is symptomatic but cystectomy or diversion may be necessary.

Hunner's ulcers cannot be seen on radiographic examinations, such as cystography or excretory urography. Radiographic examinations are nonspecific.

CHEMICAL CYSTITIS

Cyclophosphamide (Cytoxan) Cystitis

Byproducts of cyclophosphamide excreted in urine are cytotoxic to bladder mucosa, causing necrosis, swelling, and hemorrhagic cystitis. This is probably due to prolonged contact of the chemicals with the mucosa. Preventive measures include bladder irrigation or dose adjustment. In severe cases the renal pelvis may also be involved. Radiological findings are nonspecific. Thickening of the bladder wall (Fig. 19–26), and blood clots are associated with hematuria (Fig. 19–27). In chronic stage, depending on the extent of the damage, bladder wall fibrosis may ensue, resulting in small capacity bladder (Fig. 19–28), frequency, dysuria, and urinary tract infections.[40,41]

Cystitis Caused by Caustic Substances

Self-introduction of caustic substances such as acids, plumbing cleaning liquids, or inadvertent instillation of concentrated formalin and silver nitrate may result in necrosis of bladder mucosa and functional destruction of the entire organ.

BLADDER HERNIAS

Some 5% of inguinal and femoral hernias contain a part of the bladder. Some of these may be seen as "bladder ears" on a prone radiograph. In the majority of patients this finding is inconsequential. To see a large part of the bladder in the inguinal or scrotal hernia is unusual (Fig. 19–29).[42–45] These patients may complain of scrotal fullness, which may persist on bladder emptying (Fig. 19–30). Manual expression of urine from the herniated bladder may be necessary. Incisional hernias of the anterior abdominal wall are usually easily recognized (Fig. 19–31) although this is not always so (Fig. 19–32).[46]

BLADDER DIVERTICULUM

Acquired Bladder Diverticulum

Acquired bladder diverticulum is an outpouching of the bladder mucosa between the muscle bundles

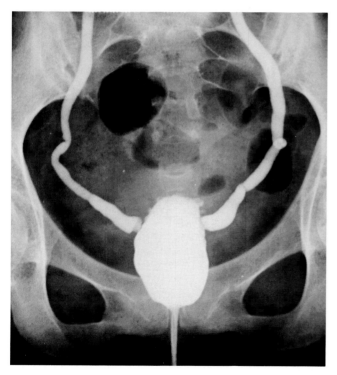

Figure 19–25. Cystogram in a patient with severe interstitial cystitis demonstrates small bladder capacity and severe bilateral vesicoureteral reflux.

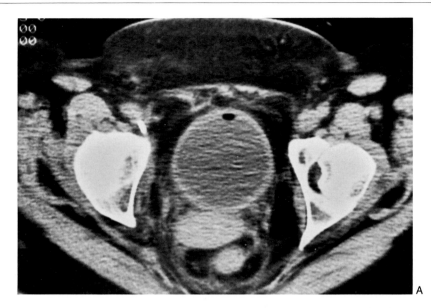

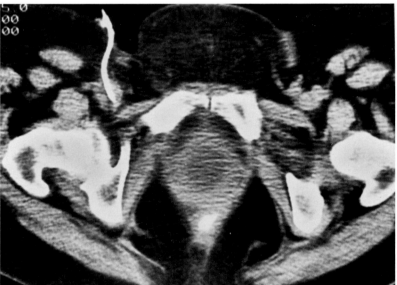

Figure 19–26. **(A)** Unenhanced CT scan through the bladder demonstrates somewhat thickened bladder wall in a patient with early clinical manifestations of cyclophosphamide cystitis. **(B)** Hyperalimentation venous catheter is seen entering the femoral vein.

caused by increased intravesical pressure (Fig. 19–33). The wall is therefore made of mucosa and serosa and is smooth compared with the surrounding trabeculated bladder. Since it lacks muscular layers, bladder diverticulum is frequently seen to contain urine or contrast on postvoid examinations (Fig. 19–34). Neck of the bladder diverticulum may be wide or, more commonly, narrow. Transitional cell and other carcinomas may originate in the diverticulum and present as a filling defect.[47–49] If the neck is narrow, it may be impossible for the urologist to visualize or biopsy the tumor. All diverticula therefore should be scrutinized no matter what imaging modalities are employed. Bladder calculi and blood clots may also present as filling defects within the saccule.

Spontaneous rupture of the bladder diverticulum may occur. Posterior bladder diverticula may give a peculiar appearance to the bladder on frontal projection (Figs. 19–35, 19–36).

Unusually high incidence of acquired diverticula in children with kinky hair (Menkes') syndrome have been described.[50]

Hutch Diverticulum

An acquired bladder diverticulum near the ureterovesical junction may weaken the detrusor muscle

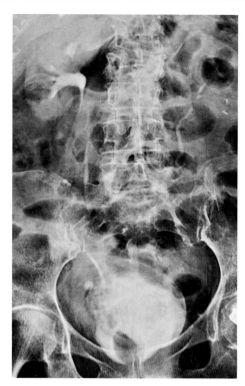

Figure 19–27. Large blood clots are present in the bladder in a patient with acute manifestations of cyclophosphamide cystitis.

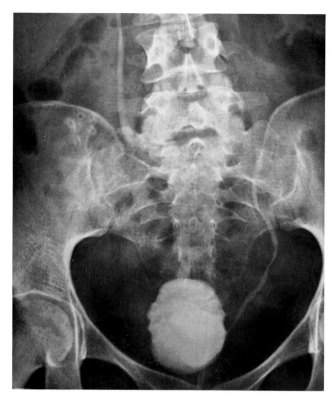

Figure 19–28. End-stage cyclophosphamide cystitis. Note changes in the right iliac crest from repeated bone biopsies.

under the intramural ureter. This weakening may be the cause or contribute to the *vesicoureteric reflux,* which is the hallmark of Hutch diverticulum. The diverticulum originates above and lateral to the ureteral orifice.[51]

Congenital Bladder Diverticula

Congenital bladder diverticula are extremely rare and may be confused with "bladder ears" or partially patent urachus. They commonly originate posterior to the bladder just behind the trigone and contain all the components of the bladder wall.

BLADDER TUMORS

Transitional Cell Carcinoma of the Bladder

Etiology. Unknown, analine dyes, cigarette smoking, infection, cyclophosphamide.[52]

Incidence. Most common in sixth and seventh decades of life. There is male preponderance. Three

percent of patients with bladder carcinoma will develop upper tract tumor, and 50–80% of patients with upper tract TCC at some time will develop bladder carcinoma.

Pathology. Malignancy of the transitional epithelium. Metastasis into lymph nodes, liver, lung, bones,

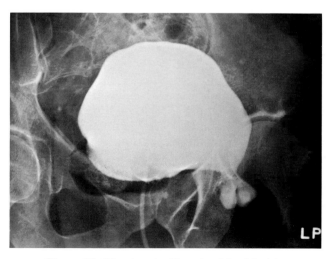

Figure 19–29. Inguinal hernia of the bladder.

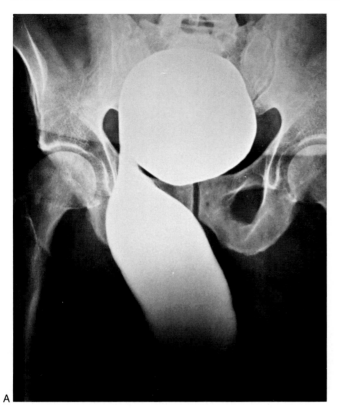
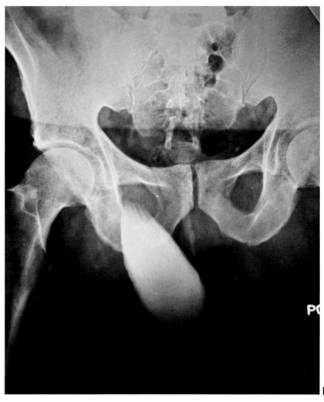

A   B

Figure 19–30. (A) Large scrotal bladder hernia. (B) On the postvoid radiograph there is large residual within the hernia.

and local extension. Morphologically, the tumor may be: a) noninvasive (in situ); b) papillary; or c) infiltrating. Four grades of cellular differentiation are recognized.

Clinical Presentation. Hematuria, frequency, ureteral obstruction, metastases.

Laboratory Findings. Malignant cells in urine, hematuria.

Radiological Findings

Diagnosis. Diagnosis of bladder carcinoma is and always will be made by cystoscopy and biopsy. Biopsy allows for cellular differentiation, grading, establishment of cellular type, number of lesions, morphological characteristics, and depth of wall invasion.

As far as diagnosis is concerned all imaging methods are ancillary. The diagnosis may be suggested on an excretory urogram or other contrast examinations if a "filling" defect or irregularity of the bladder wall is seen (Fig. 19–37). In fact, any asymmetry of the bladder on these examinations should raise suspicion for TCC (Fig. 19–38). TCC at the ureteral orifice

may produce a pseudoureterocele (Fig. 19–39). At other times TCC may present as a large mass (Fig. 19–40). A perfectly smooth bladder and lack of filling defect does not exclude malignancy, however. A radiology consultation request such as: "Hematuria, rule out bladder carcinoma," should be treated accordingly.

Other lesions may also produce bladder filling defects. Among them are clots, bladder calculi, fungus balls, malakoplakia, ureterocele, sloughed papilla, localized edema. Even extrinsic impression may on occasion cause peculiar mimicry of an intraluminal mass when none is present.

In the presence of a bladder tumor it is important to determine if the ureteral orifice is involved by the tumor and if there is resultant hydronephrosis (Fig. 19–41). On occasion, the ureteral orifice is not visible on cystoscopic examination and excretory urography may provide the answer (Fig. 19–42). At times, bladder carcinoma may exhibit retrograde growth into the ureter (Fig. 19–43).

Staging. While imaging may be secondary in detecting the tumor, its real value is in staging (Fig. 19–44). Over the years, many imaging techniques have been

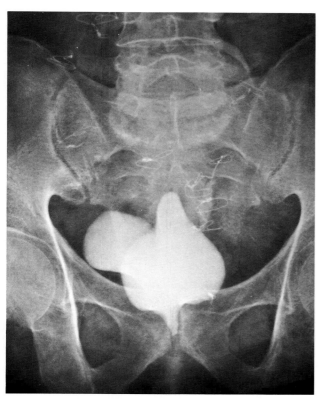

Figure 19–31. Large incisional bladder hernia causing symptoms of frequency and dysuria.

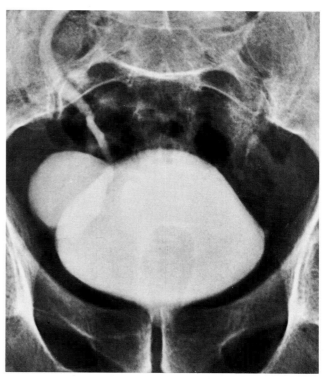

Figure 19–33. Acquired bladder diverticulum. Depending on its location, the diverticulum may displace the distal ureteral segment medially.

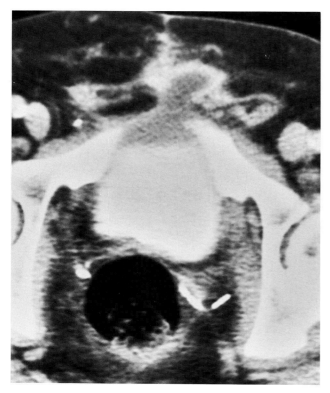

Figure 19–32. Small incisional ventral bladder hernia detected only on CT in a patient with radical prostatectomy.

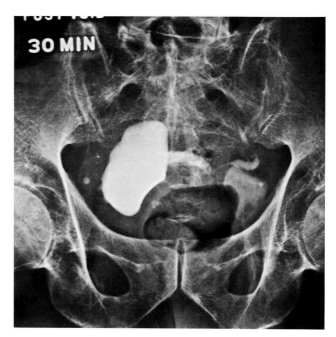

Figure 19–34. Postvoid radiograph shows residual contrast within the bladder diverticulum while the rest of the bladder is empty. Note "J" hooking of the ureter, diagnostic for prostatic enlargement.

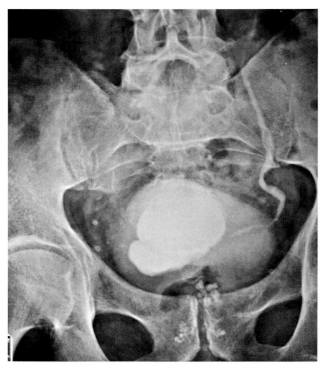

Figure 19–35. Posterior dependent bladder diverticulum is preferentially filled with contrast before the bladder fills. This is because the specific gravity of the contrast is greater. The implication is that more ventral diverticula will remain unopacified the longest if the patient remains in the supine position (See Fig. 19–32).

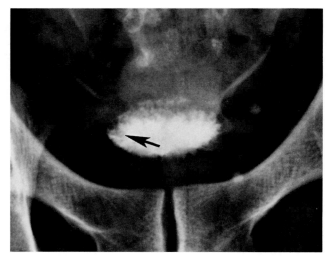

Figure 19–37. TCC seen as a minimal irregularity (arrow) only on a postvoid radiograph in a patient with hematuria. This finding may be simply overlooked or mistaken for edema due to a recently passed ureteral calculus.

employed toward this goal. Endoperivesical gas insufflation (with and without angiography), fractional cystography, double contrast cystography, and suprapubic ultrasound are some of the modalities tried and abandoned.

Three modalities remain and are still tested against each other.

CT Imaging. Even without intravenous contrast, papillary tumor is clearly visible (Fig. 19–45).[53] However, administration of intravenous contrast at a rapid rate may facilitate the staging process.[54–56]

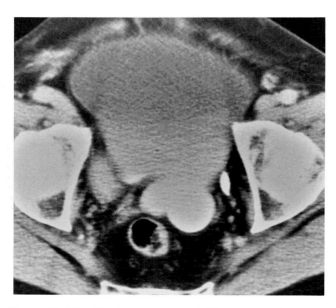

Figure 19–36. Contrast-enhanced CT scan showing contrast layering in a posterior bladder diverticulum.

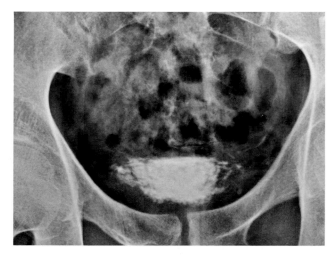

Figure 19–38. A small "filling" defect representing a TCC is seen on a postvoid radiograph on the left. This is easier to appreciate if both lateral parts of the bladder are compared.

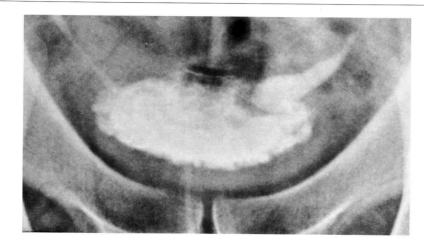

Figure 19–39. A pseudoureterocele is produced by a small carcinoma at the orifice, which can be discerned as a small "filling" defect.

Extension into the bladder wall may be judged by local bladder wall thickness. Extension outside the wall and local infiltration are judged by loss of fat planes and by detecting a mass outside of the expected bladder wall contour (Fig. 19–46). Lymph nodes larger than 1 cm in any dimension are indicative of possible metastatic disease (Fig. 19–47). Hydronephrosis and hydroureter may also be identified. Metastases in the bones are usually osteolytic (Fig. 19–48), although mixed lesions are seen in a relatively large number of patients (Fig. 19–49). Since CT imaging provides many pertinent answers as to local, lymph node, and distant spread, it is the modality of choice (Fig. 19–50).

The disadvantage of CT is its inability to thoroughly examine long tubular structures, such as ureters and pelvocalyceal system. Since TCC is a multicentric disease, the upper tract should be scrutinized for small filling defects representing other

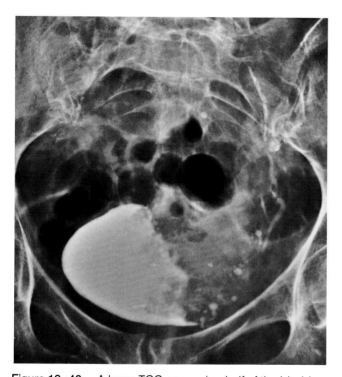

Figure 19–40. A large TCC occupying half of the bladder.

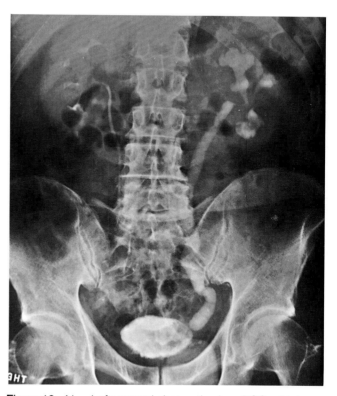

Figure 19–41. Left ureteral obstruction by a TCC, which can be recognized as a "filling" defect. Peculiar appearance of left collecting system and concomitant presence of ureteral obstruction should raise the possibility of renal tuberculosis, but none was present.

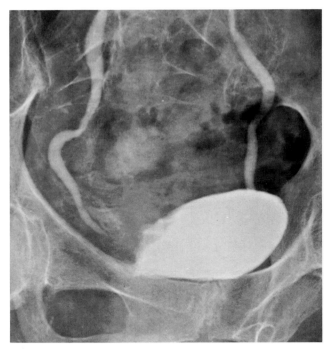

Figure 19–42. Ureteral orifice was invisible on cystoscopy. EXU demonstrates no obstruction and there is no involvement of the ureter.

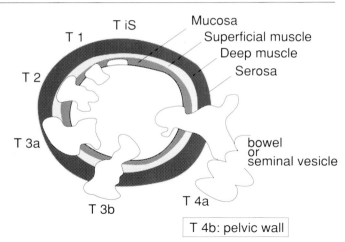

Figure 19–44. TNM classification of bladder carcinoma. Tis: carcinoma in situ; T1: infiltration of lamina propria; T2: extension to superficial muscle layer; T3a: extension to deep muscle layer; T3b: infiltration of perivesical fat; T4a: invasion of neighboring organs (uterus, vagina, prostate); T4b: invasion of pelvic or abdominal wall.

carcinomas. Excretory urogram still seems to be the examination of choice in this regard. Perhaps the ideal situation is a combined CT and excretory urogram done at the same time. A problem, however, is the oral contrast given to outline the intestines and help differentiate these from other mass lesions. This contrast interferes with excretory urography.

The second disadvantage of CT is the difficulty one may encounter in examining rounded structures. Unless the tumor is perpendicular to the beam, extension through the wall may not easily be detected.

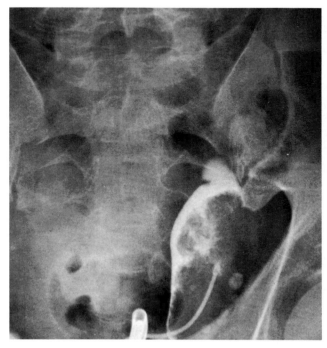

Figure 19–43. Retrograde pyelogram demonstrates retrograde growth of a large bladder carcinoma into the ureter. This has resulted in obstruction and hydronephrosis.

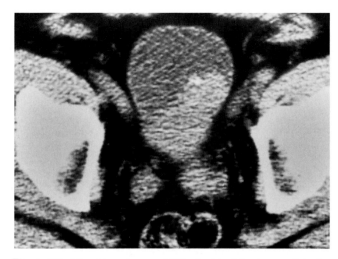

Figure 19–45. Unenhanced CT of a bladder tumor. Intraluminal portion of the tumor is nicely seen and there is clearly no invasion of the perivesical fat. What is difficult to judge is the depth of wall invasion.

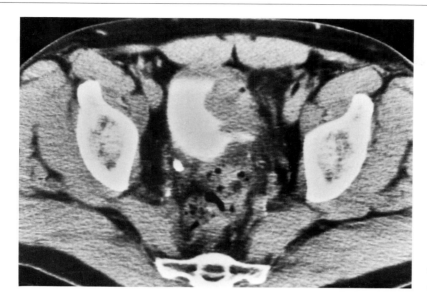

Figure 19–46. Bladder tumor, which has penetrated the serosa and begun infiltrating perivesical fat.

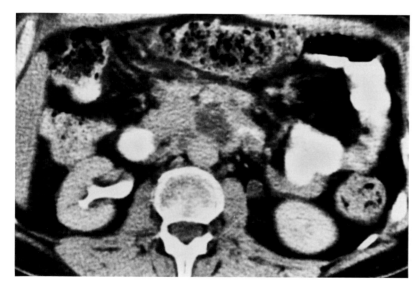

Figure 19–47. Matted lymph node metastases from TCC appear radiolucent after treatment. Note dilated left ureter, which has not filled with contrast because of distal obstruction.

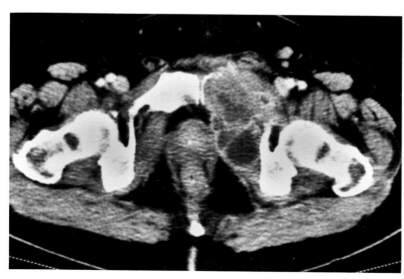

Figure 19–48. Osteolytic bone metastasis from carcinoma of the bladder. Metastasis has destroyed the bone and is growing into the adjacent soft tissues.

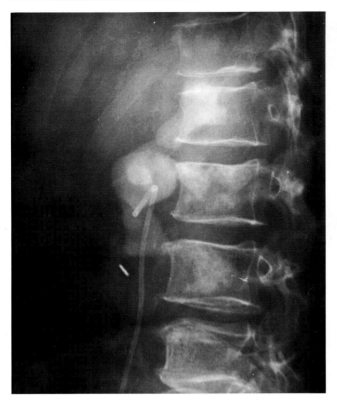

Figure 19–49. While osteolytic bone metastases from TCC are more common, in this case osteoblastic component is dominant.

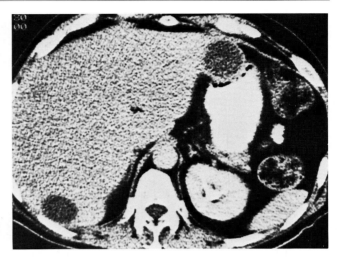

Figure 19–50. Liver metastases from TCC of the bladder.

MR Imaging. Staging of bladder tumors by this imaging modality offers some advantages over CT imaging. Any imaging plane may be chosen so that the study may be customized, depending on the direction of tumor spread. Different imaging sequences display the tumor and the bladder wall, and the different signal intensities make extension easily recognizable.[57] T2-weighted spin echo sequences display the tumor as relatively hyperintense (bright) compared to the hypointense (dark) bladder wall (Fig. 19–51).[58,59] Lymph node enlargement is seen as easily as on CT and so are skeletal metastases. Involvement of the adjacent organs may be seen somewhat better than on CT. Hydronephrosis can be recognized but small multicentric tumors elsewhere in the upper urinary tract system cannot be seen.

Enhancement with paramagnetic contrast material, such as gadolinium DTPA, have been tested and appear promising. T1-weighted sequences are employed which have inherently less noise and therefore provide better resolution than comparable T2-weighted sequences. The tumor always enhances on the postcontrast scan and is inhomogeneous in the presence of necrosis. The bladder wall also enhances so that an estimate of deep muscle wall invasion may prove to be difficult (Fig. 19–52). Layering of the contrast in the dependent parts of the bladder may obscure the tumor in the area.[60]

Intravesical Ultrasound. Radial ultrasound probes have been developed for intravesical use similar to the transrectal probe for prostate examination. The probe is introduced into the bladder during cystoscopy. The study may be somewhat difficult to perform, but it appears to be excellent for evaluation of depth of mural extension. The shortcoming of this examination is the inability to evaluate nodal enlargement, skeletal changes, and concomitant lesions elsewhere.[61,62]

Figure 19–51. Schematic drawing of a bladder neoplasm seen on T1-weighted spin echo sequence (left) and T2-weighted sequence (right).

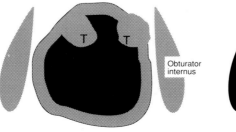
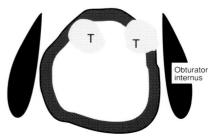

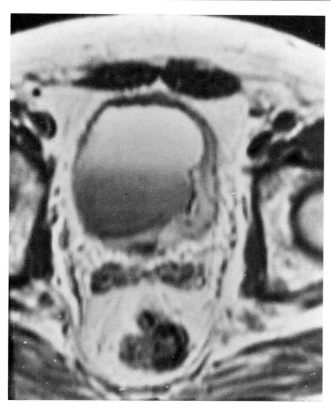

Figure 19–52. Bladder tumor seen on Gd-DTPA-enhanced T1-weighted sequence. Both the tumor and the bladder wall enhance.

Conventional Urography. Urogram is useful in evaluating the upper urinary tract for the presence of synchronous lesions and for evaluating ureteral obstruction.[63,64] Also, this is the examination of choice for follow-up of the upper tract system for development of new lesions every 2 years.[65]

Interventional Radiology in Bladder Carcinoma. On occasion, bladder tumors may hemorrhage and require repeated transfusions. Transcatheter embolization is the appropriate method to control intractable blood loss. The branches of the hypogastric artery should be selectively catheterized as close to the bleeding site as possible, preferably beyond the takeoff of the gluteal branches.[66]

Leukoplakia

Pathology. Squamous metaplasia of the transitional epithelium with hyperkeratosis. The lesion is usually a slightly elevated membranous yellowish/whitish patch. Rarely, the lesion may become big and present as a mass lesion within the bladder. Leuko-

plakia is a precancerous condition and squamous cell carcinoma may arise from these lesions.[67–69]

Clinical Presentation. There is male preponderance. Frequent urinary tract infections, long-standing urinary tract calculi, outflow bladder obstruction, strictures. The disease is not to be confused with malakoplakia.

Radiologic Findings. Poorly defined filling defects in the bladder, ureter, and pelvocalyceal system. The lesion may become large and fill most of the bladder and it may occur in the renal pelvis. Cystoscopy and biopsy are diagnostic.

Squamous Cell Carcinoma of the Bladder

Incidence. Three to 6% of all bladder neoplasms.

Etiology. Associated with chronic urinary tract infection, calculi, and strictures.[70,71] Common neoplasm in patients with schistosomiasis.

Pathology. Infiltrative squamous cell carcinoma preceded by squamous metaplasia. Cellular differentiation graded I–IV.

Clinical Presentation. Weight loss, pelvic pain, back pain, outflow bladder obstruction, chronic urinary tract infections. Poor prognosis.

Radiological Findings. Differentiation of this tumor from transitional cell carcinoma is impossible by current imaging methods. History of chronic urinary tract infection, presence of bladder calculi, history of radiological findings pointing to schistosomiasis make the diagnosis more likely. Filling defect, wall infiltration, nodal involvement, bone or other distant metastases are looked for.[72–74]

Disruption of curvilinear bladder schistosomiasis calcification likely represents growing tumor.

Adenocarcinoma of the Bladder

Incidence. Rare, less than 1% of all bladder neoplasms. There is male predominance. High association with bladder exstrophy and cystitis glandularis.[75–77]

Pathology. Papillary or solid mucin-producing adenocarcinoma. Origin is from remnants of hindgut epithelium or urachus.

Radiological Findings. Perhaps the only finding that makes this rare neoplasm somewhat different is the occasional presence of calcification within the tumor.[78] Calcification in general is easier to detect on CT scan than by any other imaging modality. However, the presence of calcification has no particular diagnostic or prognostic significance and can also be seen in other neoplasms (Fig. 19–53).

Bladder Lymphoma

PRIMARY BLADDER LYMPHOMA

This is a rare disease that may present with hematuria and is diagnosed at biopsy. Radiologically, it is indistinguishable from transitional cell carcinoma. Radiological workup involves staging.[79]

SECONDARY BLADDER LYMPHOMA

Involvement of the urinary tract is more common in non-Hodgkin's lymphoma than in Hodgkin's disease. Kidney and adrenal gland are affected more commonly compared with the bladder and testis. At the time bladder lymphoma is diagnosed, multiple organ involvement is already present in the majority of patients. Symptoms of bladder obstruction may be present. Irregularities, thickening of the bladder wall, and nodular pattern are nonspecific radiological findings.[80,81]

Rare Bladder Malignancies

Metastases should be considered in patients with lower urinary tract symptoms and primary malignancy elsewhere. Other rare bladder tumors include small cell carcinoma,[82] malignant mesenchymoma,[83] and leiomyosarcoma.

RHABDOMYOSARCOMA OF THE BLADDER (SARCOMA BOTRYOIDES)

Rare neoplasm, although the most common soft tissue sarcoma in children. After head and neck, the bladder and prostate are the most frequent sites. A subtype of this tumor has morphological appearance of grape cluster projecting intraluminally into the bladder and urethra and is referred to as *sarcoma botryoides* (Fig. 19–54). Large intravesical masses may be discovered with local invasion of periprostatic tissues and ischiorectal fossa.[84]

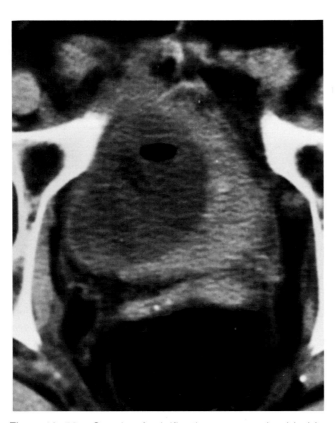

Figure 19–53. Specks of calcifications are seen in a bladder tumor on the left. Also some calcifications are seen in seminal vesicles. The two are not related.

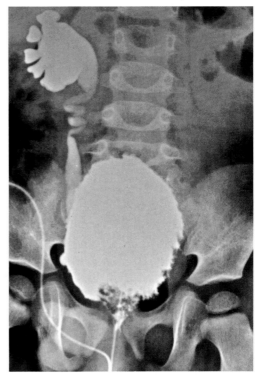

Figure 19–54. Rhabdomyosarcoma of the bladder and prostate. Grapelike "filling" defects are seen at the base of the bladder and in the proximal urethra. Outflow bladder obstruction has resulted in high bladder pressures, reflux, and parenchymal atrophy.

BENIGN BLADDER TUMORS

Benign bladder tumors are very rare. Few if any can be differentiated by imaging alone. Some have characteristic clinical presentation such as bladder pheochromocytoma (paroxysmal hypertension, sweating, headaches during micturition), bladder endometriosis (cyclic urinary symptoms), but most present with no specific complaint. Intraluminal filling defect, bladder asymmetry, thickening of the bladder wall, ureteral obstruction, outflow bladder obstruction, displacement, etc., may be seen in almost all instances, depending on tumor size and location.

Hemangioma

Hemangioma is the most common benign bladder tumor and is frequently associated with skin hemangiomas elsewhere. Frequent bleeding episodes, sometimes severe, are encountered (Fig. 19–55).[85,86] Filling defects in the bladder may disappear, since the lesion is compressible. Biopsy may be disastrous. Angiography and transcatheter embolization may be indicated on occasion (Fig. 19–56).[87]

Leiomyoma

Leiomyomas are the most common mesothelial benign bladder tumors.[88,89] They may become large and pedunculated but are usually asymptomatic. Only 160 cases have been reported. Leiomyomas may occur anywhere in the urinary tract. They have been described in the renal parenchyma, renal pelvis, ureter, prostate, epididymis, spermatic cord, testis, and seminal vesicles.[90,91]

Pheochromocytoma

Cystoscopy and retrograde cystogram may induce paroxysmal hypertension. The tumor is hypervascular on angiography. Malignant pheochromocytoma originating from the bladder has been described.[92,93]

Neurofibroma

Associated with von Recklinghausen's disease. Hypertrophy of the clitoris may be seen.[94,95]

Nephrogenic Adenoma

Rare benign bladder tumor seen in young men. Tubular epithelium found in the tumor resembles convoluted and collecting renal tubules.[96–98]

Bladder Polyp

Rare lesion, pedunculated, on stalk.

Endometriosis

Bladder involvement with endometriosis is rare. Filling defect or bladder displacement may be seen.[99–101] Ureteral obstruction may occur, depending on the site of involvement.

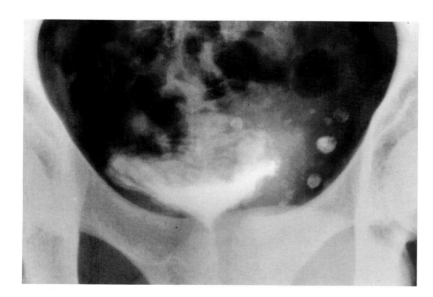

Figure 19–55. Filling defect in the bladder associated with a mass effect and several phleboliths were diagnostic features, suggesting bladder hemangioma in a young boy presenting with gross intermittent hematuria.

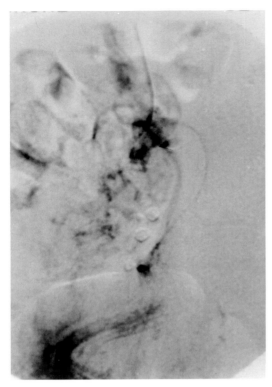

Figure 19–56. Selective angiography and embolization of the inferior vesical artery brought hemorrhage under control. A cluster of vessels is seen in the area of the tumor.

Inverted Papilloma

Usually arising from the trigone. Has characteristic histological appearance.[102,103]

Pseudotumors

Extra-articular rheumatoid nodule has been reported in a patient with rheumatoid arthritis.[104] Condylomata acuminata rarely involve the bladder, mostly in immunosuppressed patients (Fig. 19–57). At times some findings cannot be explained (Fig. 19–58).

UNUSED BLADDER

Two groups of patients may have unused bladder for prolonged periods of time: patients who for various reasons have been diverted but whose bladder was left in place, and those anephric patients maintained on dialysis.

To evaluate size, urethral anatomy, and vesicoureteral reflux, unused bladder may be examined

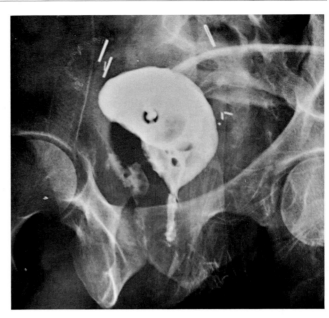

Figure 19–57. Condylomata acuminata involving the bladder and resulting in outflow bladder obstruction requiring suprapubic catheter for drainage.

by cystography prior to undiversion or prior to renal transplantation. After a prolonged dormant period, heavily trabeculated neuropathic bladder may become smooth and normal in appearance. Intramural extravasation of contrast material may be seen on occasion but is apparently an inconsequential finding.[105–107] Bladder perforation is rare.

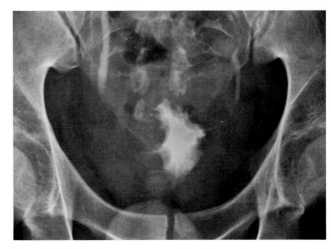

Figure 19–58. A young man without symptoms relating to the bladder was discovered to have a very irregular bladder with filling defects. Cystoscopy was performed solely on the basis of the radiographic appearance within 24 hours and bladder was found to be perfectly normal.

PELVIC LIPOMATOSIS

Incidence. Rare. More common in blacks.

Pathology. Abundant fatty proliferation displacing bladder and rectum. May cause ureteral obstruction. May be associated with cystitis cystica.

Clinical Presentation. Symptoms are related to outflow bladder obstruction. Prostate is displaced cephalad and may be difficult to palpate. Ureteral obstruction is rare. Although rectum is also displaced and elongated, symptoms related to gastrointestinal tract are never present. Cystoscopy with rigid instruments may be difficult or impossible.

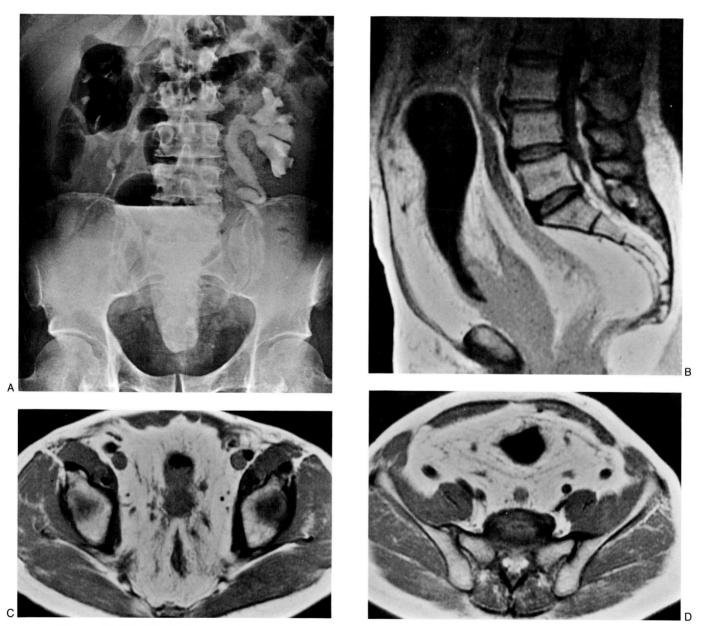

Figure 19–59. Pelvic lipomatosis and emphysematous cystitis. **(A)** Diagnosis is obvious on upright AP projection. "Inverted pear-shaped" bladder with an air-fluid level due to cystitis by gas-producing organisms. Radiolucent areas in the true pelvis represent abundant fatty tissue. **(B)** Sagittal T1-weighted sequence clearly shows why it may be very difficult to perform cystoscopy. **(C)** On axial images the bladder becomes recognizable at the cut just above femoral heads and extends way out from the true pelvis. **(D)** High signal intensity fatty tissues surround the bladder base and affect not only the bladder, but also the prostate, seminal vesicles, and rectum.

Radiological Findings. On plain radiograph, radiolucencies in the pelvis are suggestive of abundant fat. Contrast examinations of the bladder will disclose cephalad displacement and narrowing of the bladder base. This appearance resembles an upside-down pear, hence the name *pear-shaped* or *teardrop sign*.[108] Fatty tissue is particularly well seen on CT or MR imaging (Fig. 59). Differential diagnosis includes perivesical hematoma, edema due to inferior vena cava occlusion, enlarged pelvic lymph nodes, and lymphocysts.

REFERENCES

1. Mallikarjunaiah GS, Solomon B, Ramamurthy BS. Lateral displacement of the bladder. Australas Radiol 1986; 30:46–48.
2. Madayag MA, Seliger G. Inferior vena cava occlusion: characteristic radiographic changes on excretory urography and barium enema examination. AJR 1977; 128:39–42.
3. Chang SF. Pear-shaped bladder caused by large iliopsoas muscles. Radiology 1978; 128:349–350.
4. Jorulf H, Lindstedt E. Urogenital schistosomiasis: CT evaluation. Radiology 1985; 157:745–747.
5. Pollack HM, Banner MP, Martinez LO, et al. Diagnostic considerations in bladder wall calcifications. AJR 1981; 136:791–797.
6. Miller SW, Pfister RC. Calcifications in uroepithelial tumors of the bladder. Report of 5 cases and survey of the literature. Am J Roentgenol 1974; 121:827–831.
7. Verguts L, Deconick K, Mortelmans LL. Alkaline encrusting cystitis. Urol Radiol 1987; 9:53–54.
8. Nesbit RM, Bromme W. Double penis and double bladder. Am J Roentgenol 1933; 30:497–502.
9. Cacciarelli AA, Lucas B, McAlister WH. Multichambered bladder anomalies. Am J Roentgenol 1976; 126:642–646.
10. Mallikarjunaiah GS, Solomon B, Reddy DG. Double bladder (report of two unusual cases). Australas Radiol 1986; 30:51–52.
11. Kapoor R, Saha MM. Complete duplication of the bladder, urethra and external genitalia in a neonate—a case report. J Urol 1987; 137:1243–1244.
12. Mirk P, Calisti A, Fileni A. Prenatal sonographic diagnosis of bladder exstrophy. J Ultrasound Med 1986; 5:291–292.
13. Spataro RF, Davis RS, McLachlan MSF, et al. Urachal abnormalities in the adult. Radiology 1983; 149:659–663.
14. Goldman IL, Caldamone AA, Gauderer M, et al. Infected urachal cysts: a review of 10 cases. J Urol 1988; 140:375–378.
15. Thomas AJ, Pollack MS, Libshitz HI. Urachal carcinoma: evaluation with computed tomography. Urol Radiol 1986; 8:194–195.
16. Brick HS, Friedman AC, Pollack HM, et al. Urachal carcinoma: CT findings. Radiology 1988; 169:377–381.
17. Nesbith JA, Walter PJ. Computed tomographic imaging of microscopic dystrophic calcification in urachal adenocarcinoma. Urology 1986; 27:184–186.
18. Narumi Y, Sato T, Kuriyama K, et al. Vesical dome tumors: significance of extravesical extension on CT. Radiology 1988; 169:383–385.
19. Bates CP, Arnold EP, Griffiths DJ. The nature of the abnormality in bladder neck obstruction. Br J Urol 1975; 47:651–656.
20. Presman D, Ross LS, Nicosia SV. Fibromuscular hyperplasia of the posterior urethra: a cause for lower urinary tract obstruction in male children. J Urol 1972; 107:149–153.
21. Seymore SH, El-Mahdi AM, Schellhammer PF. Effect of prior transurethral resection of the prostate on postradiation urethral strictures and bladder neck contractures. Int J Radiat Oncol Biol Phys 1986; 12:1597–1600.
22. Faingold JE, Hansen CO, Rigler LG. Cystitis emphysematosa: four cases. Radiology 1953; 61:346–354.
23. Bohlman ME, Fishman EK, Oesterling JE, Goldman SM. CT findings in emphysematous cystitis. Urology 1988; 32:63–64.
24. Bartkowski DP, Lanesky JR. Emphysematous prostatitis and cystitis secondary to Candida albicans. J Urol 1988; 139:1063–1065.
25. Kauzlaric D, Barmeir E. Sonography of emphysematous cystitis. J Ultrasound Med 1985; 4:319.
26. Morse HD. Etiology and pathology of pyelitis cystica, ureteritis cystica and cystitis cystica. Am J Pathol 1928; 4:33–50.
27. Erturk E, Erturk E, Sheinfeld J, Davis RS. Metaplastic cystitis complicated with Von Brunn nests, cystitis cystica, and intestinal type of glandular metaplasia. Urology 1988; 32:165–167.
28. Walther MM, Campbell WG Jr, O'Brien DP 3d, et al. Cystitis cystica: an electron and immunofluorescence microscopic study. J Urol 1987; 137:764–768.
29. Susmano D, Rubenstein AB, Dakin AR, et al. Cystitis glandularis and adenocarcinoma of the bladder. J Urol 1971; 105:671–674.
30. Yalla SV, Ivker M, Burros HM, et al. Cystitis glandularis with perivesical lipomatosis: frequent association of two unusual proliferative conditions. Urology 1975; 5:383–386.
31. Rao KG. Cystitis glandularis causing bilateral ureteric obstruction and hydronephrosis. Br J Urol 1975; 47:398.
32. Kauzlaric D, Barmeir E, Campana A. Diagnosis of cystitis glandularis. Urol Radiol 1987; 9:50–52.
33. Palubinskas AJ. Eosinophilic cystitis: case report of eosinophilic infiltration of the urinary bladder. Radiology 1960; 75:589–591.
34. Kessler WO, Clarke PL, Kaplan GW. Eosinophilic cystitis. Urology 1975; 6:499–501.
35. Hassel DR, Glasier CM, McConnell JR. Granulomatous cystitis in chronic granulomatous disease: ultrasound diagnosis. Pediatr Radiol 1987; 17:254–255.
36. Gillenwater JY, Wein AJ. Summary of the National Institute of Arthritis, Diabetes, Digestive and Kidney Diseases Workshop on Interstitial Cystitis, National Institutes of Health, Bethesda, Maryland, August 28–29, 1987. J Urol 1988; 140:203–206.
37. Messing EM. The diagnosis of interstitial cystitis. Urology 1987; 29(Suppl):4–7.
38. Holm-Bentzen M, Lose G. Pathology and pathogenesis of interstitial cystitis. Urology 1987; 29(4 Suppl):8–13.

39. Hunner GL. A rare type of bladder ulcer in woman: report of cases. Boston Med Surg J 1915; 172:660–664.
40. Phillips FS, Sternberg SS, Cronin AP, Vidal PM. Cyclophosphamide and urinary bladder toxicity. Cancer Res 1961; 21:1577.
41. Watson NA, Notley RG. Urologic complications of cyclophosphamide. Br J Urol 1973; 45:606.
42. Bernstein JE, Meyer K. Groin hernia with inguino-scrotal herniation of the urinary bladder. Clin Nucl Med 1987; 12:155–156.
43. Lee HK, Skarzynski J. Bladder herniation in inguinal hernia detected during bone imaging. Clin Nucl Med 1986; 11:740–741.
44. Lee TA III, Siddiqui AR. Urinary bladder herniation into the scrotum seen on bone imaging. Clin Nucl Med 1986; 11:435.
45. Morano JU, Burkhalter JL. Bladder hernia simulating osseous metastatic lesion on radionuclide bone scan. Urol Radiol 1987; 9:183–184.
46. Calabro A, Di Prima F, Aragona F, et al. Bladder herniation through abdominal wall: exceptional complication of retropubic prostatic adenomectomy. Urol Radiol 1987; 9:56–57.
47. Montaque DK, Boltuch RL. Primary neoplasms in vesical diverticula: report of 10 cases. J Urol 1976; 116:41–42.
48. Nanbu A, Tsukamoto T, Kumamoto Y, et al. Squamous cell carcinoma of bladder diverticulum with initial symptoms produced by metastasis to maxillary sinus. Eur Urol 1988; 15:285–286.
49. Williams MJ, Gooding GAW. Sonographic diagnosis of a neoplasm in a bladder diverticulum. J Ultrasound Med 1985; 4:203–204.
50. Harcke HT, Capitanio MA, Grover WD, Valdes-Dapena M. Bladder diverticula and Menkes' syndrome. Radiology 1977; 124:459–461.
51. Hutch JH. Vesico-ureteral reflux in the paraplegic. Cause and correction. J Urol 1952; 68:457–465.
52. Brenner DW, Schellhammer PF. Upper tract urothelial malignancy after cyclophosphamide therapy: a case report and literature review. J Urol 1987; 137:1226–1227.
53. Amendola MA, Glazer GM, Grossman HB, et al. Staging of bladder carcinoma. MRI-CT-surgical correlation. AJR 1986; 146:1179–1182.
54. Sager EM, Fossa SD, Kaalhus O, et al. Contrast-enhanced computed tomography in carcinoma of the urinary bladder: use of different injection methods. Acta Radiol 1987; 28:67–72.
55. Bryan PJ, Butler HE, Lipiuma JP, et al. CT and MR imaging in staging bladder neoplasms. JCAT 1987; 11:96–100.
56. Koss JC, Arger PH, Coleman BG, et al. CT staging of the bladder carcinoma. AJR 1981; 137:359–362.
57. Buy JN, Moss AA, Guinet C, et al. MR staging of bladder carcinoma: correlation with pathologic findings. Radiology 1988; 169:695–700.
58. Fisher MR, Hricak H, Tanagho EA. Urinary bladder MR imaging. Part II. Neoplasm. Radiology 1985; 157:471–477.
59. Rholl SK, Lee JKT, Heiken JP, et al. Primary bladder carcinoma: evaluation with MR imaging. Radiology 1987; 163:117–121.
60. Neuerburg JM, Bohndorf K, Sohn M, et al. Urinary bladder neoplasms: evaluation with contrast-enhanced MR imaging. Radiology 1989; 172:739–743.
61. Abu-Yousef MM, Narayana AS, Franken EA Jr, Brown RC. Urinary bladder tumors studied by cystosonography. I. Detection. Radiology 1984; 153:223–226.
62. Abu-Yousef MM, Narayana AS, Brown RC, Franken EA Jr. Urinary bladder tumors studied by cystosonography. II. Staging. Radiology 1984; 153:227–231.
63. Elliott S, Davies P. Urographic appearances of ureteric obstruction secondary to bladder carcinoma. Clin Radiol 1986; 37:495–498.
64. Yousem DM, Gatewood OMB, Goldman SM, Marshall FF. Synchronous and metachronous transitional cell carcinoma of the urinary tract: prevalence, incidence, and radiographic detection. Radiology 1988; 167:613–618.
65. Smith H, Weaver D, Barienbruch OBA, et al. Routine excretory urography in follow-up of superficial transitional cell carcinoma of the bladder. Urology 1989; 34:193–196.
66. Lang EK, Deutch JS, Goodman JR, et al. Transcatheter embolization of hypogastric branch arteries in the management of intractable bladder hemorrhage. J Urol 1979; 121:30–36.
67. O'Flynn JD, Mullaney J. Vesical leukoplakia progressing to carcinoma. Br J Urol 1974; 46:31–37.
68. Roehrborn CG, Teigland CM, Spence HM. Progression of leukoplakia of the bladder to squamous cell carcinoma 19 years after complete urinary diversion. J Urol 1988; 140:603–604.
69. Witherington R. Leukoplakia of the bladder: An 8-year follow-up. J Urol 1974; 112:600–602.
70. Bessette RL, Abell MR, Herwig KR. A clinicopathological study of squamous cell carcinoma of the bladder. J Urol 1974; 112:66–67.
71. Wyman A, Kinder RB. Squamous cell carcinoma of the bladder associated with intrapelvic foreign bodies. Br J Urol 1988; 61:460.
72. Desai PG, Khan SA, Jayachandran S, Ilardi C. Paraneoplastic syndrome in squamous cell carcinoma of urinary bladder. Urology 1987; 30:262–264.
73. Stricker PD, Grant AB. Solitary metastasis of squamous cell carcinoma of the bladder to the myocardium. J Urol 1987; 137:113–114.
74. Nanbu A, Tsukamoto T, Kumamoto Y, et al. Squamous cell carcinoma of bladder diverticulum with initial symptoms produced by metastasis to maxillary sinus. Eur Urol 1988; 15:285–286.
75. Jacobo E, Loening S, Schmidt JD, et al. Primary adenocarcinoma of the bladder: a retrospective study of 20 patients. J Urol 1977; 117:54–56.
76. Abenoza P, Manivel C, Fraley EE. Primary adenocarcinoma of urinary bladder. Clinicopathologic study of 16 cases. Urology 1987; 29:9–14.
77. Blute ML, Engen DE, Travis WD, Kvols LK. Primary signet ring cell adenocarcinoma of the bladder. J Urol 1989; 141:17–21.
78. Summers EH, Gittes RF. Calcified tumor of the urinary bladder: sonographic diagnosis and distinction from the bladder calculus. J Ultrasound Med 1985; 4:681.
79. Binkovitz LA, Hattery RR, LeRoy AJ. Primary lymphoma of the bladder. Urol Radiol 1988; 9:231–233.
80. Miyake O, Namiki M, Sonoda T, Kitamura H. Secondary involvement of genitourinary organs in malignant lymphoma. Urol Int 1987; 42:360–362.

81. Bruneton JN, Drouillard J, Normand F, et al. Non-renal urological lymphomas. Fortschr Rontgenstr 1987; 146:42–46.

82. Swanson PE, Brooks R, Pearse H, Stenzel P. Small cell carcinoma of urinary bladder. Urology 1988; 32:558–563.

83. Terada Y, Saito I, Morohoshi T, Niijima T. Malignant mesenchymoma of the bladder. Cancer 1987; 15, 60:858–863.

84. Baker ME, Silverman PM, Korobkin M. Computed tomography of prostatic and bladder rhabdomyosarcomas. J Comput Assist Tomogr 1985; 9:780–783.

85. Pakter R, Nussbaum A, Fishman EK. Hemangioma of the bladder: sonographic and computerized tomography findings. J Urol 1988; 140:601–602.

86. Gupta AK, Bhargava S. Bladder hemangioma: ultrasonographic demonstration. Urol Radiol 1987; 9: 181–182.

87. Esguerra A, Carvajal A, Mouton H. Pelvic arteriography in diagnosis of hemangioma of the bladder. J Urol 1973; 109:609–611.

88. Wenz W, Sommerkamp H, Dinkel E. Leiomyoma of the bladder. Urol Radiol 1986; 8:114–115.

89. Illescas FF, Baker ME, Weinerth JL. Bladder leiomyoma: advantages of sonography over computed tomography. Urol Radiol 1986; 8:216.

90. Bramwell SP, Pitts J, Goudie SE, Abel BJ. Giant leiomyoma of the bladder. Br J Urol 1987; 60:178.

91. Jacobs MA, Bavendam T, Leach GE. Bladder leiomyoma. Urol 1989; 34:56–57.

92. Javaheri P, Raafat J. Malignant pheochromocytoma of the urinary bladder—report of two cases. Br J Urol 1975; 47:401–404.

93. Lenders JW, Sluiter HE, Rosenbusch G, Thien T. A pheochromocytoma of the urinary bladder. Eur J Radiol 1987; 7:274–275.

94. Carlson DH, Wilkinson RH. Neurofibromatosis of the bladder in children. Radiology 1972; 105:401–405.

95. Deniz E, Shimkus GJ, Weller CG. Pelvis neurofibromatosis: localized von Recklinghausen's disease of the bladder. J Urol 1966; 96:906–909.

96. Lukkarinen O, Autio-Harmainen H. Nephrogenic adenoma of the bladder. Ann Chir Gynaecol 1988; 77:45–46.

97. Gonzalez JA, Watts JC, Alderson TP. Nephrogenic adenoma of the bladder: report of 10 cases. J Urol 1988; 139:45–47.

98. Zingas AP, Kling GA, Crotte E, et al. Computed tomography of nephrogenic adenoma of the urinary bladder. J Comput Assist Tomogr 10:979–980.

99. Buka NJ. Vesical endometriosis after cesarean section. Am J Obstet Gynecol 1988; 158:1117–1118.

100. Sircus SI, Sant GR, Ucci AA Jr. Bladder detrusor endometriosis mimicking interstitial cystitis. Urology 1988; 32:339–342.

101. Shook TE, Nyberg LM. Endometriosis of the urinary tract. Uroloy 1988; 31:1–6.

102. Mattelaer J, Leonard A, Goddeeris P, et al. Inverted papilloma of bladder: clinical significance. Urology 1988; 32:192–197.

103. Schultz RE, Boyle DE. Inverted papilloma of renal pelvis associated with contralateral ureteral malignancy and bladder recurrence. J Urol 1988; 139:111–113.

104. Berman HH, Wilets AJ. Rheumatoid pseudotumor of urinary bladder simulating carcinoma. Urology 1977; 9:83.

105. Caroline DF, Pollack HM, Banner MP, Schneck C. Self-limiting extravasation in the unused urinary bladder. Radiology 1985; 155:311–312.

106. Day DL. Extravasation of contrast material from unused bladders during voiding cystourethrography. Radiology 1985; 155:105–106.

107. Matsumoto AH, Clark RL, Cuttino JT Jr. Bladder mucosal tears during voiding cystouretrography in chronic renal failure. Urol Radiol 1986; 8:81–83.

108. Ambos MA, Bosniak MA, Lefleur RS, et al. The pear-shaped bladder. Radiology 1977; 122:85–88.

20

Voiding Dysfunction

INTRODUCTION

Normal Anatomy

Sphincteric mechanism is composed of three distinct components. *Internal sphincter* is made of smooth muscle and extends throughout the length of the female urethra. *Intrinsic sphincter* is intramural striated sphincter which in the female is most prominent in the mid-urethra. The male intramural striated sphincter extends from the verumontanum inferiorly to become most prominent at the membranous urethra. *Extrinsic sphincter* is voluntary striated muscle of the urogenital diaphragm. This sphincter is somewhat incomplete in females while it completely encompasses the urethra at the membranous portion in males (Fig. 20–1).

Definitions

Vesical accommodation: In the normal bladder there is little rise in detrusor pressure upon gradual filling and there is no detrusor contraction.

Intravesical pressure: Sum of detrusor and intra-abdominal pressure.

Detrusor pressure: Pressure produced by detrusor contraction alone. It is derived by subtracting intra-abdominal (rectal) pressure from intravesical pressure.

Unstable bladder: Occurrence of involuntary phasic detrusor contraction during bladder filling, resulting in true detrusor pressure of 15 cm H_2O or more, usually by the time 120 cc are instilled.

Uninhibited bladder: Occurrence of involuntary (hyperreflexic) detrusor contractions associated with *neurogenic bladder*.

Normal urine peak flow rate: In men under the age of 40 years the normal peak flow rate is over 22 ml/sec

and it decreases somewhat with age. In women over 25 it is 25 ml/sec. Lower than normal peak flow rates are most likely caused by outflow obstruction, hyporeflexic bladder, or both.

Bladder compliance: Change in bladder volume divided by change in bladder pressure. Decreased compliance is suggested when on filling there is steady and inappropriate rise in intravesical pressure without detrusor contraction.

Sensory urgency: Sensation without concomitant involuntary detrusor contraction.

Motor urgency: Sensation with concomitant detrusor contraction.

Detrusor/sphincter dyssynergia: Inappropriate contraction of the external sphincter (striated muscle) or internal sphincter (smooth muscle) at the time of detrusor contraction.

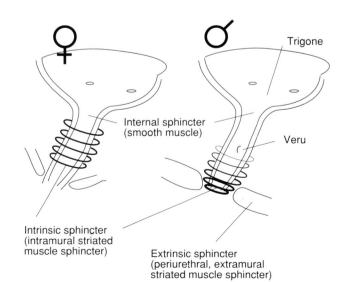

Figure 20–1. Schematic drawing of the urethral sphincters.

387

Urodynamic and Videourodynamic Evaluation

Urodynamics is the functional study of the lower urinary tract. Its purpose is to reproduce the presenting symptoms while performing simultaneous cystometry and uroflowmetry. This is accomplished by introducing small pressure transducer-fitted catheters into the bladder and rectum. The rectal transducer reflects intra-abdominal pressure while the bladder transducer measures combined bladder and intra-abdominal pressure. When electronically subtracted, the resultant *true detrusor pressure* is derived and displayed on a volume/pressure graph. Simultaneously, as urine passes through the uroflowmeter, flow rate is displayed on a time/volume-flow graph.

Videourodynamic evaluation adds simultaneous fluoroscopic observation and image recording of the bladder and urethra to the urodynamic measurements. This evaluation is helpful, for example, in patients with stress incontinence. Although a VCUG may demonstrate incontinence and urethral prolapse without knowing the detrusor pressure, it is difficult to exclude presence of unstable contractions, which may be the underlying cause for incontinence. Or, in another example, a simple VCUG cannot provide information as to why a particular patient cannot void, since there is no objective way to determine if the bladder is contracting or not (Figs. 20–2, 20–3).

Videourodynamic evaluation may be made even more sophisticated by adding simultaneous display of filling rate, urethral pressure profile, and electromyographic activity of the periurethral striated sphincter, all of which may be useful in evaluating detrusor/sphincter dyssynergia.

Linear transrectal ultrasound transducer may be used instead of fluoroscopic observation and is favored by some investigators.[1,2]

There are several classifications of voiding dysfunction. The one presented here is modified from Wein.[3,4] Every functional bladder disorder is easily placed in its proper category even if the causes for such dysfunction are not immediately clear (Table 20–1).

OUTFLOW BLADDER OBSTRUCTION

Etiology.   Causes for outflow bladder obstruction are presented in Table 20–2.

Pathology.   Prolonged outflow bladder obstruction results in hypertrophy of the smooth muscles, thickening of the bladder wall, and bladder diverticula.

High bladder pressures are reflected into the upper system. Hydroureter, hydronephrosis, and vesicoureteral reflux result. Renal function deteriorates over a period of time, eventually resulting in end-stage kidney disease.

Clinical Presentation.   Decreased stream, frequency, urgency, nocturia, incontinence, large postvoid residual urine in the bladder. Unstable bladder is a common end result of outflow obstruction and may persist even after obstruction is corrected. Urinary tract infection is common.

Radiological and Urodynamic Findings.   Bladder wall thickening may be seen on all radiological contrast examinations, CT, ultrasound, and MR imaging. Trabeculation of the bladder wall, when visible on radiological studies, is already significant (Fig. 20–4). Investigation of bladder mucosa between hypertrophied bundles of smooth muscle may produce multiple diverticular outpouches. Large diverticula may develop. Bladder stones in this setting are frequent and should be looked for diligently.

Large amounts of residual urine in the bladder after voiding imply deterioration of detrusor function. Estimation of residual urine is best done using ultrasound, since it is the least invasive. In many instances the patient will have undergone one of the contrast examinations and it is prudent to obtain a postvoid radiograph at that time.

High intravesical pressure is eventually transmitted to the upper urinary tract system. Hydronephrosis and hydroureter become evident and may eventually lead to deterioration of renal function (Fig. 20–5). Vesicoureteral reflux may develop, adding to renal demise.

Decreased urine flow rate and detrusor contractions are demonstrated on pressure-flow study. Unstable bladder contractions may also be present. Sphincteric dysfunction is frequent in patients with neurological disorder (see below).

MALE URINARY INCONTINENCE

Etiology.

1. Damage to external/intrinsic sphincter complex, usually as a complication of transurethral prostatectomy or other trauma.

2. Detrusor instability caused by outflow bladder obstruction or infection.

3. Neurogenic bladder dysfunction.

Treatment.   Depending on circumstances, either medical or surgical treatment may be needed. Surgi-

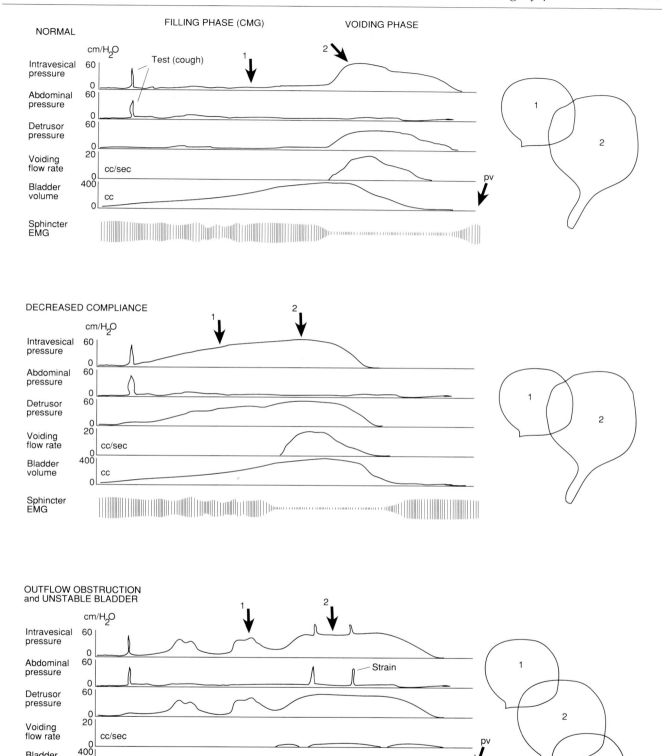

Figure 20–2. Examples of videourodynamic evaluation in a normal bladder, bladder with poor compliance, and unstable bladder with outflow bladder obstruction. Displayed at left are the basic urodynamic measurements. Arrows indicate the points in time at which the images on the right were selected. EMG of the sphincteric activity is obtained only in selected cases of neurogenic bladder and is presented here for clarity.

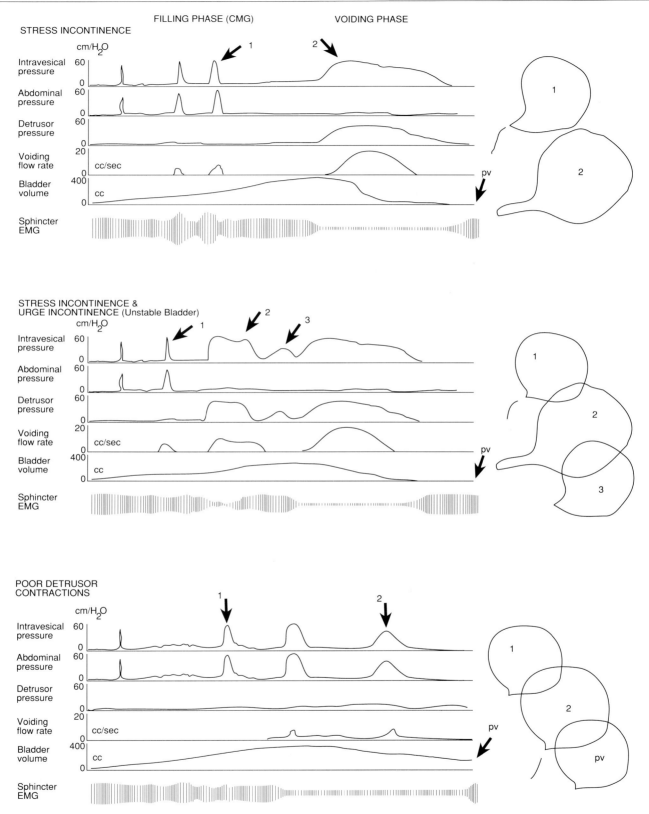

Figure 20–3.   Examples of videourodynamic evaluation in patient with pure stress incontinence, combined stress incontinence, and an atonic bladder with poor contractions. By observing the multichannel recordings, it is instantly obvious whether the increase in the intravesical pressure is due to abdominal strain or detrusor contraction.

Table 20-1. Classification of Voiding Dysfunction*

I. Failure to store
  A. Because of the bladder
    Detrusor hyperactivity
      Involuntary contractions
        Uninhibited contractions
        Unstable contractions
      Decreased compliance
        Fibrosis
      Sensory urgency
      Inflammatory
      Neurological
  B. Because of the outlet
    Stress incontinence
    Incompetent bladder neck
    Urethral instability
II. Failure to empty
  A. Because of the bladder
    Neurological
    Myogenic
    Psychogenic
  B. Because of the outlet
    Anatomical
      BPH, stricture, neoplasm
    Functional
      Sphincter dyssynergia

*Modified from Wein.[3,4]

cal procedures include placement of various anti-incontinence prostheses.

Radiological and Urodynamic Findings. Videourodynamic study determines the presence of bladder instability, atony, or normal detrusor function. Incontinence may be demonstrated and graded on a straining upright cystogram (Fig. 20–6).

Table 20-2. Causes of Outflow Bladder Obstruction

In all:	Bladder (malignant and benign tumors, diverticulum)
	Neuropathic bladder dysfunction (detrusor/sphincter dyssynergia)
In men:	Prostate (BPH, carcinoma, prostatitis, abscess, lymphoma)
	Urethra (strictures, metastases, neoplasm, prosthesis)
	Bladder (idiopathic bladder neck obstruction)
In women:	Urethra (oversuspension, diverticulum, neoplasm)
In boys:	Prostate (sarcoma botryoides)
	Bladder (idiopathic bladder neck obstruction)
	Urethra (anterior and posterior valves, stricture, meatal stenosis, polyp, prune belly syndrome)
	Ureter (prolapsed or large ectopic ureterocele)
In girls:	Cloacal anomaly
	Female hypospadia
	Female intersex
	Ureter (prolapsed or large ectopic ureterocele)

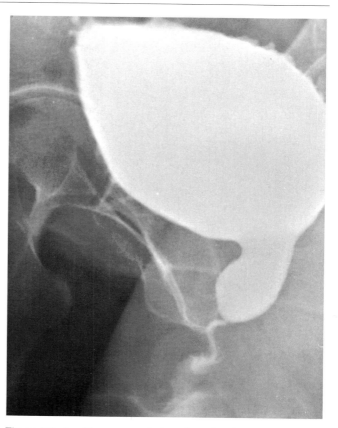

Figure 20–4. Rare example in a female of outflow obstruction caused by a mid-urethral stricture. Trabeculation is evident upon scrutinizing bladder outline.

Evaluation of Anti-incontinence Prostheses. Various devices have been devised over the years to prevent involuntary loss of urine in male patients.[5] These range from external devices, such as perineal truss and penile clamps, internal devices, such as Kaufman I and II (Fig. 20–7), and inflatable prostheses, such as Rosen and Scott.[6]

Inflatable prostheses are now in common use. These consist of an inflatable cuff, which is usually placed around bulbous urethra (occasionally around prostatic urethra) and creates outflow obstruction. The cuff is connected via subcutaneously placed tubing with a small pump in the scrotum. By squeezing the pump, fluid from the cuff is transferred into an expandable balloon reservoir placed extraperitoneally into anterior abdominal wall. By deflating the cuff, outflow obstruction is eliminated and the patient can urinate. A time-release valve in the scrotal pump allows the cuff to automatically refill within a minute or two, reestablishing continence. Fluid in the prosthesis is isotonic contrast (around 14% ionic radiographic contrast), making the prosthesis readily identifiable on plain radiographs (Figs. 20–8, 20–9, 20–10).

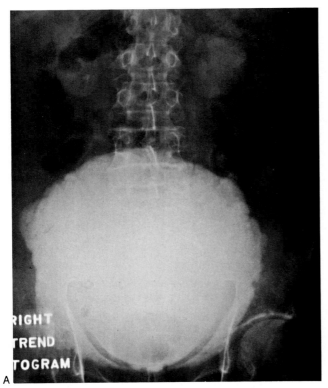
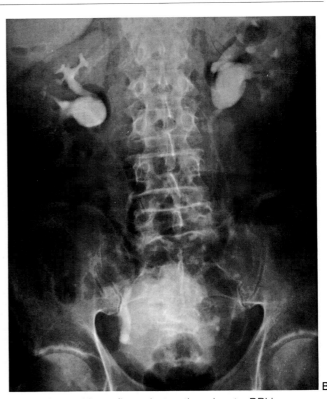

Figure 20–5. **(A)** Grade III hydronephrosis is present in a patient with outflow obstruction due to BPH. Cystogram delineates decompensated large bladder with moderate trabeculation. **(B)** After decompression with a Foley catheter the collecting system is returning to normal.

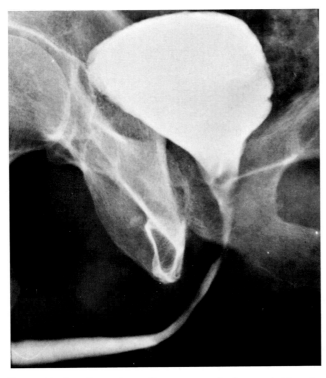

Figure 20–6. Gross incontinence on relaxing upright radiograph during VCUG in a patient after TURP. A filling defect within the prostatic urethra is either an incompletely resected or regrowing adenoma.

The prosthesis usually malfunctions because of a kink in the connecting tubing, contrast leak from the prosthesis, or because air was not purged during implantation. One or two plain radiographs of the pelvis in different projections will usually suffice to demonstrate the kink (Fig. 20–11), absence of radiographic contrast in the prosthesis, or radiolucencies in the system.[7] Pre- and postactivation radiograph may also pinpoint the cause of malfunction.

Bladder catheterization and retrograde urethrography should be done while the cuff is deflated.

Pressure exerted on the urethra may cut off the vascular supply and on occasion urethral stricture (Fig. 20–12), or erosion is the result. On urethrography, the cuff is seen surrounded by contrast (Fig. 20–13). Infection and abscess around the prosthesis are rare (Fig. 20–14).

FEMALE URINARY INCONTINENCE

Physiology

To understand female urinary incontinence, it is necessary to understand natural factors contributing to continence.

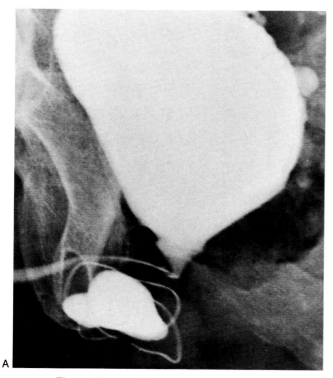

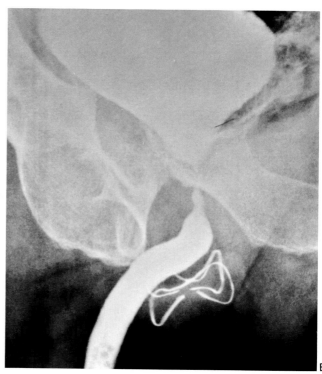

A   B

Figure 20–7. **(A)** Kaufman I prosthesis causing too much outflow obstruction and **(B)** one causing too little. Eventually the prosthesis had to be anchored to the bone by large staples.

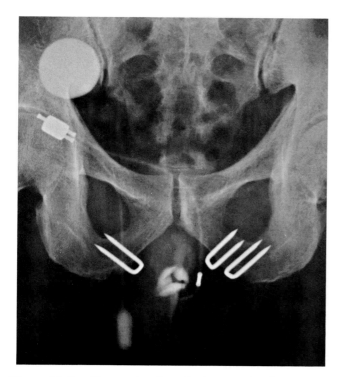

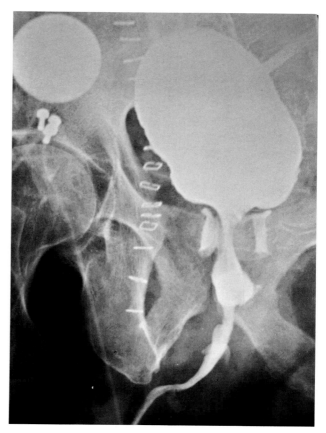

Figure 20–8. Remnants of anchoring staples from failed Kaufman II prosthesis and a modern pump prosthesis in place. Reservoir is on top right and time release valve just below it. Connecting tubing is seen leading to scrotal pump and cuff around the bulbous urethra. Note the folds and protuberances at the inside of the cuff that may produce uneven compression on the urethra and cause erosion.

Figure 20–9. A high prosthesis around prostatic urethra is unusual, although indicated in special circumstances.

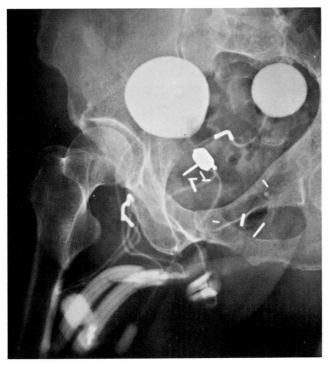

Figure 20–10. Anti-incontinence and anti-impotence prostheses are frequently seen together.

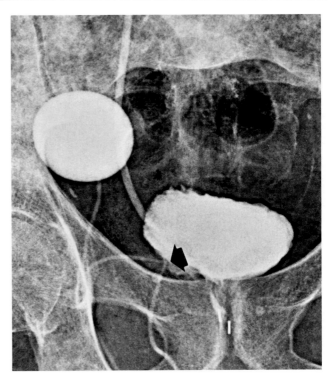

Figure 20–11. Kink in the tube (arrow).

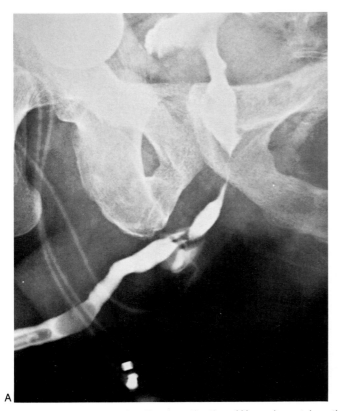

A

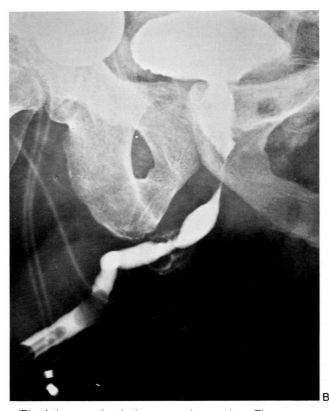

B

Figure 20–12. Predeactivation **(A)** and postdeactivation **(B)** of the prosthesis by manual pumping. The contrast from the cuff is transferred to the reservoir. Urethral stricture is present under the cuff.

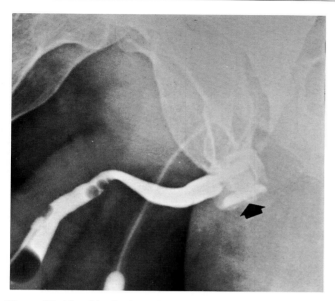

Figure 20–13. Urethral erosion by the cuff allows contrast to escape the urethral lumen and surround the cuff (arrow).

1. *Urethral length.* Normal urethra is about 4.5 cm long (Fig. 20–15). A short urethra lacks the necessary smooth muscle fibers to prevent urine leak during sudden increases in bladder pressure.

2. *Closing urethral pressure.* Intrinsic urethral pressure is the function of the external sphincter and smooth muscle fibers of the internal sphincter.

The female urethra has a thick submucosal layer containing a rich venous plexus. Turgor within submucosa helps maintain continence and is sometimes referred to as the mucosal sphincter. The integrity of the mucosal sphincter is to some extent hormonally dependent. Atrophy and some decrease of closing urethral pressure may develop with age.

3. *Intra-abdominal pressure.* Unlike the male urethra (encircled by external sphincter), the female urethra is incompletely surrounded by striated muscle fibers of the pelvic floor.

That part of the female urethra above the urogenital diaphragm is affected by intra-abdominal pressure. A sudden rise in pressure, such as can occur while lifting a heavy object, is transmitted not only to the bladder, but also to the intra-abdominal portion of the urethra. This phenomenon of transmittal of intra-abdominal pressure on the urethra greatly contributes to continence. A corollary to this anatomical setup is an inflated balloon. No matter what magnitude of external pressure one places on the balloon, a miniscule amount of external pressure at the mouthpiece is needed to keep the balloon from deflating.

4. *Bladder neck competence.* Funneling of the bladder neck occurs: a) during bladder contraction (high bladder pressure), proximal urethral fibers are pulled apart; b) "poor anatomy," the proximal urethra is gaping open even without bladder contraction (low detrusor pressure) to pull it apart. Among other reasons, videourodynamic evaluation was developed to clarify bladder neck funneling, i.e., is it due to detrusor contraction or is it just "poor anatomy?"

5. *Normal bladder enervation and function.* Uninhibited bladder contractions such as seen in hyperreflexia (neurogenic bladder) or bladder instability may contribute to loss of urine.

SUMMARY

Contributing to continence are the functional external and internal sphincters, turgor of the urethral mucosa, adequate urethral length, high position of the urethra (so that it is subject to the beneficial influence of intra-abdominal pressure), "proper anatomy" of the bladder neck, and normal bladder function. Deficiency in one or several of these factors may lead to incontinence.

Stress Incontinence

Definition. Involuntary loss of urine during straining *without* detrusor contraction.[8]

Etiology. Weak pelvic floor muscles, mostly related to delivery trauma.

Mechanism

1. Urethra prolapses and is no longer under the beneficial influence of intra-abdominal pressure. A sudden increase in intra-abdominal pressure is transmitted to the bladder while there is no simultaneous corresponding counterbalancing pressure transmitted to the urethra.

2. Urethra is too short (Fig. 20–16).

3. Bladder neck (internal sphincter) is deficient.

4. Mucosal sphincter is atrophied.

5. Intrinsic smooth muscle sphincter is defective.

Clinical Presentation. Involuntary loss of urine during straining, such as lifting, climbing stairs, and laughing.

Treatment. Surgical suspension (Pereyra, Birch, Marshall-Marchety, Pereyra-modified by Raz, Stamey). All are designed to bring the urethra back into the abdomen and under the influence of intra-abdominal pressure.

Radiological Findings. Videourodynamic voiding cystourethrogram is the examination of choice. Incontinence is observed while simultaneous pressure

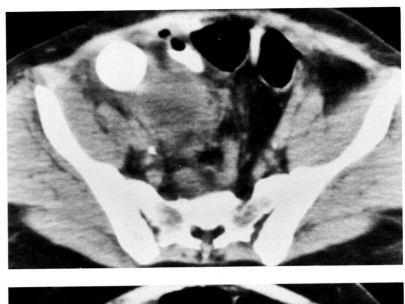

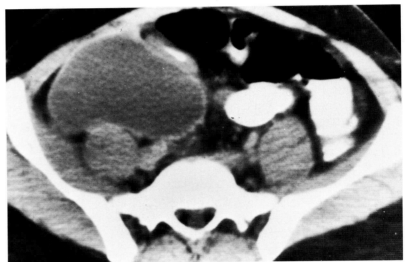

Figure 20–14. Extraperitoneal abscess originates around the reservoir **(A)** and extends cephalad **(B)**.

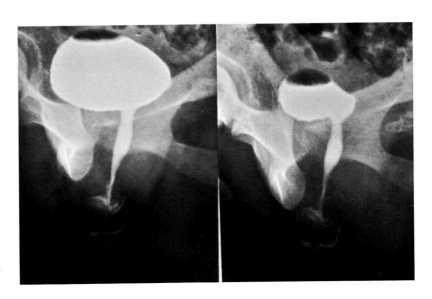

Figure 20–15. Normal female urethra. The urethra is high above urogenital diaphragm. During voiding the urethra is seldom uniformly distended.

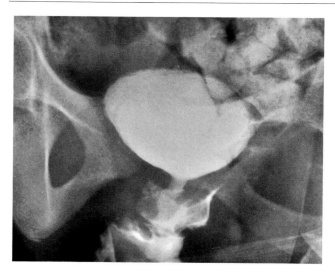

Figure 20–16. Short urethra.

recordings objectively demonstrate lack of detrusor contraction (Fig. 20–17).

In the lateral upright projection the urethra is seen prolapsed below the inferior margin of symphysis pubis. Because the more distal urethra is relatively firmly fixed to the pubic bone by the urethropubic ligament, the vertical urethral angle is greater than 35°. In fact, the prolapse may be so severe that the posterior urethra is pointing cephalad (Fig. 20–18). Odd as it sounds, outflow obstruction and stress incontinence may coincide (Fig. 20–19). Prolapse of the trigone also involves prolapse of the ureters, which may result in bilateral ureteral obstruction (Fig. 20–20A,B).

Radiological Findings after Suspension. A properly suspended urethra has almost vertical axis or even points backward (Fig. 20–21). Posterior urethra is now well above the inferior margin of the symphysis pubis, since it is brought back into the abdominal cavity. Oversuspension may cause outflow bladder obstruction. This may result in large postvoid residual urine, detrusor instability, and bladder trabeculation. At times, peculiar indentation at the bladder base is evident (Fig. 20–22).

Occasionally, bony changes are seen on top of the pubic ramus caused by suspension sutures (Fig. 20–23). Changes due to osteitis pubis are rarely present.

Urge Incontinence

Definition. Involuntary loss of urine without strain, *caused by idiopathic inappropriate detrusor contraction,* also referred to as bladder or detrusor *instability.* This entity is not to be confused with hyperreflexic bladder, a term reserved for bladder dysfunction associated with some types of neurogenic bladder dysfunction.

Incidence. Detrusor instability increases with age. Ten percent of women under the age of 50 years, and 30–40% of women above the age of 50 years are affected. The severity of urgency varies, however. The majority experiences only mild symptoms. In a few, symptoms are pronounced and incapacitating.

Clinical Presentation. Urgency and frequency. Sensation of urge is brought by uninhibited contrac-

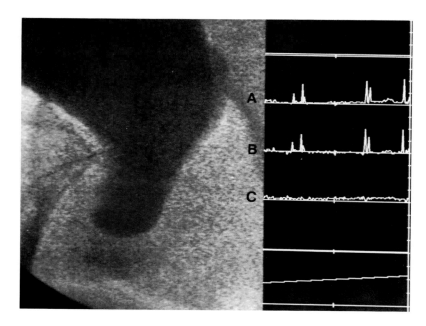

Figure 20–17. (A) Intravesical pressure and (B) intra-abdominal pressure show spikes due to coughing and straining during examination. (C) The curve representing detrusor pressure remained flat.

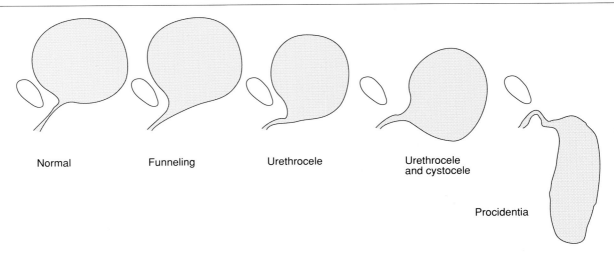

Figure 20–18. Schematic drawing of various stages of urethral prolapse in the lateral upright projection. In funneling there is loss of posterior urethrovesical angle. This finding may be associated with stress incontinence as well as with unstable bladder. As the urethra prolapses, the angle between the urethral axis and a vertical line becomes greater than the normal 35°. The prolapse may be associated with a cystocele. When there is significant bladder prolapse, the proximal urethra points cephalad.

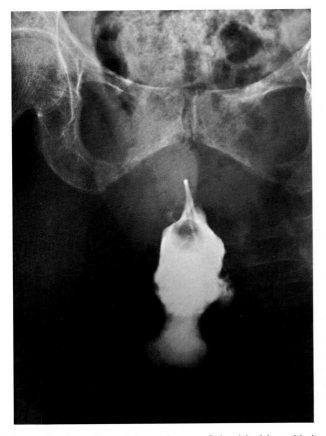

Figure 20–19. Complete prolapse of the bladder with incomplete emptying requiring catheter drainage.

tions, resulting in loss of urine. The triggering event may be exposure to cold or other stimuli.

Treatment. Medical therapy with bladder relaxants.

Radiological Findings. Videourodynamic voiding cystourethrogram is the examination of choice. Pressure recordings objectively demonstrate involuntary detrusor contraction occurring simultaneously with loss of urine. Involuntary contractions during bladder filling, which result in true detrusor pressure above 15 cm H_2O are diagnostic of *unstable bladder* (Fig. 20–2).

Bladders in patients with significant bladder instability may be recognized on simple voiding cystourethrogram because of their small capacity, somewhat trabeculated wall, and because of the patient's inability to interrupt micturition (Fig. 20–24).

Bladder instability may be caused by partial outflow obstruction. Under such circumstances some postvoid residual urine may be detected.

Variations

In some instances stress and urgency incontinence are present simultaneously, each requiring different treatment.

Many women with urethral prolapse are continent.

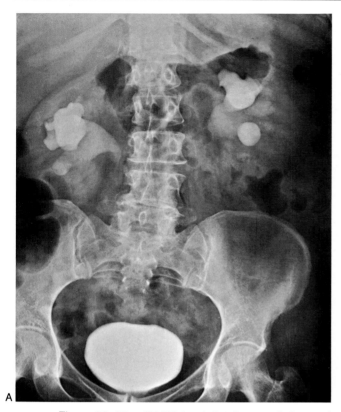 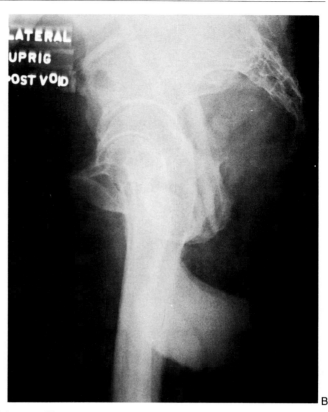

Figure 20–20. **(A)** Bilateral distal ureteral obstruction. This case illustrates the need for including the inferior pubic rami in the field of view. **(B)** Major prolapse is seen in the upright lateral projection. Ureters are seen inferior to the ischial tuberosity.

Some women with urethral prolapse may have urge rather than stress incontinence and do not require urethral suspension.

History of urinary frequency, although characteristic for urge incontinence, may also be obtained from patients with stress incontinence. Women with stress incontinence have learned that an empty bladder is less likely to leak and their frequent visits to the bathroom are preventive in nature.

Some women are still incontinent after surgical suspension.

Complications related to suspension surgery include loss of urethral compliance, total or partial outflow bladder obstruction, and periurethral abscess and fistulas.

OTHER CAUSES FOR URINARY INCONTINENCE

Fistulas

Vesicovaginal, ureterovaginal, ureterocutaneous, and vesicocutaneous fistulas may be encountered as causes of involuntary loss of urine (Fig. 20–25). Most fistulas are inadvertent surgical complications, usually a result of pelvic surgery (Figs. 20–26, 20–27). A fistula may also be the end result of an inflammatory or malignant process (Fig. 20–28). Constant dribbling or wetness is suggestive of diagnosis, particularly after recent surgery, difficult childbirth, or presence of an inflammatory or malignant disease. Otherwise, a congenital cause should be suspected.

Urethral Diverticulum in Females

Urethral diverticulum may be complicated by infection and induce bladder instability and a constant sense of urgency and dysuria (Fig. 20–29). Diverticula may be multicompartmental (Fig. 20–30). Large diverticula may retain urine, which may dribble slowly (Fig. 20–31). Most diverticula are located posterior to the mid-urethra and are probably a result of urethral trauma during vaginal delivery. Some contain stones (Fig. 20–32). More distal diverticula are probably abscessed Skene's glands. Most, if not all diverticula are identified on simple VCUG. Occlusive urethrogram using two balloons and a

Incontinence

| | Normal | Urgency | Stress | After suspension |

straining
LATERAL

relaxing
RPO

straining
RPO

voiding
RPO

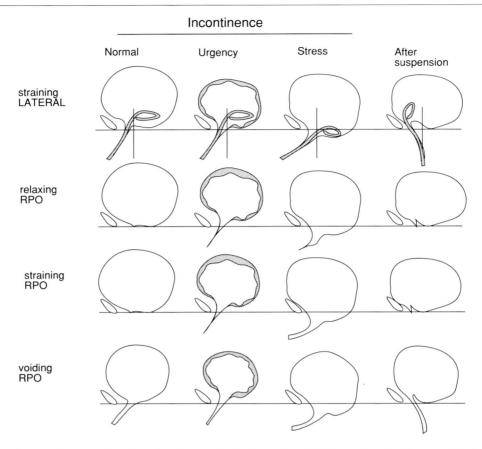

Figure 20–21.   Schematic drawing of radiographic findings in upright lateral and oblique projection in urge and stress incontinence compared with normal bladder. Note that funneling may be present in both stress and urge incontinence. Note also peculiar appearance of the urethra after suspension. If suspension is too high, patient may develop outflow bladder obstruction.

mid-urethral port is seldom necessary for diagnostic purposes.[9]

Congenital Causes of Incontinence

Congenital causes of incontinence include ectopic ureteral insertion into the urethra or vagina, bladder exstrophy, and congenital short urethra. Constant dribbling or wetness is also the principal finding.

Congenital Wide Bladder Neck Anomaly in Children

Bladder neck is opened at a time when there is no bladder contraction.[10,11] Wide bladder neck without any corresponding rise in detrusor pressure is seen during voiding urodynamic study. This is believed to be a true congenital anomaly. All patients have failure of normal "milk back" during interruption of

flow. Twenty-one percent of children with daytime incontinence may have this anomaly.[12]

Spinning Top Urethra

This is a term used to describe a wide posterior urethra seen mainly in girls on voiding cystourethrogram. Until recently, it was considered a normal variant.[13] Videourodynamic studies show, however, that spinning top urethra in children is almost always associated with unstable bladder or wide bladder neck anomaly (Fig. 20–33).[14] Involuntary uninhibited contractions raise bladder pressure. This increase in bladder pressure is resisted by a voluntary increase in distal urethral sphincter tension, allowing distention of the posterior urethra (spinning top urethra). If the patient also has wide bladder neck anomaly, the distention of the posterior urethra is maximal.

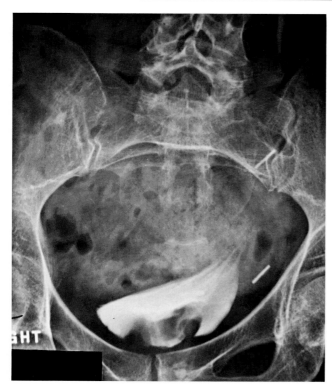

Figure 20–22. Indentation at the bladder base after Marshall-Marchety suspension and psoas hitch.

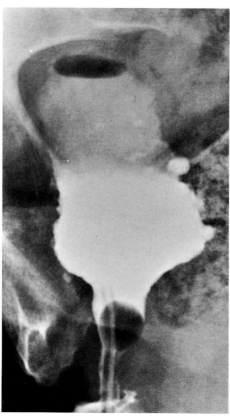

Figure 20–24. The end result of severe bladder instability for over 10 years. This patient had no neurological disorder or prior surgical procedures and had urge incontinence during this entire time. The bladder is small with thickened walls and small diverticula.

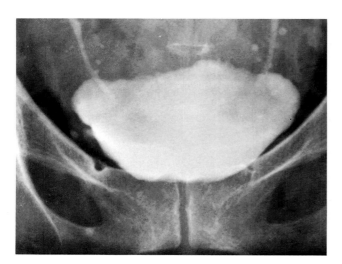

Figure 20–23. Notches in the superior rami of the symphysis pubis are due to suspension sutures that run from the anterior abdominal wall to endopelvic fascia. This is a transvaginal suspension introduced by Pereyra and unlike Marshall-Marchety does not require transperitoneal approach.

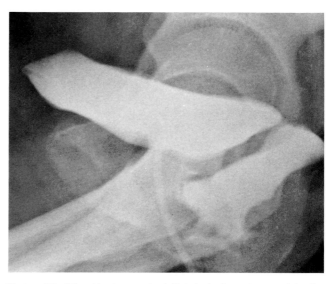

Figure 20–25. Vesicovaginal fistula is best imaged in the lateral projection. Catheter is in the bladder, which is anterior. Fistula is at the most dependent part of the bladder. Note the well-suspended urethra.

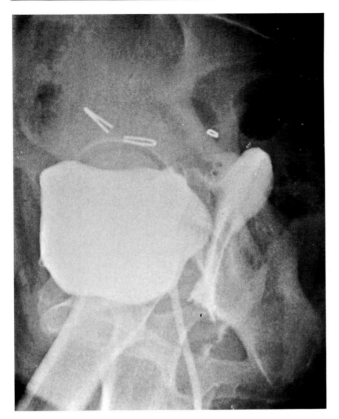

Figure 20–26.   Vesicovaginal fistula following pelvic surgery.

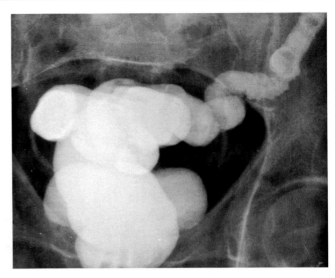

Figure 20–28.   Vesicorectal fistula.

Non-Neurogenic Neurogenic Bladder (The Hinman Syndrome)

Functional bladder disorder in neurologically normal children is characterized by failure to inhibit detrusor contraction and by overcompensation of the external sphincter. Urinary tract infection, reflux, trabeculated bladder, and hydronephrosis are common. Increased sphincter activity is present (electromyography) during unstable or normal bladder contraction.[15]

Diabetes Insipidus

Etiology.   Posterior pituitary insufficiency. Diminished production of antidiuretic hormone.

Nephrogenic diabetes insipidus. Deficiency of tubular cell antidiuretic hormone receptors.

Pathophysiology.   Massive water excretion may produce volume distention of the bladder, bladder instability, increased detrusor pressures, hydronephrosis, and, possibly, deterioration of renal function.

Clinical Presentation.   Polyuria and polydipsia. Symptoms due to bladder instability may be the initial finding. Circumstances may not allow frequent visits to the bathroom, such as in school. Urgency and frequency are common.

Radiological Findings.   Hydronephrosis and large trabeculated bladder are easily detected by any imaging modality. Changes typical for bladder instability

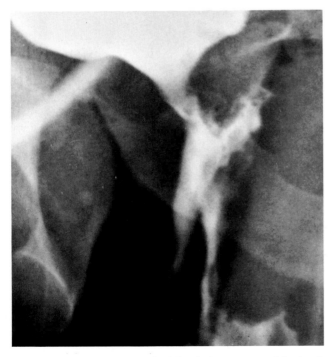

Figure 20–27.   Urethrovaginal fistula becomes evident only during voiding part of the study.

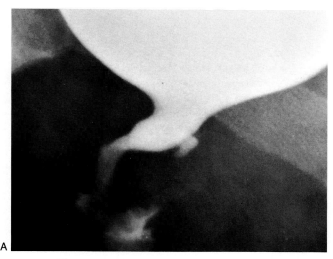 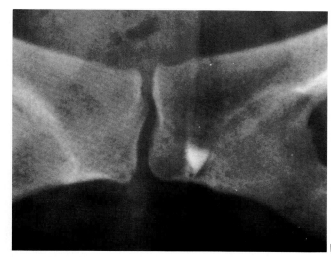

Figure 20–29. (A) Small symptomatic urethral diverticulum. (B) Contrast is retained within the diverticulum on the postvoid film.

are present on videourodynamic studies. Vesicoureteral reflux is common.

NEUROGENIC BLADDER

Hyperactive Detrusor

Synonyms. Hyperreflexic detrusor, reflex neurogenic bladder, upper motor neuron lesion bladder.

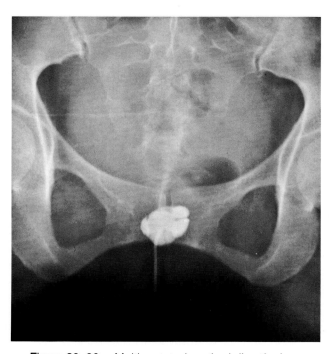

Figure 20–30. Multiseptated urethral diverticulum.

Definition. Functional bladder disorder caused by interruption in upper neural pathways and characterized by inappropriate, involuntary bladder contractions usually associated with sphincteric dysfunction.

Incidence. Most common and clinically most significant neuropathic bladder disorder.

Etiology. Brain tumor, cerebrovascular accident, brain abscess, multiple sclerosis, Parkinson's disease, spinal cord transection, spinal cord compression.

Clinical Presentation. If the offending neurologic lesion is above the pons, detrusor contraction and sphincter complex relaxation are usually coordinated. Uninhibited detrusor contractions are present and synchronous relaxation of the proximal smooth sphincter results in incontinence. Only if the sensation of urgency is preserved, may the patient be able to control sphincter function. There is usually no postvoid residual urine.

Complete or incomplete cord transection not only produces hyperreflexic detrusor, but there is also a lack of synergistic relaxation of striated muscle (external) sphincter. On the contrary, at the time of uninhibited detrusor contraction, an inappropriate contraction of the external sphincter occurs simultaneously, creating outflow obstruction and increase in intravesical pressure. This abnormal activity is commonly referred to as *detrusor-striated sphincter dyssynergia*. Working against resistance, the detrusor hypertrophies, eventually causing a trabeculated bladder. Incontinence ensues when during an uninhibited contraction high intravesical pressure over-

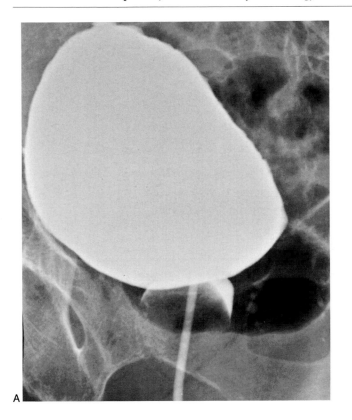

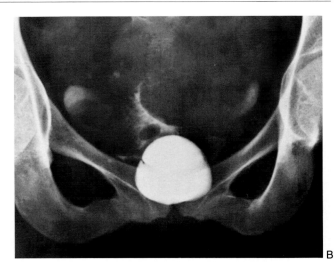

Figure 20–31A,B.   (A) Foley balloon catheter is inadvertently inflated within a large urethral diverticulum without consequence. (B) Retained contrast in the diverticulum on postvoid film. Some contrast is also present in the vagina where it outlines the cervix.

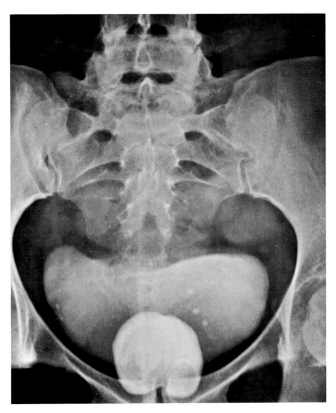

Figure 20–32.   Urethral diverticulum containing a large laminated stone.

comes sphincteric resistance. When the detrusor contraction is over, the sphincter resumes its normal tone, preventing further bladder emptying. Increase in postvoid residual urine is the result.

A spinal cord lesion above T12 may induce discordant activity of the sphincteric smooth muscle sphincter or *detrusor-smooth sphincter dyssynergia.* This event may occur either as an isolated finding or in combination with striated sphincter dyssynergia.

Although sphincter hyperactivity is most commonly expressed as an inappropriate contraction, it may occasionally result in an inappropriate relaxation, which, together with uninhibited bladder contraction, leads to incontinence.

Radiological and Videourodynamic Findings. Typically, the bladder is of small capacity, trabeculated, and frequently assumes a *Christmas tree* appearance on VCUG (Fig. 20–34) or urogram (Fig. 20–35). In patients who have coordinated sphincter activity, mostly those with suprapontine lesions, the bladder usually empties completely, as seen on the postvoid radiograph. Moderate postvoid residual implies sphincter dyssynergia, which usually implies that the lesion is below the pons. In some patients the progression of the disease from suprapontine to infrapontine areas may be suspected if there is a change from no residual to moderate residual.

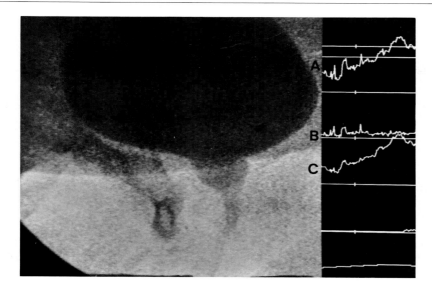

Figure 20-33. Videourodynamic evaluation in a patient with a classic "spinning top" urethra. **(A)** Intravesical pressure. **(B)** Abdominal pressure. **(C)** True detrusor pressure. Without a doubt there are inappropriate detrusor contractions.

Postvoid residual and high intravesical pressure are a setup for urinary tract infection and urolithiasis (Fig. 20-36). In general, renal function is below that of matched normal population.

Radiological and urodynamic evaluation are designed to appraise whether there is discordant activity (dyssynergia) between hyperactive detrusor contraction and sphincter complex.

VCUG. A major problem with VCUG is that after the bladder is filled with contrast, patients are usually unable to initiate voiding. Because the sensation of fullness is frequently absent, they are also unable to tell the examiner if there is a sense of urgency, i.e., an uninhibited hyperreflexic bladder contraction. Since it is detrusor contraction that initiates sphincteric activity, be it normal coordinated relaxation or inappropriate contraction, it is only during active voiding that fluoroscopy and spot filming of the sphincter complex should be performed to evaluate its function (Fig. 20-37). To be sure, there are tricks to trigger an uninhibited contraction, by extrinsic stimulation, for instance, but by and large this is relatively insufficient. Thus, a considerable amount of time may be spent in fluoroscopy, with rather unsatisfactory results and unnecessary radiation to the patient.

Functional Retrograde Urethrogram (RUG) in Males. This technique was proposed to circumvent technical difficulties associated with VCUG.[16] A small balloon catheter is placed in the fossa navicularis after being purged of air. Bladder is filled with contrast in increments with a 50 cc glass syringe. When uninhibited bladder contraction occurs and is of sufficient magnitude to overcome the sphincter, the plunger of the glass syringe is seen moving. It is at that moment the spot film is obtained, eliminating unnecessary fluoroscopy and assuring that sphincteric activity is captured on film. During the act of voiding, a coordinated sphincter will open while a dyssynergic external (or internal) sphincter will not. This method is

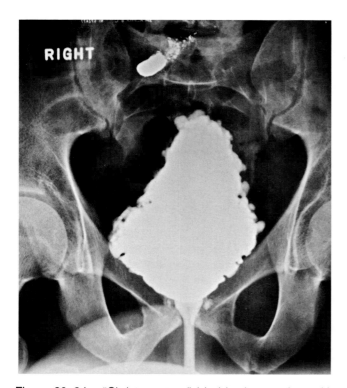

Figure 20-34. "Christmas tree" bladder in a patient with spinal cord transection. The outflow obstruction is most likely due to detrusor/external sphincter dyssynergia, since the proximal urethra is dilated.

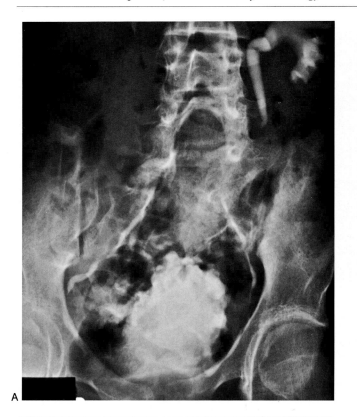

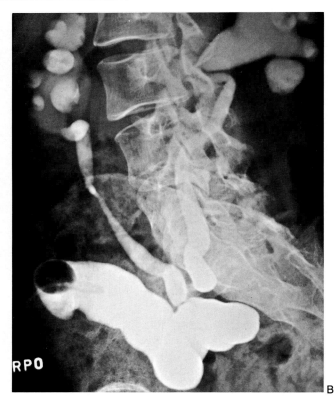

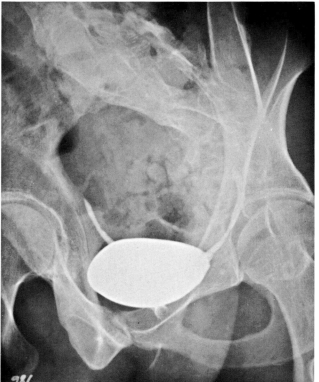

Figure 20–35. This case illustrates the detrimental effect of detrusor/sphincter dyssynergia on the bladder wall. **(A)** Typical trabeculated, thick wall bladder, almost Christmas tree in appearance in a patient with neurogenic bladder. **(B)** At the time, diversion was a common method for treatment of neurogenic bladder and an ileal loop diversion was created. **(C)** Some 10 years later, much was learned about management of neurogenic bladder and the patient was evaluated for possible undiversion. Cystogram shows complete lack of trabecular pattern after 10 years of inactivity.

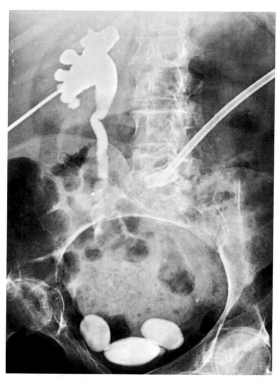

Figure 20–36. Bladder and ureteral calculi in a patient with multiple sclerosis and large postvoid residual urine. Nephrostomy tube is present on right, gastrostomy on left.

preferred over VCUG because it allows *controlled* functional assessment of sphincter action and morphological evaluation of the bladder (Fig. 20–38).

Transrectal Sonography. This technique may eliminate the need for fluoroscopy and radiography. Sphincter activity is observed using a rectal linear probe aimed at the bladder base, prostate, and external sphincter. The bladder is filled with a small catheter and simultaneous urodynamic evaluation is performed.[2,17–19] In addition, by using this technique, previously unsuspected findings, such as posterior ledge at the bladder neck,[20] and beneficial effect on striated sphincter by suprapubic tapping whereby striated sphincter becomes exhausted and thereafter relaxed, have been described (Fig. 20–39).[21]

Videourodynamic Evaluation. Videourodynamic VCUG integrates in one study imaging, dynamic pressure-flow measurements, and electromyography of the external sphincter. The sensation of fullness, true detrusor pressure during uninhibited contraction, electrical activity of the sphincter during uninhibited contraction, bladder compliance, visual confirmation of sphincter activity, and morphological appearance of the bladder are all evaluated in one session (Fig. 20–40).

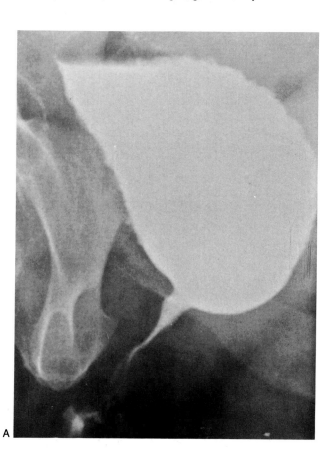

A

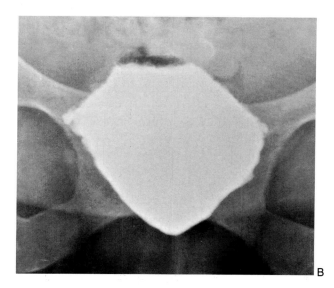

B

Figure 20–37. **(A)** Spot film obtained in the voiding phase demonstrates opened bladder neck and abnormally narrow distal urethra (compare with Fig. 20–14) in a patient with multiple sclerosis. **(B)** Large postvoid residual and trabeculated bladder are present.

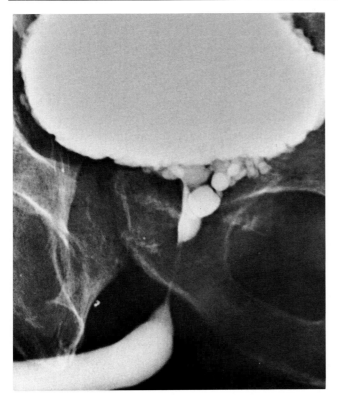

Figure 20–38. Functional RUG. Spot film is obtained during detrusor contraction. Both internal and external sphincter are narrow. There is reflux of contrast into dilated ejaculatory duct and seminal vesicle, implying chronic presence of high pressure in the proximal prostatic urethra.

Special Precautions. Vesicoureteral reflux is frequent in patients with hyperreflexic and areflexic bladders. Any retrograde examination should be terminated if reflux is observed (Fig. 20–41). None of the above studies should be performed in the presence of unchecked urinary tract infection.

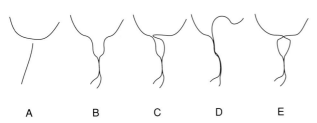

Figure 20–39. Midsagittal plane obtained with linear transrectal transducer. This drawing depicts expected findings regarding proximal urethra and sphincteric action. **(A)** Closed sphincter. **(B)** Detrusor/striated muscle dyssynergia. **(C)** Posterior ledge at the bladder neck. **(D)** BPH with prominent middle lobe. **(E)** Circumferential stricture at the bladder neck.

Detrusor Normoflexia Associated with Sphincter Dysfunction

Definition. Functional sphincteric disorder caused by sympathetic or pudendal nerve interruption.

Incidence. The rarest of neuropathic bladder-sphincter disorders.

Etiology. Bilateral sympathectomy at L2 and retroperitoneal lymphadenectomy may sever sympathetic supply to intrinsic smooth muscle sphincter.

Pudendal nerve disruption and lesions in the spine at the S2, S3, and S4 level interrupt enervation of the striated muscles to the external sphincter.

Clinical Presentation. Isolated dysfunction of the sphincteric mechanism is usually clinically silent or may result in retrograde ejaculation. Outflow bladder obstruction due to hyperactive sphincter without bladder dysfunction is likewise rare.

Areflexic and Hyporeflexic Detrusor

Definition. A functional bladder disorder caused by interruption in lower motor or sensory neural pathways and characterized by absence of bladder contractions. There is associated sphincteric dysfunction.

Incidence. Second most common neuropathic bladder disorder.

Etiology. Diabetes mellitus, disc herniation, multiple sclerosis, syringomyelia, tabes dorsalis, and pernicious anemia result in sensory denervation by affecting the pathways in the posterior spinal column and produce *sensory paralytic bladder.*

Radical pelvic surgery, major trauma, disc herniation, and conus tumor may result in *motor paralytic bladder.*

More commonly, both sensory and lower motor pathways are involved, resulting in *autonomous bladder.*

Clinical Presentation. Sensation of bladder fullness is usually lacking. Over time, due to infrequent emptying, the bladder becomes chronically overdistended, atonic, and of large capacity.

When motor nerves are severed or damaged, the voiding reflex is interrupted. These patients are able to sense bladder fullness, but are unable to initiate micturition.

Although most bladders with interrupted lower motor pathways are large, not all are atonic. Some postganglionic parasympathetic fibers are still func-

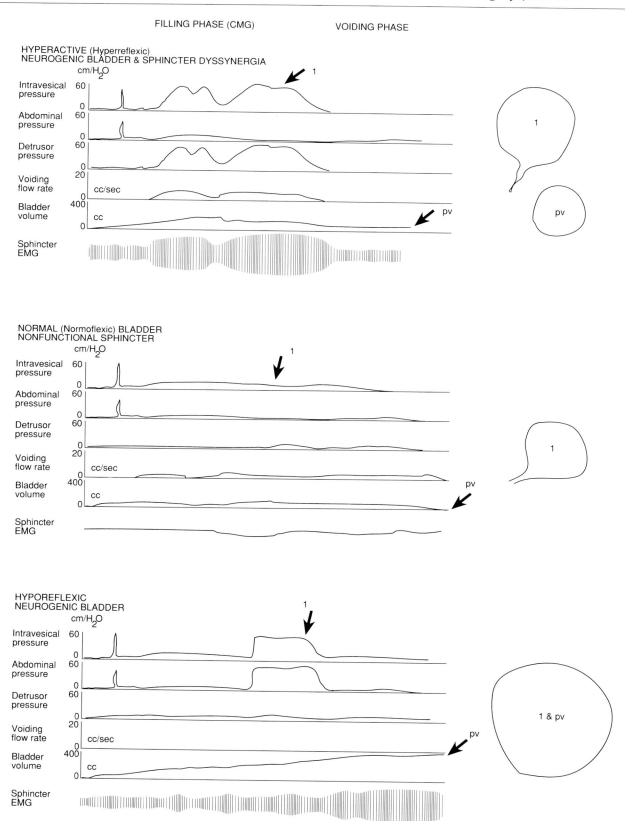

Figure 20–40. Schematic presentation of expected urodynamic findings during voiding associated with hyperreflexic, normoflexic bladder with nonfunctional sphincter, and hyporeflexic bladder. Sphincteric dyssynergia is evident as increased sphincter activity on EMG during uninhibited detrusor contraction.

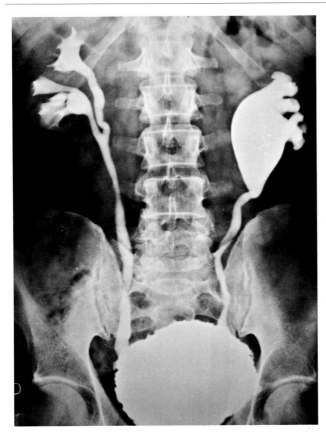

Figure 20–41. VCUG in a patient with neurogenic bladder. There is gross vesicoureteral reflux and the bladder is heavily trabeculated.

tional and considerable bladder tonicity may still be present in some cases.

If sphincteric enervation is preserved, excessively high intravesical pressures may develop. This is because the normally enervated sphincters cannot relax without an initiating concurrent bladder contraction.

Occasionally, sympathetic enervation of the smooth muscle sphincter is intact while the striated sphincter is denervated. Continence is maintained by the internal smooth muscle sphincter only. High intravesical pressures do not develop since the smooth muscle resistance is easy to overcome.

If both sphincters are denervated by the same mechanism as the bladder, little resistance to the outflow is provided. Such incompetent urethra results in continuous incontinence.

Radiological and Videourodynamic Findings. Most patients with coordinated sphincteric mechanism have a large bladder, large postvoid residual, and usually empty the bladder by means of overflow incontinence. Since there is no detrusor contraction to initiate sphincter relaxation, there is no other method of bladder emptying.

VCUG may demonstrate competent sphincter mechanism in patients with intact enervation. Again, these patients also have difficulty in initiating voiding and one could spend hours observing the moment of overflow incontinence under fluoroscopic control.

Patients with altered enervation to the sphincter complex have an incompetent, wide-open urethra. There is leaking around the catheter during the filling phase.

Vesicoureteral reflux in these patients is as common as in patients with hyperreflexic bladder.

Urodynamic evaluation usually demonstrates low detrusor pressure with discordant sphincter activity (Fig. 20–40).

AUTONOMIC DYSREFLEXIA

Etiology. Autonomic dysreflexia is a pathologic autonomic reflex that occurs only in patients with spinal cord lesion above T7. Triggering mechanism is distention of the bladder, urethra, or rectum and may also be induced by angiography.[22,23]

Clinical Presentation. Subjective symptoms are sudden onset of severe headache, flushing of the face and neck, and difficulty in breathing caused by mucosal swelling of the nasal passages. The severity and type of symptoms may vary. Bradycardia and markedly elevated systolic and diastolic blood pressure are present. Face and neck are red and flushed. The lower torso and legs are pale and cold.

Pathophysiology. Distention of the bladder (such as during cystography) or other viscera trigger the reflex, which is transmitted via spinothalamic tracts and dorsal column. The impulses excite the sympathetic neurons of the interomedial lateral horns, which results in vasoconstriction of the splanchnic vascular bed, kidney, skin, and legs. The net result is dramatic elevation of blood pressure.

Response of a Normal Individual. The normal individual regulates blood pressure rise via baroceptors in the carotid sinus and aortic wall, which send informative messages to the medulla. Inhibitory impulses are generated from vasomotor center in the medulla which slow the heart rate and dilate splanchnic and skin vessels, and thereby effectively balance the sympathetic excitation caused by bladder distention.

Response of a Patient with a Cord Lesion Above T7. In the patient with a high cord lesion (e.g., transection), the inhibitory impulses from the vasomotor center cannot reach the splanchnic circulation so that sympathetic excitation and vasoconstriction in the abdominal viscera, lower torso, and extremities continue uncontrolled. Legs remain pale and cold while hypertension continues.

The inhibitory impulses from the vasomotor center reach their target in the upper part of the body and cause vasodilatation in the head and neck, inducing flushed face, stuffy nose, and perspiration in this area. This response, however, is insufficient to control marked hypertension.

For vasomotor center, the only alternative left to control elevated blood pressure is to decrease the heart rate via the vagus. It is this reflex that induces bradycardia. Still, decreased heart rate only minimally decreases blood pressure.

In addition, there are increased levels of epinephrine and norepinephrine in the blood, suggesting stimulation of the adrenal glands.

Severity. The severity of dysreflexia is unpredictable. In general, the higher the lesion the more pronounced the symptoms. In some patients it may manifest itself with the most severe symptoms on one occasion and be absent on other occasions. The patient should be questioned regarding symptoms, blood pressure, and pulse rate monitored during examinations such as cystography, voiding cystourethrography, rectal ultrasound, barium enema, or angiography.

Treatment. Dangerously high blood pressure may cause retinal or cerebral hemorrhage. The bladder should be emptied immediately. If symptoms persist, 5–10 cc of 1% lidocaine hydrochloride (Xylocaine, Astra) may be introduced into the bladder, thereby breaking the afferent limb of the dysreflexia.

REFERENCES

1. Perkash I, Friedland GW. Principles of modern urodynamic studies. Invest Radiol 1987; 22:279–289.
2. Shabsigh R, Fishman TJ, Krebs M. Combined transrectal sonography and urodynamics in the evaluation of detrusor-sphincter dyssynergia. Br J Urol 1988; 62:326–330.
3. Wein AJ. Classification of voiding dysfunction. Am Urol Assoc Update Series 1986; 6:1–8.
4. Wein AJ. Overview of voiding function and dysfunction: relevant anatomy, physiology, pharmacology, classification, definitions. In: Clinical Urography (Pollack HM, ed). Philadelphia: Saunders, 1990. Sec 8: 1926–1934.
5. Siegel SW. History of the prosthetic treatment of urinary incontinence. Urol Clin North Am 1989; 16:99–104.
6. Scott FB. The artificial urinary sphincter. Experience in adults. Urol Clin North Am 1989; 16:105–117.
7. Rose SC, Hansen ME, Webster GD, et al. Artificial urinary sphincters: plain radiography of malfunction and complications. Radiology 1988; 168:403–408.
8. Blaivas JG, Olsson CA. Stress incontinence: classification and surgical approach. J Urol 1988; 139:727–730.
9. Greenberg M, Stone D, Cochran ST, et al. Female urethral diverticula: double balloon catheter study. AJR 1981; 136:259–264.
10. Stanton L, Williams DI. Wide bladder neck in children. Br J Urol 1973; 45:60–64.
11. Murray K, Nurse D, Borzykowski M, Mundy AR. The "congenital" wide bladder neck anomaly: a common cause of incontinence in children. Br J Urol 1987; 59:533–535.
12. Borzykowski M, Mundy AR. Video urodynamic assessment of diurnal urinary incontinence. Arch Dis Child 1987; 62:128–131.
13. Shophner CE, Hutch JA. The normal urethrogram. Radiol Clin North Am 1968; 6:165–189.
14. Saxton HM, Borzykowski M, Mundy AR, Vivian GC. Spinning top urethra: not a normal variant. Radiology 1988; 168:147–150.
15. Hinman F Jr. Non-neurogenic neurogenic bladder (the Hinman syndrome)—15 years later. J Urol 1986; 136:769–777.
16. McCallum RW. The radiological assessment of the lower urinary tract in paraplegics—a new method. J Can Assoc Radiol 1974; 25:34–38.
17. Shapeero LG, Friedland GW, Perkash I. Transrectal sonographic voiding cystourethrography. Studies in neuromuscular bladder dysfunction. AJR 1983; 141: 83–90.
18. Shabsigh R, Fishman TJ, Krebs M. The use of transrectal longitudinal real-time ultrasonography in urodynamics. J Urol 1987; 138:1416–1419.
19. Perkash I, Friedland GW. Catheter induced hyperreflexia in spinal cord injury patients. Diagnosis by sonographic voiding cystourethrography. Radiology 1986; 159:453–455.
20. Perkash I, Friedland GW. Posterior ledge at the bladder neck: the crucial diagnostic role of ultrasonography. Urol Radiol 1986; 8:175–183.
21. Perkash I, Friedland GW. Using transrectal sonography to teach patients with spinal cord injuries to retrain their bladders. Radiology 1984; 152:228–229.
22. Barbaric ZL. Autonomic dysreflexia in patients with spinal cord lesions: Complication of voiding cystourethrography and ileal loopography. Am J Roentgenol 1976; 127:293–295.
23. Black J. Autonomic dysreflexia/hyperreflexia in spinal cord injury. AUAA J, 1988; 8:12.

ADDITIONAL READING

1. Yalla SV, McGuire EJ, Elbadawi A, Blaivas JG (eds). Neurourology and Urodynamics: Principles and Practice. New York: Macmillan, 1988.
2. Wein AJ, Barett DM. Voiding Function and Dysfunction: A Logical and Practical Approach. Chicago: Year Book Medical Publishers, 1988.
3. Urol Clin North Am 1985; 12.
4. Pollack HM ed. Clinical Urography. Philadelphia: Saunders, 1990. Sec 8: 1926–2075.

21

Prostate

ANATOMY

The prostate gland is chestnut-sized, surrounded by a capsule, with apex pointing inferiorly. Anteriorly, there is a retropubic space that contains fat as well as the ramified plexus from the dorsal vein of the penis. This area is very richly vascularized and is frequently a site of intraoperative bleeding.

Traditionally, the prostate has been grossly subdivided into four lobes (median, anterior, and two lateral).

Prostatic urethra is divided into proximal and distal at the verumontanum. These two segments form a 145° angle. *Periurethral glands* surround the proximal prostatic urethra and drain directly into it. Smooth muscular sphincter surrounds both segments of the prostatic urethra and periurethral glands. Striated muscle gradually appears in the distal prostatic urethra and eventually blends with the external sphincter.

The prostate is composed of one nonglandular and three different glandular regions, which are referred to as zones.[1-3] The largest is the *peripheral zone,* which contains 70% of all glandular tissues, followed by the *central zone* with 25%, and the *transition zone* with 5%. Anteriorly, a nonglandular region contains fibromuscular stroma (Fig. 21–1).

There is a natural anatomic weakness of the capsule at the point of entrance of the seminal vesicles

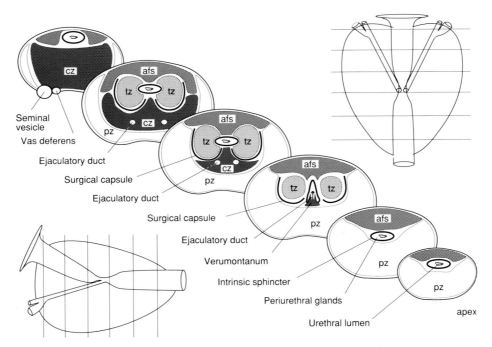

Seminal vesicle
Vas deferens
Ejaculatory duct
Surgical capsule
Ejaculatory duct
Surgical capsule
Ejaculatory duct
Verumontanum
Intrinsic sphincter
Periurethral glands
Urethral lumen
apex

Figure 21–1. Zonal anatomy of the prostate. pz: peripheral zone; cz: central zone; tz: transition zone; afs: anterior fibromuscular stroma.

and vas deferens.[1] As ejaculatory ducts are formed, they transverse the central zone and empty into the verumontanum.

Most prostatic carcinomas originate within the peripheral zone, while benign prostatic hypertrophy has its origins from the periurethral glands. Peripheral and central zones are separated from the transition zone by the *surgical capsule,* which prevents tumor spread. No such capsule exists between peripheral and central zones; only a thin band of connective tissues separates them.

On T1-weighted sequences, the entire prostate is of uniform medium signal intensity and the zonal anatomy cannot be appreciated. On T2-weighted sequences, the outer peripheral zone exhibits high signal intensity (bright), while the central zone is of medium to low signal intensity (dark gray) (Fig. 21–2).[4,5]

Seminal vesicles are usually symmetrical, fluid filled, and of high signal intensity (bright) on T2-weighted sequences.

Transrectal ultrasonography (TRUS) is well suited for examination of the prostate, at least for directing the biopsy needle in the suspicious area. Either transverse (Fig. 21–3) or sagittal images are obtained, depending on probe. On sonography, the central zone is usually more echogenic compared with the peripheral zone. This is ascribed to larger and more reflective glands found in the central zone.

ACUTE PROSTATITIS AND PROSTATIC ABSCESS

Etiology. *E. coli, Proteus, Klebsiella, Enterobacter,* enterococci, *Mycobacterium tuberculosis, Neisseria gonorrhoeae.*

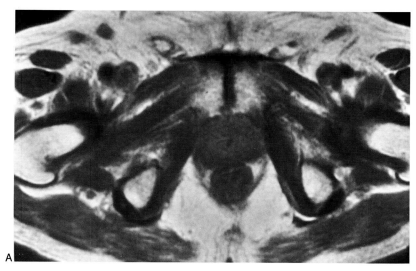

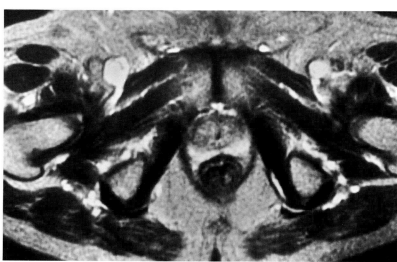

Figure 21–2. T1- **(A)** and T2-weighted **(B)** sequences show marked change in signal intensities from the peripheral zone.

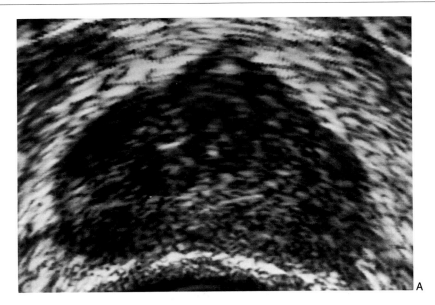

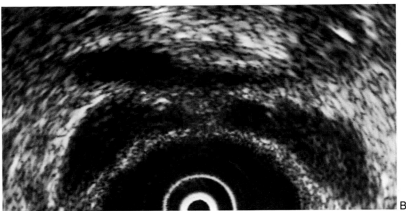

Figure 21–3. Transverse TRUS of the prostate **(A)** and seminal vesicles **(B)**.

Pathology. Acute suppurative process, prostatic abscesses, septicemia.

Clinical Presentation. Fever, back pain, perineal pain, frequency, urgency, dysuria, outflow bladder obstruction. The diagnosis is usually obvious on physical examination.

Laboratory Findings. Urine and prostatic fluid smear and culture positive for offending organism, leukocytosis.

Radiological Findings. Prostate may be enlarged on any of the radiographic examinations. Prostatic abscess may be identified as a hypoechoic area on transrectal sonography.[6] On CT and MR imaging, the abscess may be seen as a radiolucent or dark (low signal) lesion on T1-weighted image and bright (high signal) compared with the normal prostatic tissue on T2-weighted sequence (Fig. 21–4).[7,8] Drained or ruptured abscess may leave a permanent cavity (see Fig.

22–23). Imaging is usually unnecessary, since the diagnosis is clear on physical examination.

CHRONIC PROSTATITIS

Incidence. Common infection of middle-aged men.

Etiology. *E. coli, Proteus, Klebsiella, Enterobacter,* enterococci, *Mycobacterium tuberculosis, Neisseria gonorrhoeae.*

Clinical Presentation. Pain, dysuria, urgency, frequency, outflow obstruction.

Laboratory Findings. Tenfold increase in number of colonies from expressed prostatic secretions (prostatic massage) compared to voided urine.

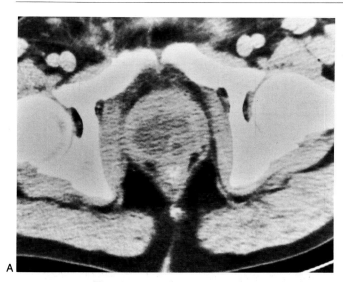
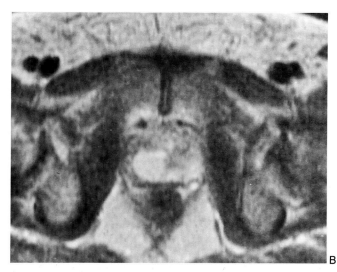

Figure 21–4. Acute prostatic abscess seen on CT **(A)** and T2-weighted **(B)** spin echo sequence.

Radiological Findings. Radiographic findings in this common disease are nonspecific.[9,10] Concomitant benign prostatic hypertrophy may be present. Prostatic calcifications may be seen more frequently.

PROSTATIC CALCIFICATIONS

Prostatic calcifications are a common finding on imaging studies of the pelvis and abdomen. These are small calculospherules within the prostatic ductules. On urethroscopic examination, prostatic calculi are seen as tiny black dots in the region of the prostatic urethra. Increase in the number is seen in chronic prostatitis and granulomatous prostatitis. Mostly, however, prostatic calcifications are clinically silent and an insignificant finding. As expected, they are the most visible on CT scan because of excellent contrast differentiation of this modality.

On rectal ultrasound, as with any other calcification, marked echogenicity and acoustical shadowing will be present.

Calcification never develops within a benign prostatic adenoma but is rather displaced posteriorly by the enlarging mass.

BENIGN PROSTATIC HYPERTROPHY

Incidence. Rare before 50 years of age. Between the ages of 60 and 70, 60% have benign prostatic hypertrophy (BPH). Above the age of 80, 80% have the disease. Fifteen to 20% develop obstructive symp-

toms and require intervention. In the United States, 500,000 transurethral prostatectomies are performed annually for this disease.

Pathology. Hyperplasia of the glandular tissues in the transition zone or periurethral glands. Proliferation of periductal, periacinar, and periurethral stroma involving both connective tissue and smooth muscle fibers. Hyperplastic glandular growth also occurs. Large portions of the lateral lobes, median lobe, or subcervical glands of Albarran may be enlarged alone or in any combination.

Clinical Presentation. Nocturia, frequency, decreased stream, hematuria. Outflow bladder obstruction may result in hydronephrosis and diminished renal function. Anuria and massive bladder enlargement are possible if significant outflow obstruction is present.

Treatment. Expectant, transurethral prostatectomy (TURP), suprapubic and retropubic prostatectomy, transurethral balloon dilatation. Evaluation of oral drugs, hyperthermia, and sclerotherapy is ongoing.

Radiological Findings. There are two principal reasons to subject the patient with suspected BPH to imaging procedures. One is to determine the amount of postvoid residual and the second is to evaluate other parts of the urinary tract system when symptoms are unclear or may be associated with other diseases (hematuria, for example). On occasion, it is useful to determine the true size of the prostate in absolute number values either for treatment response assessment or deciding on surgical approach.

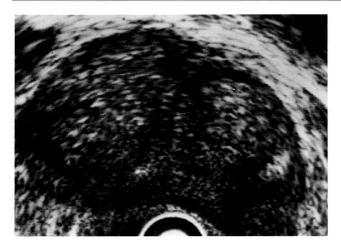

Figure 21–5. TRUS showing BPH. The enlargement involves periurethral glands and transitional zone.

Sonography. Transrectal ultrasound most accurately determines prostatic size (Fig. 21–5). Suprapubic sonography most easily and cheaply determines postvoid residual (Fig. 21–6).

Urogram, VCUG, and RUG. Prostatic enlargement is evident if there is "J" hooking of the ureter as the trigone is displaced cephalad (Fig. 21–7, 21–8). Impression upon the bladder base is associated with moderate enlargements and is generally easier to detect on oblique projections. The extent of an adenoma may be at times clarified on RUG (Fig. 21–9).

CT and MR Imaging. On MR imaging, the ratio between hyperintense peripheral zone and inner zone changes with age. BPH cannot be reliably differentiated from prostatic carcinoma.[11] CT demonstrates globally enlarged prostate (Fig. 21–10).

Enlarged median lobe expands into the bladder and is seen as a "filling defect" originating at the bladder base (Fig. 21–11).

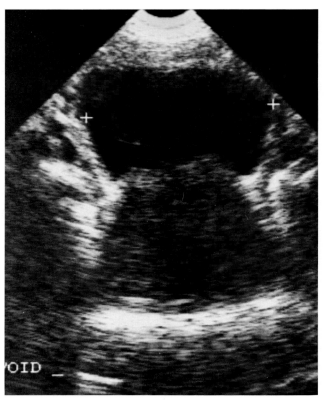

Figure 21–6. Prostatic enlargement seen on suprapubic scan. Bladder serves as an acoustical window.

Transurethral Dilatation of the Prostate

After urethrography for localization purposes, the balloon-carrying catheter is introduced into the urethra and the balloon is positioned in the prostatic urethra. Care is taken to position the balloon above the membranous urethra so that the external sphincter is not dilated. The balloon is inflated to 2 cm in diameter. Forceful distention of unyielding adenomatous tissues ruptures the prostatic capsule. The

Figure 21–7. Left: "J" hooking of the distal ureters seen during an excretory urogram. Only the most dependent part of the bladder (patient supine) is filled. Right: Postvoid radiograph from the same study. Contrast is now admixed with urine and the entire lumen is visualized. There is obvious postvoid residual. Trabeculated bladder wall and diverticula are seen.

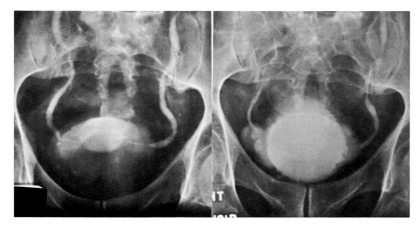

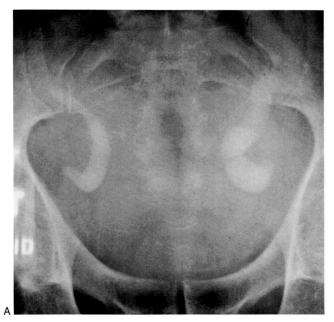
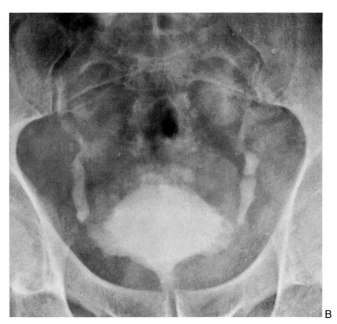

A   B

Figure 21–8. **(A)** Distal ureteral segments may assume unusual reverse "J" hooking in BPH. **(B)** After transurethral prostatectomy (TURP), the ureters assume more normal appearance. Just below the bladder base, contrast fills the area of the cavity created by TURP.

combination of capsular rupture and compression results in improved stream at least for the short term.[12] Long-term results are still unknown. The procedure is painful but can be performed under sedation and analgesia. Moderate postprocedural urethral bleeding is the rule and is controlled with a Foley catheter.

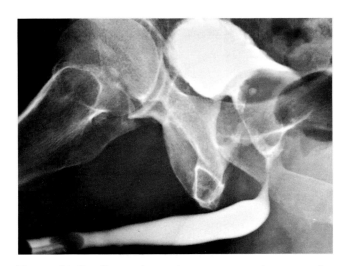

Figure 21–9. Regrowing adenoma several years after TURP. A "filling" defect is seen in the posterior urethra.

PROSTATIC CYST

Etiology. Unknown.

Clinical Presentation. Usually asymptomatic. May cause urinary retention.

Radiological Findings. Most cysts are detected on cross-sectional imaging. On ultrasound, there should be no internal echoes, the walls are sharp, and there is through transmission.[13] On CT, the attenuation value is between 0 and 20 HU. On MR imaging, simple cysts are of low signal intensity on T1-weighted sequences and of high signal intensity on T2-weighted sequences.

CARCINOMA OF THE PROSTATE

Incidence. Thirty percent of men over 50 years of age have foci of adenocarcinoma within the prostate and 28,000 die from prostatic carcinoma annually with 96,000 new cases discovered each year. Prostatic carcinoma is the second most common malignancy and the third most common cause of cancer death in American men.

Pathology. Adenocarcinoma. Origins: peripheral zone, 70%; transition zone, 20%; central zone, 10%.

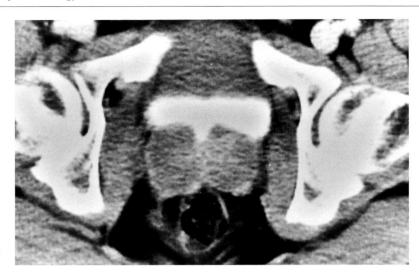

Figure 21–10. BPH appearance on CT.

Locally, the tumor may penetrate the capsule, invade the seminal vesicle, urethra, bladder, ureter, and rectum. Distant metastases to bone, lymph nodes, lungs, spine (via Batson's plexus), ureter.

Clinical Presentation. Asymptomatic in early stages. Later symptoms depend on the extent of the disease. Hematuria, ureteral obstruction, outflow bladder obstruction, bone pain, hematospermia, weight loss, CNS symptoms if metastases are present. Many carcinomas are latent and well differentiated.

Laboratory Findings. Prostate-specific antigen (PSA) is present in serum of men with normal or malignant prostatic tissues. Following prostatectomy, PSA should be at the female serum level. Presence of PSA after radical prostatectomy implies recurrence of prostatic carcinoma. Somewhat elevated serum levels may be found in patients with benign prostatic hypertrophy, prostatic carcinoma, prostatic biopsy, prostatitis, urinary retention, etc.[14]

Treatment. Controversial. Some studies show no difference in survival between placebo and surgically treated groups. Others show radiation therapy to produce similar results to radical prostatectomy for tumors confined to the prostate (stages A and B).[15] Staging is therefore one of the most important tasks of imaging (Fig. 21–12).

Radiological Findings

Transrectal Ultrasound (TRUS). Two different types of transrectal probes have been developed. The radial probe demonstrates prostate and seminal vesicles in an axial plane, while the linear transrectal probe demonstrates prostate and seminal vesicles in the sagittal or oblique sagittal projections.

Prostatic carcinoma is most commonly seen as a hypoechoic lesion compared with the echo texture of the surrounding normal prostatic tissues (Fig. 21–13).[16–18] However, the tumor may be isoechoic, hyperechoic, or even of mixed echogenicity compared with the normal prostate (Fig. 21–14). The reason for this varied appearance is believed to be stromal fibrosis, which may vary in different tumors. Also,

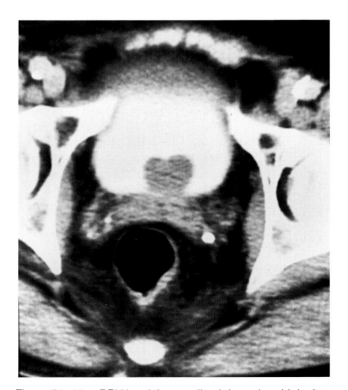

Figure 21–11. BPH involving median lobe only, which characteristically expands into the bladder.

TNM STAGING

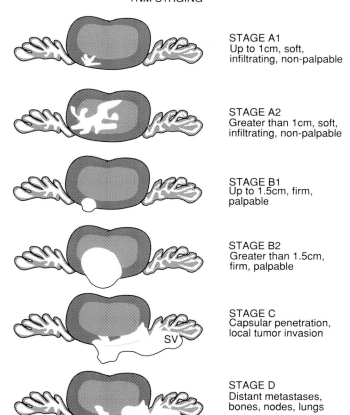

STAGE A1
Up to 1cm, soft,
infiltrating, non-palpable

STAGE A2
Greater than 1cm, soft,
infiltrating, non-palpable

STAGE B1
Up to 1.5cm, firm,
palpable

STAGE B2
Greater than 1.5cm,
firm, palpable

STAGE C
Capsular penetration,
local tumor invasion

SV

STAGE D
Distant metastases,
bones, nodes, lungs

Figure 21–12. Schematic drawing of the staging system for carcinoma of the prostate.

lower grade and less uniform tumors tend to appear hyperechoic, possibly because of increased tissue interfaces. The implication, of course, is that iso-echoic lesions may be missed unless there is distortion of the prostatic contour. Other benign diseases such as infarct, inflammation, and benign prostatic hyperplasia may present as hyperechoic, hypo-echoic, and mixed nodular lesions.

Specificity and sensitivity of this examination are well above 80% for evaluating local extension,[19] although not as impressive in other series.[20] Biopsy of the suspected nodules either by a skinny needle or a

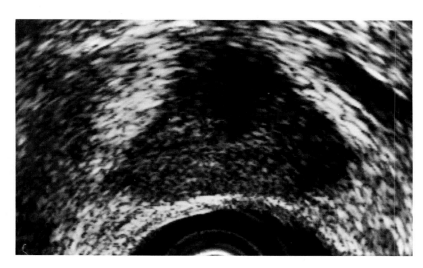

Figure 21–13. Hypoechoic 1 cm area in left lateral section of the posterior zone.

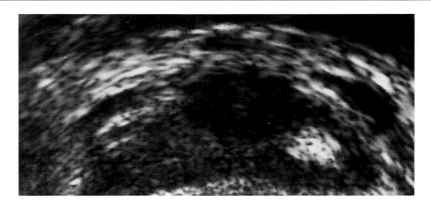

Figure 21–14.   Hyperechoic lesion on the left.

larger prostatic biopsy needle, as well as the aspiration of seminal vesicles with the guidance of the transrectal probe is fairly simple.[21]

CT. Diagnosis of prostatic carcinoma on CT is made by judging the size, abnormalities in contour, difference in attenuation values, symmetrical appearance of the seminal vesicles and their enlargement, calcification within the prostate, and detection of enlarged lymph nodes or bony metastases. Although CT appears to be a much better staging modality than physical examination, it has significant deficiencies. Changes in contour, for instance, are usually seen only in the advanced stages of disease, while in early stages the tumor may be imperceptible. Invasion or breakthrough of the capsule is very difficult to detect unless it is gross (Fig. 21–15, 21–16, 21–17). Likewise, invasion of the seminal

vesicle must be significant before it is detectable. Since the only criterion for lymph node metastases is lymph node enlargement, a significant number of metastases are missed. Furthermore, CT is ill-suited for separating prostatic carcinoma from BPH.

MR Imaging. Appearance of prostatic carcinoma depends on the strength of the magnetic field. In high field magnets the peripheral zone (where 70% of carcinomas originate) is of high signal intensity (bright). The tumor is of somewhat lower signal intensity and may be identified as a gray area within the bright peripheral zone (Fig. 21–18).

In low field magnets the signal intensity of the tumor is greater than the peripheral zone. The tumor is of high signal within medium signal peripheral zone.[22,23]

The detection and local staging of carcinoma of the

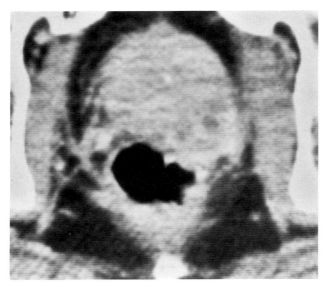

Figure 21–15.   CT of prostatic carcinoma that originates in the left posterior zone and has extended through the capsule. Fat plane in that area is obliterated.

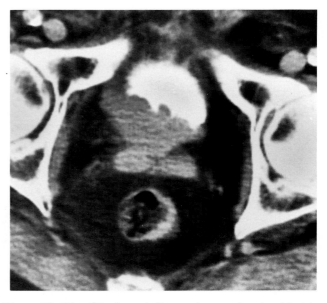

Figure 21–16.   CT of prostatic carcinoma showing bladder invasion.

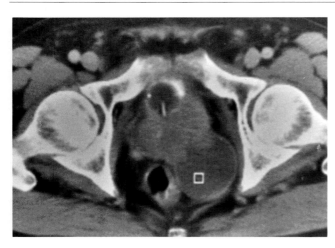

Figure 21–17. Unusual cystic component associated with prostatic carcinoma involving much of the prostate and causing bladder outflow obstruction.

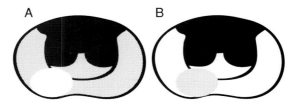

Figure 21–18. Schematic drawing of carcinoma of the prostate as it may appear on T2-weighted sequences in low field (**A**) and high field magnet (**B**).

prostate may be greatly improved by the use of an inflatable intrarectal surface coil.[24,25]

Metastases

Lymph Nodes. Metastases to the regional lymph nodes are difficult to detect by any imaging modality (Fig. 21–19). By CT criteria, a lymph node is considered normal if less than 1 cm in its longest axis (Fig. 21–20). Up to 1.5 cm is a gray indeterminate area, and above that it is definitely abnormal. Needless to say, many metastatic lymph nodes will be normal in size either on CT or MR imaging. A surprisingly high incidence of malignancy was found at random transperitoneal thin needle biopsy of normal-appearing lymph nodes as determined by lymphangiography.[26] In clinical (physical examination)

stage A 5 to 25% of the nodes may already be metastatic. These numbers are higher for clinical stages B (8–45%), C (40–80%), and D (100%). It is no wonder that radical prostatectomy is preceded by radical lymph node dissection and microscopic examination.

The particular value of cross-sectional radiological imaging is the upstaging of the clinical stage by demonstrating one or more enlarged lymph nodes (Fig. 21–21). These may be biopsied percutaneously.

Bones. Osteoblastic metastases predominate. Osteolytic metastases are extraordinarily rare and are likely to represent other rare types of prostatic malignancy, carcinoma of the ejaculatory duct, for example. Bone scan is the examination of choice (Fig. 21–22). Bone window facilitates detection on CT (Fig. 21–23). On MR imaging, replacement of high signal fat by low signal osteoblastic tumor on T1-weighted sequence is evident. Differential diagnosis includes other numerous causes of "white bone," the most common being the "bone island." Comparison with any previous studies (as always) usually clarifies the issue. It is possible, however it is rare, for the bone island to be "hot" on the nuclear medicine bone scan.

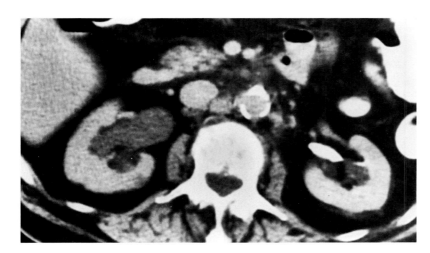

Figure 21–19. A lymph node of 1.5 cm is wedged between the aorta and inferior vena cava. Right kidney is obstructed.

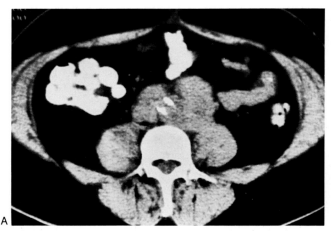
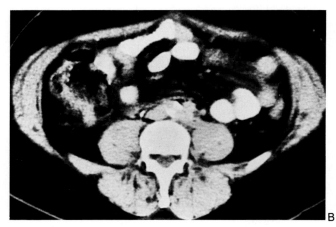

Figure 21–20. Lymph node metastases from carcinoma of the prostate **(A)** disappear after chemotherapy and orchiectomy **(B)**.

Lungs. Small nodular metastases are slow in growing and tend to creep up imperceptibly from one chest radiograph to the next. It is essential to dig into the film jacket for older chest radiographs for comparison.

Other. Metastases from the prostate may be found in subdural areas in the spine. The mode of propagation is thought to be via the Batson's plexus of veins. Compression upon the cord may cause neurological deficit, including paralysis. MR is the imaging modality of choice.

Distant ureteral metastases probably propagate in similar fashion along the periureteral plexus of veins (Fig. 21–24).

Radiation Therapy Planning. CT is invaluable in calculating the radiation dose distribution and establishing the radiation ports.

Postoperative Evaluation. Disruption and urine leak at the anastomotic site after radical prostatectomy can be determined even without removing the large Foley catheter (Fig. 21–25).

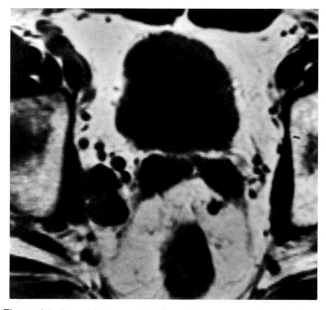

Figure 21–21. Metastasis in the obturator lymph node. Normal seminal vesicles.

OTHER MALIGNANT DISEASES OF THE PROSTATE

Endometrioid Carcinoma (Papillary Carcinoma)

Endometrioid or papillary carcinoma of the prostate is rare. The tumor is usually difficult to detect by palpation. Unlike prostatic carcinoma, papillary carcinoma frequently arises or extends to the central zone of the prostate.[27]

Sarcoma

Sarcoma of the prostate is rare. The most common type is myosarcoma, followed by lymphosarcoma, spindle cell sarcoma, and other forms (Fig. 21–26 A,B). Metastases are to lungs and bones. Rhabdomyosarcoma (sarcoma botryoides [Fig. 21–27]) is discussed elsewhere (p. 380).

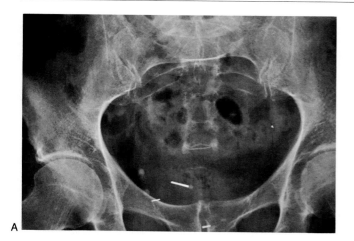

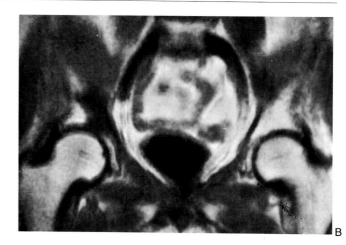

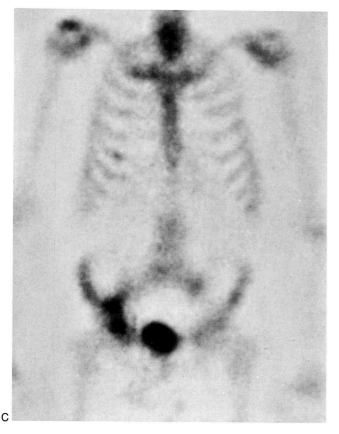

Figure 21–22.   (A) Plain radiograph of the pelvis fails even in retrospect to detect bone metastases. (B) T1-weighted sequence in the coronal plane unequivocally demonstrates replacement of normal high signal fatty bone marrow with medium to low signal metastasis in the right acetabular roof (compare with the opposite side). (C) Bone scan is also "hot" in that area.

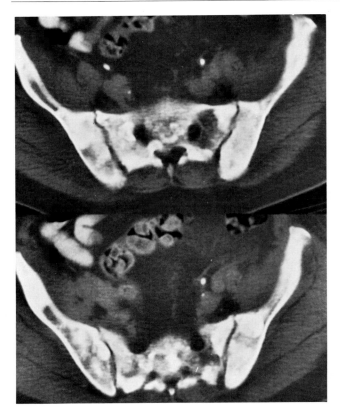

Figure 21–23. Bone window in the region of the sacroiliac joints demonstrates many osteoblastic bone metastases.

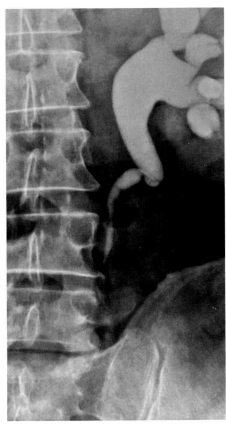

Figure 21–24. Mid-ureteral distant metastasis from carcinoma of the prostate.

Lymphoma

Primary and *secondary lymphoma* involving the prostate are rare.[28] Outflow bladder obstruction may be the presenting symptom (Fig. 21–28). Diagnosis is made by biopsy.

VAS DEFERENS, SEMINAL VESICLES, AND EJACULATORY DUCT

Normal anatomy is presented in Figure 21–29.

Seminal Vesiculography. The procedure may be performed by antegrade or retrograde method. Retrograde method involves endoscopic catheterization of ejaculatory ducts at verumontanum.

Antegrade method is preferred. A small scrotal incision is made; vas deferens is identified and cannulated using a 25 gauge needle. Radiographic contrast (preferably nonionic) is slowly injected, during which time radiographic exposures are made. The main indication for this procedure is to demonstrate

patency or occlusion of the vas deferens in infertile patients.

Vas Deferens Calcification

Most commonly seen in patients with diabetes mellitus. Rarely, it has been described in nondiabetics as well. It is of no clinical significance (Fig. 21–30).

Seminal Vesicle

Seminal Vesicle Agenesis. Diagnosis is made by transrectal ultrasound or MR imaging if suspected as a cause of infertility. May be associated with cryptorchidism.

Seminal Vesicle Cyst. Ipsilateral renal agenesis or dysgenesis is present in most patients. Other congenital anomalies such as agenesis of vas deferens or ejaculatory duct and ectopic insertion of the ureter may also be present. The cyst may become very large

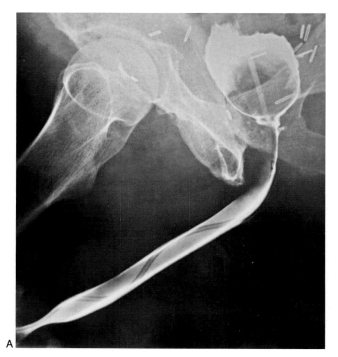

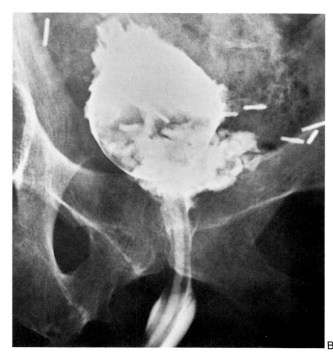

Figure 21–25. Retrograde urethrogram is performed by introducing a small feeding tube along the side of the larger Foley catheter into the bulbous urethra. Mild distal occlusion is created by manual compression and contrast is gently injected. **(A)** Normal postradical prostatectomy study. **(B)** Leak at the anastomotic site between bladder and urethra.

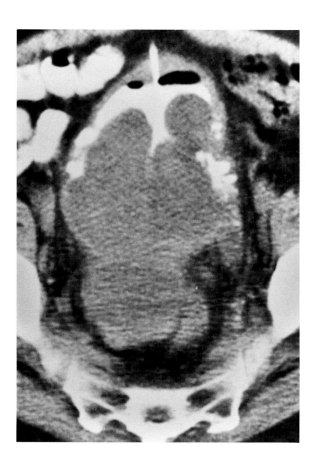

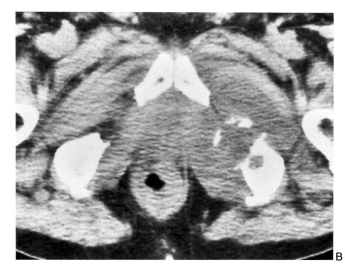

Figure 21–26. Sarcoma of the prostate extending into the bladder **(A)** and left ischial bone **(B)**.

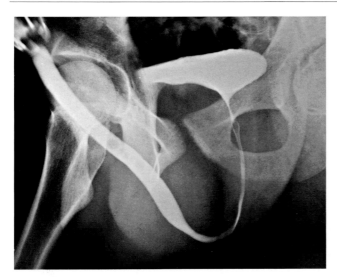

Figure 21–27. Rhabdomyosarcoma presents as a mass that displaces and elongates prostatic, membranous, and bulbous urethra.

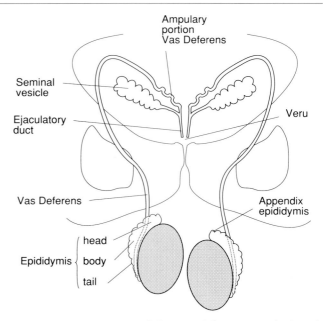

Figure 21–29. Anatomy of the vas deferens, seminal vesicle, ejaculatory duct.

and symptomatic. Cystic nature is easily determined by ultrasound, CT, or MR imaging.[29–31]

Seminal Vesicle Calcification. Calcification of the seminal vesicle is seen less commonly compared with calcification of vas deferens. Diabetes mellitus is the most common cause. May be seen in schistosomiasis and tuberculosis.

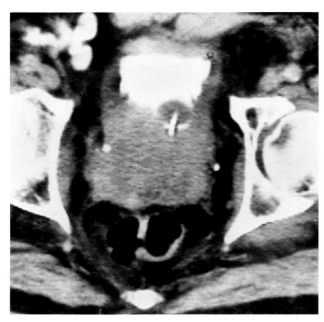

Figure 21–28. Lymphoma of the prostate. (Photograph courtesy of A. Augustine.)

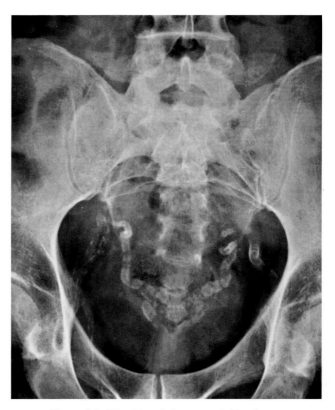

Figure 21–30. Vas deferens calcifications.

Seminal Vesiculitis. Symptoms are similar to those of chronic prostatitis. Diagnosis may be made if semen cultures are positive. Transrectal ultrasound may be used to aspirate seminal vesicle contents and antibiotics could be administered via the same route.

Abscess. Rare. May be diagnosed by transrectal ultrasound or CT and MR imaging.[32,33]

Carcinoma of the Seminal Vesicle. Extremely rare. May be confused with prostatic carcinoma on physical examination.[34]

REFERENCES

1. Lee F, Torp-Pedersen ST, Siders DB, et al. Transrectal ultrasound in the diagnosis and staging of prostatic carcinoma. Radiology 1989; 170:609–615.
2. McNeal JE. Regional morphology and pathology of the prostate. Am J Clin Pathol 1968; 49:347–357.
3. Fornage BD. Normal US anatomy of the prostate. Ultrasound Med Biol 1986; 5:101–103.
4. Hricak H, Dooms GC, McNeal JE, et al. MR imaging of the prostate gland: normal anatomy. AJR 1987; 148: 51–54.
5. Schnall MD, Lenkinski RE, Pollack HM, et al. Prostate: MR imaging with an endorectal surface coil. Radiology 1989; 172:570–574.
6. Lee F Jr, Lee F, Solomon MH, et al. Sonographic demonstration of prostatic abscess. J Ultrasound Med 1986; 5:101–102.
7. Thornhill BA, Morehouse HT, Coleman P, et al. Prostatic abscess: CT and sonographic findings. AJR 1987; 148:899–991.
8. Dennis MA, Donohue RE. Computed tomography of prostatic abscess. J Comput Assist Tomogr 1985; 9:201–202.
9. Wasserman NF, Lapointe S, Eckmann DR, Rosel PR. Assessment of prostatism: role of intravenous urography. Radiology 1987; 165:831–834.
10. Talner LB. Routine urography in men with prostatism. AJR 1986; 147:960–964.
11. Ling D, Lee JKT, Heiken JP, et al. Prostatic carcinoma and benign prostatic hyperplasia: inability of MR imaging to distinguish between the two diseases. Radiology 1986; 158:103–107.
12. Castaneda F, Reddy PK, Wasserman N, et al. Benign prostatic hypertrophy: retrograde transurethral dilatation of the prostatic urethra in humans: work in progress. Radiology 1987; 163:649–652.
13. Hamilton S, Fitzpatric JM. Ultrasound diagnosis of a prostatic cyst causing acute urinary retention. J Ultrasound Med 1987; 6:385–386.
14. Brawer MK, Lange PH. Prostate-specific antigen in management of prostatic carcinoma. Urology 1989 33(Suppl):11–16.
15. Hanks GE. External beam radiation therapy for prostate gland clinically confined to the gland. Urology 1989; 33(Suppl):21–26.
16. Rifkin MD, McGlynn ET, Choi H. Echogenicity of prostate cancer correlated with histologic grade and stromal fibrosis: endorectal US studies. Radiology 1989; 170:549–552.
17. Rifkin MD, Choi H. Implications of small peripheral hypoechoic lesions in endorectal US of the prostate. Radiology 1988; 166:619–622.
18. Lee F, Torp-Pedersen ST, Siders DB. Use of transrectal ultrasound in diagnosis, guided biopsy, staging, and screening of prostate cancer. Urology 1989; 33 (Suppl):7–12.
19. Salo JO, Kivisaari L, Rannikko S, Lehtonen T. Computerized tomography and transrectal ultrasound in the assessment of local extension of prostatic cancer before radical retropubic prostatectomy. J Urol 1987; 137:435–438.
20. Hardeman SW, Causey JQ, Hickey DP, Soloway MS. Transrectal ultrasound for staging prior to radical prostatectomy. Urology 1989; 34:175–180.
21. Resnic MI. Transrectal ultrasound guided versus digitally directed prostatic biopsy: a comparative study. J Urol 1988; 139:754–757.
22. Hricak H, Dooms GC, Jeffrey RB, et al. Prostatic carcinoma staging by clinical assessment, CT, and MR imaging. Radiology 1987; 162:331–336.
23. Biondetti PR, Lee JKT, Ling D, Catalona WJ. Clinical stage B prostate carcinoma; staging with MR imaging. Radiology 1987; 162:325–329.
24. Martin JF, Hajek P, Baker L, et al. Inflatable surface coil for MR imaging of the prostate. Radiology 1988; 167:268–270.
25. Schnall MD, Lenkinski RE, Pollack HM, et al. Prostate: MR imaging with an endorectal surface coil. Radiology 1989; 172:570–574.
26. Gothlin JH, Hoiem L. Percutaneous fine-needle biopsy of radiographically normal lymph nodes in the staging of prostatic carcinoma. Radiology 1981; 141:351–354.
27. Wernert N, Luchtrach H, Seeliger H, et al. Papillary carcinoma of the prostate, location, morphology, and immunohistochemistry: the histogenesis and entity of so-called endometrioid carcinoma. Prostate 1987; 10:123–131.
28. Fell P, O'Connor M, Smith JM. Primary lymphoma of prostate presenting as bladder outflow obstruction. Urology 1987; 29:555–556.
29. Kneeland JB, Auh YH, McCarron JP, et al. Computed tomography, sonography, vesiculography, and MR imaging of a seminal vesicle cyst. J Comput Assist Tomogr 1985; 9:964–966.
30. Heaney JA, Pfister RC, Meares EM Jr. Giant cyst of the seminal vesicle with renal agenesis. AJR 1987; 149: 139–141.
31. King BF, Hattery RR, Lieber MM, et al. Seminal vesicle imaging. Radiographics 1989; 9:653–676.
32. Lee SB, Lee F, Solomon MH, et al. Seminal vesicle abscess: diagnosis by transrectal ultrasound. J Clin Ultrasound 1986; 14:546.
33. Zagoria RJ, Papanicolaou N, Pfister RC, et al. Seminal vesicle abscess after vasectomy: evaluation by transrectal sonography and CT. AJR 1987; 149:137–138.
34. Sussman SK, Dunnick NR, Silverman PM, et al. Carcinoma of the seminal vesicle: CT appearance. J Comput Assist Tomogr 1986; 10:519.

22

Male Urethra

ANATOMY

The male urethra is conveniently divided into the anterior and posterior urethra (Fig. 22–1).[1,2]

The *posterior urethra* consists of prostatic urethra and membranous urethra. Numerous prostatic ductules open into the prostatic urethra. At the posterior aspect of the midportion of the prostatic urethra, there is a protuberance called the verumontanum. Ejaculatory ducts and utricle have their openings at this mound. Posterior urethra is lined with transitional cell epithelium.

Anterior urethra is divided into bulbous urethra and pendulous urethra. Bulbocavernosus muscle is on the inferior aspect of the urethra (Fig. 22–2). Cowper's gland ducts, sometimes 4.5 cm long, have their openings in the bulbous urethra. Numerous small glands of Littré empty into the anterior urethra. Fossa navicularis is a 1 cm long bulbous dilatation on the very distal end of the anterior urethra. The entire anterior urethra is surrounded by corpus spongiosum. Anterior urethra is lined with squamous epithelium.

URETHROGRAPHY

Retrograde Urethrography

Drip Infusion Method. Over the years, several methods have gained and declined in popularity. The method that uses a small 10 F Foley catheter seems to work best. After cleansing the area, the catheter is connected to a 30% contrast drip, purged of air, and placed so that the balloon inflates in the fossa navicularis. Only a few milliliters of fluid need to be introduced into the balloon. Since the fossa navicularis is wider in lumen than the meatus, the balloon anchors the catheter and seals the urethra for contrast infusion. Patient is in the supine position and 35°–45° oblique projection. Dependent leg should be bent at the knee and hip to equalize radiographic density in this projection. Contrast is infused and either spot films under fluoroscopic control or overhead radiographs are obtained. Low radiation dose to the examiner is the main advantage of this method.

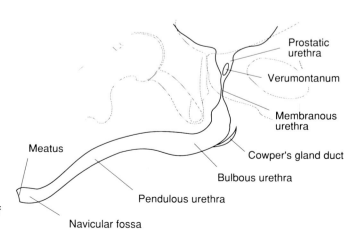

Figure 22–1. Schematic drawing of male urethral anatomy.

Prostatic urethra

Verumontanum

Membranous urethra

Cowper's gland duct

Bulbous urethra

Pendulous urethra

Meatus

Navicular fossa

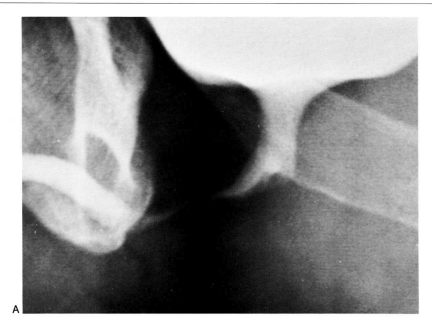

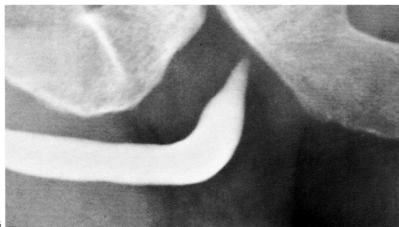

Figure 22–2. **(A)** A spot radiograph during a voiding cystourethrogram (VCUG) demonstrates a severe narrowing of the bulbous urethra, which could easily be mistaken for a stricture. **(B)** Retrograde urethrogram (RUG) conclusively demonstrates that the narrowing is due to spasm of the bulbocavernosus muscle. The posterior urethra is now well distended all the way back to the external sphincter.

Hand Injection. Again, the Foley catheter may be employed. Urologists sometimes prefer one of several clamps, such as Brodney (Fig. 22–3) or Knutson, or a newly developed rubber catheter with a Velcro cage for fixation and effective seal. Radiation dose to the examiner is higher.

Special Circumstances. After radical prostatectomy or urethral trauma, it may be necessary to demonstrate urethral integrity without removing an already present large Foley catheter. A small pediatric feeding tube may be inserted alongside the large catheter and contrast infused. The small feeding tube may also be used in meatal stenosis or distal urethral stricture.

Precautions. The study should not be performed immediately following cystoscopy. Small mucosal laceration may lead to moderate urethrocorpus spongiosum "intravasation." This complication may result in sepsis and prophylactic antibiotics are recommended (Figs. 22–3, 22–4).

Antegrade Urethrography

Voiding Cystourethrogram (VCUG). On this examination, normal urethra never distends to the degree seen on a retrograde examination (Fig. 22–5). Therefore important pathological processes may remain undetected. However, in situations where some resistance to the flow of urine exists (stricture, for example), urethra above the point of obstruction is dilated.

Resistance Voiding Urethrogram. Artificial obstruction may be placed at distal urethra using Zippser

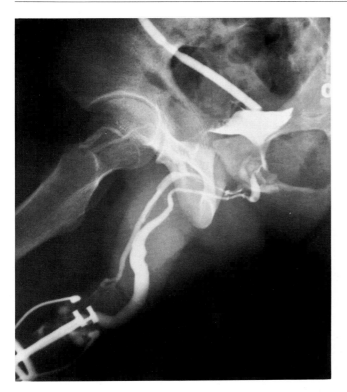

Figure 22–3. RUG with Brodney clamp affixed to the glans. Unfortunately, there is intravasation of contrast material into the dorsal vein of the penis. The entire posterior urethra is narrow.

clamp (Fig. 22–6) or a similar device.[3] Distention of the urethra is usually adequate to permit diagnosis. Patient can control the device and remove it if there is any discomfort. Adequate visualization of the urethra is possible even without catheterization (after excretory urography, for example).

CONGENITAL ANOMALIES OF THE URETHRA

Most congenital anomalies of the male urethra result in significant outflow bladder obstruction. Following birth, there may be rapid progression of renal failure. Most congenital anomalies are discovered in early childhood.

Posterior Urethral Valves

Posterior urethral valves are mucosal flaps in the posterior urethra that interfere with normal flow of urine and frequently produce a moderate to marked degree of outflow obstruction.[4,5] Large, usually trabeculated bladder, dilated ureters, and vesicoureteral reflux are thus commonly found, as are hydronephrotic and dysplastic kidneys. Decreased urine stream is usually present, although occasionally the stream may be well preserved. Three types are described:

- Type I: mucosal flaps extend below the verumontanum and the small opening is posterior or anterior.
- Type II: mucosal flaps are above the verumontanum and extend to the internal orifice.
- Type III: there is a web with a central opening.

VCUG is the examination of choice. Usually, the mucosal flaps present no obstacle to retrograde bladder catheterization. Characteristic finding is dilatation of the proximal posterior urethra (Fig. 22–7). Hyperreflexic dilated or trabeculated bladder may be seen with reflux. Reflux is apparently rare or nonexistent in blacks.[6] Many of the findings may be

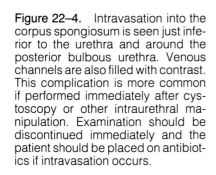

Figure 22–4. Intravasation into the corpus spongiosum is seen just inferior to the urethra and around the posterior bulbous urethra. Venous channels are also filled with contrast. This complication is more common if performed immediately after cystoscopy or other intraurethral manipulation. Examination should be discontinued immediately and the patient should be placed on antibiotics if intravasation occurs.

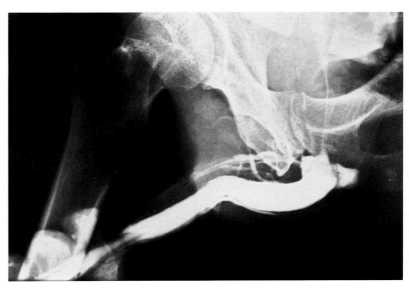

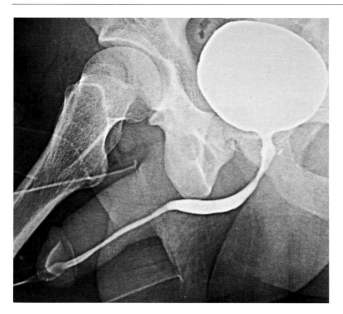

Figure 22–5. Normal voiding cystourethrogram (VCUG). The external sphincter never distends as much as the bulbous urethra. Even the pendulous urethra appears narrow. Reflux into the utricle is seen just posterior to the relatively radiolucent filling defect representing the verumontanum. The urine receptacle is almost radiolucent. No part of the receptacle should compress the urethra during voiding.

identified by sonography.[7] Primary treatment is by endoscopic fulguration. Temporary, and sometimes permanent, diversion may be necessary.[8]

Urethral valves should be suspected as the cause of fetal hydronephrosis discovered by sonography in utero.

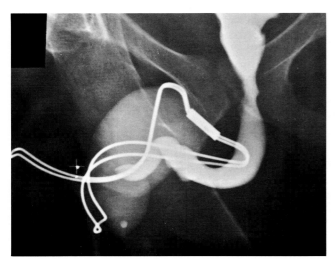

Figure 22–6. Resistance voiding urethrogram. The urethra is well distended once the artificial outflow obstruction is created at the distal end with an external soft clamp.

Anterior Urethral Valves

Although less common,[9] anterior urethral valves may present a significant diagnostic problem if the entire urethra is inadequately examined during the voiding part of the study (Fig. 22–8). Radiologically it may be difficult at times to differentiate anterior urethral valves from wide mouth urethral diverticulum (Fig. 22–9).

Congenital Diverticulum

Wide mouth congenital diverticula are seen in the pendulous urethra.[10,11] Anterior flap may interfere with the normal flow of urine and cause outflow bladder obstruction. Utricle may also develop into a diverticulum (Fig. 22–10). Other types of urethral diverticula are usually acquired (Fig. 22–11).

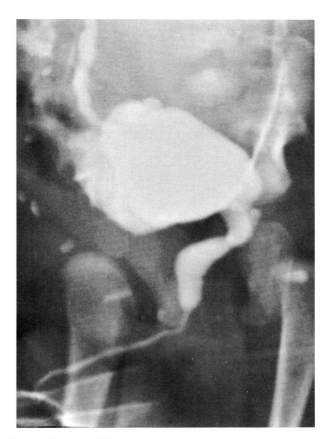

Figure 22–7. VCUG in a patient with posterior urethral valves. Dilatation of the posterior urethra and bladder trabeculation are reflection of outflow bladder obstruction. Vesicoureteral reflux is also present. (Photograph courtesy of Dr. M. Ines Boechat.)

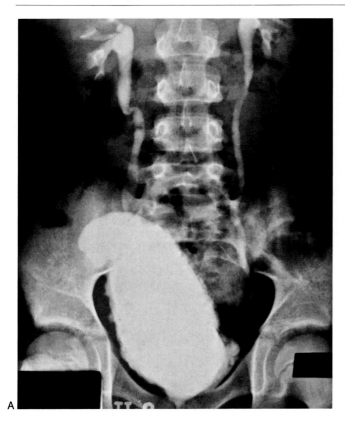

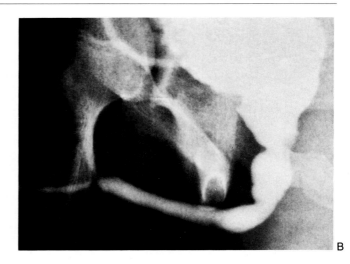

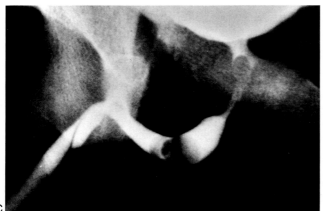

Figure 22–8. **(A)** EXU in 9-year-old boy demonstrates moderate bladder thickening and trabeculation. Repeated VCUGs and cystoscopies (elsewhere) failed to disclose the cause. None of the VCUGs, however, had distal urethra in the field of view. **(B)** Repeated VCUG, now with a suprapubic tube in place, demonstrates dilatation of the proximal and bulbous urethra. In the pendulous urethra there is an abrupt change in urethral caliber and mucosal flap can be strongly suggested. **(C)** RUG clearly demonstrates valve in the pendulous urethra. Orientation of the anterior valve is such that retrograde catheterization can be easily achieved and yet there is serious impediment to the antegrade flow of urine. Filling defects in the bulbous urethra are bubbles of air (inadvertently introduced during retrograde contrast installation), and verumontanum in the prostatic urethra.

Congenital Strictures

Congenital strictures are short and weblike, can cause significant outflow obstruction and are simple to correct.[12]

Urethral Duplication

Urethral duplication is a rare congenital anomaly (Fig. 22–12).[13,14] Urinary tract infection is a common presentation. Urethral duplications have been classified into three groups (Fig. 22–13):[15]

- Type I: Complete duplication with separate external and bladder orifices.
- Type II: Variable external openings, originate from dominant urethra.
- Type III: Perineal opening, originating from the bladder or dominant urethra.

Meatal Stenosis

Tip of the urethra should always be included on the retrograde or antegrade contrast examination (Fig.

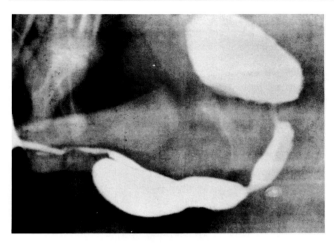

Figure 22–9. Urethra proximal to the anterior urethral valve may dilate to the extent it cannot be differentiated from a urethral diverticulum. Diverticulum may also create outflow obstruction by extending beneath the urethral mucosa so as to create a mucosal flap that may act as a valve.

22–14). The length of stenosis needs to be determined.[16]

Megalourethra

Megalourethra is characterized by the absence of corpus spongiosum.[17] Wide and elongated urethra is seen on the contrast study (Fig. 22–15).[18,19]

Müllerian Duct Cyst

Müllerian duct cysts originate from fused müllerian ducts.[20] Peak incidence is in the third decade of life.

The cyst may extend outside the prostate, compress the urethra and ejaculatory ducts, and could produce symptoms of outflow bladder obstruction, hematuria, pain, and infertility. Cystic fluid may be clear, mucoid, purulent, or hemorrhagic. MR imaging may be the imaging modality of choice, since intraprostatic anatomy and the ability to obtain images in different planes can help localize the lesion more precisely.[21] May contain calculi.

URETHRAL STRICTURES

Inflammatory Strictures

If left untreated, gonococcal infection involving periurethral glands results in scarring of the periurethral tissues (Fig. 22–16). Increased intraurethral pressures proximal to the obstruction may produce mucosal injuries causing secondary strictures to develop (Fig. 22–17). Secondary infections in these areas may result in diverticula, abscesses, fistulas, etc.

Urethral strictures may be divided into hard and soft.[2] The urethra involved with soft strictures may be quite distensible, and it is of some importance in planning treatment to radiographically document their extension (Figs. 22–18, 22–19). This is particularly important if the soft stricture involves the external sphincter.

Strictures may be diffuse, or localized (Figs. 22–20, 22–21). Areas of normal urethra may be present between strictured segments. Localized bulbous urethral stricture may mimic normal external sphincter (Figs. 22–22, 22–23).

Inflammatory strictures of the prostatic urethra

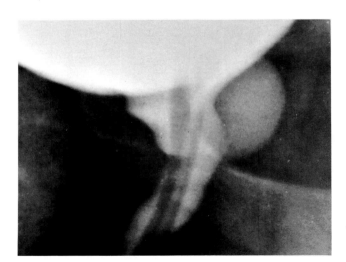

Figure 22–10. Diverticulum of the utricle.

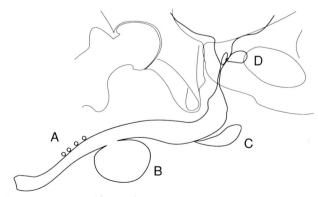

Figure 22–11. Schematic drawing of congenital and acquired urethral diverticula. **A:** Abscessed glands of Littré in chronic urethritis; **B:** Congenital or acquired diverticula of the pendulous urethra; **C:** Diverticular dilatation of the Cowper's gland duct; **D:** Diverticulum of the utricle.

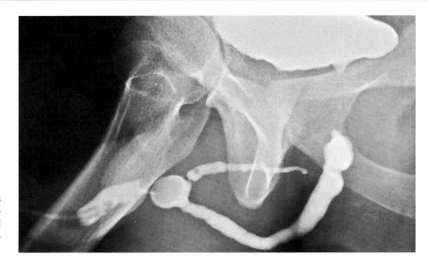

Figure 22–12. RUG demonstrates a urethral duplication, which is difficult to classify because of several prior apparently unsuccessful surgeries in the area.

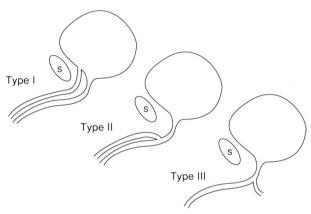

Figure 22–13. Schematic drawing of three types of congenital urethral duplication.

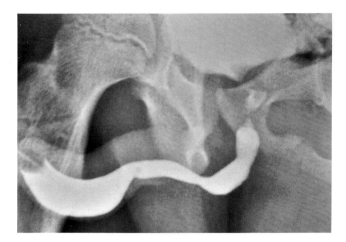

Figure 22–15. RUG in a patient with megalourethra. Urethra is abnormally distended due to lack of support from corpus spongiosum, which is absent in this congenital anomaly.

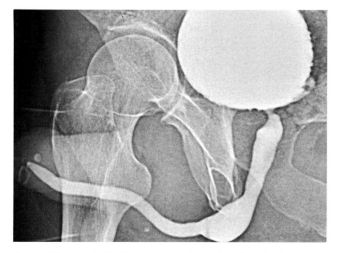

Figure 22–14. VCUG in meatal stenosis. Bladder is trabeculated and urethra is distended all the way to the meatus. The bladder neck normally need not be seen fully opened at all times.

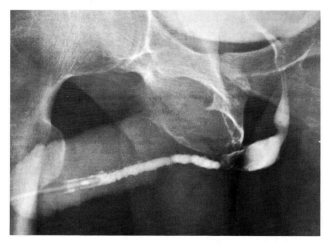

Figure 22–16. RUG in a patient with chronic urethritis, multiple strictures involving all but very posterior aspect of the bulbous urethra. Glands of Littré are abscessed and fill with contrast in a retrograde manner.

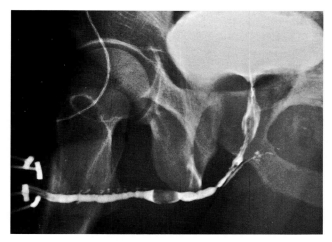

Figure 22-17. Diffuse involvement of the entire urethra with chronic urethritis and strictures. There is reflux into Cowper's gland duct and gland. Reflux into these structures by itself is not an abnormal finding.

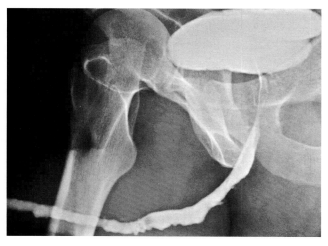

Figure 22-19. RUG demonstrates irregularities along the ventral aspect of the bulbous and along the entire pendulous urethra. There is a lack of distention of the bulbous urethra. The stricturing process is far advanced, yet there is no functionally significant narrowing of the urethral lumen.

are practically unheard of. The urethra in this area may be narrowed due to extrinsic pressure caused by acutely inflamed prostate or prostatic neoplasm.

Uncommon causes of inflammatory strictures include tuberculosis[22] and schistosomiasis.

Post-Traumatic Strictures

The most common post-traumatic stricture of the male urethra is related to iatrogenic injury during

transurethral prostatectomy,[23] followed by strictures resulting from urethral transection or urethral tear associated with pelvic trauma. If the urethral stricture is complete, retrograde urethrogram cannot demonstrate the superior extension. Since suprapubic tube will always be present under these circumstances, a combined retrograde urethrogram and antegrade suprapubic cystogram will clearly demonstrate the extent of the lesion.[24]

Balloon dilatation of urethral strictures (Fig. 22-24) has some apparent advantages over traditional dilatation with stiff urethral dilators.[25,26]

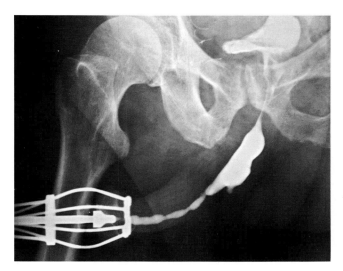

Figure 22-18. Is it or isn't it? Besides detecting and determining the morphological characteristic of urethral strictures, the most important role of urethrography is to determine whether the external sphincter area is involved with the stricture process or not. Smooth cone at the inferior margin, as seen in this case, excludes the presence of a stricture. Most anterior urethra in this patient is involved with severe strictures.

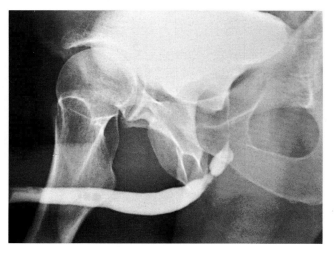

Figure 22-20. Localized stricture in the bulbous urethra. There is also an apparent prostatic enlargement.

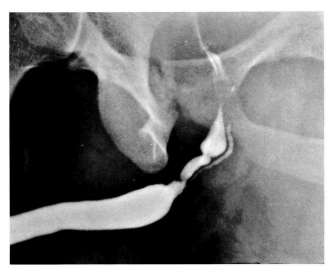

Figure 22-21. Moderate stricture involving the bulbous urethra extending for about 2 cm. Reflux into the Cowper's gland duct is present.

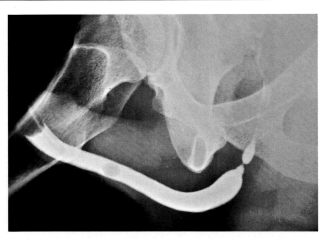

Figure 22-22. Localized stricture involving posterior aspect of bulbous urethra. Clues that this is not a membranous urethra, normally underdistended on RUG, are: a) Membranous urethra is located along the horizontal line crossing the inferior margin of the obturator foramen. The stricture is 1 cm below that line; b) the cone at the stricture is not perfect. The perfect cone is found 1 cm above the stricture at the horizontal line mentioned above, representing the external sphincter.

False Passages

False passages are usually seen in patients with urethral strictures and are created during instrumentation (Fig. 22-25). The false passage may end blindly or may reenter the bladder.

Acquired Diverticula

Acquired urethral diverticula may result as a complication of urethral surgery (Fig. 22-26) or prolonged presence of an external anti-incontinence clamp (Fig. 22-27).

Inflammatory Papilloma and Condyloma Accuminatum

Both may present as filling defects in the urethra (Fig. 22-28). Radiological findings are nonspecific. Differential diagnosis includes primary urethral carcinoma or metastases.

NEOPLASTIC DISEASES OF MALE URETHRA

Congenital Polyp

This rare epithelialized fibrous tumor originates in the region of verumontanum in the posterior urethra.[27] Outflow bladder obstruction may be the

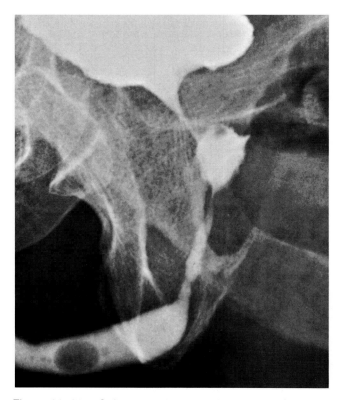

Figure 22-23. Stricture at the posterior aspect of the bulbous urethra masquerading as normal external sphincter. Using criteria described in Figure 22-22, it becomes apparent that the external sphincter is higher than the narrowing. The lack of any cone suggests the external sphincter may also be included in the stricture. A prostatic abscess cavity draws attention away from this important area, a factor that may contribute to misdiagnosis.

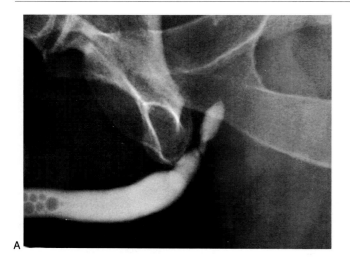

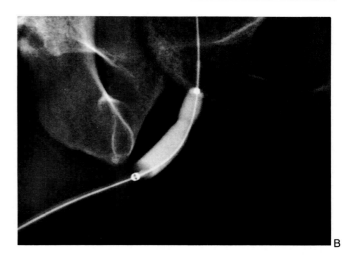

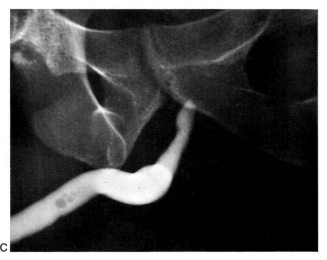

Figure 22–24. **(A)** Severe stricture of the bulbous urethra. **(B)** A balloon-catheter is positioned across the stricture and inflated. Radial distention with the balloon may be less injurious compared with that of urethral dilators. **(C)** Appearance of the stricture after dilatation.

presenting symptom. Usually discovered by 8 years of age as a filling defect in the posterior urethra (Fig. 22–29). Ultrasound may be used to differentiate polyp from a urethral calculus or a clot.[28]

Metastases to Urethra

Metastases appear as multiple filling defects (Fig. 22–30). This is a late finding as the patient is likely to have distant metastases from primary disease discovered elsewhere by the time urethral metastases become clinically apparent.

Urethral Carcinoma

Neoplastic processes involving the urethra are rare. Squamous cell carcinoma is the most common, usually involving bulbous urethra and usually occurring in patients with previously known strictures. Transi-

tional cell carcinoma originates from posterior urethra. Adenocarcinoma and melanoma constitute the rest of these rare tumors.

Penile bleeding is a common presentation. Radiographically, this neoplasm is difficult to differentiate from simple stricture (Fig. 22–31). Urethroscopy and biopsy are the only reliable means of establishing the presence of a neoplastic process.

MR imaging may prove useful in determining tumor extension and in separating neoplastic tissue from fibrous.

TRAUMA

Trauma to the urethra is described in Chapter 17. Three important facts should be reiterated. First, retrograde urethrography is a simple, quick, and accurate method for establishing the degree and the

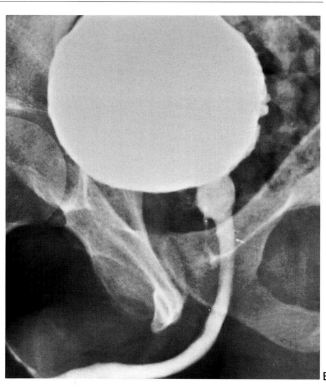

A

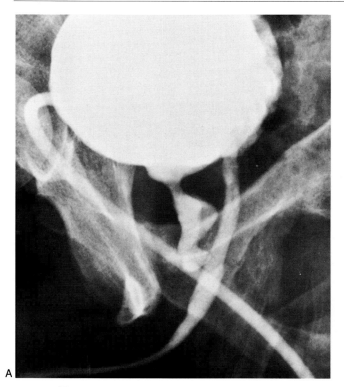

B

Figure 22–25.   False passage in a patient with urethral strictures. **(A)** False passage is seen posterior to the prostatic urethra. Prostatic urethra is easily recognized because of radiolucent filling defect representing verumontanum. Suprapubic catheter crosses the field of view and is likely to draw attention away from the area of interest. **(B)** Several months later the false passage is now the dominant draining channel. Partially collapsed prostatic urethra is barely seen anterior to the false channel.

location of urethral injury. Second, bladder catheterization should be attempted only by an experienced physician because a partial urethral tear could be inadvertently made worse. Third, a long-standing indwelling catheter is likely to cause accumulation of urethral secretions, particularly in bulbous urethra, resulting in infection and stricture. Catheter bend at the penoscrotal junction can cause necrosis and subsequent stricture.

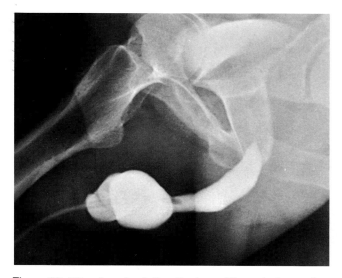

Figure 22–26.   Acquired diverticulum of the anterior urethra at the penoscrotal junction.

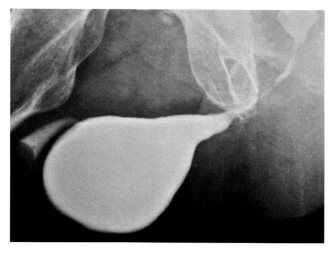

Figure 22–27.   Acquired urethral diverticulum from an external penile clamp used to control urinary incontinence.

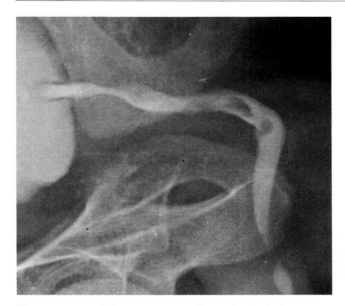

Figure 22–28. Inflammatory papilloma in the bulbous urethra. (Photograph courtesy of Dr. Milton Kunin.)

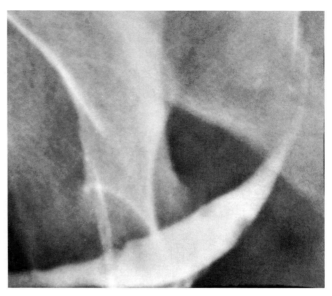

Figure 22–30. Metastases to the urethra from carcinoma of colon. Multiple small filling defects are seen on RUG.

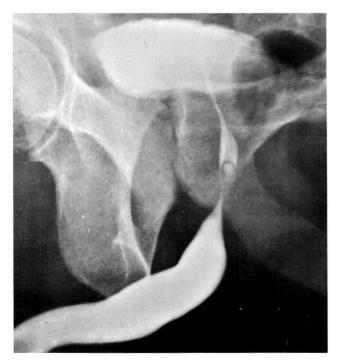

Figure 22–29. Small congenital polyp in the posterior urethra may be misdiagnosed as normal verumontanum.

POSTSURGICAL FINDINGS

Surgical techniques for urethral repair are of interest because of the postoperative radiographic findings. Two-stage urethroplasty is a technique whereby a perineal opening is created during the first stage of repair of distal urethral strictures so that the male patient has to squat to empty his bladder (Fig. 22–32). Later an end-to-end anastomosis is made to the more anterior repaired urethra. Another technique bypasses strictured membraneous urethra by creating end-to-side anastomosis of the bulbous to prostatic urethra (Fig. 22–33).

A significant percentage of urethral trauma is iatrogenic. Some complications of transurethral surgery or catheterization are false passage, urethral strictures, urethral fistulas (Fig. 22–34), incontinence, and bladder perforation.

Urinary incontinence is a common complication of transurethral prostatectomy. This is almost always because of injury to the distal urethral sphincter mechanism.

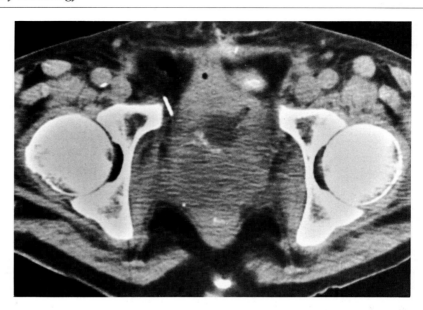

Figure 22–31. Recurrent carcinoma of the urethra extending cephalad into the true pelvis.

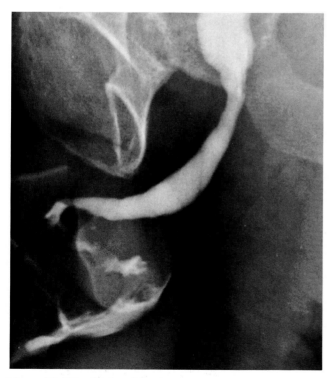

Figure 22–32.   Perineal fistula after first stage urethroplasty.

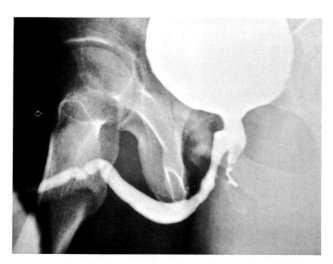

Figure 22–33.   Bulbous urethra is brought through the urogenital diaphgram and anastomosed through the anterior prostate with the prostatic urethra. Symphysis pubis may or may not be resected. Continence is maintained by internal sphincter.

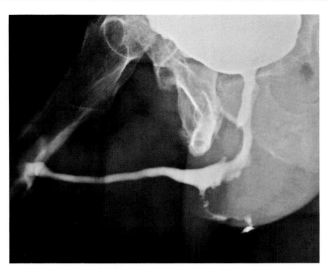

Figure 22-34. Urethroperineal fistula complicating urethral surgery. This may be seen in rare cases of urethral tuberculosis where multiple sinus tracts lead from the urethra to the perineum.

REFERENCES

1. McCallum RW, Colapinto V. Urological Radiology of the Adult Male Lower Urinary Tract. Springfield, Ill: Charles C Thomas, 1976.
2. McCallum RW. The adult male urethra. Radiol Clin North Am 1979; 17:227–244.
3. Fitts FB, Mascatello VG, Mellins HZ. The value of compression during excretion voiding urethrography. Radiology 1977; 125:53–56.
4. Macpherson RI, Leithiser RE Jr, Gordon L, Turner WR. Posterior urethral valves: update and review. Radiographics 1986; 6:753–768.
5. Hulbert WC, Duckett JW. Current views on posterior urethral valves. Pediat Ann 1988; 17:31–36.
6. Nancarrow PA, Lebowitz RL. Primary vesicoureteral reflux in blacks with posterior urethral valves: does it occur? Pediatr Radiol 1988; 19:31–35.
7. Cremin BJ. Review of the ultrasonographic appearances of posterior urethral valve and ureteroceles. Pediatr Radiol 1986; 16:357–360.
8. Mininberg DT, Genvert HP. Posterior urethral valves. Role of temporary and permanent urinary diversion. Urology 1989; 33:205–208.
9. Scherz HC, Kaplan GW, Packer MG. Anterior urethral valves in the fossa navicularis in children. J Urol 1987; 138:1211–1213.
10. Smith AEW. Unexpected anterior urethral diverticula. Clin Radiol 1986; 37:55.
11. Zaontz MR, Kaplan WE, Maizels M. Surgical correction of anterior urethral diverticula after hypospadias repair in children. Urology 1989; 33:40–42.
12. Rao KG. Congenital proximal bulbar stricture in adults. Urology 1975; 6:576–579.
13. Effman EL, Lebowitz RL, Colodny AH. Duplication of the urethra. Radiology 1976; 119:179–185.
14. Gyrtrup HJ, Kure HH. Duplication of the upper and lower urinary tract. Br J Urol 1989; 63:217–218.
15. Das S, Brosman SA. Duplication of the male urethra. J Urol 1977; 117:452–454.
16. Allen JS, Summers JL. Meatal stenosis in children. J Urol 1974; 112:526–527.
17. Nesbitt TE. Congenital megalo-urethra. J Urol 1955; 73:839–842.
18. Appel RA, Kaplan GW, Brock WA, Streit D. Megalourethra. J Urol 1986; 135:747.
19. Schrom SH, Cromie WJ, Duckett JW Jr. Megalourethra. Urology 1981; 17:152:1981.
20. Felderman T, Schellhammer PF, Devine CJ, Stecker JF. Müllerian duct cysts: conservative management. Urology 1987; 29:31–34.
21. Thurnher S, Hricak H, Tanagho EA. Müllerian duct cyst: diagnosis with MR imaging. Radiology 1988; 168:25–28.
22. Symes JM, Blandy JP. Tuberculosis of the male urethra. Br J Urol 1973; 45:432–436.
23. Lentz HC Jr, Mebust WK, Foret JD, et al. Urethral stricture following transurethral prostactomy. Review of 2223 resections. J Urol 1977; 117:194–196.
24. Bissada NK, Redman JF. Simultaneous retrograde and antegrade urethrography in urethral strictures. Urology 1975; 6:493.
25. Acunas B, Acunas G, Gokmen E, Celik L. Balloon dilatation of iatrogenic urethral strictures. Eur J Radiol 1988; 8:214–216.
26. Daughtry JD, Rodan BA, Bean WJ. Retrograde balloon dilatation of urethra. (Letter.) Urology 1989; 33:257.
27. Kimche D, Lask D. Congenital polyp of the prostatic urethra. J Urol 1982; 127:134–135.
28. Caro PSA, Rosenberg HK, Snyder HM III. Congenital urethral polyp. AJR 1986; 147:1041.

23

Impotence

Physiology of Cavernosal Erection. The initiating process of cavernosal erection is the relaxation of smooth muscles in the walls of the cavernosal sinusoids. Relaxation is mediated by parasympathetic release of acetylcholine, possibly by an intestinal polypeptide, and possibly by an endothelium-derived relaxing factor (EDRF).

Relaxed cavernosal sinusoids distend with blood and simultaneously compress small peripheral outflow venous tributaries against unyielding tunica albuginea. The venous outflow from the corpora is thus severely restricted. This veno-occlusive mechanism plays a crucial role in erection.

Arterial flow is also markedly increased until cavernosal pressure approaches systolic.

Incidence. Ten million middle-aged or elderly men in the United States.[1]

Etiology. Psychogenic, 50%; organic, 50%. Vasculogenic impotence is the most common form of organic impotence and is divided almost equally among *arteriogenic impotence, venogenic impotence,* and *combined venogenic-arteriogenic impotence.* Trauma and diabetes are frequent causes of vasculogenic impotence.

Clinical Presentation. Psychogenic impotence: presence of nocturnal erection. Organic impotence: absence of noctural erection.

Radiological Findings

Arteriogenic Impotence (Failure to Fill). Arteriogenic impotence is defined as bilateral and functionally significant arterial occlusion usually seen in diabetics (Fig. 23–1). Cavernosal arteries may be evaluated with duplex scanning before and after intracavernosal injection of papaverine-phentolamine (60 mg papaverine mixed with 1 mg phentolamine). Lack of increase in caliber and flow through the cavernosal arteries suggests the presence of arterial occlusion.[2]

Penile angiography may disclose arterial occlusion at any level, but the most common site is at the distal internal pudendal artery. Nonionic contrast is used for selective[3] or nonselective arterial[4] injection. Intracavernosal injection of papaverine-phentolamine is necessary to augment arterial flow and to produce veno-occlusive phenomen.

Treatment may consist of angioplasty, bypass surgery, arterialization of the dorsal penile vein, etc.

Venogenic Impotence (Failure to Store). Defective veno-occlusive mechanism prevents pressure buildup in the corpora. This veno-occlusive insufficiency is referred to as a *venous leak.* Presence of venous leak and the degree of venous insufficiency is determined by subjecting the patient to cavernosography and cavernosometry.

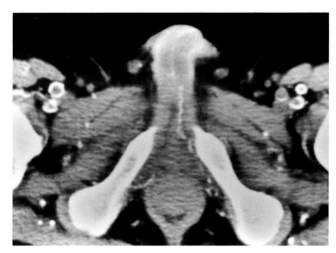

Figure 23–1. Calcification of the left internal pudendal and dorsal artery of the penis is present in a patient with diabetes and arteriogenic impotence. Other vessels are calcified as well.

CAVERNOSOGRAPHY AND CAVERNOSOMETRY

Cavernosography is a radiological procedure designed to render corpora and draining penile veins radiopaque (Fig. 23–2). This is accomplished by infusion of diluted contrast via direct needle puncture into the corpora at the rate of 2 ml/sec. Infusion into only one side opacifies both corpora, spongiosum, and glans. All the penile veins are usually visualized. These include dorsal penile vein, superficial penile veins, external pudendal veins, and crural perforators.

Cavernosometry is a method of determining cavernosal pressure during the infusion of diluted contrast (or normal saline). This is accomplished by placing a needle into the opposite corpus cavernosum and connecting to a pressure recorder. Infusion at a fast rate of 2 ml/sec will raise intracavernosal pressure to only 45 mm Hg.

In normal subjects after intracavernosal injection of papaverine-phentolamine, the penile veins are no longer visualized. Cavernosal pressure rises above 100 mm Hg and the infusion rate needed to maintain it drops to only 2–12 ml/min.[5]

If venous leak is present, infusion rate must be increased to maintain pressures above 100 mm Hg, despite papaverine-phentolamine injection. Leakage of 25–45 ml/min is significant in the presence of arterial insufficiency. Leakage of 45 ml/min or more is always associated with impotence.[6]

The site of venous leakage is evident on pharmaco-cavernosograms. The most common are abnormal filling of deep dorsal penile vein (Fig. 23–3) and crural perforators. The deep dorsal vein forms plexus of Santorini in the retropubic space (space of Retzius). Crural perforators drain into pudendal veins. Superficial veins may also fill and drain into the external pudendal veins.

One of the complications associated with papaverine-phentolamine intracavernosal injection is priapism. Treatment should be instituted after several hours of continuous erection. Cavernosal aspiration and intracavernosal injection of 10–15 µg of epinephrine should produce detumescence.

Treatment for venogenic impotence may consist of ligation of leaking veins. Dorsal vein ligation is relatively easy while ligation of crural perforators is not yet feasible. Exact anatomy provided by pharmaco-cavernosography is therefore important for treat-

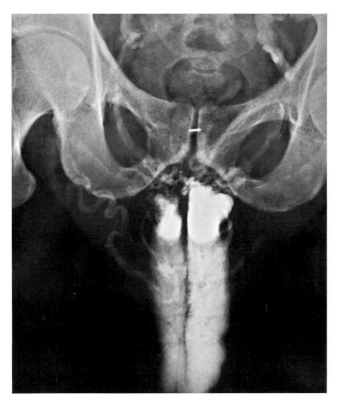

Figure 23–2. Cavernosogram in a patient with venogenic impotence. Injection into one corpus cavernosum will opacify both. Venous outflow is a normal finding unless papaverine and phentolamine are also injected into the corpus cavernosum. Then visualization of veins becomes an abnormal finding and is known as "venous leak."

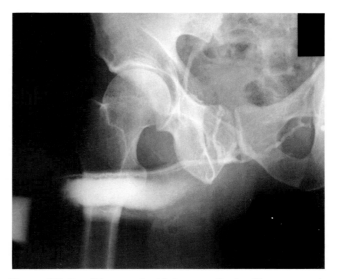

Figure 23–3. "Venous leak" in a patient with venogenic impotence. Despite intracorporeal injection of papaverine-phentolamine, there is filling of the dorsal vein of the penis and flow into the plexus of Santorini. Infusion rate had to be increased to 45 ml/min to maintain intracavernosal pressure of 100 mm Hg. (Photograph courtesy of Drs. J. Rafer and M. Mehringer.)

ment planning. Occlusion using angiographic techniques also seems possible.

END-ORGAN DISEASE

Peyronie's Disease

Sexually disabling disease characterized by fibrous plaques developing in the fascial layers of the penis. The plaques may be painful or they may ossify and calcify (Fig. 23–4). Depending on location, the plaques may interfere with erection. If calcification is detected on CT scan, implication is that the plaque is ossified and surgery is preferred over expectant therapy.

Priapism

Etiology. Idiopathic, sickle cell anemia, leukemia, spinal cord lesions, intracavernosal pharmacotherapy, trauma.

Pathophysiology. In sickle cell disease decreased oxygen tension during erection may induce sickling. Stasis, thrombosis, and calcifications may ensue, eventually resulting in impotence (Fig. 23–5). Following penile trauma, increased arterial inflow may be present, resulting in priapism.

Penile Prosthesis

Surgical implantation of penile prosthesis is a common method of treatment for all types of impotence

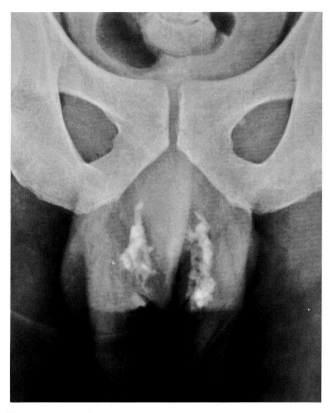

Figure 23–5. Calcified corpora in a patient with sickle cell disease which has resulted in end-organ failure.

(Fig. 23–6). Two main types of prostheses are noninflatable and inflatable.

NONINFLATABLE PROSTHESIS

These consist of paired semirigid or malleable rods that are inserted into the corpora cavernosa (Fig.

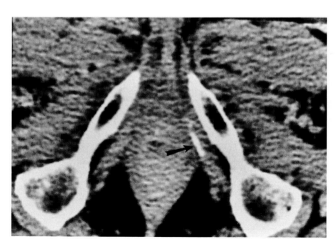

Figure 23–4. Calcified plaque in the left crus in a patient with Peyronie's disease.

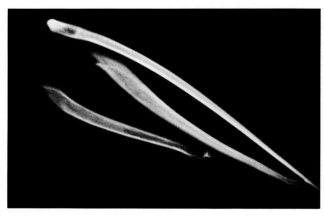

Figure 23–6. Penile bone radiographs of deer (top), wolf (middle), and bear (bottom). These served as inspirations to urologists in the development of penile prostheses.

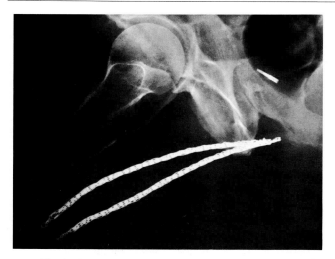

Figure 23–7. Jonas malleable penile prosthesis.

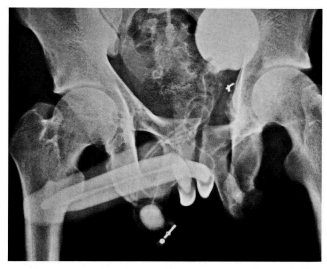

Figure 23–8. Inflatable penile prosthesis. Manual operation of the pump in the right hemiscrotum transfers fluid from extraperitoneal reservoir (top left) into a pair of cylinders. Extensive old healed fractures are also present, suggesting severe trauma as a possible cause for impotence.

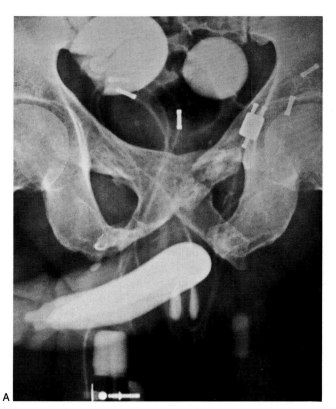

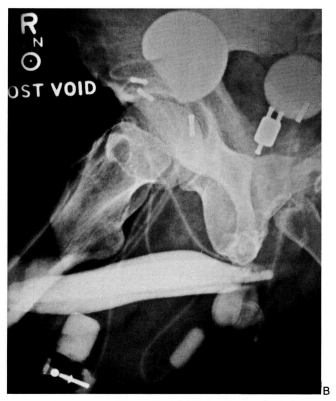

A

B

Figure 23–9. Both an inflatable penile prosthesis and an anti-incontinence prosthesis are present **(A)**. Evaluation as to the cause of malfunctioning prosthesis may be that much more difficult because of overlapping hydraulic connecting tubing and reducing valves. It may be necessary to obtain one or two different projections to accomplish this task **(B)**. This patient also has evidence of old healed fractures.

23–7). There are many manufacturers. The most comprehensive pictorial and radiographic atlas is found in Hovsepian and Amis.[7]

INFLATABLE PROSTHESIS

Unlike the semirigid prosthesis, the inflatable prosthesis is made rigid when erection is called for. This is accomplished by transferring fluid (usually isotonic contrast) from an extraperitoneal reservoir to inflatable cylinders in the corpora (Fig. 23–8).[8–11] Fluid transfer is accomplished via a palpable hydraulic intrascrotal pump and connecting tubing (Fig. 23–9).

In some types the scrotal pump also serves as the reservoir.

The newest inflatable prostheses are self-contained. Reservoir is at the proximal end of the single-cylinder prosthesis. Fluid transfer to the middle cylinder, which makes the prosthesis rigid, is accomplished via a pump in the distal end of the prosthesis.

MECHANICAL PROSTHESIS

Mechanical prostheses are made of plastic segments interconnected with a spring cable. Slight shortening of the cable tightens the plastic segments, making the prosthesis rigid.

Radiological Findings. Evaluation of a malfunctioning penile prosthesis requires pelvic radiography, usually in two different projections:

1. *Leaks.* Decreased amount of fluid (isotonic contrast) in reservoir is detected on pelvic radiograph (Fig. 23–10).[12] Leaks may occur anywhere in the closed hydraulic system (Fig. 23–11). Connecting tubing should be scrutinized, looking for separation.
2. *Aneurysmal dilatation.* May result in deviated and asymmetric erections and gradual loss of rigidity. Easily detected on pelvic radiograph (Fig. 23–12).
3. *Kinks.* Two projections may be needed to demonstrate a kink in the connecting tubing.

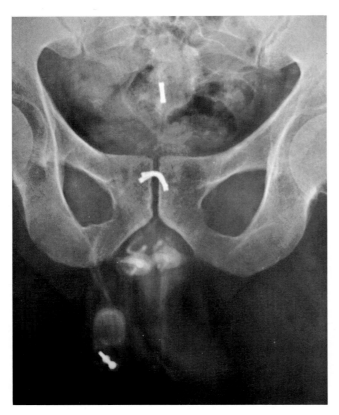

Figure 23–10. Empty system signifies a leak in the system. Contrast is reabsorbed from the soft tissues and is not detected.

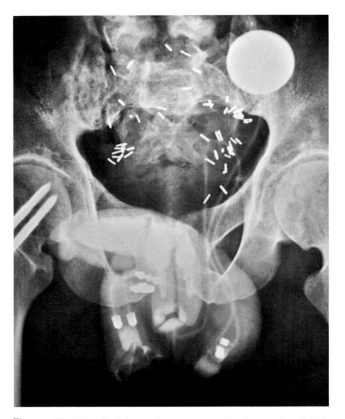

Figure 23–11. Anti-incontinence prosthesis on the left is intact. Inflatable penile prosthesis is partially empty, signifying a leak. The reservoir and the pump in this particular type of prosthesis are in the scrotum.

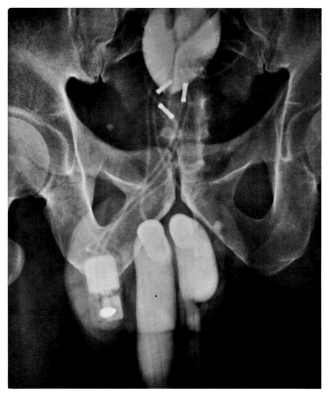

Figure 23–12. Incomplete dilatation of the distal end and aneurysmal dilatation of the proximal end of the left cylinder.

4. *Pump malfunction.* Should be suspected if cylinders and reservoir are normal and no kink is detected.

5. *Erosion.* Erosion results from ischemia, most likely caused by compression of the adjacent tissues by the prosthesis. Migration of the reservoir into adjacent organs[12–14] (bladder, ileal loop, sigmoid colon, and peritoneal cavity) may occur and

is difficult to diagnose unless it is clearly seen dislocated from its former position.

REFERENCES

1. Mayo Clinic health letter: Impotence in America. Rochester, MN: Mayo Clinic, May 1986:1–8.
2. Lue TF, Hricak H, Marich KW, Tanagho EA. Vasculogenic impotence evaluated by high resolution ultrasonography and pulsed Doppler spectrum analysis. Radiology 1985; 155:777–781.
3. Bookstein JJ, Valji K, Parsons L, Kessler W. Pharmacoarteriography in the evaluation of impotence. J Urol 1987; 137:333–337.
4. Schwartz AN, Freidenberg D, Harley JD. Nonselective angiography after intracorporeal papaverine injection: an alternative technique for evaluating penile arterial integrity. Radiology 1988; 167:249–253.
5. Bookstein JJ. Cavernosal venoocclusive insufficiency in male impotence: evaluation of degree and location. Radiology 1987; 164:175–178.
6. Bookstein JJ. Penile angiography: the last angiographic frontier. AJR 1988; 150:47–54.
7. Hovsepian DM, Amis ES. Penile prosthetic implants: a radiographic atlas. Radiographics 1989; 9:707–716.
8. Furlow WL, Goldwasser B, Gundian JC. Implantation of model AMS 700 penile prosthesis: long term results. J Urol 1988; 139:741–742.
9. Merill DC. Clinical experience with the Mentor inflatable penile prosthesis in 301 patients. J Urol 1988; 140:1424–1427.
10. Krane RJ. Penile prosthesis. Urol Clin North Am 1988; 15:103–109.
11. Kirschenbaum A, Mitty HA. Penile prosthesis. Urol Radiol 1988; 10:160–165.
12. Cohan RH, Dunnick NR, Carson CC. Radiology of penile prosthesis. AJR 1989; 152:925–931.
13. Furlow WL, Goldwasser B. Salvage of the eroded inflatable penile prosthesis: a new concept. J Urol 1987; 138:312–314.
14. Dupont MC, Hochman HI. Erosion of an inflatable penile prosthesis into the bladder, presenting as the bladder calculi. J Urol 1988; 139:367–368.

24

Scrotum

CONGENITAL ANOMALIES

Anorchism and Monorchism

Absence of one or both testes is rare and is included in the differential diagnosis of undescended testes. Testis is absent in 4% of patients in whom a testis cannot be palpated in the inguinal canal.

Undescended Testicle (Cryptorchidism)

Incidence. Premature neonates, 33%; full-term neonates, 3%; boys and young adults, 1%. Bilateral in 10%.

Clinical Presentation. In 80–90% of patients with empty scrotum or hemiscrotum testis is palpable in the inguinal canal. Incidence of malignancy is ten times the lifetime risk in normal men. The risk of malignancy is increased to the undescended testicle, to the undescended testicle after orchiopexy, and to the normally placed contralateral testis.

Treatment. Orchiopexy at 1 year of age. Orchiectomy between puberty and 32 years of age. Surgery is not indicated after 32 years of age.

Imaging Methods for Localization. There is a good argument for disproving any imaging techniques used for the purpose of localizing or even establishing the existence of an impalpable testicle.[1] All imaging modalities have unacceptably low sensitivity in determining whether a high undescended testicle is present, or if an impalpable testicle is entirely absent. The surgical approach is therefore not influenced by imaging. Most surgeons will explore the inguinal canal and continue exploration until the testicle is found or proved absent.

Others believe MR imaging is the method of choice.[2,3] The testicle is isointense (gray) to the soft tissues on T1-weighted sequence and hyperintense (bright) on T2-weighted images. With this imaging modality, it is possible to identify a low-lying undescended testis with a high degree of accuracy. Higher up in the abdominal cavity differentiation from loops of bowel may be difficult or impossible. Also, an atrophied testicle need not have very strong signal intensity on T2-weighted image. While this is a prognostic factor, it may interfere with recognition of the testis.

CT scanning is as good as MR imaging in locating a low-lying undescended testicle. There is a radiation dose to be concerned with. One should image the inguinal area first and, failing to see the testicle, proceed to examine the rest of the abdomen.[4,5]

Retrograde spermatic venography is an older method that is occasionally useful if everything else fails.[6,7] This examination depends on identifying the plexus pampiniformis, which even in an undescended testicle remains in close proximity to the organ.

Ultrasound may be used for initial detection of the testis in the inguinal canal but is otherwise unreliable.[8]

Imaging Methods for Follow-Up. Because of increased incidence of testicular malignancy, the undescended testicle in patients over 32 years of age should be periodically imaged. The frequency with which this should be carried out has not been determined.

Ultrasound should be used to periodically image the testis after orchiopexy as well as the normal contralateral testicle. The incidence of malignancy is increased in both.

CT is the imaging method of choice for staging and follow-up imaging should malignancy develop.[1]

448

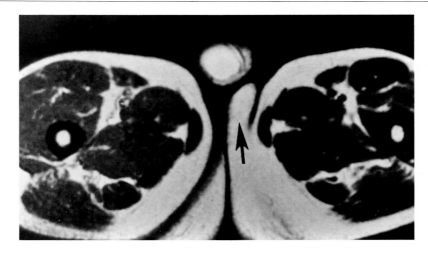

Figure 24–1. T2-weighted sequence in a patient with empty left hemiscrotum and impalpable testicle. High signal intensity right testicle is in the scrotum. Ectopic testicle is in the soft tissues of the perineum (arrow).

Ectopic Testicle

Ectopia must be considered in differential diagnosis of the undescended testis. Common ectopic sites are femoral triangle and perineum (Fig. 24–1). Ectopic testicle is usually readily diagnosed on physical examination.

Scrotal Transposition

A rare anomaly. Scrotum may be located anterior to the phallus (Fig. 24–2). Frequently associated with hypospadia.[9,10]

Polyorchidism

Supernumerary testes are rare and of no particular clinical significance. However, they should not be confused with a neoplasm. Ultrasound and MR imaging are excellent methods of diagnosis.[11,12] The testes, tunica albuginea, and epididymis are readily identified.

Cystic Dysplasia

This is a rare anomaly. On ultrasound, a cystic mass or testicular enlargement is present. Small cysts from 2 to 8 mm are present in the rete testis.[13] Renal agenesis or dysplasia may be associated findings.

EXTRATESTICULAR PATHOLOGICAL CONDITIONS

Fluid Collections

Hydrocele. A simple hydrocele is an abnormal collection of serous fluid in the tunica vaginalis. An infantile hydrocele is a collection of fluid in the funicular process that failed to close.

Fluid is either the result of overproduction or poor reabsorption. The hydrocele may be a reaction to an inflammatory process in the testicle or the epididymis.

Pyocele. A pyocele is an infected hydrocele.

Spermatocele. A spermatocele is an abnormal collection of proteinaceous fluid that contains immobile spermatocytes. Its cause is obstruction to the sperm flow, usually in the epididymis at the globus major (head), and is a common finding after vasectomy.

Hematocele. Hemorrhage in the tunica vaginalis may be spontaneous (diabetes, neoplasm) or post-traumatic (blunt trauma, surgery, birth injury).

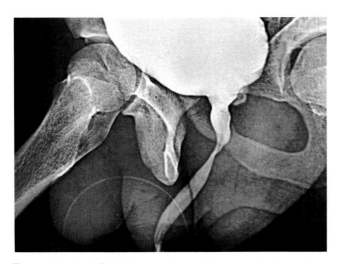

Figure 24–2. VCUG in a patient with scrotal transposition. Scrotum is seen anterior to the urethra.

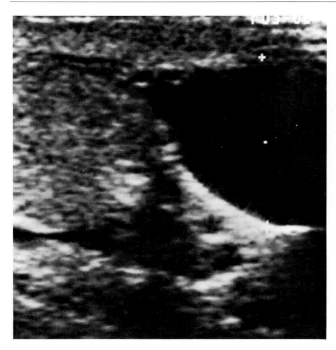

Figure 24–3. Anechoic large left hydrocele. (Photograph courtesy of D. Choe.)

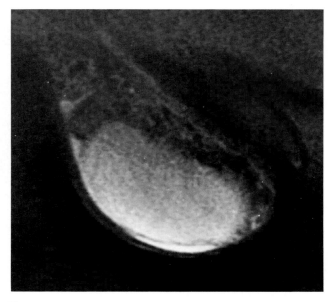

Figure 24–4. T2-weighted sequence using surface coil. Testicle is seen in the sagittal plane. A small high signal hydrocele is seen as a crescent just below the testicle. Note epididymis at the posterior surface of the testicle.

Imaging Modalities. Sonography is the method of choice in the initial evaluation of a hydrocele or other fluid collections.[14,15] The presence of fluid is easily established in ambiguous cases (Figs. 24–3, 24–4). Detection of an underlying cause such as an impalpable neoplasm or inflammatory disease is common. Infected hydroceles and hematoceles may contain numerous internal echoes that can shift and be seen floating and changing with changes in the patient's position, or may contain septa and loculi.

On MR imaging, the hydrocele has low signal intensity on T1- and high signal intensity on T2-weighted images (Fig. 24–5).[16,17] Depending on age, hemorrhagic fluid is usually of high signal intensity (bright) on both imaging sequences. Infected hydrocele may appear as a nonuniform mass.

Scrotal Calculi (Scrotal Pearl)

Scrotal calculi are calcified loose bodies in the tunica vaginalis and are extremely rare. They form either from fibrinous debris following inflammation of the tunica vaginalis or from the torsion of the appendix

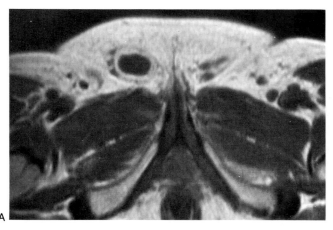

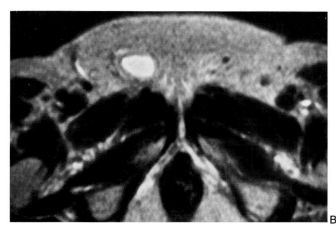

Figure 24–5. T1- **(A)** and T2-weighted **(B)** sequences demonstrate ascites extending into the funicular process.

testis. If sufficiently calcified, they may be identified on CT or plain radiograph. Sonography will demonstrate the calculus within a hydrocele.[18,19]

ACUTE SCROTUM

Testicular Torsion

Types. *Intravaginal torsion:* torsion of the testicle within the tunica vaginalis.

Extravaginal torsion: a testis and tunica vaginalis both turn, twisting the spermatic cord.

Incidence. Intravaginal torsion is most common in adolescents from 12 to 18 years of age, but can occur at any age. Extravaginal torsion is primarily a disease of newborns and represents only 6% of all torsions. At the time of diagnosis, the torsion is bilateral in 5% of patients.

Etiology. Capacious tunica vaginalis, which more completely envelops the testis than usual, is what permits intravaginal torsion. Loose attachment of the tunica vaginalis to the scrotum permits development of extravaginal torsion.

Pathology. The vascular supply to the testicle is interrupted. First venous occlusion causes enlargement and passive venous stasis, followed by interruption of arterial flow and ischemic necrosis. Extratesticular hemorrhage may be present.[20]

Clinical Presentation. *Intravaginal torsion* may be insidious, over several hours, or acute after strenuous exercise. Groin pain, increasing in severity, is the principal complaint. Testis is swollen and tender. Scrotum may become red and edematous. Elevation of testicle does not relieve pain; on the contrary, it may actuate more pain. Testis may be in a higher than normal position.

Extravaginal torsion in neonates is relatively asymptomatic. Relatively nontender hard mass is palpated.

Treatment. Immediate surgical intervention.

Radiological Findings. The principal indication for imaging in this condition is to confirm torsion and exclude other causes of acute testicular pain, such as epididymitis, epididymo-orchitis, or torsion of the appendix testis or appendix epididymis. Imaging, of course, is unnecessary if the clinical findings are clear-cut. In many instances, however, clinical presentation is unclear. If imaging studies are contemplated, they must be performed within a reason-able period of time. Salvage rate is high 2 to 6 hours after onset of symptoms but decreases to less than 20% after 12 hours. Differentiation from acute inflammatory disease and hernia is not always possible.[21]

Radionuclide scintigraphy using an intravenous bolus of Tc-99m-pertechnetate is the imaging modality of choice.[22] A dose between 3 and 7 mCi is adjusted to body weight. Normal perfusion of the testes is present in cases of epididymitis, while hypoperfusion of the affected side is expected in cases of testicular torsion. One should keep in mind that the study is not always accurate. An abscessed epididymo-orchitis, for instance, may also exhibit hypoperfusion.[23]

Sonography may demonstrate generalized testicular hyperechogenicity.[24] Color flow duplex sonography may have an important role in the future, and so may MR imaging.[25]

Torsion of the Appendix Testis and Appendix Epididymis

Torsion of appendix testis or appendix epididymis may present with similar symptoms and physical findings as those of patients with torsion. In some instances radionuclide imaging may provide a clue as to the diagnosis.[26] Testicular perfusion is unaffected and the process is self-limiting (Fig. 24–6).

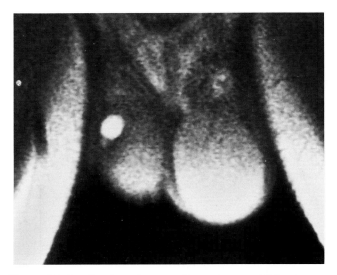

Figure 24–6. Torsion of appendix testis or epididymis was the clinical diagnosis. T1-weighted sequence in the coronal plane demonstrates a high signal lesion a few millimeters in diameter in the region of the head of the right epididymis.

Epididymitis

Incidence. Common in adults.

Etiology. Unknown (nonspecific), trauma, reflux in vas deferens during straining and micturition, *E. coli, Neisseria gonorrhoeae.* Rarely, *Treponema pallidum* and *Mycobacterium tuberculosis.*

Clinical Presentation. Pain, tenderness, and enlargement of the epididymis. Pain may be eased by elevating the testicle. Pyuria may be present while massaging the prostate. Must be differentiated from testicular torsion and orchitis. Commonly induces a hydrocele.

Radiological Findings. There is rarely a need for imaging. Differentiation from other diseases causing acute scrotum, particularly testicular torsion, is the primary goal of imaging. Duplex ultrasound may demonstrate normal pulsatile flow through the testicle, but, more importantly, an enlarged epididymis or a part thereof implies an extratesticular process (Fig. 24–7).[27–30]

BENIGN INTRASCROTAL MASSES

Hyperechoic Tumors

Benign tumors or tumorlike conditions that usually appear hyperechoic on sonography are spermatic granuloma, benign mesothelioma, lipoma, and ade-

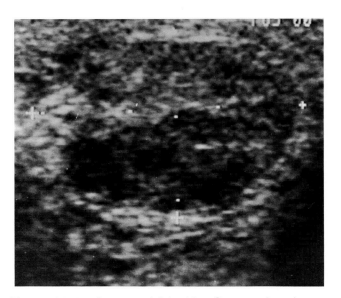

Figure 24–7. Acute epididymitis. Sonography demonstrates an enlarged epididymis. (Photograph courtesy of D. Choe.)

nomatoid tumors of the epididymis, testicular tunic, and spermatic cord.[31–33]

Testicular Cyst

Cysts may originate from the tunica albuginea or rete testis. Those originating from the tunica albuginea are usually palpable. The rete testis cysts are located in the mediastinum testis and may not be palpable on physical examination. Benign cysts are hypoechoic and exhibit through transmission.[34,35] There should be no septations, internal echoes, or filling defects. They may be differentiated from cystic testicular neoplasms by employing these criteria together with a thorough physical examination and reasonable follow-up examinations. Some may be confused with markedly hypoechoic seminoma.

Epididymal Cyst

Epididymal cyst is seen as an extratesticular hypoechoic mass and should be readily differentiated from intratesticular pathology.

Vasectomy—Postoperative Findings

After vasectomy, 45% of patients have persistent changes in the epididymis. These consist of enlargement, cysts, and an inhomogeneous echo pattern. These findings are usually not associated with symptoms.[36]

MALIGNANT TESTICULAR TUMORS

Incidence. The most common cancer in late adolescents and young adults. May occur at any age, including infants and males over 50 years of age. Relatively rare in blacks. Represents 1 to 2% of all malignant diseases in men.

Etiology. Unknown. Carcinogens, trauma, undescended testicle, inflammatory disease, and familial predisposition have been implicated.

Pathology. Testicular malignancies are either a mix of germ cell or stromal tumors (Table 24–1).

Clinical Presentation. Usually painless but sometimes painful (5%) testicular mass is detected by patient or examining physician. Palpable lymph node metastases in the supraclavicular region or abdomen may be the first presenting symptom.

Table 24-1. Pathological Classification of Testicular Malignant Neoplasms

A. Germ cell tumors
  1. Seminoma comprises 50% of all testicular tumors
  2. Nonseminomatous tumors are:
    a. Teratocarcinoma (teratoma and embryonal carcinoma), 20 to 30%
    b. Embryonal carcinoma, 20% of all testicular tumors
    c. Teratoma, 5 to 10% of all testicular tumors
    d. Choriocarcinoma. Rare
    e. Mixed choriocarcinoma and embryonal carcinoma, 3%
B. Stromal tumors
  Leydig cell tumor, Sertoli cell tumor, and gonadoblastoma are all rare
C. Others
  Primary carcinoid, plasmocytoma, and metastases

Weight loss and pulmonary symptoms are seen with mediastinal and lung metastases. Gynecomastia may be present (Leydig cell).

Laboratory Findings. Elevated serum markers alpha-fetoprotein (AFP) and beta human chorionic gonadotropin (β-hCG) are present in 60 to 70% of patients with nonseminomatous carcinoma at staging. Elevated serum markers are also found in about the same percentage in patients with recurrent tumor.

Serum markers are generally not elevated in pure seminoma.

Staging. Staging is local and clinical (Table 24–2).

Imaging of Scrotal Contents. Most testicular tumors, but not all,[37] are palpable and require no direct imaging. A firm testicular mass is explored. Imaging is used when diagnosis of an intratesticular mass and differentiation from an extratesticular lesion is uncertain. Sonography is the examination of choice.

Table 24-2. Local and Clinical Stages of Testicular Malignant Neoplasms

Local staging	
Stage T0	No evidence for primary tumor
Stage T1	Confined to the testis
Stage T2	Extends beyond tunica albuginea
Stage T3	Involves rete testis or epididymis
Stage T4a	Invades spermatic cord
Stage T4b	Invades scrotal wall
Clinical staging	
Stage I	Confined to the testis
Stage II	Retroperitoneal lymph node metastases
Stage III	Supradiaphragmatic node metastases or retroperitoneal/supradiaphragmatic node metastases
Stage IV	Metastases to parenchymal organs

Intratesticular mass can be easily differentiated from extratesticular masses, such as epididymitis, hydrocele, spermatocele, and scrotal calculi.

Almost all testicular tumors are moderately to mildly hypoechoic in comparison to normal testicles. Seminomas in particular tend to be moderately hypoechoic.[38,39] Very few nonseminomatous tumors may be isoechoic or even somewhat hyperechoic to the surrounding parenchyma. While seminomas tend to be relatively homogeneous, nonseminomatous tumors tend to be more inhomogeneous. The majority of nonseminomatous tumors may have some cystic components, particularly teratocarcinomas. Also in nonseminomatous tumors bright echogenic foci are frequently seen in the presence of focal calcification, immature bone elements, cartilage, and scarring.

On MR imaging, testicular tumors demonstrate a spectrum of findings. Usually testicular neoplasms exhibit lower signal and appear somewhat darker compared with the surrounding normal testicular parenchyma on T2-weighted images (Fig. 24–8).[40–43]

For intrascrotal staging of testicular tumors, both ultrasound and MR imaging are disappointing, but in no way influence management.[44] Surgical explo-

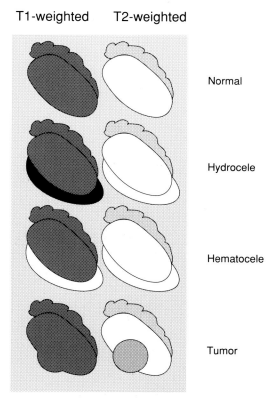

T1-weighted   T2-weighted

Normal

Hydrocele

Hematocele

Tumor

Figure 24–8. Schematic drawing of normal testicle, hydrocele, hematocele, and testicular tumor on spin echo sequences.

ration by the inguinal approach is required regardless of the local tumor stage.

Imaging Staging for Extrascrotal Disease. CT imaging is the examination of choice for staging purposes (Fig. 24–9).[45,46] One centimeter contiguous slices through the pelvis, abdomen, and thorax will demonstrate most enlarged lymph nodes.[47,48] Unfortunately, a pathological lymph node may be diagnosed only if it is enlarged. Small metastatic deposits are unrecognized. In general, if the lymph node is larger than 1 cm in any diameter, it is considered pathological. Inflammatory lymph node enlargement cannot be differentiated from malignant enlargement. Other organs may harbor metastases as well (Fig. 24–10). Overall accuracy of CT staging is around 80%.

In at least one study abdominal lymph node enlargement could be readily detected by ultrasound.[49] Using the 1 cm criterion, overall accuracy of this staging procedure was 96% and positive predictive value was 100%.

Imaging for Follow-Up and Detection of Recurrence. CT is the imaging modality of choice. CT is better than plain chest radiography, excretory urography, or lymphangiography for detecting recurrence either in the retroperitoneum, mediastinum, or lungs (Fig. 24–11). In combination with elevated β-hCG, AFP, and CT imaging, most, if not all, recurrent disease in nonseminomatous tumors is discovered.[50]

Radiopaque testicular prosthesis may be discovered (Fig. 24–12) and, depending on the type of prosthesis, varying MR signal characteristics will be encountered.

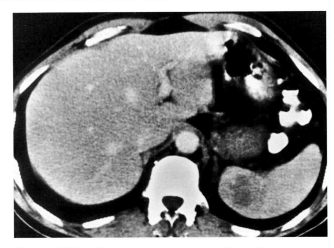

Figure 24–10.   Splenic metastasis in patient with seminoma.

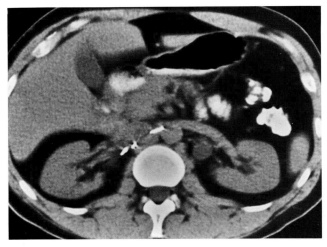

Figure 24–11.   Recurrence of testicular carcinoma in a retroperitoneal lymph node just posterior to the left renal vein some time after lymphadenectomy.

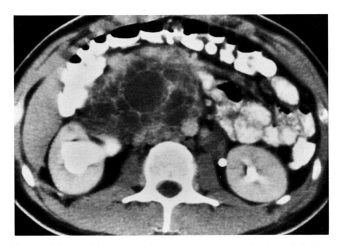

Figure 24–9.   Mature testicular teratoma metastatic into the retroperitoneum.

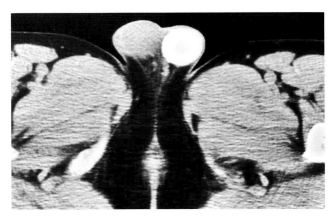

Figure 24–12.   Testicular prothesis.

TESTICULAR LEUKEMIA AND LYMPHOMA

Testicular involvement by lymphoma and leukemia is usually seen in the generalized form of the disease. Testes are usually enlarged due to diffuse infiltration by the lymphoma cells. On ultrasound examination, the areas of infiltration are seen as hypoechoic areas compared to the normal testicular tissues.[51,52] Diffuse infiltration may present difficulties in appreciating widespread echogenicity.

SCROTAL VARICOCELE

Definition. *Clinical varicocele* is dilatation of plexus pampiniformis which is palpable in the upright position. *Subclinical varicocele* cannot be palpated and is diagnosed by other means, usually by sonography, Doppler sonography, or retrograde spermatic vein venography.

Incidence. Clinical varicocele is found in up to 17% of fertile males and in up to 40% of infertile males. Subclinical varicocele is found in up to 44% of fertile males.[53] While by far more common on the left side, right and bilateral varicoceles are present in a substantial number of men (Fig. 24–13).

Pathology. Defective and incompetent valves of the spermatic veins allow development of abnormal dilatation of the plexus pampiniformis under increased hydrostatic pressure.

Effect on Spermatogenesis. Varicocele appears to be more common in males with impaired spermatogenesis and infertility. Increased scrotal temperature in the presence of varicocele and other factors have been implicated as the cause of impaired spermato-

genesis. Sixty to 80% of those with varicocele and impaired spermatogenesis show improvement in their semen quality following surgical ligation, and 30 to 55% of those undergoing ligation are likely to initiate pregnancy. Eleven percent of surgically corrected varicoceles recur.

Since subclinical varicocele is so common in fertile men, its effect on spermatogenesis is at best questionable.[53]

Radiological Findings. Most varicoceles are readily apparent on physical examination. Imaging may be indicated when the varicocele is the suspected cause of impaired spermatogenesis and yet is not apparent on physical examination (subclinical varicocele). Imaging is indispensable in determining the exact site of recanalization following unsuccessful surgery.

Venography used to be the imaging method and served as "the gold standard." Sonography may detect the dilated venous structures, particularly if the examination is performed in the upright position (Fig. 24–14). Duplex Doppler may become the examination of choice.[54] Thermography and MR imaging are of passing interest (Fig. 24–15).

Varicocele may be graded, depending on the extent of retrograde flow in the spermatic vein as seen on venography or Doppler sonography.[54] The vessel is usually enlarged, several parallel channels are identified and dilated, and tortuous pampiniform plexus of veins is identified. Cross-connection with the opposite hemiscrotum is unusual.

Treatment. Surgical ligation and transcatheter venous occlusion are two competing treatment methods. Retrograde venography is necessary to evaluate causes for surgical failure (Fig. 24–16). There are several different angiographic techniques, but basically occlusion of the spermatic vein is achieved by depositing a detachable balloon, steel

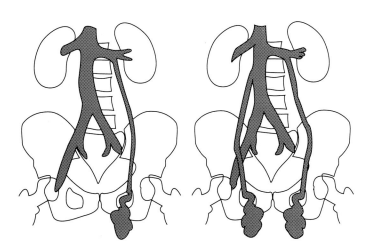

Figure 24–13. Schematic drawing of left and bilateral varicocele.

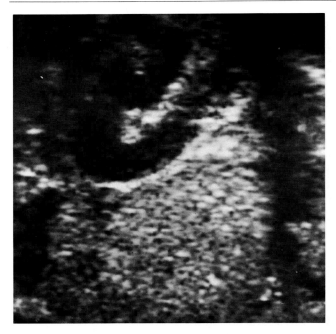

Figure 24–14. Spermatic vein varicocele seen adjacent to the normal testicle.

coil, sclerosing agent, or even hot contrast into the lower part of the spermatic vein.[55–61] Care is exercised to include all visible parallel collateral channels and thus prevent recurrence. Occlusive material should be placed above the inguinal ligament so that it does not interfere with venous outflow from the varicocele via cremasteric and inferior epigastric vein. The procedure is performed on an outpatient basis and the patient may resume normal activity the following day. Results appear to be as good as with surgical ligation (Fig. 24–17).[62]

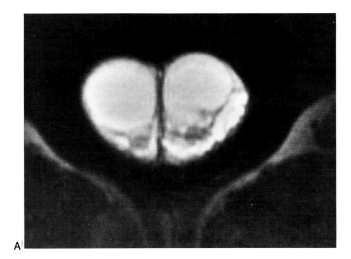

A

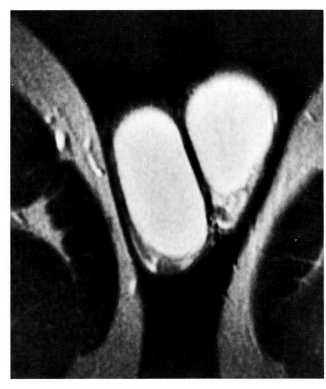

B

Figure 24–15. (A) Large left spermatic vein varicocele seen on T2-weighted sequence appears of high signal intensity. (B) Normal scrotum on same sequence is given for comparison.

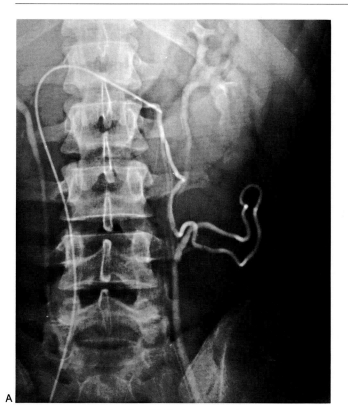
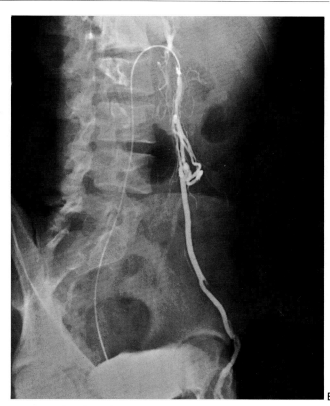

Figure 24–16. **(A)** Left spermatic venogram demonstrates recanalization of the vessel via a large retroperitoneal collateral. **(B)** LPO projection.

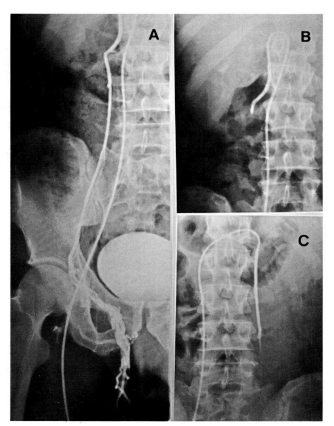

Figure 24–17. **(A)** Right spermatic varicocele before and **(B)** after transcatheter occlusion. **(C)** Left spermatic venogram demonstrates a competent valve and no evidence of a varicocele.

REFERENCES

1. Friedland GW, Chang P. The role of imaging in the management of impalpable undescended testis. AJR 1988; 151:1107–1111.
2. Kier R, McCarthy S, Rosenfield AT, et al. Nonpalpable testis in young boys: evaluation with MR imaging. Radiology 1988; 169:429–433.
3. Fritzsche PJ, Hricak H, Kogan BA, et al. Undescended testis: value of MR imaging. Radiology 1987; 164:169–173.
4. Wolverson MK, Houttuin E, Heiberg E, et al. Comparison of computed tomography with high resolution real-time ultrasound in localization of the impalpable undescended testis. Radiology 1983; 146:133–136.
5. Lee JKT, McClennan BL, Stanley RJ, Sagel SS. Utility of computed tomography in the localization of the undescended testis. Radiology 1980; 135:121–125.
6. Glickman MG, Weis RM, Itzchak Y. Testicular venography for undescended testes. AJR 1977; 129:67–70.
7. Weis RM, Glickman MG. Venography of the undescended testicle. Urol Clin North Am 1982; 9:387–395.
8. Weis RM, Carter AR, Rosenfield AT. High-resolution real-time ultrasonography in the localization of the undescended testis. J Urol 1986; 135:936–938.
9. Yamaguchi T, Hamasuna R, Hasui Y, et al. 47,XXY/48,XXY,+21 chromosomal mosaicism presenting as hypospadias with scrotal transposition. J Urol 1989; 142:797–798.
10. Nonomura K, Koyanagi T, Imanaka K, et al. One-stage total repair of severe hypospadias with scrotal transposition: experience in 18 cases. J Pediatr Surg 1988; 23:177–180.
11. Baker LL, Hajek PC, Burkhard TK, et al. Polyorchidism: evaluation by MR. AJR 1987; 148:305–306.
12. Goldberg RM, Chilcote W, Kay R, et al. Sonographic findings in polyorchidism. JCU 1987; 15:412–413.
13. Cho CS, Kosek J. Cystic dysplasia of the testis: sonographic and pathologic findings. Radiology 1985; 156:777–778.
14. Leopold GR, Woo VL, Scheible FW, et al. High resolution ultrasonography of scrotal pathology. Radiology 1979; 131:719–722.
15. Carroll BA, Gross DM. High frequency scrotal sonography. AJR 1983; 140:511–515.
16. Baker LL, Hajek PC, Burkhard TK, et al. MR imaging of the scrotum: normal anatomy. Radiology 1987; 163:89–92.
17. Baker LL, Hajek PC, Burkhard TK, et al. MR imaging of the scrotum: Pathologic conditions. Radiology 1987; 163:93–98.
18. Linkiwski GD, Avellone A, Gooding GAW. Scrotal calculi: sonographic detection. Radiology 1985; 156:484.
19. Doherty FJ, Mullins TL, Sant GR, et al. Testicular microlithiasis: unique sonographic appearance. J Ultrasound Med 1987; 6:389–391.
20. Vick CW, Bird K, Rosenfield AT, et al. Extratesticular hemorrhage associated with torsion of the spermatic cord: sonographic demonstration. Radiology 1986; 158:401–403.
21. Wood MJ. Hernia mimicking testicular torsion. Clin Nucl Med 1987; 12:142–144.
22. Dunn EK, Macchia RJ, Chauhan PS, et al. Scintiscan for acute intrascrotal conditions. Clin Nucl Med 1986; 11:381–386.
23. Vieras F. Evolution of acute epididymitis to testicular infarction: scintigraphic demonstration. Clin Nucl Med 1986; 11:158–161.
24. Chinn DH, Miller EI. Generalized testicular hyperechogenicity in acute testicular torsion. J Ultrasound Med 1985; 4:495–497.
25. Bretan PN Jr, Vigneron DB, Hricak H, et al. Assessment of testicular metabolic integrity with P-31 MR spectroscopy. Radiology 1987; 162:867–870.
26. Fischman AJ, Palmer EL, Scott JA. Radionuclide imaging of sequential torsions of the appendix testis. J Nucl Med 1987; 28:119–121.
27. Doble A, Taylor-Robinson D, Thomas BJ, et al. Acute epididymitis: a microbiological and ultrasonographic study. Br J Urol 1989; 63:90–94.
28. See WA, Mack LA, Krieger JN. Scrotal ultrasonography: a predictor of complicated epididymitis requiring orchiectomy. J Urol 1988; 139:55–56.
29. Archer A, Choyke PL, O'Brien W, et al. Scrotal enlargement following inguinal herniorrhaphy: ultrasound evaluation. Urol Radiol 1988; 9:249–252.
30. Martin B, Conte J. Ultrasonography of the acute scrotum. JCU 1987; 15:37–44.
31. Aquino NM, Vazquez R, Matari H. Ultrasound demonstration of benign mesothelioma of tunica vaginalis testis. JCU 1986; 14:310–311.
32. Ramanathan K, Yaghoobian J, Pinck RL. Sperm granuloma. JCU 1986; 14:155–157.
33. Hertzberg BS, Mahony BS, Bowie JD, et al. Sonography of an intratesticular lipoma. J Ultrasound Med 1985; 4:617–619.
34. Gooding GAW, Leonhardt W, Stein R. Testicular cysts: US findings. Radiology 1987; 163:537–538.
35. Hamm B, Fobbe F, Loy V. Testicular cysts: differentiation with US and clinical findings. Radiology 1988; 168:19–23.
36. Jarvis LJ, Dubbins PA. Changes in the epididymis after vasectomy: sonographic findings. AJR 1989; 152:531–534.
37. Stoll S, Goldfinger M, Rothberg R, et al. Incidental detection of impalpable testicular neoplasm by sonography. AJR 1986; 146:349–353.
38. Grantham JG, Charboneau JW, James EM, et al. Testicular neoplasms studied by high-resolution US. Radiology 1985; 157:775–779.
39. Schwimer SR, Jacobson E, Lebovic J. Seminoma in a atrophic testis: ultrasound evaluation. J Ultrasound Med 1987; 6:97–99.
40. Seidenwurm D, Smathers RL, Lo RK, et al. Testes and scrotum: MR imaging at 1.5T. Radiology 1987; 164:393–396.
41. Baker LL, Hajek PC, Burkhard TK, et al. MR imaging of the scrotum: normal anatomy. Radiology 1987; 163:89–92.
42. Baker LL, Hejek PC, Burkhard TK, Dicapua L, Landa HM, Leopold GR, Hesselink JR, Mattrey RF. MR imaging of the scrotum: pathologic conditions. Radiology 1987; 163:93–97.
43. Rholl KS, Lee JKT, Ling D, Heiken JP, Glazer HS. MR imaging of the scrotum with a high-resolution surface coil. Radiology 1987; 163:99–103.
44. Thurnher S, Hricak H, Carroll PR, et al. Imaging the testis: comparison between MR imaging and US. Radiology 1988; 167:631–636.
45. Bradey N, Johnson RJ, Read G. Abdominal computed tomography in teratoma of the testis: its accuracy in

stage I disease and an assessment of the distribution of retroperitoneal lymph node metastases in other stages of the disease. Br J Radiol 1987; 60:487–491.

46. O'Brien WM, Choyke PL, Lynch JH, Zeman RK. Invasion of the inferior vena cava by testicular seminoma: demonstration by computed tomography and venography. Urol Radiol 1986; 8:108.

47. Williams MP, Husband JE, Heron CW. Stage I nonseminomatous germ cell tumors of the testis: radiologic follow-up after orchidectomy. Radiology 1987; 164:671–674.

48. Poskitt KJ, Cooperberg PL, Sullivan LD. Sonography and CT staging nonseminomatous testicular tumors. AJR 1985; 144:939–945.

49. Schwerk WB, Schwerk WN, Rodeck G. Testicular tumors: prospective analysis of real-time US patterns and abdominal staging. Radiology 1987; 164:369–374.

50. Stomper PC, Jochelson MS, Garnick MB, et al. Residual abdominal masses after chemotherapy for nonseminomatous testicular cancer: correlation of CT and histology. AJR 1985; 145:743–747.

51. Lupetin AR, King W III, Rich P, Lederman RB. Ultrasound diagnosis of testicular leukemia. Radiology 1983; 146:171–172.

52. Rayor RA, Scheible W, Brock WA, Leopold GR. High resolution ultrasonography in the diagnosis of testicular relapse in patients with acute lymphoblastic leukemia. J Urol 1982; 128:602–603.

53. Kursh ED. What is the incidence of varicocele in a fertile population? Fertil Steril 1987; 48:510–511.

54. Annoni F, Colpi GM, Marincola FM, Negri L. Doppler examination in varicocele. A standard method of evaluation. J Androl 1988; 9:248–252.

55. Marsman JWP. Clinical vs subclinical varicocele: venographic findings and improvement of fertility after embolization. Radiology 1985; 155:635–638.

56. White RI Jr, Kaufman SL, Barth KH, et al. Occlusion of varicoceles with detachable balloons. Radiology 1981; 139:327–334.

57. Sayferth W, et al. Percutaneous sclerotherapy of varicocele. Radiology 1981; 139:335–340.

58. Morag B, Rubinstein ZJ, Goldwasser B, et al. Percutaneous venography and occlusion in the management of spermatic varicoceles. AJR 1984; 143:635–640.

59. Shuman L, White RI Jr, Mitchell SE, et al. Right-sided varicocele: technique and clinical results of balloon embolotherapy from the femoral approach. Radiology 1986; 158:787–791.

60. Smith TP, Hunter DW, Cragg AH, et al. Spermatic vein embolization with hot contrast material: fertility results. Radiology 1988; 168:137–139.

61. Fobe F, Hamm B, Sorensen R, Felsenberg D. Percutaneous transluminal treatment of varicoceles: where to occlude internal spermatic vein. AJR 1987; 149:983–987.

62. Bach D, Bahren W, Gall H, Altwein JE. Late results after sclerotherapy of varicocele. Eur Urol 1988; 14:115–119.

25

Female Pelvis

UTERINE LEIOMYOMA

Incidence. Common. Large number of patients (35%) never become pregnant.

Pathology. Smooth muscle predominates. Sharply demarcated from surrounding myometrium by a pseudocapsule. Pseudocapsule is either areolar tissue or compressed myometrium. Frequently multiple and of varying size. May be complicated by intratumoral hemorrhage and hyaline degeneration. Heavy calcification is common. Sarcomatous malignant transformation is possible.

Clinical Presentation. Pelvic mass. May be a cause of decreased fertility and interfere with gestation and delivery.

Radiological Findings. Imaging is commonly done as a part of the routine workup of a newly found pelvic mass. Ultrasound is more than adequate for this purpose. If the imaging is done to assess the size and relative location of the tumor prior to myomectomy, MR appears to be the imaging modality of choice.

Because of high fibrous tissue content and occasional presence of calcification, these tumors are relatively hypointense to normal myometrium on T1- and T2-weighted sequences (Fig. 25–1).[1] If complicated by hemorrhage, varying signal intensities may be discovered (Fig. 25–2).[2] Leiomyomas may be submucosal, subserosal, or endocervical and they are frequently multiple (Fig. 25–3). Their size, location, and relation to the endometrial cavity are determined more accurately with MR imaging than with ultrasound, which may be of importance if myomectomy is considered.[3]

Because leiomyoma is well demarcated, differentiation from adenomyosis (see below) is highly accurate on MR.

On CT (Fig. 25–4) and plain radiograph (Fig. 25–5) pelvic masses may be discovered with or without heavy calcification. Hysterosalpingography will occasionally demonstrate a tumor projecting into the endometrial cavity (Fig. 25–6) or endocervical canal.

ADENOMYOSIS

Incidence. Common. Occurs during menstrual life.

Pathology. Benign invasion of the endometrium into the myometrium (endometrial islands, myome-

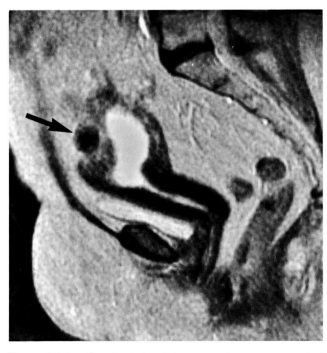

Figure 25–1. Small uterine leiomyoma is seen as a dark nodular mass at the fundus, which is well demarcated from myometrium (arrow) (T2-weighted sequence).

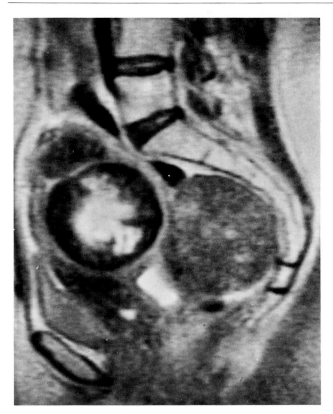

Figure 25–2. Several uterine leiomyomas are present. Hemorrhage in one of these is recognized as area of high signal intensity.

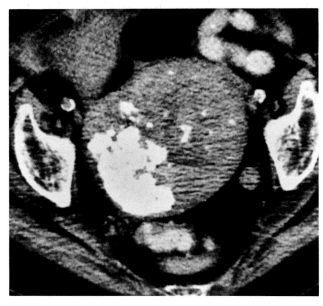

Figure 25–4. Heavily calcified uterine leiomyoma seen on CT.

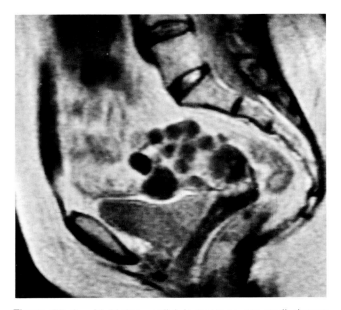

Figure 25–3. Multiple small leiomyomas are well demarcated and scattered throughout the uterus.

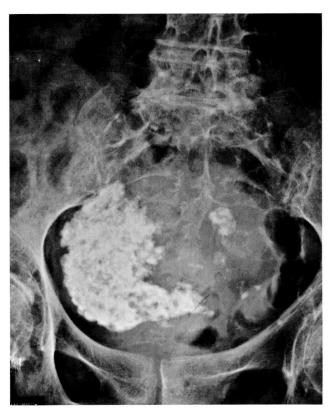

Figure 25–5. Heavily calcified uterine leiomyoma on plain radiograph.

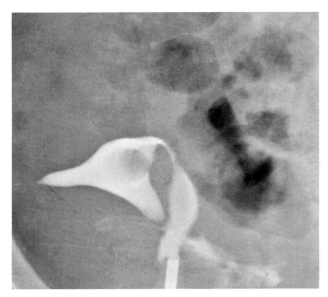

Figure 25–6. Small submucosal fibroid is seen as a filling defect within the contrast at hysterosalpingography. (Photograph courtesy of Dr. Barbara M. Kadell.)

trial endometriosis), promoting diffuse overgrowth and condensation of the smooth muscle in the area. Unlike leiomyomas, there is no pseudocapsule and no demarcation with normal myometrium.

Clinical Presentation. Dysmenorrhea and menorrhagia.

Treatment. Unlike leiomyoma, which in some instances may be treated by myomectomy, adenomyosis requires hysterectomy. Differentiating these two entities is important if myomectomy is planned.

Radiological Findings. MR is the imaging modality of choice. The bulk of the mass lesion is of relatively low signal intensity equal to that of junctional zone. The differentiating finding from leiomyoma is in that the leiomyoma has a very distinct and well-demarcated border with the myometrium while adenomyosis does not.[4-6] Within the mass bright areas representing small islands of endometrium may be detected. If functional bleeding occurs within the islands, these appear hyperintense on both T1- and T2-weighted sequences.

Diagnosis by sonography may be difficult.[7,8]

CERVICAL CARCINOMA

Etiology. Human papillary virus (HPV) is implicated. Smoking.

Incidence. In the United States there are 14,000 new cases and 7,000 deaths per year. More common in sexually active women with multiple partners. Rare in those sexually inactive.

Pathology. Squamous cell carcinoma, locally invasive. Adenocarcinoma is less common.

Treatment. Treatment depends on tumor volume and stage of the disease.[9] Radiation therapy, surgery, or both may be used for stage I and limited stage IIA disease.[10] For more advanced stages, radiation therapy is the method of choice. Determining parametrial extension (stage IIB) is important, as are assessment of the lymph nodes and presence of ureteral obstruction.[11,12]

Staging. FIGO staging classification (Fig. 25–7, Table 25–1).

MR Imaging. Because the cervix is mostly composed of connective tissues, it is of low signal intensity (dark) on T2-weighted sequences. Relatively high signal intensity (bright) carcinoma of the cervix is readily apparent on this sequence. Unlike CT imaging where it is difficult to differentiate the tumor from normal uterus, the precise tumor volume is clearly apparent on MR. Parametrial involvement is also recognizable, as is invasion of the bladder wall.[11] Perhaps more important is high predictve value of MR imaging for determining the absence of bladder, parametrial (Fig. 25–8), or vaginal involvement.

Overall staging accuracy of MR imaging is reported to be 81%; accuracy for determination of vaginal extension, 93%; and parametrial extension, 88%.[11]

CT Imaging. CT is perhaps better than MR in demonstrating hydronephrosis, hydroureter, and lymph node enlargement (Fig. 25–9).[13,14] Recurrence is also usually obvious (Fig. 25–10), as is invasion of the pelvic wall (Fig. 25–11). Biopsy under CT control may be indispensable (Fig. 25–12). Skeletal involvement is usually by local extension (Fig. 25–13).

ENDOMETRIAL CARCINOMA

Incidence. Fourth most common malignancy in females.

Predisposing Factors. Obesity, hypertension, diabetes, late menopause, nulliparity. Patients with endometrial cancer are at increased risk of developing breast cancer.

AXIAL PLANES   SAGITTAL PLANE

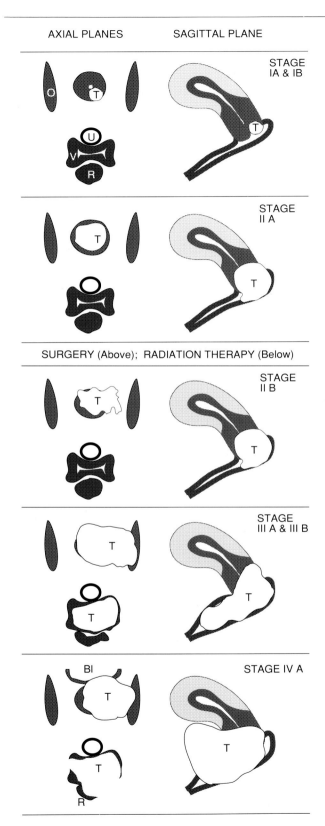

STAGE IA & IB

STAGE II A

SURGERY (Above); RADIATION THERAPY (Below)

STAGE II B

STAGE III A & III B

STAGE IV A

Figure 25–7. Cervical carcinoma. Schematic drawing of various stages of the disease as it may be seen on MR imaging using T2-weighted sequences.

Table 25–1. FIGO Staging of Cervical Carcinoma*

Stage	0	Carcinoma in situ
Stage	IA	Preclinical carcinoma confined to the cervix
	IB	Confined to cervix (may extend to uterus)
Stage	IIA	Extension into the upper vagina. No parametrial involvement
	IIB	Parametrial involvement and/or extension into the upper vagina
Stage	IIIA	Extension to the lower third of the vagina
	IIIB	Extension to the pelvic wall and/or hydronephrosis
Stage	IVA	Spread to the adjacent organs (rectum, bladder)
	IVB	Spread to distant organs

*From American Joint Commmitee on Cancer.[9]

Staging.   FIGO staging classification (Fig. 25–14, Table 25–2).

Radiological Findings.   On MR imaging, the uterus is usually enlarged and endometrial cavity expanded. Endometrial cavity is filled with high signal intensity endometrium or endometrial secretions. Carcinoma is seen as variously sized nodules of intermediate signal intensity (gray) within the cavity.

Because endometrial cavity is so well visualized, particularly on T2-weighted sequences, endometrial carcinoma may be detected in 84% of cases.[15,16]

Endometrial carcinoma cannot be differentiated from adenomatous hyperplasia or blood clots, however. These may also appear as intermediate signal intensity (gray) lesions within the endometrial cav-

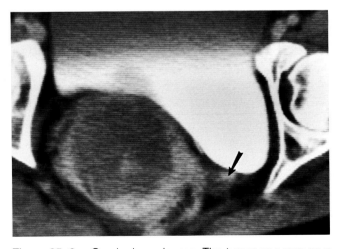

Figure 25–8. Cervical carcinoma. The tumor appears as a low density mass expanding the cervix. To the left it is difficult to determine whether there is extension into the parametrium (arrow). Under these circumstances MR imaging appears to be the superior imaging modality.

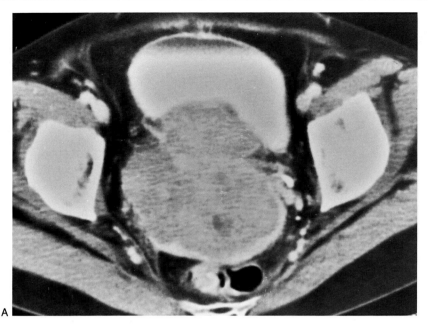

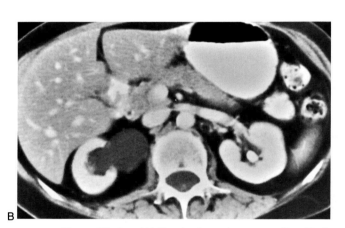

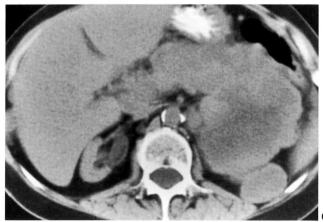

Figure 25–9. **(A)** Cervical carcinoma confined to the pelvis is seen as a large inhomogeneous mass. **(B)** At the same time, hydronephrosis of the left kidney is discovered but otherwise there is no evidence for nodal involvement. **(C)** Months later a CT slice at the same level demonstrates huge retroperitoneal metastases involving the lymph nodes, pancreas, and left adrenal.

ity. Histological diagnosis following curettage is therefore essential.

Correct staging may play a significant role in choosing appropriate therapy. Overall staging accuracy may reach 92%, while accuracy in determining the depth of myometrial extension may reach 82%.[15]

GESTATIONAL TROPHOBLASTIC NEOPLASMS

Incidence. One in 2000 deliveries, or one in 1200 pregnancies.

Pathology. Spectrum of tumors ranging from hydatidiform mole (most common), locally invasive moles (less common), to choriocarcinoma (rare). Epithelial neoplasm characterized by proliferation of cytotrophoblast and syncytiotrophoblast. Arteriovenous shunting and hypervascularity are present.[16] Metastases are to lung, liver, and brain (choriocarcinoma). Theca lutein cysts are frequently present and may persist even after therapy.

Clinical Presentation. Threatened miscarriage in second trimester, larger than expected uterus, ab-

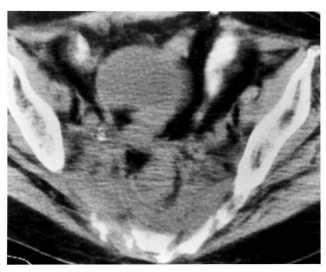

Figure 25–10. Cervical carcinoma with invasion of both piriformis muscles. The fat plane outlining the muscles is obliterated by inhomogeneous and irregular mass.

sence of fetal heart motion, and transvaginal passage of vesicles. Pulmonary emboli and high-output cardiac failure are rare.

Laboratory Findings. Serologic marker is β-human chorionic gonadotropin (hCG). Serum levels drop, reflecting positive response to therapy.

Radiological Findings. Presence of metastatic disease to the lung is detected on chest radiography, elsewhere by CT scan.[17] Uterine involvement is probably best imaged by MR. Uterine zonal anatomy is

obliterated by inhomogeneous hypervascular mass.[18] MR imaging may be indicated if the use of radiographic contrast is contraindicated or if it becomes necessary to exclude the presence of the tumor within the uterus.

OVARIAN CYSTIC TERATOMAS (DERMOID CYST)

Incidence. Twenty percent of all ovarian neoplasms. Most occur during reproductive years. May be multiple or bilateral.

Pathology. Cyst lined by squamous epithelium resembling keratinized epidermis. Sebaceous and sweat glands are present. Fatty liquid (sebum), matted hair, and cellular debris are found in the cyst. The debris may be floating or forming fluid-fluid interphase. Besides ectoderm, tissues from the other two germ layers are also present. Malignant transformation may occur in 2–3%, the most common being squamous cell carcinoma. The common site for malignancy is in the dermoid plug, also known as Rokitansky protuberance, which projects from the wall into the cyst. Torsion is a common complication.

Treatment. Conservative surgery.

Imaging. As in all pelvic tumors, ultrasound is the imaging method of choice.[19,20] Only if the diagnosis is uncertain and clinical situation warrants it is additional imaging necessary. On CT, fatty liquid is seen as a radiolucent mass, usually more lucent than

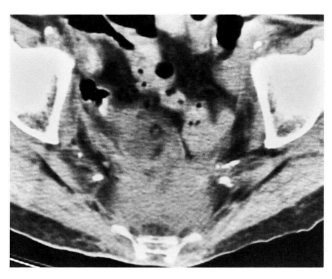

Figure 25–11. Recurrence of the tumor in the true pelvis and extension to the sacrum.

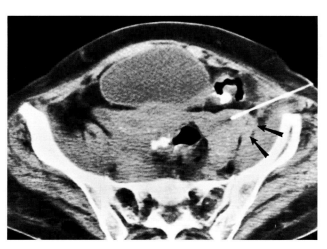

Figure 25–12. Aspiration biopsy of enlarged iliac lymph nodes. CT is very useful in guiding the biopsy. Large vessels (arrows) and intestine can be avoided.

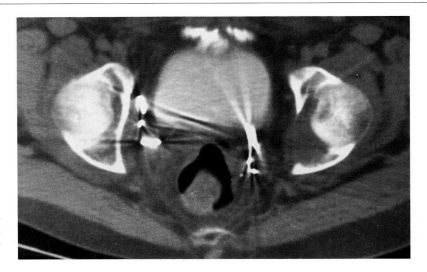

Figure 25–13. Lytic skeletal metastasis involving left acetabular wall developed sometime after tumor resection.

retroperitoneal fat (Figs. 25–15, 25–16).[21,22] CT has the advantage in detecting minute calcifications and is considered by some to be better in depicting these tumors than ultrasound or MR.[23] Thickened cyst wall may be observed associated with torsion due to edema and hemorrhage.[24]

Fatty liquid is of high signal intensity on both T1- and T2-weighted sequences on MR imaging.[25] Fluid layers or intraluminal masses representing floating proteinaceous debris may be seen (Fig. 25–17). Fluid-fluid interphase need not be present in every instance. On MR, differential diagnosis includes hemorrhagic fluid such as seen in endometrial cysts, for example. Fatty content of the tumor typically displays a chemical shift artifact, a finding apparently not seen in hemorrhagic cysts.[26]

Plain radiography is insensitive except in those instances where a tooth or an unquestionable radiolucent mass can be seen.

ENDOMETRIOSIS

Incidence.   Twenty-five percent of women in their third and fourth decades.

Pathology.   External endometriosis refers to ectopic endometrial implants outside of the uterus. The common sites are the ovary, serosal surface of the uterus, uterosacral ligament, and the cul-de-sac. Bladder, vagina, and other sites in the pelvis may be involved. Ectopic endometrial implants respond to cyclic ovarian hormonal stimulation with internal hemorrhage. Marked fibrotic reaction ensues, producing encapsulated hemorrhagic cysts and adhesions. Diffuse multiple implants are more common than a solitary endometrioma. Endometrial cysts of the ovary are rarely larger than 10 cm and are frequently bilateral. Intrauterine endometriosis (adenomyosis) is discussed elsewhere.

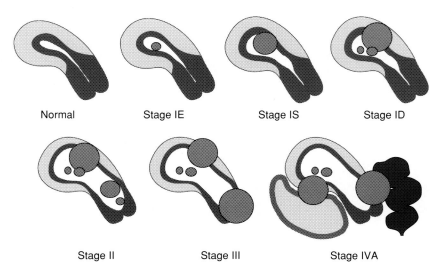

Normal   Stage IE   Stage IS   Stage ID

Stage II   Stage III   Stage IVA

Figure 25–14. Endometrial carcinoma. Schematic drawing of various stages of the disease as it may appear on MR imaging on T2-weighted sequences.

Table 25–2.   FIGO Staging of Endometrial Carcinoma

Stage	I	Confined to corpus
	IA	Uterine cavity is less than 8 cm long
	IB	Uterine cavity is longer than 8 cm
Stage	II	Corpus and cervix involved, tumor confined to uterus
	III	Extension outside uterus but not outside true pelvis
Stage	IV	Extension outside true pelvis or mucosal involvement of bladder or rectum
	IVA	Spread to the adjacent organs
	IVB	Spread to distant organs

Although rare, malignant transformation is possible. Endometrioid carcinoma arising from ovarian endometrial cyst is the most common malignancy.

Clinical Presentation.   Premenstrual pain, dysmenorrhea, abnormal uterine bleeding.

Radiological Findings.   Mass lesions may be detected on both ultrasound and CT, but the findings are nonspecific.[27,28]

On MR imaging, the diagnosis of endometrioma may be strongly suggested, since hemorrhagic fluid has relatively predictive behavior. Usually an indistinct multilocular cyst, hyperintense on T1- and T2-weighted sequences, is seen. However, similar to hemorrhagic renal cysts, a combination of different signal intensities is possible, including low signal intensity on T2-weighted sequences. Encapsulating thick fibrotic wall presents as a dark ring on T2-weighted sequence and because of adherence to adjacent organs, these organs become difficult to outline. Differentiation from hemorrhagic cysts may be difficult. These are usually homogeneous, unilocular, and distinct.

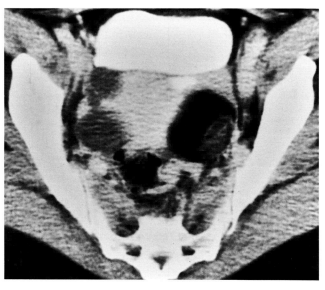

Figure 25–15.   Cystic teratoma. Multiple low density pelvic masses are present. Most are of water density except the one on the left, which measures −60 HU, indicating presence of fat. Within it there is a soft tissue protrusion (Rokitansky protuberance).

Smaller foci of endometriosis, as are found in the more common diffuse form, are not readily apparent by any imaging technique, including MR.[29,30]

Endometriosis arising from a cesarean section scar has been imaged by MR.[31]

At the present time, none of the imaging methods, including MR, can compete with laparoscopy in definitive diagnosis or staging of endometriosis.[30,32] Its use may be in monitoring treatment response instead of laparoscopy after the diagnosis has been established.

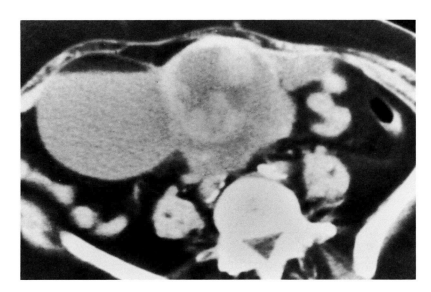

Figure 25–16.   Cystic teratoma discovered 10 years after menopause. Fat-fluid level is present in the right-sided cystic mass. (Photograph courtesy of Dr. David Cho.)

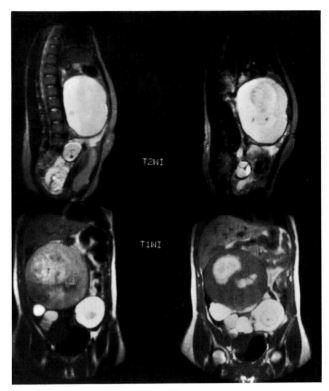

Figure 25–17. Large cystic teratoma seen in sagittal plane on T2-weighted sequence (upper row) and coronal plane on T1-weighted sequence (lower row). (Photograph courtesy of Dr. Lee Chiu.)

Bladder and ureteral involvement are possible and may result in ureteral obstruction.[33–35]

OVARIAN CARCINOMA

Incidence. Ovarian carcinoma is the most common cause of death from gynecological malignancy and the fourth most common cause of cancer death in women (after breast, colon, and lung). Peak occurrence is in the immediate postmenopausal years.

Pathology. Epithelial or mesothelial. Cystic or solid. Depending on size, areas of degeneration and hemorrhage develop. Papillary serous and mucinous cystadenocarcinoma make up a high proportion of cases. Less common are endometrioid, clear cell, and undifferentiated tumors. Psammomatous calcifications are present in 30%. Peritoneal implants at diaphragmatic peritoneum on the right and omentum are very common. Anterior mediastinal lymph node metastases are probably from peritoneal implants absorbed by diaphragmatic lymphatics. Ascites may be found in early and advanced stages.

Distant metastases are to liver, lungs, bone, and lymph nodes.

Clinical Presentation. Most patients present with advanced disease, pelvic masses, ascites, pleural effusion accompanied by shortness of breath or intestinal symptoms. Adnexal mass may be detected on physical examination.

Radiological Findings

Primary Tumor. Findings are usually nonspecific. On plain radiographs (Fig. 25–18) and urography (Fig. 25–19), a mass may be discovered at times with psammomatous calcifications (Fig. 25–20). On CT, mass may be inhomogeneous or cystic (Fig. 25–21). Calcifications (Fig. 25–22) and thick septa may be identified (Fig. 25–23).

Metastases. CT may demonstrate ascites, peritoneal metastases larger than 2 cm in diameter, and liver metastases (Fig. 25–24).[36,37] Calcified peritoneal plaques adjacent to the liver or in hepatorenal fossa may become evident even without ascites or mass effect *("perihepatic calcification sign")* (Fig. 25–25).[38] Psammomatous calcifications may be detected in the abdominal and mediastinal lymph nodes (Fig. 25–26).

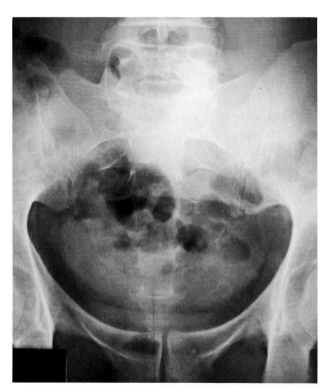

Figure 25–18. Ovarian carcinoma. On plain radiograph a nonspecific mass is identified. Perivesical fat stripe is present, leading one to conclude the mass is not the bladder.

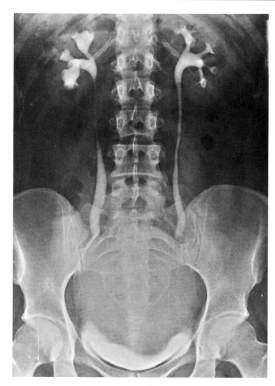

Figure 25–19. Ovarian carcinoma seen on EXU. The bladder is effaced and both ureters are displaced laterally. There is minimal hydronephrosis and the ureters are dilated above the pelvic brim.

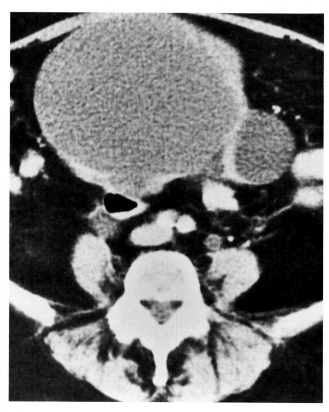

Figure 25–21. Cystadenocarcinoma of the ovary with thick wall.

Other Ovarian Neoplasms

These are usually of low malignant potential and include dysgerminomas, Brenner tumor, embryonal carcinomas, teratomas, struma ovarii, and carcinoid tumors. Fibroma may be associated with ascites and pleural fluid, a finding known as Meigs' syndrome. Except for cystic teratomas (see above), none has characteristic imaging qualities.

Metastases to the ovary are from the breast (Fig.

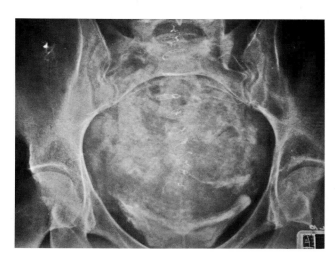

Figure 25–20. Psammomatous calcifications in cystadenocarcinoma of the ovary.

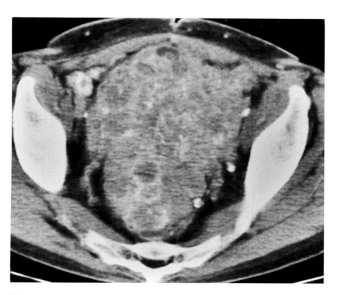

Figure 25–22. Cystadenocarcinoma of the ovary with psammomatous calcifications.

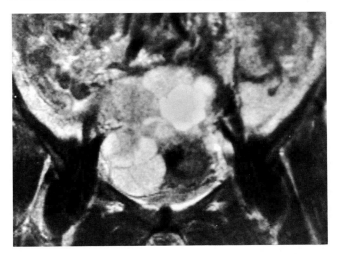

Figure 25–23. Cystadenocarcinoma of the ovary (proton density) in the coronal plane.

25–27), stomach, lungs, liver, pancreas, contralateral ovarian neoplasm, bladder, and uterus. The Kruken-berg tumor is a metastatic tumor to the ovary with predominant sarcomatous elements and signet-ring cells.

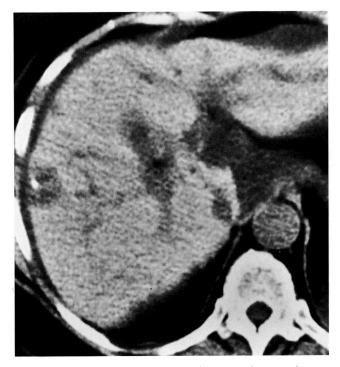

Figure 25–24. Liver metastases from ovarian carcinoma. Upon close scrutiny small amount of perihepatic intraperitoneal fluid is evident. The larger metastasis contains calcium.

VAGINA

Vaginal Agenesis (Mayer-Rokitansky-Kuster-Hauser Syndrome)

Vaginal agenesis is a rare congenital anomaly that may be partial or complete. Symptoms and treatment depend on the presence or absence of the cervix and functioning endometrium. In the presence of functioning endometrium, symptoms are related to acute hematometra shortly after menarche.[39,40] In the absence of functioning endometrium, the presenting symptom is primary amenorrhea. Associated congenital anomalies of other organ systems, particularly in the urinary tract and skeleton, are frequent.

MR is the imaging method of choice. Absence of the vagina (Fig. 25–28), absence or presence of the cervix, and hematometra with its rather characteristic appearance are readily diagnosed.[41]

Vaginal Neoplasms

MR appears to be the imaging modality of choice (Fig. 25–29A,B). On T2-weighted sequences, vaginal neoplasms are seen as infiltrating lesions of relatively high signal intensity (bright). As such, they cannot be differentiated from inflammatory process without biopsy. However, with the positive histological diagnosis at hand, it is possible to determine with high accuracy the extent of the disease. Furthermore, MR is excellent in excluding vaginal involvement by adjacent neoplasm.[42] Recurrent tumor is easily differentiated from postoperative fibrosis, since fibrotic tissues are of low signal intensity (dark) on T2-weighted sequences.

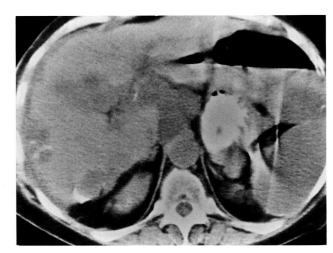

Figure 25–25. Calcified perihepatic metastases and ascites in subdiaphragmatic area and Morison's pouch.

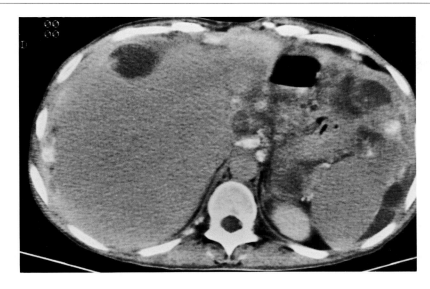

Figure 25–26. Liver metastasis and perihepatic calcification sign in a patient with mucinous cystadeno-carcinoma of the ovary. Perisplenic calcifications are also present and so are psammomatous calcifications in the lymph nodes.

Cystic lesions such as Gartner duct cysts are also hyperintense on T2-weighted sequences and usually well delineated.[42]

FEMALE PELVIS AFTER SURGERY AND RADIATION THERAPY

Pelvic Exenteration

Pelvic exenteration is an operation intended for cure of cervical, vaginal, vulvar, endometrial, rectal, and anal carcinomas that have invaded adjacent organs but are still confined to the pelvis. There are three types:

1. Total pelvic exenteration: Bladder, rectum, anus, uterus, vagina, and adnexa are removed.
2. Anterior pelvic exenteration: Rectum and anus are left intact. Bladder, uterus, vagina, and adnexa are removed. Ureters are diverted.
3. Posterior pelvic exenteration: Bladder is left intact. Rectum, anus, uterus, vagina, and adnexa are removed. Colostomy is created.

Omental flap may be brought down to cover pelvic walls, support the intestine, and promote reabsorption of exudates. Neovagina may be created from

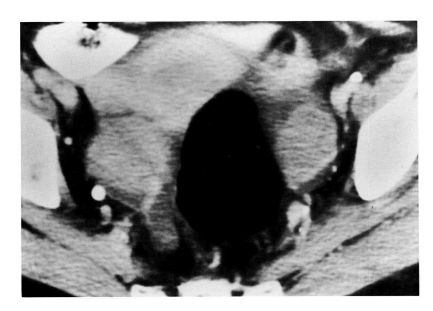

Figure 25–27. Bilateral metastases to the ovaries from the breast.

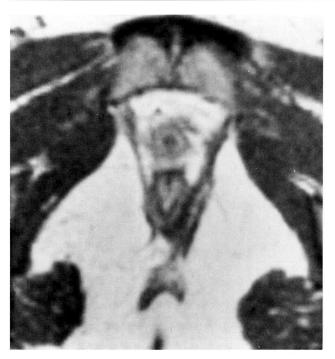

Figure 25–28. Vaginal agenesis. Urethra and rectum are clearly identified with small amount of fatty tissues instead of vagina between the two.

gracilis muscles and a cutaneous flap. This also helps support the intestine and fill the empty space.

Radiological Findings. A CT scan 2 months after pelvic surgery should be obtained for baseline, and routinely at 6-month intervals thereafter.

Tumor recurrence is detected in about 50% of patients. Neoplastic process must be differentiated from other mass effects usually associated with pelvic surgery. These include postoperative fibrosis, fluid collections, and abscess.

A common finding is soft tissue thickening in the presacral region.[43] This may be due to recurrent neoplasm, omental flap, dense postoperative fibrosis, or edema. CT is relatively nonspecific in establishing the definitive diagnosis. MR imaging has some use in these circumstances. Six months after surgery, fibrotic tissues are usually of very low signal intensity (dark) on T2-weighted sequences, while recurrent tumor is usually of high signal intensity (bright) (Fig. 25–30). Erosion of the sacrum has been observed only in association with recurrent tumor.

In many instances needle biopsy may be necessary to establish the diagnosis. Posterior approach under CT guidance is relatively easy to perform. Care should be taken to avoid injury to the sciatic nerve.

Fluid collections in the pelvic cavity may be symptomatic and require drainage. If gas is present, diagnosis of an abscess is likely. Low-lying loop of bowel may mimic tumor or an abscess. Bowel and ureteral obstruction may be found.

Urinary Fistulas

Urinary fistulas in patients with incurable pelvic malignancy are most commonly associated with cervical carcinoma, but may also be a complicating factor in vaginal and endometrial carcinoma. Occurrence rate is increased after radiation therapy alone or combined with surgery.

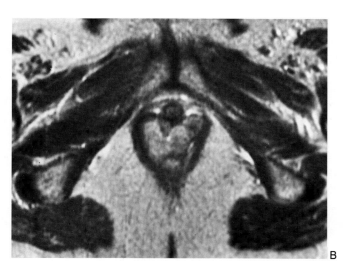

Figure 25–29. Primary carcinoma of the vagina. **(A)** CT is unable to differentiate neoplasm from the vaginal wall, urethra, and rectum. **(B)** All these structures are distinct from the tumor on MR imaging (T2-weighted sequence). The depth of vaginal wall invasion can be judged, since the neoplasm is of high signal intensity and the muscular vaginal wall is of low signal intensity.

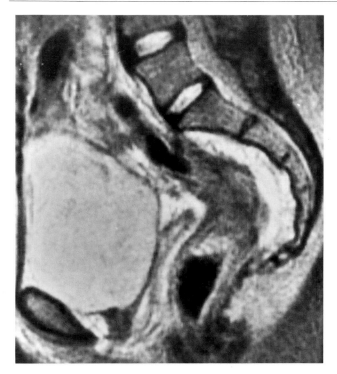

Figure 25–30. Bright signal in the presacral region on T2-weighted sequence represents metastatic carcinoma of the colon in a 30-year-old patient.

The most common is vesicovaginal fistula (see Chapter 20), followed by urethrovaginal, vesicoenteric, ureterovaginal, ileal loop-perineal, continent pouch-perineal, and vaginoperineal fistulas (Fig. 25–31).

The diagnosis is usually established by a VCUG or loopogram. Excretory urogram and retrograde (or antegrade) pyelogram may be required to diagnose ureteral fistulas.

Many of these patients with terminal disease are not surgical candidates. Their lives are made miserable with constant urine leak, skin irritation, and infection. Urinary diversion, such as percutaneous nephrostomy, may or may not be sufficient to dry out the fistula. A method of permanent ureteral occlusion is needed in addition to nephrostomy. Several antegrade percutaneous methods have been tested, including ureteral balloons,[44] butyl-2-cyanoacrylate glue,[45] plugs,[46] external ureteral clipping via a percutaneous tract,[47] endoscopic fulguration,[48] and endoureteral electrocautery using balloon electrocautery.[49]

Injury to the ureter occurs perhaps as commonly as in 0.5% of all pelvic surgery (Figs. 25–32, 25–33). Pelvic hematoma (Fig. 25–34) and lymphoceles (Fig. 25–35) may also cause ureteral obstruction.

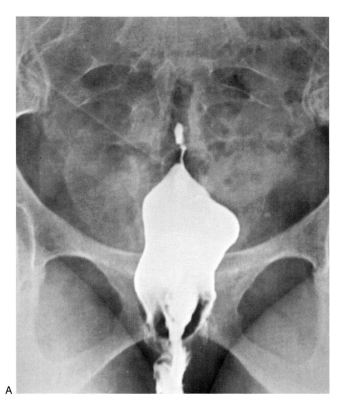
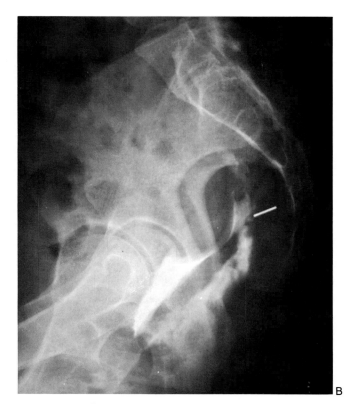

A

B

Figure 25–31. Vaginogram in a patient with vesicoperineal fistula **(A)** AP projection and **(B)** lateral projection. Vagina is anterior to the fistulous tract. Cervix can be identified as a protrusion in the upper vagina.

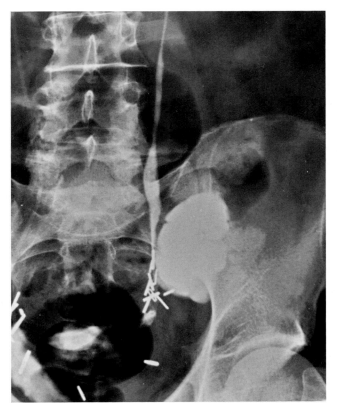

Figure 25–32. Ureteral clipping resulting in obstruction and ureteral fistula after pelvic surgery.

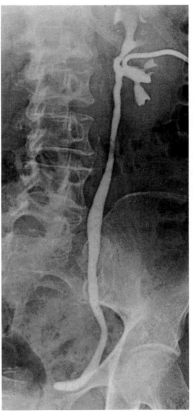

Figure 25–33. Ureteral ligation during suspension.

Intrauterine Devices

Most intrauterine devices (IUD) are detected by sonography. Abdominal radiograph may be required if IUD is not found in the uterus (Fig. 25–36).

PELVIC PAIN SYNDROME

Intractable pelvic pain in females with otherwise normal gynecological examination is a common entity. It has been shown that many of these patients have pelvic varicosities and stasis within the pelvic veins (Fig. 25–37). Both ovarian veins are usually enlarged, and retrograde flow through these vessels is frequently present and can be easily demonstrated by retrograde ovarian vein venography. Despite the fact that several studies have documented the presence of venous varicosities in the pelvis in this patient population, no serious research has been pursued to determine the cause and relationship. Treatment consists of prolonged psychological counseling.[50]

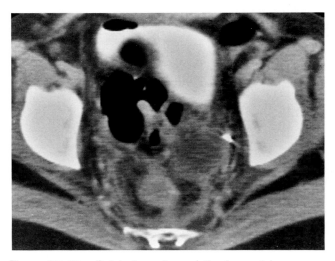

Figure 25–34. Pelvic hematoma following pelvic surgery. Collection around the left ureter was causing obstruction.

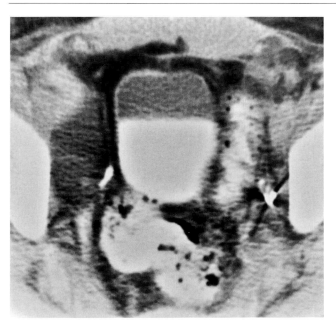

Figure 25–35.   Low density lymphocele is present along the right pelvic wall displacing the right ureter medially.

INFERTILITY

Contrast Hysterosalpingography

Hysterosalpingography is a radiological procedure designed to evaluate patients with infertility and recurrent abortions. The most important part of the examination is determination of tubal patency. The study is preferably taken during preovulatory phase. The procedure is performed with the patient in lithotomy position. Cervix is cleansed with povidone-iodine solution and os is cannulated with one of several cannulas (Leech-Wilkins, Rubens, Margolin, Foley catheter).[51–53] Some cannulas require grasping of the anterior cervical lip with a tenaculum in order to stabilize the uterus prior to insertion. The procedure causes mild discomfort, rarely requiring sedation or analgesia. Use of the tenaculum makes the procedure somewhat more painful.

Once cannulation is complete, contrast is delivered slowly, under mild pressure, and under fluoroscopic

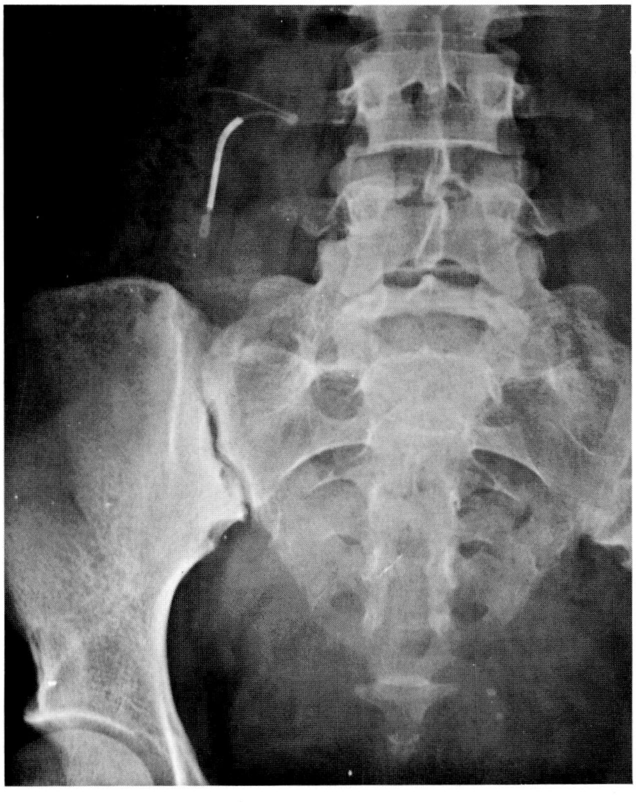

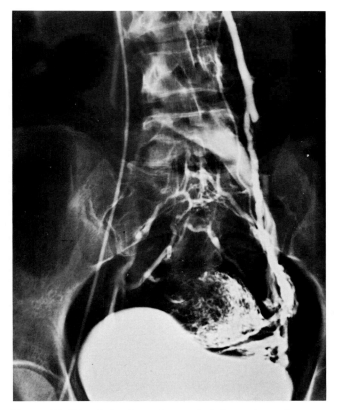

Figure 25–37.   Selective retrograde left ovarian vein venogram. Ovarian veins exit the broad ligament close to the ovary. Venous outflow from the uterus is via ovarian and uterine veins, the latter emptying into internal iliac veins. This cross-communication is well demonstrated here. Stasis in the pelvic vein is evident if there is delay in emptying.

Figure 25–36.   IUD has migrated outside the uterus.

control. Oblique views are obtained if necessary and the uterus may be gently manipulated with the cannula to profile the uterine cavity.

The type of contrast used for examination has received much attention in the literature. Meglumine ionic contrast seems the best and the least irritating. Some radiologists prefer more viscous contrast material such as Sinografin (diatrizoate meglumine 52.7% and iodipamide meglumine 26.8%, Squibb). Others use Ethiodol (Savage) which is an iodinated (37%) compound made from ethyl esters of the fatty acids of poppy seed oil.[54] It is claimed that oily contrasts have therapeutic effect and promote pregnancy.[55]

Postprocedural antibiotics should be considered in patients with a demonstrated tubular inflammatory process but are otherwise unnecessary. Venous embolization with oily contrast material is possible should intravasation occur (Fig. 25–38).[56] Fluoroscopic observation during the procedure is obviously necessary. Small peritoneal foreign body granulomas may be seen, particularly if oily contrasts are used (Fig. 25–39). Bleeding, recent pelvic inflammatory disease, recent instrumentation, and pregnancy are contraindications to the procedure.

Radionuclide Hysterosalpingography

Unlike contrast hysterosalpingography where contrast is injected under some pressure into the uterine cavity, in radionuclide hysterosalpingography the radioactive particles are deposited into the vagina. The natural retrograde migration of the radioactive particles via the uterus, ovarian tubes, into the peritoneal cavity is recorded on serial images at 15-minute intervals by a 30° caudally angulated gamma camera. One millicurie Tc-99m human serum albumin microspheres (Tc-99m HAM) is the radiopharmaceutical used.[57] The calculated dose to the ovary is similar to radiographic examination.

Spillage into the peritoneal cavity may be demonstrated, as well as complete obstruction, or pooling into the dilated and obstructed tubes. Unlike contrast hysterosalpingography which demonstrates tubal anatomy, radionuclide hysterosalpingography is said to reveal functional status of the fallopian tubes.

Interventional Procedures

An obstructed fallopian tube may be recanalized by selective ostial catheterization and passage of minute guidewire through the tube.[58–60]

Abnormal Findings

Congenital Anomalies. Bicornuate (Fig. 25–40), unicornuate, and arcuate uterus, as well as uterus didelphys, constitute congenital anomalies (Fig. 25–41).

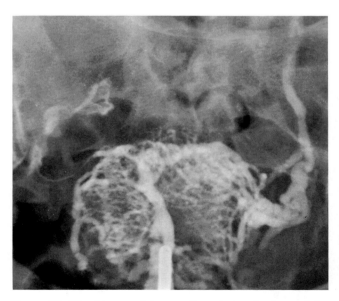

Figure 25–38. Venous intravasation during hysterosalpingography. (Photograph courtesy of Dr. Barbara Kadell.)

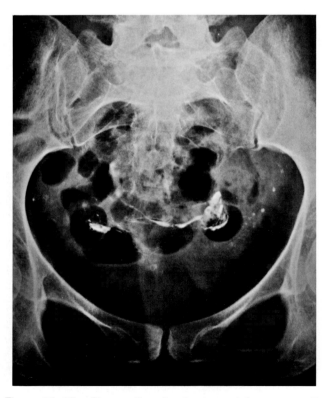

Figure 25–39. Six months after hysterosalpingogram, oily contrast is still seen in the peritoneal cavity.

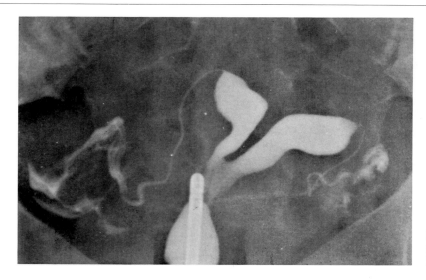

Figure 25–40. Bicornuate uterus. (Photograph courtesy of Dr. Barbara Kadell.)

Salpingitis Isthmica Nodosa (SIN). Seen in at least 4% of patients undergoing hysterosalpingography, it probably represents sequelae of an inflammatory process. Histologically, there is overgrowth of tubular epithelium forming inclusion nests in the thickened muscular wall. Many of these inclusions are seen as typical 1–2 mm diverticular outpouches in the proximal and mid-part of the fallopian tube on hysterosalpingography (Fig. 25–42).[61,62]

Tubal Obstruction. May be the result of adhesions or mucosal plug. Differential diagnosis includes spasm. Selective tubal catheterization or gentle manipulation together with spasmolytics may be necessary to differentiate mechanical obstruction from tubal spasm.

Hydrosalpinx. End result of pelvic inflammatory disease. Clubbing of the fimbrial end and dilatation are present (Fig. 25–43A,B). SIN and peritubular adhesions may coexist.

Intrauterine Adhesions (Asherman's Syndrome). Intrauterine synechiae are sequelae of intrauterine trauma usually induced by instrumentation (Fig. 25–44).[63]

Filling Defects. Benign and occasionally malignant processes present as "filling defects" within the uterine cavity. These include: polyps, myomas (Fig. 25–6), blood clots, foreign bodies, air bubbles, retained products of conception, adenomyosis, and neoplasms, such as endometrial carcinoma.

Anomalies from Diethylstilbesterol (DES) Exposure. A large number of women exposed to DES develop a hypoplastic, T-shaped uterus with irregular cavity contour and cervical stenosis (Fig. 25–45).[64]

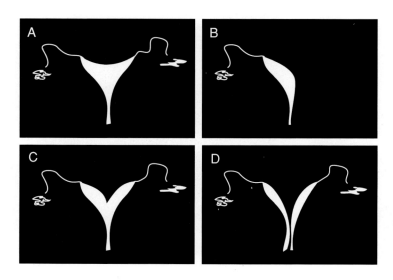

Figure 25–41. Schematic drawing of congenital anomalies. **A:** Arcuate uterus; **B:** unicornuate uterus; **C:** bicornuate uterus; **D:** uterus didelphys.

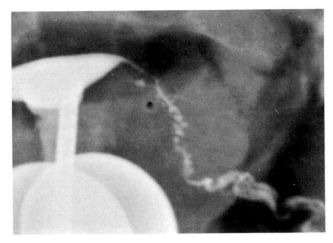

Figure 25–42.   Salpingitis isthmica nodosa. Small diverticular outpouches are typical for this disease. (Photograph courtesy of Dr. Barbara Kadell.)

RADIOLOGY IN PREGNANCY

Physiologic Changes in the Urinary Tract

During pregnancy, there is increase in renal blood flow (RBF) and glomerular filtration rate (GFR) up to 30% above baseline. There is corresponding increase in renal size and weight. Tubular reabsorptive mechanism may be overwhelmed by increased GFR so that occasional glucosuria and aminoaciduria may be detected.

Collecting system and ureter dilate and exhibit decreased peristaltic activity. This laxity of the smooth muscle is most likely a progesterone effect. Ureteral compression upon the pelvic brim by an enlarged uterus, and compression by enlarged ovarian veins, contribute to the dilatation of the collecting system.

It takes several weeks in the postpartum period for uterus, collecting system, ureters, and gonadal veins to return to their normal size.

Urinary Tract Obstruction

Obstruction in pregnancy is most likely caused by a ureteral calculus. It is, of course, the most difficult diagnosis to make. Ultrasound is practically useless, since grade I or II hydronephrosis is already present in normal pregnancy (Fig. 25–46). Certainly, ultrasound should be used initially, searching for the telltale sign of a hyperacoustic calculus accompanied by shadowing anywhere along the expected course of the ureter. Negative predictive value, however, must be poor.

Failing the discovery of an obstructing calculus by ultrasound, the choices are few. One has to be concerned with the radiation dose to the fetus (and mother), yet the presence, cause, location, and severity of the obstruction need to be determined if appropriate treatment is to be instituted.

Limited and tailored excretory urogram seems to

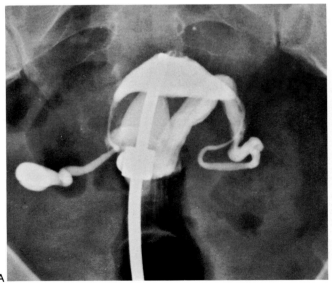
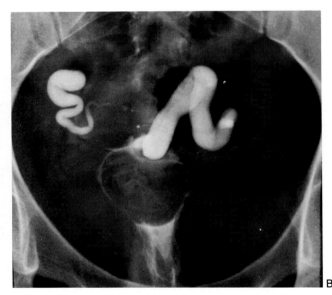

A   B

Figure 25–43.   Hydrosalpinx. **(A)** Bilateral dilatation and clubbing are present. There is no intraperitoneal spill even on delayed film **(B)**. (Photograph courtesy of Dr. Barbara Kadell.)

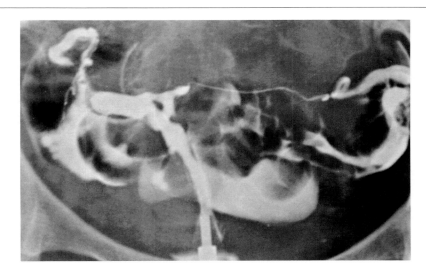

Figure 25–44. Intrauterine synechiae. Irregularity and intraluminal "filling defect" are present. Both tubes are patent. (Photograph courtesy of Dr. Barbara Kadell.)

be the only alternative. Radiographic contrasts carry a disclaimer concerning their use in pregnancy so that risks versus benefits have to be carefully considered.

The excretory urogram in pregnancy consists of a scout radiograph which is scrutinized for ureteral calculi. Contrast material is slowly injected intravenously. Since the object is to determine site and cause of obstruction, the next radiograph should be a delayed one. Just how delayed is a good question. In the presence of a really significant obstruction it may take several hours for the contrast to reach the site of obstruction. Two hours after the injection is a good bet, but usually the examining radiologist buckles under the pressure of uncertainty and obtains a radiograph after 1 hour. If there is an increased and discrepant nephrogram on the affected side, obstruction is probably present. The normal side may be washed out by then, but this is irrelevant. If the ureter is still not visualized, another delayed radiograph is obtained using the radiologist's best judgment. With three or four exposures, it is possible therefore to diagnose the obstruction and accomplish the goals set initially. By using rare earth film-screen combination, exposure would equal the dose received during pelvimetry.

The obstruction may be treated with a double "J" ureteral stent or percutaneous nephrostomy until delivery. After delivery, appropriate therapy is instituted.

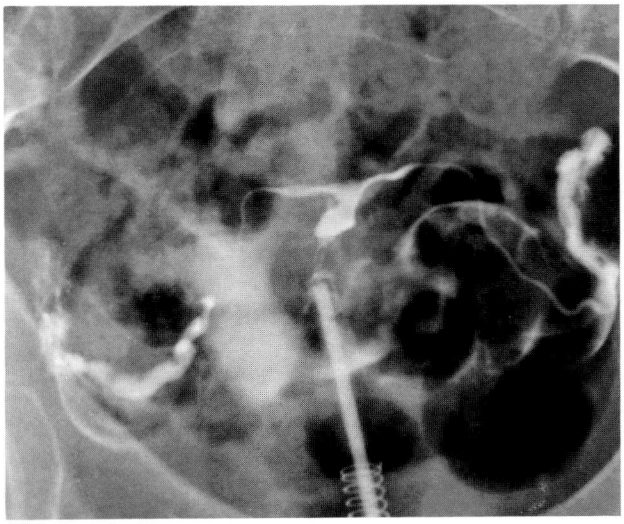

Urinary Tract Infection

Asymptomatic bacteriuria is common in first antenatal urinalysis and is seen in 6–7% of expectant mothers. Two to 3% of all pregnant women develop symptomatic urinary tract infection, 20–50% involving upper urinary tract.

Obstetrical Renal Failure

Renal failure associated with pregnancy is becoming very rare in industrially developed countries with readily available medical care. In developing countries renal failure is commonly seen following septic abortion in the first trimester of pregnancy, whereas in late pregnancy renal failure is precipitated by eclampsia, preeclampsia, hemorrhage, and puerperal sepsis.[65]

Acute tubular necrosis (ATN) is the most common cause of renal failure and is usually reversible. Acute

Figure 25–45. DES exposure in utero. T-shaped uterus with cervical stenosis. (Photograph courtesy of Dr. Barbara Kadell.)

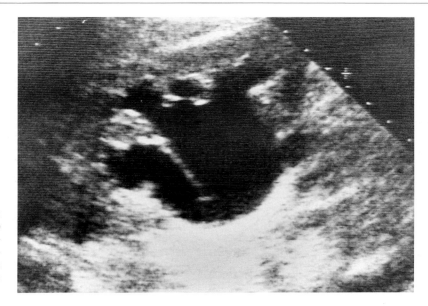

Figure 25–46. Renal sonogram in 21-week pregnant woman with two bouts of acute pyelonephritis. Moderate dilatation of the collecting system is present, but some dilatation is expected at this stage. Is obstruction present?

cortical necrosis (ACN) has been reported as an infrequent cause of postabortion and late pregnancy renal failure.

Pelvimetry

Once a common radiological procedure, pelvimetry is now seldom used. Several different techniques have been described (Colcher-Sussman, Borell-Fern-ström, etc.) (Fig. 25–47).[66,67] Lately, CT method has gained in popularity because of its simplicity, fast cursor-electronic measurement technique, and, above all, because of decreased exposure to the fetus and mother (Fig. 25–48).[68–70] Ultrasound and even MR imaging, with the advantage of lack of radiation, are vying for attention.[71–73]

The main indication for pelvimetry is in determining whether cephalopelvic disproportion exists that may account for abnormal labor. The presence of such disproportion may well influence whether vaginal delivery or cesarean section is implemented and avoid prolonged unsuccessful labor trials. However, there is growing evidence that pelvimetry is of no clinical use in uncomplicated labor,[74,75] nor is it necessary in the majority of patients who have previously undergone cesarean section.[76]

Estimating Fetal Size in Diabetic Women

The risk of shoulder dystocia during vaginal delivery is increased in infants born to diabetic mothers. This is because these infants are larger than normal at birth, frequently weighing more than 4000 g. Accu-

racy of birthweight prediction by sonography, pelvimetry, or physical examination is limited.[77,78]

Measurement of fetal shoulder width with CT appears the most promising.[79] Scoutogram (topogram) is obtained in frontal and lateral projections and immediately inspected. A single axial section is ob-

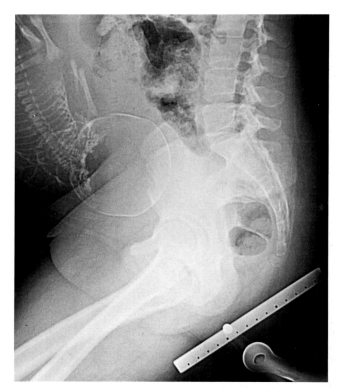

Figure 25–47. Lateral projection from a pelvimetry. Perforated 1 cm ruler is elevated on a stand so that midplane of the patient and the ruler exhibit same magnification.

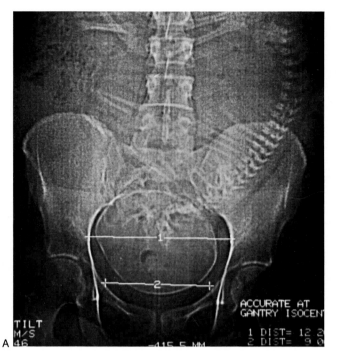

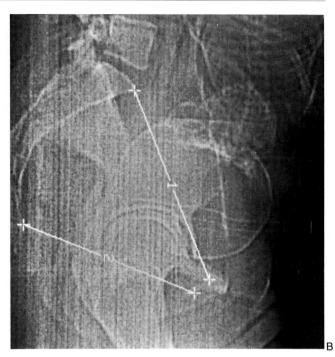

Figure 25–48. (A) Scoutogram in the frontal projection shows the points between the distances are measured. Transverse diameter of the pelvic inlet is the larger of the two. Bispinous diameter is smaller. (B) On the lateral scoutogram, points to measure sagittal diameter of the pelvic inlet and outlet are shown.

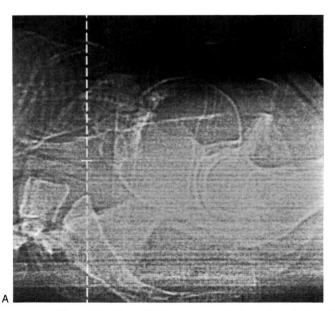

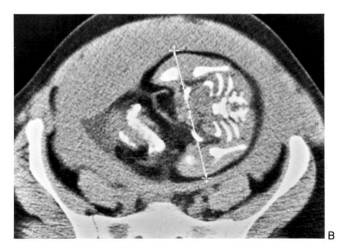

Figure 25–49.   (A) Scoutogram in lateral projection is examined and a cursor placed between two shoulders (dotted line). If necessary, the line may be slanted and the gantry tilted accordingly for subsequent axial slice. (B) One or two axial cuts are obtained immediately after the scoutogram. The cursor is placed at the outer edge of subcutaneous fat of the fetus at shoulder level, which is easily identified by humeral heads and scapulas. Shoulder width of more than 14 cm indicates fetal weight of more than 4200 gm.

tained through the shoulders of the fetus. The gantry may have to be tilted slightly to ensure both proximal humeri are on the axial slice. Thereafter, the greatest distance between outer margin of the soft tissues, including subcutaneous fat, is measured electronically, with a cursor (Fig. 25–49).

Shoulder width measuring more than 14 cm is abnormal. This width is also a good predictor of fetal weight, as in all instances infants with this measurement or greater weighed 4200 g or more.

Postpartum Ovarian Vein Thrombosis and Thrombophlebitis

Enlarged ovarian vein, usually right, is detected to contain thrombus. On contrast-enhanced CT scans the thrombus is seen as a low-density radiolucent filling defect propagating along the expected course of the ovarian vein. Duplex Doppler sonography is particularly useful in this regard.[80,81] Thrombus may be seen protruding into the inferior vena cava. In the presence of suppurative thrombophlebitis patients present with pain, fever, and a very rapid pulse rate.

Lithopedion

Calcified contents of ectopic pregnancy are occasionally discovered. At times, the dead fetus may be recognized.

REFERENCES

1. Hricak H, Tscholakoff D, Heinrichs L. Uterine leiomyomas: correlation of MR, histopathologic findings and symptoms. Radiology 1986; 158:385–391.
2. Hamlin DJ, Petterson H, Fitzsimmons J, Morgan LS. MR imaging of uterine leiomyomas and their complications. J Comput Assist Tomogr 1985; 9:902–907.
3. Dudiak CM, Turner DA, Patel S, et al. Uterine leiomyomas in the infertile patient: preoperative localization with MR imaging versus US and hysterosalpingography. Radiology 1988; 167:627–630.
4. Togashi K, Nishimura K, Itoh K, et al. Adenomyosis: diagnosis with MR imaging. Radiology 1988; 166:111–114.
5. Togashi K, Ozasa H, Konishi I, et al. Enlarged uterus: differentiation between adenomyosis and leiomyoma with MR imaging. Radiology 1989; 171:531–534.
6. Mark AS, Hricak H, Heinrichs LW, et al. Adenomyosis and leiomyoma: differential diagnosis with MR imaging. Radiology, 1987 May, 163:527–529.
7. Siedler D, Laing FC, Jeffrey RB Jr, Wing VW. Uterine adenomyosis. A difficult sonographic diagnosis. J Ultrasound Med, 1987; 6:345–349.
8. Bohlman ME, Ensor RE, Sanders RC. Sonographic findings in adenomyosis of the uterus. AJR, 1987; 148:765–766.
9. American Joint Committee on Cancer. Manual for staging cancer. 2nd ed. Philadelphia: Lippincott, 1983; 135–137.
10. Rubens D, Thornbury JR, Angel C, et al. Stage IB cervical carcinoma: comparison of clinical, MR, and pathologic staging. AJR 1988; 150:135–138.
11. Hricak H, Lacey CG, Sandles LG, et al. Invasive cervical carcinoma: comparison of MR imaging and surgical findings. Radiology 1988; 166:623–631.
12. Lee JKT. The role of MR imaging in staging of cervical carcinoma (editorial). Radiology 1988; 166:895–896.
13. Vick CW, Walsh JW, Wheelock JB, Vrewer WH. CT of the normal and abnormal parametria in cervical cancer. AJR 1984; 143:597–603.
14. Whitley NO, Brenner DE, Francis A, et al. Computed tomographic evaluation of carcinoma of the cervix. Radiology 1982; 142:439–446.
15. Hricak H, Stern JL, Fisher MR, et al. Endometrial carcinoma staging by MR imaging. Radiology 1987; 162:297–305.
16. Worthington JL, Balfe DM, Lee JKT, Gersell DJ, et al. Uterine neoplasms: MR imaging. Radiology 1986; 159:725–730.
17. Miyasaka Y, Hachiya J, Furuya Y, et al. CT evaluation of invasive trophoblastic disease. J Comput Assist Tomogr 1985; 9:459–462.
18. Hricak H, Demas B, Braga CA, et al. Gestational trophoblastic neoplasm of the uterus: MR assessment. Radiology 1986; 161:11–16.
19. Laing FC, Van Dalsem VF, Marks WM, et al. Dermoid cysts of the ovary: their ultrasonographic appearances. Obstet Gynecol 1981; 57:99–104.
20. Quinn SF, Erickson S, Black WC. Cystic ovarian teratomas: the sonographic appearance of the dermoid plug. Radiology 1985; 155:477–478.
21. Friedman AC, Pyatt RS, Hartman DS, et al. CT of benign cystic teratomas. AJR 1982; 138:659–665.
22. Skaane P, Heubener KH. Computed tomography of cystic ovarian teratomas with gravity-dependent layering. J Comput Assist Tomogr 1983; 7:837–841.
23. Buy JN, Ghossain MA, Moss AA, et al. Cystic teratoma of the ovary: CT detection. Radiology 1989; 171:697–701.
24. Feldberg MAM, Van Waes PFGM, Hendricks MJ. Direct multiplanar CT findings in cystic teratoma of the ovary. J Comput Assist Tomogr 1984; 8:1131–1135.
25. Mitchell DG, Mintz M, Spritzer CE, et al. Adnexal masses: MR imaging observations at 1.5 T, with US and CT correlation. Radiology 1987; 162:319–324.
26. Togashi K, Nishimura K, Itoh K, et al. Ovarian cystic teratomas: MR imaging. Radiology 1987; 162:669–673.
27. Sandler MA, Karo JJ. The spectrum of ultrasonic findings in endometriosis. Radiology 1978; 127:229–231.
28. Fishman EK, Scatarige JC, Saksouk FA, et al. Computed tomography of endometriosis. J Comput Assist Tomogr 1983; 7:257–264.
29. Nishimura K, Togashi K, Itoh K, et al. Endometrial cysts of the ovary: MR imaging. Radiology 1987; 162:315–318.
30. Arrivé L, Hricak H, Martin MC. Pelvic endometriosis: MR imaging. Radiology 1989; 171:687–692.

31. Wolf GC, Kopecky KK. MR imaging of endometriosis arising in cesarean section scar. J Comput Assist Tomogr, 1989; 13:150–152.
32. Zawin M, McCarthy S, Scoutt L, Comite F. Endometriosis: appearance and detection on MR imaging. Radiology 1989; 171:693–696.
33. Sircus SI, Sant GR, Ucci AA Jr. Bladder detrusor endometriosis mimicking interstitial cystitis. Urology, 1988; 32:339–342.
34. Appel RA. Bilateral ureteral obstruction secondary to endometriosis. Urology, 1988; 32:151–154.
35. Shook TE, Nyberg LM. Endometriosis of the urinary tract. Urology, 1988; 31:1–6.
36. Amendola MA, Walsh JW, Amendola BE, et al. Computed tomography in the evaluation of carcinoma of the ovary. J Comput Assist Tomogr 1981; 5:179–186.
37. Jeffrey RB Jr. CT demonstration of peritoneal implants. AJR 1980; 135:323–326.
38. Mitchell DG, Hill MC, Hill S, Zaloudek C. Serous carcinoma of the ovary: CT identification of metastatic calcified implants. Radiology 1986; 158:649–652.
39. Rosenberg HK, Sherman NH, Tarry WF, et al. Mayer-Rokitansky-Kuster-Hauser syndrome: US aid to diagnosis. Radiology 1985; 161:815–819.
40. Togashi K, Nishimura K, Itoh K, et al. Vaginal agenesis: classification by MR imaging. Radiology 1987; 162:675–677.
41. Hricak H, Chang YCF, Thurnher S. Vagina: evaluation with MR imaging. Part I. Normal anatomy and congenital anomalies. Radiology 1988; 169:169–174.
42. Chang YCF, Hricak H, Thurnher S, Lacey CG. Vagina: evaluation with MR imaging. Part II. Neoplasms. Radiology 1988; 169:175–179.
43. Pan G, Shirkhoda A. Pelvic exenteration: role of CT in follow-up. Radiology 1987; 164:665–670.
44. Gunther RW, Klose KJ, Alken P, Bohl J. Transrenal ureteral occlusion using a detachable balloon. Urol Radiol 1984; 6:210–214.
45. Gunther R, Margerger M, Klose K. Transrenal ureteral embolization. Radiology 1979; 132:317–319.
46. Sanchez R, Quinn SF, Morrisseau PM, et al. Urinary diversion by using a percutaneous ureteral occlusion device. AJR 1988; 150:1069–1070.
47. Darcy MD, Lund GB, Smith TP; et al. Percutaneously applied ureteral clips: treatment of vesicovaginal fistula. Radiology 1987; 163:819–821.
48. Reddy PK, Moore L, Hunter D, Amplatz K. Percutaneous ureteral fulguration: a nonsurgical technique for ureteral occlusion. J Urol 1987; 138:724–726.
49. Kopecky KK, Sutton GP, Bihrle R, Becker GJ. Percutaneous transrenal endoureteral radiofrequency electrocautery for occlusion: case report. Radiology 1989; 170(2):1047–1048.
50. Beard R, Reginald P, Pearce S. Psychological and somatic factors in women with pain due to pelvic congestion. Adv Exp Med Biol 1988; 245:413–421.
51. Margolin FR. A new cannula for hysterosalpingography. AJR 1988; 151:729–730.
52. Winfield AC, Wentz AC. Techniques and complications of hysterosalpingography. In: Diagnostic Imaging of Infertility. (Winfield AC, Wentz AC, eds). Baltimore: Williams & Wilkins, 1987: 1–9.
53. Wolf DM, Spataro RF. The current state of hysterosalpingography. Radiographics 1988; 8:1041–1058.
54. Loy RA, Weinstein FG, Seibel MM. Hysterosalpingography in perspective: the predictive value of oil-soluble versus water-soluble contrast media. Fertil Steril 1989; 51:170–172.
55. Rasmussen F, Justesen P, Tonner Nielsen D. Therapeutic value of hysterosalpingography with Lipiodol ultra fluid. Acta Radiol (Stockh) 1987; 28:319–322.
56. Nunley WC Jr, Bateman BG, Kitchin JD 3d, Pope TL Jr. Intravasation during hysterosalpingography using oil-base contrast medium—a second look. Obstet Gynecol, 1987; 70:309–312.
57. Angtuaco TL, Boyd CM, London SN, et al. Technetium-99m hysterosalpingography in infertility: an accurate alternative to contrast hysterosalpingography. Radiographics 1989; 9:115–128.
58. Thurmond AS, Novy M, Uchida BT, Rosch J. Fallopian tube obstruction: selective salpingography and recanalization. Work in progress. Radiology 1987; 163:511–512.
59. Thurmond AS, Rösch J, Patton PE, et al. Fluoroscopic transcervical fallopian tube catheterization for diagnosis and treatment of female infertility caused by tubal obstruction. Radiographics 1988; 8:621–636.
60. Rösch J, Thurmond AS, Uchida BT, Sovak M. Selective transcervical fallopian tube catheterization: technique update. Radiology 1988; 168:1–6.
61. Thomas ML, Rose DH. Salpingitis isthmica nodosa demonstrated by hysterosalpingography. Acta Radiol (Diagn) (Stockh) 1973; 14:295–304.
62. Creasy JL, Clark RL, Cuttino JT, Groff TR. Salpingitis isthmica nodosa: radiologic and clinical correlates. Radiology 1985; 154:597–600.
63. Berquist CA, Rock JA, Jones HW. Pregnancy outcome following treatment of intrauterine adhesions. Int J Fertil 1981; 26:107–110.
64. Kaufman RH, Adam E, Noller K, et al. Upper genital tract changes and infertility in diethylstilbestrol exposed women. Am J Obstet Gynecol 1986; 154:1312–1318.
65. Chugh KS, Kjellstrand CM. The changing epidemiology of acute renal failure: patterns in economically advanced and developing countries. In: International Yearbook of Nephrology. (Andreucci VE, ed). Boston: Kluwer Academic Publishers, 1989: 213–215.
66. Colcher AE, Sussman WA. A practical technique for roentgen pelvimetry with a new positioning. AJR 1944; 51:207.
67. Borell U, Fernström I. Radiologic pelvimetry. Acta Radiol (Stockh) 1960; Suppl 191.
68. Federle MH, Cohen M, Rosenwein M, et al. Pelvimetry by digital radiography: a low dose examination. Radiology 1982; 143:733–735.
69. Lotz H, Ekelund L, Hietala SO, Eriksson L, Wiklund DE, Wickman G. Low dose pelvimetry with biplane digital radiography. Acta Radiol (Stockh) 1987; 28:577–580.
70. Dobson J, Nelson J. CT pelvimetry: replacing conventional with digital. Radiology 1988; 54:18–19.
71. Deutinger J, Bernaschek G. Vaginosonographical determination of the true conjugate and the transverse diameter of the pelvic inlet. Arch Gynecol 1987; 240:241–246.
72. Stark DS, McCarthy R, Filly R, et al. Pelvimetry by magnetic resonance imaging. AJR 1985; 144:947–950.
73. Woerner H, Brill G, Frenzel T, Stoll H, Tesseraux M. Pelvimetry using magnetic resonance tomography. ROFO 1988; 149:378–382.
74. Floberg J, Belfrage P, Ohlsen H. Influence of pelvic

outlet capacity on labor. A prospective pelvimetry study of 1,429 unselected primiparas. Acta Obstet Gynecol Scand 1987; 66:121–126.

75. Barton JJ, Garbaciak JA, Ryan GM Jr. The efficacy of x-ray pelvimetry. Am J Obstet Gynecol 1982; 143:304–311.

76. Lao TT, Chin RK, Leung BF. Is X-ray pelvimetry useful in a trial of labour after caesarean section? Eur J Obstet Gynecol Reprod Biol 1987; 24:277–283.

77. Thurnau GR, Morgan MA. Efficacy of the fetal-pelvic index as a predictor of fetal-pelvic disproportion in women with abnormal labor patterns that require labor augmentations. Am J Obstet Gynecol 1988; 159:1168–1172.

78. Morgan MA, Thurnau GR. Efficacy of the fetal-pelvic index in patients requiring labor induction. Am J Obst Gynecol 1988; 159:621–625.

79. Kitzmiller JL, Mall JC, Gin GD, et al. Measurement of fetal shoulder width with computed tomography in diabetic women. Obstet Gynecol 1987; 70:941–945.

80. Baran GW, Frisch KM. Duplex Doppler evaluation of puerperal ovarian vein thrombosis. AJR 1987; 149:321.

81. Savader SJ, Otero RR, Savader BL. Puerperal ovarian vein thrombosis. Evaluation with CT, US, and MR imaging. Radiology 1988; 167:673.

Index

Citations contained in tables and figures are indicated in this index by the italic letters *t* and *f* following page numbers.